HANDBOOK
OF TOXICOLOGY

HANDBOOK OF TOXICOLOGY

Edited by

Thomas J. Haley
University of Arkansas for Health Sciences

William O. Berndt
University of Nebraska Medical Center

⦿ **HEMISPHERE PUBLISHING CORPORATION**, Washington
A subsidiary of Harper & Row, Publishers, Inc.

Cambridge   New York   Philadelphia   San Francisco
London   Mexico City   São Paulo   Singapore   Sydney

HANDBOOK OF TOXICOLOGY

1 2 3 4 5 6 7 8 9 0   B R B R   8 9 8 7 6

This book was set in Press Roman by Hemisphere Publishing Corporation. The editors were
Christine Flint Lowry, Eleana Cornejo-de-Villanueva, and Elizabeth Dugger; the production
supervisor was Peggy M. Rote; and the typesetter was Sandra F. Watts.
Braun-Brumfield, Inc. was printer and binder.

Library of Congress Cataloging in Publication Data

Handbook of toxicology.

  Includes bibliographies and index.
  1. Poisons—Physiological effect. 2. Toxicology.
I. Haley, Thomas J. II. Berndt, William O.
[DNLM: 1. Poisons. 2. Toxicology. QV 600 H235]
RA1220.H36 1987   615.9   86-7670
ISBN 0-89116-403-0

Contents

Contributors

WILLIAM O. BERNDT, PhD
University of Nebraska Medical Center
Omaha, Nebraska

ALLEN BRANDS, RAdm (Ret),
 DSc
Assistant Surgeon General (Ret) USPHS
Washington, D.C.

C. JELLEFF CARR, PhD
Life Sciences Research Office, FASEB
Bethesda, Maryland

WALTER J. DECKER, PhD
Toxicology Consultant Services
El Paso, Texas

WILLIAM F. DURHAM, PhD, USEPA
Research Coordination Office
Research Triangle Park, North Carolina

BRUCE A. FOWLER, PhD
Laboratory of Pharmacology
National Institute of Environmental
 Health Sciences
National Institutes of Health
Research Triangle Park, North Carolina

PETER L. GOERING, PhD
Laboratory of Pharmacology
National Institute of Environmental
 Health Sciences
National Institutes of Health
Research Triangle Park, North Carolina

THOMAS J. HALEY, PhD
University of Arkansas for Health
 Sciences
Little Rock, Arkansas

I. K. HO, PhD
Department of Pharmacology and
Toxicology
University of Mississippi Medical
Center
Jackson, Mississippi

BETH HOSKINS, PhD
Department of Pharmacology
and Toxicology
University of Mississippi
Medical Center
Jackson, Mississippi

CAROL K. KELLOGG, PhD
Departments of Psychology
and Pharmacology
University of Rochester School
of Medicine and Dentistry
Rochester, New York

JEROLD A. LAST, PhD
University of California
California Primate Research Center
Davis, California

CHARLES L. LITTERST, PhD
Laboratory of Medicinal Chemistry
and Pharmacology
Division of Cancer Treatment
National Cancer Institute
National Institutes of Health
Bethesda, Maryland

HARIHARA M. MEHENDALE, PhD
Department of Pharmacology
and Toxicology
University of Mississippi
Medical Center
Jackson, Mississippi

RICHARD K. MILLER, PhD
Departments of Obstetrics/Gynecology/
Pharmacology and Division
of Toxicology
University of Rochester School
of Medicine and Dentistry
Rochester, New York

PRAKASH MISTRY, PhD
Laboratory of Pharmacology
National Institute of Environmental
Health Sciences
National Institutes of Health
Research Triangle Park, North Carolina

R. V. REDDY, PhD
Toxicology Program
Utah State University
Logan, Utah

RISA A. SALTZMAN, Ph.D.
Departments of Obstetrics/Gynecology
and Division of Toxicology
University of Rochester School
of Medicine and Dentistry
Rochester, New York

R. P. SHARMA, PhD
Toxicology Program
Utah State University
Logan, Utah

M. J. TAYLOR, PhD
Toxicology Program
Utah State University
Logan, Utah

HANSPETER WITSCHI, MD
Biology Division
Oak Ridge National Laboratory
Oak Ridge, Tennessee

Preface

Since humans first discovered the medicinal properties of plants, we have known that these same plants can also have toxic effects. Hippocrates cautioned his followers on the adverse effects of *veratrum album*. Galen pointed out the toxic effects of lead, opium, mandragora, and hyocyamus, while the Arabs discussed the toxicity of mercury vapor. Paracelsus pointed out that dose determined the difference between therapeutic efficacy and toxicity of a given chemical. Indeed, the earliest texts on toxicology were those written by Maimonides in the twelfth century and Orfilia in the eighteenth century.

More recently, developments in analytical chemistry have advanced and specialized the field of toxicology. The analytical chemical approach to toxicology has altered our thinking. We have become able to recognize smaller and smaller quantities of more and more chemicals. At times it would appear that this analytical approach has blunted our perception of the biological aspects of toxicology, whereas in reality newer developments in our discipline have afforded us broader insights and a wider range of concerns that are emphasized in this state-of-the-art text. Such concerns include the study of birth defects and chemical effects on the immune system; the worldwide use of pesticides, rodenticides, herbicides, and fungicides for increasing food production and permitting protection from various insects and animals that has resulted, in many instances, in human population poisonings; studies on the neurotoxicity and tolerance to the organophosphates in an effort to better understand these important chemicals, and develop better modalities to counter their adverse effects; and target organ toxicity involving the liver, kidney, and lungs. The development of a better understanding of biotransformation of chemicals by tissues, whereby through oxidation and reduction reactions parent compounds are converted to active species, has projected an entirely new concept into toxicology. Furthermore, the importance of conjugation processes in both activation and detoxication of chemicals has shed light on the overall handling of various toxic chemicals.

The book considers not only the student and clinician, but also the active practitioner of toxicological investigations. A broad, but focused view of toxicology is presented by experts in the field, with particular emphasis on specific target organs and the current state-of-the-art concerns already mentioned, rather than on subjects such as carcinogenesis and mutagenesis that are thoroughly covered in numerous other texts. This unique text will serve to narrow the gaps in the existing knowledge base, gaps that must continue to be filled by ongoing and future research, thus expanding our collective knowledge of biological aspects of toxicology.

Thomas J. Haley
William O. Berndt

Chapter 1

Introduction and History

Walter J. Decker

Toxicology is considered by many to be a very recently developed scientific discipline. On the contrary, observation of harmful effects of chemical substances on living organisms is rooted in prehistory. Even the ancient peoples sought antidotes for poisons.

Prehistoric humans, in their constant search for food, observed that certain fruits, berries, or roots had an injurious rather than a nourishing effect. Similarly, it was noted that the bite of some insects or reptiles was likewise followed by severe illness or even death. Attempts to cure ailments probably led to still further experimentation with plants and minerals, some of which were found to produce harmful results even in healthy persons.

While mankind's original quest was for foods and other materials of a beneficial nature, these observations of potently destructive substances must have stirred one's imagination. Poisons were used for hunting and fishing, particularly by the more ingenious peoples. Why should a hunter waste many valuable arrows in mortally wounding his quarry, when a single arrow tipped with deadly curare would produce the same effect? The use of poisoned arrows presented the added advantage that the wounded animal would not be able to run very far before the paralyzing effect of the venom brought it down; the hunter was thus saved an often long and troublesome search for his wounded prey. Likewise, in fishing, it was much easier to throw a basketful of fishberries into the lake and haul out the paralyzed fish than to catch them singly by spearing or hooking. The focus of early toxicology quickly became the murder of fellow beings. Prehistoric man must have realized that those substances that made him ill or that had such a potent effect on animals could also be used to destroy human life. Poison was a great boon to those who were timid or physically weak. To remove an enemy in combat, particularly if that enemy were stronger or more skilled in the use of weapons, presented a serious problem. A trap or ambush could be laid, but not without some personal hazard to the perpetrator. Poison brought the weak up to the level of the strong, the coward up to the standard of the courageous. It required no physical courage or great ability to drop a pinch of poison into a goblet of wine. Furthermore, all were equally vulnerable—prince and pauper alike.

Thwarted ambition, jealous love, or envious hate might now come into their own. Indeed, females furnished the larger number of poisoners, and in medieval Italy and France, the use of poison reached the proportions of a profession. Great was the number who, for a fee, would gladly arrange the elimination of any desired person; adept was their skill in preparing a lethal potion that would operate with time-clock precision; and crafty were they in devising ways of administering the poison without arousing fear or suspicion in their victim.

The use of arrow poisons appears to be one of the most ancient applications of this deadly art. Homer told that Odysseus went to Ephyra "to learn the direful art to taint with drugs the barbed dart." According to Ovid, the arrows of Hercules were tipped with the venom of the Lerneian serpent. This skill was developed in many peoples and in widely scattered continents, but in each case, the special mixture of poisons used was a characteristic of the group. The substances employed and the method of their preparation were often jealously guarded tribal secrets known only to the chiefs and medicine men, and passed on by them to their successors. For the most part, these poisons consisted of extracts of highly toxic plants or crushed insects mixed with snake venom and human blood serum. When used for hunting, the single requirement was that the poison be of such a nature as to leave the meat of the animal edible. For this purpose, snake venoms proved to be almost ideal, for they are practically innocuous if eaten and only exert their harmful effect if introduced into the bloodstream. To this day, the art of poisoning arrows, lance heads, and blowgun darts is practiced in many of the undeveloped areas of the world.

Translations of early Sanskrit medical writings in the Ayur Veda (about 900 B.C.) and the Shastras or commentaries thereon, written by Charaka and Sushruta (about 600 B.C.) indicate that the Hindus of that early period had a considerable knowledge of poisons. The original writings describe the effects of mineral, vegetable, and animal poisons and the bites of venomous reptiles and insects, but only vague comments are made on the prevention or treatment of such poisonings. The Shastras, however, treat more extensively the antidoting of poisons. It is of interest to note, that even at this early date, criminal poisoning was causing concern, as the following extract from the Shastras will indicate:

A person who gives poison may be recognized. He does not answer questions, or they are evasive answers; he speaks nonsense, rub the great toe along the ground, and shivers; his face is discolored; he rubs the roots of the hair with his fingers; and he tries by every means to leave the house. The food which is suspected, should be first given to certain animals, and if they die, it is to be avoided.

Three varieties of *Datura* were alleged to have been employed in India for the solution of domestic quarrels. It has been suggested that the practice of "suttee," in which a widow is burned on the funeral pyre of her husband, may have had its origin as a discouragement to conjugal homicide.

There is little doubt that the ancient Egyptians had considerable information concerning poisons, although many of the details regarding the extent of their knowledge remain vague. The Papyrus Ebers, which was written about 1500 B.C., mentions both mineral and vegetable poisons and describes the effects of lead, copper, antimony, hyoscyamus, hemlock, and opium. A cryptic exhortation to a secret cult of the Eyptian priesthood is found in an early papyrus, "Speak not of the name of I A O under the penalty of the peach." This might signify that the deadly nature of the cyanogen, amygdalin, contained in peach kernels, was known to those ancients and employed by them against those who betrayed their secrets.

Apart from references to the venom of "serpents," early Hebrew writings contain few allusions to poison. However, during the Egyptian captivity, it seems quite probable that the Hebrews acquired some knowledge of poisons from their captors. The "water of bitterness" described in the Book of Numbers as an ordeal to test the fidelity of a suspected wife must have had some toxic properties if the results were ever to indicate guilt. The "water of gall," spoken of by Jeremiah as a means of punishment for offenders against the laws of Jehovah, likewise must have been a poison. The Hebrew word "rosch," in the original manuscripts, appears to have been a generic term for poisonous herbs or plants.

Present knowledge of the use of poisons by the Greeks of the classical period may be traced back into the legendary shadows of their mythology. Hecate, who was said to have been skilled in sorcery and the preparation of poisons, imparted this information to her two daughters Circe and Medea. Circe applied her art in transforming Odysseus's men into swine, and Odysseus himself only escaped through the protective effects of an herb supplied by Hermes. Medea employed her knowledge in preparing a narcotic poison to be used by her lover Jason in subduing the dragon that guarded the Golden Fleece.

Xenophon, writing about 400 B.C., relates that the use of poison was so frequent among the Medes that it was customary for the cupbearer to taste the wine before presenting it to the king or nobles of the court.

The use of poison hemlock for political executions was common in Greece. The death of Socrates in 339 B.C. is perhaps the best-known example. The following account of the great philosopher's death, as given by Plato, is an accurate description of the progressive paralysis that hemlock, or its active principle coniine, produces:

When the fatal cup was brought, he asked what it was necessary for him to do. "Nothing more," replied the servant of the judges, "than as soon as you have drunk of the draught, to walk about until you find a heaviness in your legs. Then lie down and it will do its purpose." After drinking the cup and reproving his friends for indulging in loud lamentations, he continued to walk about as directed until he found his legs grow heavy. Then he lay down his back, and the person who had administered the poison went up to him and examined for a little time, his feet and legs. And then squeezing his foot hard, he asked if he felt it. Socrates replied that he did not. He then did the same to his legs and thighs, and proceeding upward in this way, showed us that he was growing cold and stiff. Then Socrates touched himself and said that when the poison reached his heart, he should then depart. But now the parts around the lower belly were almost cold, when uncovering himself, he said, and they were his last words, "Crito, we owe a cock to Aesculapius. Pay the debt therefore, and do not neglect it." Shortly afterwards he gave a convulsive movement. His eyes were fixed and when Crito observed this he closed his eyelids and his mouth.

Suicide by poison was not at all uncommon among Greeks. The state was the official repository of poisons, and these not only were administered to the condemned but also were provided for those who could present to the Council satisfactory evidence that life was a burden and that it were better to end it. If the reasons were deemed sufficient, a cup of hemlock was provided at public expense.

It is related that Olympias, widow of Philip of Macedon, having captured her rival Eurydice, placed her in prison and provided a sword, a rope, and a cup of hemlock, with orders to choose her mode of death.

The earliest works dealing specifically with poisons are two poems by Nikander of Colophon (185–135 B.C.), who was physician to Attalus, King of Bithynia. At court, Nikander was said to have been given special facilities for studying poisons by being allowed to experiment on condemned criminals. The first of these poems, the "Theriaca" of about a thousand lines, deals with poisonous plants and animals; the other, the "Aloxipharmaca" of some 600 lines, had to do with antidotes. He discussed the effects of snake venoms, opium, henbane, aconite, and hemlock, and recommended suitable antidotes for each. While these verses are mostly fable, there is, however, a considerable body of information that must have resulted from experience and careful observation.

The "Materia Medica" of Dioscorides, written in the 1st century A.D., contained a treatise on poisons and their antidotes. In it the then-known poisons were classified according to their origin. Those arising from animal sources were cantharides ("Spanish fly"), serpents, toads, salamanders, crustaceans, the sea hare, blood of the wild bull, and Honey of Heraclea. The plant kingdom provided mandragora, aconita, colcicum or "meadow saffron," opium, and hemlock. Minerals known to have poisonous effects were listed: arsenic, litharge, white lead, and cinnebar. This writing remained the standard work on the subject for the following 15 centuries, and although many commentaries were written on Dioscorides' work, no material additions were made. One commentator, Galen, writing in the 2nd century, apologized for the scant information given by saying, "It is imprudent to treat of poisons and to make known their composition to the common people, who could only profit from this by committing crimes."

It is noted that in Dioscorides's list there are several preparations that are not known at the present time. For example, the sea hare, often alluded to by the Greeks, was probably a large snail or mollusk. It was described by the older writers as a dreadful object, so poisonous that it could neither be touched nor even looked upon with safety. It seems very likely that its rareness and its unknown habits stimulated the imagination of amateur naturalists.

Wild bull's blood was reputed by the ancients as a very potent poison. However, unless it were permitted to putrefy or was fortified by other active poisons, it is difficult to understand how it could have possessed such harmful properties. Nevertheless, the deaths of notables have been attributed to this poison. Herodotus related that in 525 B.C., Psammenitus, a king of Egypt who was conquered by Cambyses, having revolted, was captured and forced to drink bull's blood, which caused immediate death. The deaths of Midas, of the golden touch, and of Themistocles, hero of Salamis, were attributed to it. Although Cicero ridiculed the latter account, Plutarch, in his Life of Themistocles, said, "Having decided that his best course was to put a fitting end to his life, he made a sacrifice to the gods, then called his friends together, gave them a farewell clasp of his hand, and as the current story goes, drank bull's blood—or as some say—took a quick poison, and so died." Another reference to this event is found in the "Knights" of Aristophanes—which was written in 424 B.C., a few years after Themistocles' demise. Two slaves are discussing suicide:

First Slave: "Let's die then, only and for all; that's the best way; only we must contrive to manage it nobly and manfully in a proper manner."
Second Slave: "Aye, aye. Let's do the thing manfully—that's my maxim."
"Well, there's the example of Themistocles. To drink bull's blood—that seems a manly death."

Little can be found concerning the exact composition of Honey of Heraclea mentioned by Dioscorides. It is known that it was prepared in southern Italy as well as in Bithynia and appears to have been an infusion of poisonous roots in a honey solution. Ignophen reported that some of his soldiers were poisoned with this material: "They were delirious, vomited, purged, and could not stand on their legs. Those with only a taste were drunken; those who had more seemed mad, others dying. Those that recovered were still weak and fatigued three or four days." This description is reminiscent of the signs of intoxication by wolfsbane or aconite, a poison that was well known in that period. This is further borne out by the report that aconite derived its name from Akon, a small city of Heraclea, where the roots of wolfsbane were collected and prepared.

Plutarch described a similar incident, which occurred during a campaign of Mark Anthony against the Parthians. The short rations of the Romans caused them to supplement their food supply with herbs and roots. The long tap roots of aconite were mistaken for edible parsnips, and wholesale poisonings resulted.

The interest of the ancients stimulated a concomitant search for counterpoisons or antidotes. Deriving their names from the two poems of Nikander, they are called theriacs and alexipharmics. One of the most remarkable of these was *terra sigillata* or "sealed earth"—a reddish clay found on the island of Lemnos. According to religious custom, it was only dug on one day of each year during the festival of Diana.

According to Dioscorides, the clay was made into a paste with goat's blood, and the resulting tablets were stamped or "sealed" with the image of Diana, one of the goddesses associated with healing. The elaborate precautions for identifying the authentic tablets suggest that, even at that early date, spurious preparations were being sold (the precursor to the "look-alikes"?). There may have been merits in such an antidote. In modern times, it has been observed that certain clays, such as fuller's earth and bentonite, have the property of adsorbing comparatively large quantities of vegetable poisons such as strychnine, opium, aconite, and hemlock. It seems quite possible that the "sealed earth" distributed by Diana's priestesses might have had similar properties.

It is said that Zopyrus, a physician of Alexandria in the employ of Mithridates, King of Pontus, invented a general antidote that would give protection against any known poison. Celsus wrote that it consisted of 36 ingredients, Galen gave the number as 44, and Pliny generously increased it to 54. At any rate, Mithridates, who was in constant fear of poisoning, is reported to have alternated doses of poison and antidote until he became completely immune to all toxic substances. Legend has it that when he wished to commit suicide following a disastrous defeat by Pompey, poisons had no effect and he was forced to have a mercenary dispatch him with a sword.

Antidotal mixtures were very popular throughout the Middle Ages. All were based upon the original mithridatic mixture, but new and "secret" ingredients were constantly added. Dried vipers' heads, probably crushed, were reputed to have potent properties as an antidote, probably on the homeopathic principle of *similia similibus curantur*, that "like cures like." Vipers' heads, having the property of causing poisoning, were likewise expected to cure it. Unquestionably their effect was purely psychological.

Criminal poisonings began to occur with alarming frequency in ancient Rome. Livy wrote that in the 423rd year of the Republic (331 B.C.) there were a great number of sudden deaths, all with the same peculiar symptoms. Since these did not correspond to any recognized disease, the city was thrown into a panic. A slave finally confessed that some 20 matrons had conspired to dispose of unwanted persons by the use of poisoned beverages. With great effectiveness, they had proceeded to exterminate those whose property they wished to inherit, or flagging husbands who stood in the way of more ardent lovers, or those who merely displease them. This group, surprised in the act of concocting their lethal brew, offered the defense that they were only preparing medicine. The magistrates required them to drink their preparation, with the result that all perished. Further investigation disclosed 170 accomplices who were finally convicted and punished. Livy, in his account, stated that never before had there been cases of criminal poisoning in Rome. Whether or not this was true, certainly they were not the last.

Similar cases of what appeared to be wholesale poisoning were investigated in 184 and 180 B.C. The first outbreak was traced to Bacchanalian orgies, while the second occurred during a pestilence. In both, the great number of persons who were accused of having administered poison were convicted. In view of present knowledge, it would appear that there may have been a gross miscarriage of justice, at least in the latter outbreak.

Epidemic diseases, such as cholera and plague, complicated by dysentery and the ever-present malaria, undoubtedly produced many incidents that were incorrectly attributed to toxic agents. It must be remembered that the recognition of poisoning was based on very sketchy (and often erroneous) signs and symptoms. Any suddenly developed illness in which there was vomiting, diarrhea, convulsions, or unconsciousness and paralysis was likely to be classified as a poisoning. If, after death, the body quickly developed the discolorations and distortions that normally accompany putrefaction, this was taken as certain confirmation that the deceased had been poisoned. Direct evidence was seldom obtainable; rarely was a person observed in the act of administering poison.

In a crowded city built partially on marshy ground where malarial mosquitos might be expected to thrive, where there was the ever-present hazard of dubious water supply and sewage disposal, and where refrigeration was unknown and most meat dishes had to be highly seasoned to cover up the flavor of incipient spoilage, it is not difficult to understand how a naturally occurring illness could easily be mistaken for poisoning. It was not until sensitive chemical tests for poisons were developed that the detection of poisoning could be placed on a certain and scientific basis.

By the time of the civil wars in Rome, poisoning became so common that the dictator Sulla issued an edict against such assassinations. This was the *Lex Cornelia*, the first legislative enactment against poisoning. Upon conviction, punishment consisted of banishment and confiscation of property if the poisoner were of high rank and exposure to wild animals if of low degree. This law continued in force, with certain additions and modifications, until the fall of the empire. One of the added provisions made the law applicable to pharmacists who carelessly compounded or administered poisons.

In spite of such laws, poisons continued in popularity in high places as well as among the lowly. Livia, wife of Emperor Augustus, was accused of having poisoned Marcellus, the son of Octavia, and Caius and Lucius, the children of Julia. Finally, she was reputed to have fatally poisoned her husband in order to secure the succession of her son Tiberius. Tiberius in turn is said to have disposed of Germanicus by means of poison.

About this time, poisoning began to take on a professional aspect. Agrippina, wife of Emperor Claudius, had so many toxicological problems that she hired an expert, one Locusta, to remain in residence at Court. Locusta prepared poisonous mixtures, tested their strength on both animals and humans, and supervised their administration to those persons who had been selected for destruction. In an extremely businesslike fashion, she removed all obstacles that stood in the way of Agrippina's ambition. First to go was one of Agrippina's superfluous husbands, Crispus Passiennus; then Emperor Claudius succumbed to her artful technique; and finally, Brittanicus, son of Claudius and rightful heir to the throne, was eliminated so as to secure the coveted place for Agrippina's son Nero.

The literature of the time, particularly during the period of the Roman Empire, is full of allusions to poisons. The patricians seemed to be the chief offenders, judging from the remark of Juvenal, "You will drink no aconite out of an earthenware cup; You may dread it when Setine wine sparkles in a golden bowl."

Although records during the Dark Ages are not so complete, it appears that there were plenty of poisonings during that period. Of the 83 Emperors of the East, from Valens to Constantine III, seven were known to have been poisoned. Nine of the successors of Charlemagne died of poison, and up to 1471, five popes perished in the same way.

Among the few advances in poison lore that were made during the period between the fall of the Roman Empire and the Renaissance were discovery by Arabian alchemists of the toxic properties of corrosive sublimate and the replacement of arsenic sulfide in poison preparations by white arsenic or sublimed arsenic. From the viewpoint of the poisoner, the latter represented a distinct improvement. The ease with which a person might be secretly poisoned by white arsenic opened up a new field for professionals and amateurs alike. Its discovery ushered in what might be called the Golden Age of poisoning. There are several properties of this almost ideal poison that made it so useful for secret extermination. It was potent; as little as 200 mg might well produce death. It was white in color, and dissolved readily in water to give a colorless and odorless solution having little taste. It could therefore be added in lethal amounts to foods and beverages without making its presence known. Finally, it could be used to kill quickly by giving a single large dose, or death could be accomplished more subtly and slowly by administering small daily doses over a more protracted period. When administered in this latter fashion, the symptoms of poisoning so closely resembled natural diseases that detection was almost impossible in that "pre-analytical chemistry" era.

As an example of the technique employed in using white arsenic, an attempted poisoning of the royal house of France occurred in 1384. At that time Charles the Bad, of Navarra, sent Woudreton, a minstrel, to the French court with instructions to poison Charles VI, the King's brother the Duke of Valois, and his uncles, the Dukes of Bourbon, Bourgoyne, and Berry. Woudreton received explicit instructions from his employer:

> Go thou to Paris; thou canst do great service if thou wilt do what I tell thee; I will reward thee well. Thou shalt do thus: There is a thing which is called sublimed arsenic; if a man eat a bit the size of a pea, he will never survive. Thou wilt find it in the apothecaries' shops in Pampeluna, Bordeaus, Bayonne, and in all good towns through which thou wilt pass. Take it and powder it; and when thou shalt be in the house of the king, draw near and betake thyself to the kitchen, to the larder, to the cellar or any other place where they point can best be gained, and put the powder in the soups, meats or wines, provided that thou canst do it secretly. Otherwise do it not.

The diabolical plot failed; Woudreton was detected, convicted, and quartered in the Place de Creve.

With the dawn of the Renaissance in Italy, toxicology was cultivated along with the other arts, and poisoning was employed by states as well as by individuals under the impulse of avarice, jealousy, or lust for power. Political murder by poison became so commonplace that no one believed in the natural death of princes, kings, or cardinals; they were either poignarded or poisoned. During the 15th century, Peter of Abano's handbook of poisons "De Venenis" went through no less than 14 editions. Their present rarity speaks eloquently of the hard use to which they were put.

Rings contained small receptacles to carry a small but deadly charge of poison; a wave of the hand over a goblet of wine was all that was needed to inject death into the contents. As a refinement of the arrow poisoning technique, the blades of daggers were made with depressions into which poison could be placed. Even a minor wound by such a weapon could be fatal. Knives were made with recesses in one side of the blade, so that upon cutting a peach or melon, only one portion was poisoned; the murderer allayed any fears of his victim by eating the uncontaminated portion. Everything was poisoned; not only food and wine but cups, books, incense, tapers, coins, gloves, clothing—even the cosmetic on the lips of the king's mistress.

That the use of poisons for political extermination was sanctioned during this period is evidenced by various entries found in the then secret archives of the Venetian Council of Ten. Contracts to eliminate unwanted persons were entered into and bargained for in much the same way as agreements for other dealings, such as the construction of a palace or the repair of a bridge. The following are a few excerpts from the minutes of Council meetings:

May 24, 1419. The Council signifies its agreement to a proposition of Michaletus Mudacio to poison Sigismund, King of Hungary, for a specific reward and orders that poison for this purpose shall be furnished.

Sept. 24, 1419. The Archbishop of Trebizond offers to poison Marilius of Carrara. The offer was accepted, an advance payment of 50 ducats made and a horse ordered.

Dec. 2, 1450. Council received poison in the form of balls which, when thrown into the fire, produce highly toxic fumes. Poisoning of Count Francesco Sforza considered. Efficacy of poison to be first established by experiment on a condemned prisoner.

Jan. 17, 1478. Accepts offer of one Lazarus "the Turk" to poison wells from which Turkish army obtains its water.

Just as the name of Macchiavelli carried the connotation of political perfidy and dissimulation, so the name of the contemporaneous family of Borgia has come to be almost synonymous with poisoning. One might add that both families are unfairly maligned thereby; their offense was merely one of frank and open recognition of techniques that were frequently employed, albeit surreptitiously, and generally countenanced in their time.

One of the most notorious poisonings carried out by the Borgia Pope Alexander was his skillful removal of Prince Zizim, younger son of Mohamet II and pretender to the Turkish throne. Sultan Bajazet, brother of the deceased, paid the Pope 300,000 ducats for this work of art. The Borgia assassination plan was usually quite simple. At dinner, a goblet of wine suitably treated with the notorious Borgia "cantarella" would be served, and death would result at the appointed time. The poison of the Borgias was reported to function with time-clock precision. It is said that a draught could be prepared that would kill in a day, a month, or a year, as desired. Unquestionably, the alleged delayed action of their poison was grossly exaggerated, but the fact that many victims departed this life by way of the Borgia cantarella cannot be denied.

It is reported that Pope Alexander fell victim to his own poison in 1503, in an attempt to eliminate the wealthy Cardinal Adriano of Corneto. By mistake, the cup bearer served the poisoned wine to Alexander and his son Cesare. The elderly Pope succumbed, but the more vigorous son recovered after a brief illness.

The notorious Toffana carried on a similar business in Naples. She dispensed a colorless, odorless, and tasteless solution in special vials bearing the representation of a local saint associated with a medicinal spring, the waters of which had a reputation for miraculous healing. The liquid was sold under the name of "Manna of St. Nicholas di Bari," ostensibly for improvement of the complexion by external application. But anyone who was in on the secret knew of its deadly effect when taken internally. Toffana cunningly worked on the minds of clients who were susceptible to religious or superstitious influences, and those who were unaware of the origin of her deadly "acquetta" were told that it was a miracle-working fluid that oozed from the tomb of Saint Nicholas.

During this period, the search for antidotes came to have prime importance. A potent and successful counterpoison might be all that stood between a diner and eternity. Unicorn's horn was thought to have the property of absorbing poison, and drinking cups fashioned from the horn of this mythical animal were highly prized. By their use, any drink, however poisoned, would be rendered "safe." The traffic in unicorn's horn proved highly lucrative to the racketeers of that day; it was hard on narwhals, whose tusks served as substitutes when unicorns could not be found.

Another protection against poisoning that had great popularity at that time was bezoars, concretions found in the alimentary tract of herbivores. The potency of the antidotal effect of a bezoar was held to be proportional to the rarity of the species in which it was found and the remoteness of its habitat. Bezoars, particularly those of oriental origin, were highly prized until Ambrose Pare, physician to King Charles IX, demonstrated their utter uselessness as antidotes. The demonstration resulted from a controversy between the king and his physician over a very rare and expensive bezoar that one of the courtiers had presented. Pare insisted that there was no merit to the belief in its antidotal properties. As an experiment, the king offered a condemned criminal a sporting chance to save his life. He was to be given a fatal dose of poison together with a generous dose of the King's precious bezoar. If the criminal lived, he was to be pardoned. The offer was accepted and the experiment performed as ordered. The poor wretch writhed in agony for several hours and finally expired. The remainder of the powdered bezoar was thrown away.

Poisoning as an art and profession came to France with Catherine de Medici, the Italian bride of Henry II. She undoubtedly had received excellent schooling, for it was for the Florentine court of her father that Macchiavelli wrote his famous treatise on government by murder, artifice, and intrigue. Catherine is credited with poisoning Jeanne d'Albret, Queen of Navarre, the Duc d'Anjou, and Coffe, a marshal of France.

In 1665, two Italian soldiers of fortune and a German apothecary named Glaser formed a partnership in Paris for the manufacture and sale of poisons. It appears that Glaser manufactured the preparations, which were either used or sold by his Italian confederates. A priest, who heard of the nefarious traffic through the confessional, denounced them to the civil authorities, and the two Italians were lodged in the Bastilo. Glaser was not under suspicion and retained his freedom.

During their incarceration, one of the Italians died and the other, named Exili, was placed in a cell with a cavalry captain named Sainte Croix. After a year of imprisonment, during which he learned the secrets and techniques of poisoning from his cellmate Exili, Sainte Croix was liberated. Exili also gave him Glaser's address. Sainte Croix lost no time in seeking out the German apothecary; a new business venture was established. Glaser, with Sainte Croix's help, prepared poisonous mixtures. They had a large clientele to which they supplied poisons—"powders of succession" as they were called, because they were so effective in making inheritances available.

Sainte Croix fell victim to his own wiles; he died from inhaling toxic fumes (probably arsine) while working in his laboratory.

Pressures of public opinion then forced the civil authorities in Paris to establish a special court to hear cases of alleged criminal poisoning and witchcraft. This court, which was under the immediate direction of Louvois, minister of justice, sat from 1678 to 1682. During the 3 years of its existence, it heard charges against 442 persons and imposed sentence on 282. Undoubtedly, many more investigations and convictions would have been secured if offenders of high rank had not been able to hamper the court's action.

So common was poisoning at that time that people came to look on it fatalistically as one of the ordinary hazards of life. If you were poisoned and recovered, no remonstrance was made. If the poison had a fatal effect, people shrugged their shoulders. It was quite similar to dueling; the most important thing was to exhibit good sportsmanship.

Another celebrated poisoner of that time was Catharine Deshayes, better known as La Voisine, abortionist, sorceress, and arch poisoner. Her establishment might properly be classified as big business, for her annual income amounted to over one hundred thousand francs. Not only did she dispense "powders of succession" and other poisons, but also love philters, charms, and amulets. Subsequent investigation showed that she had murdered some 2500 infants. She was apprehended and condemned. However, in tracing her accomplices and clients, the trail of crime began to involve persons close to the King. Finally, in 1682, when it was disclosed that the mistress of Louis XIV, Madam Montespan, had purchased poison from La Voisine, the King summarily dismissed Louvois's court and impounded its records to avoid further scandal. In spite of this early manifestation of the "fixing" of courts, enough of the horrible details of La Voisine's business had been aired to mobilize public opinion, and La Voisine was the last of the professional poisoners on the Continent.

Although there exist no records of professional poisoners in England, it is certain that there were many whose amateur standing would not have stood close scrutiny. One may obtain some information concerning the use of poisons during the Elizabethan period from the writings of Shakespeare. These show a wide knowledge of toxic substances and of many ways in which they might be administered. In his plays, suicide is frequently accomplished by poison. Weapons are tainted so as to produce certain death. The murder of Hamlet's father by pouring henbane into the ear seems a tale of fantasy. However, experiments on animals have shown that one of its toxic constituents, hyoscyamine, can be absorbed from the external auditory canal in sufficient amount to cause death. Thus, it seems probable that Shakespeare's usage was based more on popular knowledge than on flights of imagination.

The death blow to secret or criminal poisoning came in the middle of the 19th century. In 1836, Marsh developed an extremely sensitive test for arsenic, which would permit its identification in foods and beverages, as well as in body tissues or excreta. The application of this test raised the diagnosis of arsenical poisoning from a mere suspicion to a scientific certainty. If arsenic was the King of Poisons, one might truly say—the king is dead.

Another advance in the detection of poisons came about through a murder that was accomplished by means of nicotine. In the year 1850, Count Bocarme and his wife conspired to gain control of the family estate by disposing of her brother Gustave Fougnies. The Count set about his problem in a methodical fashion, by first studying chemistry. Later, when he had developed sufficient proficiency, he prepared nicotine from tobacco in his own laboratory. After enticing his brother-in-law to his chateau at Bitremont, nicotine was administered orally by force, as a result of which Fougnies died within 5 minutes. Although there was much circumstantial evidence available, the Belgian authorities requested the aid of Jean Servais Stas, an eminent chemist of the time, in an attempt to isolate poison from the vital organs of the deceased. Not only was Stas able to demonstrate the presence of nicotine in the stomach of the deceased, but his technique also permitted a reasonably accurate measure of the quantity of poison present.

Occasional cases of criminal poisoning still exist, but these are generally stimulated by laxity of civil authorities in the investigation of sudden or suspicious deaths.

One of the last (and outstanding) attempts at mass murder by poison occurred in Chicago on February 10, 1916. That evening, a dinner was held at the University Club in honor of Cardinal Mundelein, then Archbishop of the Chicago archdiocese. Some 300 guests attended, including clergymen, the Governor, and other officials in state and local governments, as well as many business and professional men of the community. Shortly after the soup course had been served, many of the diners suddenly developed severe symptoms of gastric irritation. The situation was so disastrous that John B. Murphy, M.D., who was among the guests, set up an emergency "field hospital" in an adjoining room. There were no fatalities, and all the victims recovered within a few days. Chemical tests revealed the presence of arsenic in the soup, apparently placed by an assistant chef, Jean Crones, who was known to be a rabid anticleric. Crones disappeared that night and was never apprehended.

In more recent times, poisoning, apart from suicides, has in large measure been a result not of criminal activity, but of ignorance, thoughtlessness, and carelessness. In our present day, poisoning through accidental exposure to toxic dusts or vapors in industry, carelessness in preparing, labeling, or prescribing medicines, or the misuse of pesticides has taken its toll.

Advances in the knowledge of chemistry led to enhanced capability in analytical methodology, which in turn sparked the evolution of toxicology as we now know it. The stage was set when Joseph Plenck wrote in his 1781 treatise, *Elementa Medicinae et Chirurgiae Forensis,* "The only certain sign of poisoning is the chemical identification of the poison in the organs of the body." Some highlights of the early development of analytical toxicology have been compiled by Dr. Kurt M. Dubowski and Dr. Sunil K. Niyogi:

1775—Scheele discovered that when zinc and acid act on arsenic, a gaseous compound is evolved, which, on burning, deposited metallic arsenic.

1821—Serullas used the decomposition of arsine for the detection of small quantities of arsenic in stomach contents and urine in poisoning cases.

1821—Mathieu Orfila proposed a division of poisons into four classes: irritants, narcotics, narcoticoacrids, and putrefiants.

1832—*Poisons and Asphyxia*, a book written by Henry Coley of New York, included mention of the testing of gastric contents by chemical means.

1836—James M. Marsh devised his test for arsenic based on Scheele's discovery.

1839—Mathieu Orfila was the first to extract arsenic from human organs other than gastrointestinal tissue.

1842—Hugo Reinsch, a German chemist, presented a new test to detect arsenic.

1844—Frensenius and von Bobo devised a method for the systemic search for all mineral poisons. They used wet ashing with chlorine. Duflos also developed it in 1838.

1850—Jean Servais Stas (1813–1891), a chemist of Brussels, developed a method of extracting alkaloids from cadavers. This led to other similar studies. Quantitative determination of metals in organs began about this time.

1852—Casper's *Vierteljahrschrift für Gerichtliche Medizin* offered only qualitative testing of copper in urine, gastric content of oxalic acid and phosphorus, and arsenic by the Marsh Test.

1853—T. Graham and A. W. Hofman noted that charcoal has the power of adsorbing strychnine from beer. This idea gave many toxicologists, in subsequent years, to develop the adsorption method in toxicological analysis work.

1856—F. J. Otto modified the Stas method, treating the final aqueous liquid, while still acid, with ether to remove fats and other nonalkaloid substances which are soluble in ether. This modification has become well known as the "Stas–Otto" method.

1862—Electrolyte deposition was first used and metals were quantified by weight of electrode deposit.

1865—Helwig first demonstrated microsublimation. Carbon monoxide qualitative tests were developed from this time to 1889 by Hoppe Seyler's spectroscopic, Salkowski's alkali and Stopczanski's dilution and tannic acid precipitation. In 1880, Fodor measured carbon monoxide quantitatively using palladium chloride and titrated with standard potassium iodide solution.

1867—Schmiedeberg decomposed chloroform in a combustion tube containing magnesium oxide and then titrated the chloride. Theodore George Wormley, an American toxicologist, published *Microchemistry of Poisons*, an important contribution to poison identification and the first American book devoted entirely to toxicology.

1868—Hofmann's isonitrile reaction for chloroform developed. Schwartz's resorcin reaction was reported in 1888. Dragendorff made a new approach and developed a systematic method of extraction and separation of nonvolatile organic compounds from biological specimens.

1870—Lieben developed an iodoform test for alcohol. Between 1852 and 1883, quantitative methods for alcohol based upon the reduction of chromic acid were devised by Cotte, Subbotin, Bodlander, and Strassmann. A micromethod was reported by Nicloux in 1906 and Widmark in 1922. Up until 1956, many quantitative methods for alcohol in blood, urine, spinal fluid, expired air and tissues had been developed by investigators including E. Bogen, J. W. Cavett, W. W. Jetter, A. O. Gettler, L. A. Greenberg, H. W. Haggard, R. N. Harger, H. A. Heise, L. D. MacLeod, C. W. Muehlberger, and T. Winnick.

1874—Selmi examined organs from putrefied bodies and found cadaveric alkaloids reported to be morphine. Crystalline derivatives of alkaloids were first prepared between 1846 and 1884. Some color reactions for alkaloids were developed in 1861–1882. Quantitative methods for alkaloids came into use in 1890.

1879—Gutzeit's method of detection of small quantity of arsenic. This method is still very useful for the quantitation of arsenic in toxicological analysis.

1880—Rudolph A. Witthaus, Prof. of Chemistry at the Cornell University Medical School, did much of the important toxicological examinations for New York City and other cases from outlying areas. He wrote a textbook on toxicology with Becker in 1911.

1881—K. L. Dey, Calcutta, India, developed the test for opium in toxicology, detecting "porphyroxin," morphia and meconic acid in opium.

1884—A. W. Blyth wrote *Poisons: Their Effects and Detection,* a valuable work in analytical toxicology.

1895—C. Kippenberger initiated the use of tannic acid and glycerol for the isolation of alkaloids and glycosides from tissue. In 1900, Kippenberger modified his own method.

Prior to the advent of chromaographic methods in the early 1950s, difficulty of separation of mixtures of drugs and lack of sensitivity posed numerous problems. Typically, the biological specimen was steam-distilled twice to yield an acidic and a basic fraction containing volatile compounds. The acid distillate contained such compounds as hydrocyanic acid, chloroform, methanol, ethanol, nitrobenzene, free iodine, iodoform, phenol, chloral hydrate, formaldehyde, carbon disulfide, acetone, turpentine, phosphorus, cresols, and carbon tetrachloride. The basic distillate contained volatile amines, ammonia, aniline, and volatile alkaloids such as nicotine and coniine. The residue in the distilling flask was then acidified and extracted four times with ethanol under reflux conditions. These extracts were combined, filtered, and evaporated to a syrupy consistency, acidified with sulfuric acid, and refrigerated to separate lipoid material. After filtration, the filtrate was extracted several times with ether to remove acid drugs, including acetanilid, acetophenetidin, antipyrine, aminopyrine, barbiturates, salicylates, sulfa drugs, caffeine, theobromine, and theophylline. The remaining aqueous solution was made alkaline with magnesium oxide and extracted several times with chloroform to remove alkaline compounds such as strychnine, brucine, nicotine, cocaine, procaine, quinine, atropine, codeine, and morphine. The three fractions—volatile, acidic, and basic—were assayed largely by "spot tests" of varying sensitivity and specificity. The cumbersome extraction procedure described took the better part of a day to perform, and the assays took up to several days to complete. Many compounds ranging from considerable to slight volatility, such as amphetamine, could not be recovered at the low concentrations normally found in urine. The spot tests used on the extract to detect morphine—that is, Marquis's, Mecke's, and Froehde's reagents—were quite sensitive. They are able to produce their characteristic colors with 20 μg morphine, but when mixture of drugs is present, their selectivities are poor.

In 1946, J. W. Jailer and Leo R. Goldbaum adapted the technique of water-immiscible solvent extraction, long used by pharmacologists to determine oil:water partition coefficients of drugs to toxicology. By this method, acidic and basic drugs could be selectively extracted from specimens by adjusting the pH. Acidic drugs were concentrated in the immiscible organic solvent by making the specimen acid, and basic drugs were likewise concentrated by making specimen alkaline. Amphoteric drugs, such as morphine, were extracted by adjusting the pH to the isoelectric point of the drug. In this manner, some separation of drugs was attained.

The next technique adapted for further separation of drugs was paper chromatography, reported by R. Munier and M. Machebouet in 1950. This did indeed improve separation; individual drugs showed up as discrete spots on the paper, but the time for analysis was very long. Using the method of descending chromatography (downward solvent flow; capillary action aided by gravity), development required at least an overnight period. Ascending chromatography (upward solvent flow; capillary action hindered by gravity) took about twice as long to accomplish. The paper was slow to dry; the use of heat was deleterious to the somewhat volatile compounds. Paper electrophoresis was a faster method, but drying was again a problem; this technique was refined by L. R. Goldbaum and Leo Kazyak in 1954.

Column adsorption chromatography was used to separate and purify alkaloids and barbiturates in the late 1940s by Abraham Stolman and C. P. Stewart, but the collection of fractions was quite cumbersome. Application of the adsorbent (silica gel) in a thin layer on a sheet of glass gave rise to the technique of thin-layer chromatography (TLC). This technique, first described in 1949, was adapted to forensic toxicology in the late 1950s by Gottfried Machata. It is much faster and more convenient than paper chromatography: development time is usually less than an hour, and air drying at room temperature is accomplished in a few minutes.

Although the use of ion-exchange resins in toxicology was described by L. Levi and C. G. Farmilo in 1952, its application to detection of drugs of abuse in the urine did not become widespread until the middle 1960s, when V. P. Dole, W. K. Kim, and I. Eglitis published their simplified method. In this technique, a piece of ion-exchange paper is soaked in the diluted urine, extracting all the commonly abused drugs. The paper is dried and sent to the laboratory for elution and analysis, obviating shipment of urine specimens and decreasing the amount of solvent required.

The development of gas chromatography (GC) in 1952 (A. T. James and A. J. P. Martin) signalled a powerful technique for the separation and identification of drugs. The first applications appeared in the literature in the late 1950s, but they were largely confined to the analyses of volatiles such as carbon monoxide and ethanol. During the 1960s, however, almost all drugs were found to be amenable to GC analysis.

A system for coupling gas chromatography and mass spectrometry (MS) was developed in 1959 by R. S. Gohlke. However, most toxicologic applications of GC/MS did not appear until the early 1970s. MS/MS has recently been promoted as an even more sensitive and specific technique.

There are several other methods in current use that have varying degrees of sensitivity and specificity. These include colorimetry, ultraviolet spectrophotometry, fluorometry, and immunoassays. Colorimetric methods for a number of drugs were developed during 1930s. These and later such tests were developed primarily for the quantification of specific drugs.

Similarly, the assays employing ultraviolet spectrophotometry were designed to quantify specific drugs or chemical classes of drugs, such as barbiturates by L. R. Goldbaum and phenytoin by Jack E. Wallace and Horace E. Hamilton. Fluorometry as a technique to detect drugs of abuse was developed during the 1940s as a result of B. B. Brodie's and Sidney Udenfriend's research, but expanded markedly during the heroin "epidemic" of the late 1960s and early 1970s. Its specificity in the detection of morphine in urine is very high.

The latest methodology to be applied to analytical toxicology is that of immunoassay. Five individual techniques have been developed: free radical assay technique (FRAT), hemagglutination inhibition (HI), enzyme-multiplied inhibition assay (EMIT), radioimmunoassay (RIA), and fluorescent immunoassay (FIA). FRAT is quite useful in detecting morphine in urine but suffers a great disadvantage in that it requires a very expensive, dedicated instrument, an electron spin resonance spectrometer. The other four systems—EMIT, HI, RIA, and FIA—are currently in quite common use.

Within the last 2 years, the techniques of apoenzyme reactivation immunoassay (ARIS) and substrate-labeled fluorescent immunoassay (SLFIA) have become commercially available.

Studies on mechanisms of poisoning were hampered until suitable measurement techniques and basic understanding of biochemical, chemical, physiological, and pathological processes became available. Even so, early observations proved invaluable to the developing field of toxicology.

Surprisingly, Cleopatra was one of the first persons recorded to have an interest in the mechanisms of poisoning. She wished to find a poison that was quick and caused a minimum of premortal suffering. Cleopatra commanded that "clinical research" be conducted on slaves (and perhaps on persons outside her favor) to find such a poison. A preparation containing strychnine (seeds of the *Nux vomica* plant) appeared to be a likely candidate, except for one aspect of its action—the distinctive grin ("risus sardonicus") that the victims took on in the final phase of their death. As history reports, Cleopatra opted for the bite of the asp, a poisonous snake indigenous to Egypt, as best satisfying her concept of an "ideal" poison.

Philippus Theophrastus Bombastus von Hohenheim, familiarly known as Paracelsus, in the early part of the 16th century not only laid the groundwork for modern concepts of chemotherapy, but also studied in detail the adverse effects of drugs available at the time. Indeed, his statements, "Poison is in everything, and no thing is without poison. The dosage makes it either a poison or a remedy," are held as valid today by most toxicologists.

In 1806, Friedrich Wilhelm Adam Setürner, a young pharmacist from Westphalia, isolated and named morphine (for the Greco–Roman god of sleep, Morpheus). He performed studies on himself and several friends; they ingested about 10 times the currently recommended dose of morphine. Setürner noted that it had a profound central nervous system depressant action (including respiration), and that complete recovery took several days to occur.

Around this time period, Francois Magendie was studying the Borneo arrow poison, *Upas tiente*, which later proved to contain strychnine as its active (convulsant) principle. In the dog and the horse, he attempted to localize the pathways of absorption and distribution, as well as the site of action. Claude Bernard, Magendie's student, showed during the mid-19th century that the paralytic effect of curare is due to its block of nerve impulse transmission at the neuromuscular junction. In addition, Bernard was the first to demonstrate that carbon monoxide combines irreversibly with hemoglobin so that oxygen cannot be carried effectively to the tissues, resulting in tissue asphyxiation. James Blake, an Englishman, also a student of Magendie, was the first scientist to report the actions of various substances injected as solutions directly into the bloodstream of dogs, and to measure the effects on respiratory or heart rate, blood pressure, gastroenteric activity, and neuromuscular responses. Blake was first to grasp the concept of target organ toxicity. Bernard's student, Paul Bert, noted oxygen toxicity at high pressure, and demonstrated that high-altitude sickness is a result of hypoxemia. John Letsom, an English physician, provided in his observations on chronic alcoholism a pioneering description of drug addiction.

A Spanish chemist and physician, Mathieu Joseph Bonaventura Orfila (1787–1853), can properly be called "the father of modern toxicology." He was the first researcher to recognize the need for quantitative toxicological data, and he proceded to amass considerable such information. Orfila proved the value of chemical analysis for evidence of poisoning, and demonstrated the antidotal effectiveness of such substances as milk, egg white, gallnuts (which contain tannins), and milk of magnesia. His two-volume work, *Traité des Poisons* (Treatise on Poisons), was the first textbook of toxicology; it was published in the English language in 1817. Magendie and Orfila were roundly criticized for their use of animals in toxicological research. "Orfila, like his contemporary Magendie, has been accused of an inordinate sacrifice of animal life in carrying out his experimental inquiries, and met with much censure thereupon" [Anonymous (1861), Analytical and Critical Review, *The British and Foreign Medico- Chirurgical Review*, 27:125]. Controversy on this subject continues today.

During the latter half of the 19th century, advances in chemistry enabled the isolation and precise identification of chemical substances. Hand in hand, knowledge of mechanisms of toxicity grew rapidly. Thus, by 1875, Ringer (of Ringer's solution fame) was able to characterize the toxic effects of atropine and scopolamine, as well as antidotal aspects. Excerpts of his work are as follows:

Atropine employed either internally or externally checks or even suppresses the secretion of the glands. This at least is true of the mammary, sudoriparous and salivary glands, and possibly of other glands. Its influence on the secretion of the submaxillary glands has been fully worked out. This gland receives branches from the chorda tympani nerve which is endowed with two sets of fibres, one acting immediately on the cells, the other causing the blood-vessels to dilate, being vaso-inhibitory. [It] acts through the nerves distributed to the cells, for after the injection of atropia, if the chorda tympani nerve is irritated, the vessels of the submaxillary gland become distended as usual, but the gland does not secrete. The paralyzing effect of atropia is antidoted by physostigma, for after the injection of physostigma, irritation of the chorda tympani causes the gland to secrete. Dropped into the eye, applied to the skin in its neighborhood, or taken by the stomach, preparations of belladonna very speedily produce extreme dilatation of the pupil. This one of the most characteristic effects of [this drug]. A full dose [of atropine] produces great dryness of the tongue and roof of the mouth, extending down the pharynx and larynx, inducing consequently some difficulty in swallowing, with hoarseness, and even dry cough; and a large dose will sometimes induce dryness of the Schneidarian membrane, and dryness of the conjunctiva, with much injection. [Atropine] often relieves colic of the intestines; and is especially serviceable in the colic of children. After a considerable dose (of atropine), the face becomes much flushed, the eye bright, dry, and injected, the pupil dilated, the sight dim and hazy, while the power of accommodation in the eye for distance is lost. The mind and senses are peculiarly affected. The ideas, at first rapid and connected, become incoherent and extravagant; there is often decided delirium, with pleasing illusions. Sometimes the patient is possessed with constant restlessness, keeps continually moving, and cannot be quieted. A kind of somnambulism is occasionally observed; thus cases are recorded where, under the influence of [atropine], the patient for a long time performs the movements customary to his occupation; thus, it is narrated of a tailor that he sat for hours moving his hands and arms as if sewing and his lips as if talking, but without uttering a word. The delirium may be furious and dangerous, requiring the patient to be restrained; nay, it is recorded of one poisoned by this drug that so violent did he become that he was ordered to be confined in a mad-house. The first effect of [atropine] on the pulse is to increase its quickness, fullness, and force to the extent even of 50 to 60 beats in the minute. . . . Meuriot is of opinion that [it] paralyses the peripheral branches of the vagal nerve, and by this means accelerates the heart's action. . . .

[Scopolamine] produces dryness of the mouth and throat, dilatation of the pupil, presbyopia, lightness and swimming in the head, delirium and hallucinations, a drunken gait, and often a strong desire to fight. Sometimes there is aphonia, and often sleepiness, with oppressive disagreeable dreams. A red rash has been observed after large doses. The pulse at first is much lessened in frequency but soon recovers itself, sometimes becoming even quicker than before medicine was taken. [Scopolamine] is generally used to produce sleep when opium disagrees. It has also been employed in neuralgia.

Chauncey Leake (1896–1978), whose toxicological research encompassed effects of war gases, toxic actions of morphine and general anesthetic agents on blood, spleen, and bone marrow, and toxicity of industrial chemicals, cited concepts in toxicology developed during the latter part of the 19th century that gave promise of significant progress during the 20th:

Chemotherapy from organometallic compounds through sulfa drugs to antibiotics;
    Analysis of the actions of and development of clinically useful autonomic drugs;
    Derivation of central nervous system stimulants, depressants, and hallucinogens, with analysis of their actions, and including psychotropic drugs and the management of their abuses;
    Recognition of the importance of enzyme mediation in drug action;
    Beginning of an appreciation of the social and ecological effects of chemical compounds; and
    Beginning of bureaucratic governmental control of drug use.

REFERENCES

Belloni, L. 1957. In *Psychotropic Drugs,* eds., S. Garattini and V. Ghetti. Amsterdam: Elsevier Publishing.

Bernard, C. 1857. *Leçons sur les Effets des Substances Toxiques et Médicamenteuses.* Paris: J. B. Balliere et Fils.

Blake, J. 1848. On the influence of isomorphism in determining the reactions that take place between inorganic compounds, and the elements of living beings. *Am. J. Med. Sci.* 15(new series):63–76.

Bowman, I. A. 1977. Experimentation with poisons. *The Bookman (University of Texas Medical Branch, Galveston)* 4(11):1–11.

Decker, W. J. 1977. Laboratory support of drug abuse control programs: An overview. *Clin. Toxicol.* 10:23–35.

Guthrie, D. A. 1946. *A History of Medicine.* Philadelphia: J. B. Lippincott.

La Wall, C. H. 1927. *Four Thousand Years of Pharmacy.* Philadelphia: J. B. Lippincott.

Leake, C. D. 1975. *An Historical Account of Pharmacology to the Twentieth Century.* Springfield, Ill.: Thomas.

Lewin, L. 1929. *Gifte und Vergiftungen.* Berlin: Stilke.

McIntyre, A. R. 1969. The influence of toxicology on pharmacology and physiology. *J. Clin. Pharmacol.* 9:1–4.

Mettler, C. C., and Mettler, F. A. 1947. *History of Medicine.* Philadelphia: Blakiston.

Niyogi, S. K. 1980. Historic development of forensic toxicology in America up to 1978. *Am. J. Forensic Med. Pathol.* 1:249–264.

Orfila, M. J. B. 1817. A general system of toxicology, or a treatise on poisons. London: Cox.

Pachter, H. M. 1961. *Paracelsus: Magic Into Science.* New York: Collier.

Ringer, S. 1875. *A Handbook of Therapeutics,* 4th ed. New York: Wood.

Thompson, C. J. S. 1931. *Poisons and Poisoners. With Historical Accounts of Some Famous Mysteries in Ancient and Modern Times.* London: Shaylor.

Dedicated to the memory of Dr. C. W. Muehlberger, toxicologist and historian, whose presentation, "The Gentle Art of Poisoning" to the Chicago Literary Club, April 23, 1945, contributed a considerable amount to this chapter.

Chapter 2

Absorption, Distribution, Biotransformation, Conjugation, and Excretion of Xenobiotics

Thomas J. Haley

INTRODUCTION

For any foreign compound (xenobiotic) to produce its deleterious effect(s) on the organism, it must be absorbed, pass into the vascular or lymphatic systems, and be distributed to the target organ(s) or tissues. The main routes of absorption are ingestion, inhalation, and dermal, but absorption may occur via the rectal mucosa, sublingually, subcutaneously, intramuscularly, intravenously, or intraarterially.

MECHANISMS OF ABSORPTION

Regulation of the size of a molecule or micelle that can pass into or out of the cell is governed by the thickness of the cell membrane, about 100 Å, and the diameter of the cell pores, 4–40 Å. Compounds with molecular weights of 100–200 or greater do not pass into the erythrocyte even if they are water-soluble. Weak electrolytes exist as ionized and unionized species; and the former cannot pass the cell membrane, and their distribution is determined by the pK_a value, the pH gradient, and active transport, resulting in concentration difference on each side of the membrane. Unionized materials are usually lipid-soluble and pass the cell membrane.

Simple Diffusion

Many toxic compound cross cell membranes by simple diffusion. Very small hydrophilic materials pass via aqueous channels and large lipophilic organic molecules both diffuse through the lipid membrane. The lipid/aqueous partition coefficient determines their rate of membrane passage, along with their concentration gradient across the membrane.

Facilitated Diffusion

Carrier transport shows selectivity, saturability, and blocking by metabolic inhibitors, but it cannot move a compound against a gradient (e.g., glucose). This process is not energy-dependent.

Active Transport

This process requires energy and enzymatic activity to cause compounds to enter cells selectively against an electrochemical or osmotic gradient. Metabolic or enzyme inhibitors block this process. The central nervous system has two active-transport systems in the choroid plexus for clearing organic acids and organic bases from the cerebrospinal fluid. There are two such systems in the kidney for elimination of xenobiotics, and the liver has three, one for organic acids, one for organic bases, and one for organic neutral compounds.

Filtration

This is the process whereby water flows across a porous membrane due to hydrostatic or osmotic force. This process is governed by pore size in the membrane and acts to exclude larger molecules (e.g., albumin) (Cohn, 1971).

ROUTES OF ABSORPTION

Concentration and solubility of the chemical in tissue fluids are major factors in the rate of absorption, along with the area of the absorbing surface, the extent of the capillary circulation, and the route of administration.

Gastrointestinal Absorption

Most toxic substances are absorbed by the gastrointestinal tract, but the degree and rate of absorption are influenced by solubility, formation of food complexes, susceptibility to the action of digestive enzymes, gastric emptying time, and, with irritants, the induction of emesis.

Absorption, to varying degrees, takes place throughout the gastrointestinal tract from the mouth to the rectum. The sublingual area, with its rich capillary circulation, readily absorbs chemicals such as nitroglycerine and bypasses the liver where such chemicals can be stored and metabolized. The acidic nature of the gastric juice in the stomach prevents the absorption of ionized chemicals, but nonionized lipid-soluble chemicals are readily absorbed.

By far the greatest absorption of chemicals occurs in the intestine with its large surface area of the villi and microvilli, particularly the proximal segment. Any agent that causes sloughing of the intestinal mucosa also increases absorption, for example, arsenic (Haley, 1984). The duodenum can absorb particulate material of varying sizes, such as azo dye (Barnett, 1959) or latex spheres (Sanders and Ashworth, 1961), with entrance into the intestinal cells via pinocytosis (Williams and Beck, 1969). Absorption from the rectal mucosa is selective and irregular but is used to administer drugs.

Pulmonary Absorption

There is a large absorbing surface in the lungs and a rich blood and lymph flow for rapidly distributing aerosols, gases, and vapors into body tissues. Particulates such as plutonium oxide (Nenot and Stather, 1979), asbestos fibers (Haley, 1975a), and lanthanides (Benjamin et al., 1975) can be engulfed by pulmonary macrophages and transported to the lymphatics or into other tissues, resulting in long-term effects culminating in neoplasia. Solvents (i.e., benzene) upon inhalation can cause liver and kidney damage and can result in death from aplastic anemia (Haley, 1977a).

The same physiological mechanisms that operate in the exchange of oxygen and carbon dioxide at the alveolar membrane also operate when exposure to carbon monoxide, cyanide, sulfur oxides, and nitrogen oxides occurs, but their toxic actions differ. Carbon monoxide and cyanide combine with hemoglobin to produce non-oxygen-carrying compounds, while sulfur and nitrogen oxides destroy pulmonary tissue by their irritant action. Exposure to paraquat aerosol results in the development of fibrosis of the alveoli, preventing oxygen exchange, and this results in death (Autor, 1977; Haley, 1979b).

Dermal

The skin is composed of the epidermis and dermis; the former has the stratum corneum, stratum granulosum, stratum spinosum, and stratum germinativum, while the latter has sweat ducts, sweat glands, sebaceous glands, blood vessels, and hair follicles. The keratinized area of the epidermis generally prevents many chemicals from penetrating into the lower skin layer and thus prevents passage into the circulation; however, the thinness of the skin in the axillary and inguinal areas allows easy penetration of toxicants into the circulation. Furthermore, vesicants, such as cantharidin or mustard gas, destroy the epidermis, creating a serous surface that readily absorbs toxicants. Solvents such as dimethyl sulfoxide increase skin permeability, allowing toxicants access to the circulation. It has also been observed that boots contaminated with mevinphos and parathion allowed penetration of the plantar surface of the foot, producing organophosphate poisoning (Reichert et al., 1978).

Special Routes

Intraarterial injection is utilized to bring a high concentration of chemical to a tissue using a smaller dose and thus reducing the possibility of adverse systemic reactions.

Intravenous injection is utilized to produce an immediate high blood chemical concentration but can cause hemolysis of erythrocytes of precipitation of blood constituents. Moreover, once injected, the chemical can only be removed by diuresis or hemodialysis. This is a route used by drug abusers to get "high" with heroin and cocaine.

Subcutaneous injection gives higher blood concentrations than oral administration but depends on lipid and aqueous solubility, extent of capillary circulation, and diffusion rates.

Intramuscular injection is similar and even more rapid.

DISTRIBUTION

After absorption, a chemical passes into the blood or lymph, then into the plasma and partially into the blood cells. From the plasma, it passes via the intracellular spaces or directly through the cells of the capillary endothelium into the intrastitial fluid and eventually to the cell walls or into the cellular fluid. This process is highly dependent on the capillary blood flow to the tissues. The ability of a particular chemical to pass through the cell membranes of various tissues determines its tissue distribution, which in many cases require special transport mechanisms. Lipid-soluble materials readily penetrate cell membranes. Only limited distribution occurs with toxicants that do not readily pass through the cell membranes whereas those that do have wide tissue distribution.

The *blood–brain barrier*, composed of the capillary endothelium and the glia cells, prevents diffusion or active transport circulating toxicants into brain cells and the intracellular spaces of the brain and spinal cord. This protective mechanism is ineffective in the presence of inflammation.

The *blood–cerebrospinal fluid barrier* is composed of cells of the choroid plexus, which are similar to the cells of the renal tubules; it prevents the passage of toxicants into and increases excretion of toxicants from the brain. This barrier is ineffective in the presence of inflammation.

STORAGE DEPOTS

Storage depots are protective mechanisms for preventing high concentrations of toxicants from reaching their sites of toxic action in sensitive tissues. However, at such sites toxicants are in equilibrium with their plasma concentrations, and any condition that results in their release results in a toxic episode. The main storage depots are the plasma proteins, liver, kidney, body fat, and bone. Although the lung is not considered a major storage depot, it does store asbestos (Haley, 1975a), plutonium compounds (Nenot and Stather, 1979), and paraquat (Autor, 1977; Haley, 1979b).

Plasma Proteins

Albumin binds many toxicants as well as naturally occurring body chemicals, such as bilirubin, which if displaced can cause severe toxic reactions. Transferrin, a β-globulin, transports iron, while ceruloplasmin transports copper. Lipid-soluble compounds—vitamins, steroids, and cholesterol—are transported by the lipoproteins.

Liver and Kidney

The liver, as the active metabolizing tissue, removes many toxicants during their first pass through the body and changes them to both less toxic and, in some cases, more toxic analogs. Cadmium is bound to metallothionein in liver and transported to the kidney for excretion (Friberg, 1978). The liver also binds lead very rapidly (Klaassen and Shoeman, 1972). Removal of toxicants from the liver and kidney requires active transport, and protein-binding and intracellular-binding proteins in both tissues concentrate and store toxicants.

Fat Depots

Body fat stores—neutral fat and myelin—store liposoluble chemicals, such as cyclodiene pesticides, and conditions that reduce fat stores release these organochlorine compounds into the general circulation, causing toxic reactions (Klemmer et al., 1977). Fat storage is a protective mechanism preventing toxic reactions in sensitive tissues. Concerning storage in the myelin sheath of nerves, it is essential that further investigations be conducted to determine the role of the organochlorine pesticides in modifying nerve conduction.

Bone

Although bone is considered an inert tissue, it is in dynamic equilibrium with the circulation of calcium, fluoride, and phosphate in the blood. Calcium in the hydroxyappetite crystal of bone can be replaced by lead, radiostrontium, radium, or plutonium. The first causes no toxic reactions unless released by administration of EDTA (Haley, 1977b); the other elements have produced osteosarcoma and other neoplasms (Martland and Humphries, 1929; Finkel, 1956; Nenot and Stather, 1979). Excessive ingestion of fluoride led to fluorosis with a mottled discoloration of the tooth enamel (Singh et al., 1963) and to skeletal fluorosis with osteosclerosis and osteomalacia. Excessive fluoride is only slowly excreted.

BIOTRANSFORMATION REACTIONS

Oxidation

The liver is the main organ for biotransforming chemicals in the body, but such reactions also occur in the kidney, brain, lungs, and skin, and oxidation is largely dependent on chemical structure. Aliphatic and aromatic alcohols are converted first to aldehydes and then to acids. Methyl groups are oxidized to carboxyl groups.

Aliphatic alcohols can be completely oxidized to carbon dioxide and water, while many aromatic compounds are converted to phenols, but rarely is the aromatic ring opened.

Reduction

Ketones are converted to secondary alcohols, while aromatic nitro compounds become amines, with hydroxylamines as intermediates. The availability of the new radical allows conjugation.

Glycuronide Conjugation

Alcoholic, phenolic hydroxyl, and some aromatic groups form glycuronides, while hydroxylamines and aliphatic carboxyls do not, except in instances where the latter group is attached to a tertiary carbon atom. Both stable ether-type and unstable ester-type glycuronides are formed, depending on the group conjugated.

Ethereal Sulfate Conjugation

Phenolic hydroxyl groups are conjugated with sulfuric acid to give aryl sulfates, while heterocyclic phenols form sulfuric acid esters.

Glycine Conjugation

Arylglycines or hippuric acids are formed by conjugation of aromatic acids with glycine. The types of carboxyl groups combining with glycine are those attached to the nucleus of benzene, naphthylene, thiophene, furane, or pyridines; carboxyl groups of phenylacetic acids; a carboxyl group separated from the aromatic ring by a vinyl group; carboxyl groups attached to tertiary carbon atoms; and those on the aliphatic side-chains of bile acids, but not the aliphatic carboxyl group per se.

Mercapturic Acid Conjugation

Cysteine and its N-acetyl derivative combine with benzene, polycyclic hydrocarbons, halogenated cyclic hydrocarbons where the halogen is attached to the nucleus, and benzyl chloride. With benzyl chloride the sulfur is attached to the methyl group, and with the other compounds to a nuclear carbon atom.

Ornithinine Conjugation

Birds utilize ornithinine instead of glycine in the conjugation of aromatic acids.

Glutamine Conjugation

Phenylacetic acid is conjugated with glutamine in humans and chimpanzees.

Acetylation

The amine groups of α-amion acids and aromatic amine groups are acetylated, but hydroxyl groups are not acetylated in vivo, and the only aldehyde acetylated is furfural.

Methylation

Pyridine and quinoline compounds are methylated at the heterocyclic nitrogen atom, but other heterocyclics containing nitrogen are not. Biologically active amines, such as epinephrine, are O-methylated in the meta position, and many sulfur compounds are S-methylated.

Thiocyanate Detoxication

The toxic CN radical is converted to the less toxic CNS radical by the enzyme rhodenase.

It is quite obvious that many of the foregoing processes can occur simultaneously as the body attempts to eliminate absorbed xenobiotics. Only three things can happen: (1) no metabolism with the compound being excreted unchanged, as for EDTA; (2) the compound is changed to several inactive compounds, as for sulfa drugs, which are hydroxylated and acetylated; or (3) the compound is changed first into an active compound, followed by further metabolism to an inactive one, as for codeine → morphine → normorphine → N-desmethylmorphine glycuronide.

ENZYMES INVOLVED
IN BIOTRANSFORMATIONS

Mitochondrial Enzymes

These organelles have two distinct membranes: an outer smooth one 7 nm thick, and an inner one, separated by an 8-nm space. The inner membrane has cristae forming incomplete septa through the matrix space. There are specialized transporter systems that can be specifically influenced by xenobiotics, many of which cause inhibition of ATP formation and block cation accumulation across the inner membrane. Xenobiotics influence the free cytosolic concentration of calcium, thereby affecting function of intracellular enzymes: for example, phosphorylase by kinase, lipases, phospholipases, and the Ca^{2+}-stimulated ATPase of the plasma membrane (Noack, 1983). Purified rat hepatic mitochondria convert the local anesthetic fomocaine to its N-oxide (Blume and Oelschalager, 1981). The liver has mono- and diamine oxidases; the former attacks short-chain monoamines, homosulfanilamide, benzylamine, furfuralamine, long-chain diamines, some tri- and tetraamines, and bioamines such as catecholamines and tryptamine, but not methylated amines. The latter attacks histamine and short-chain diamines.

Microsomal Enzymes

Axelrod (1983) discovered that xenobiotics were metabolized by a hepatic microsomal system requiring both NADPH and oxygen. Earlier, Baker and Chaykin (1960) showed nitrogen compounds were metabolized by enzymes located in hepatic endoplasmic reticulum. These enzyme systems are located in the microsomes, which make up a canal system in the cell for intracellular transport of xenobiotics, are continuous with the cell and nuclear membranes, and have small ribonucleoprotein particles. The activity is in the smooth-surfaced membranes, while the rough-surfaced membranes synthesize proteins. Only lipid-soluble compounds are metabolized and converted into more polar water-soluble compounds to assist in their excretion. Microsomes contain more than one variety of cytochrome P-450 and also cytochrome P-448, and these enzymes vary in the response to stimulators and inhibitors. Porcine hepatic microsomal preparations contain another mixed-function amine oxidase, whose spectral properties showed that it was distinct from NADPH-cytochrome c reductase, and they do not contain iron, copper, or cytochromes (Ziegler et al., 1969; Ziegler and Mitchell, 1972; Masters and Ziegler, 1972). There have been a number of reviews on the various enzyme reactions involved in the biotransformation of xenobiotics by various species (Hucker, 1973; Uehleke, 1973; Jerina and Daly, 1974; Schreiber, 1974), and these reactions will be discussed separately.

Enzyme Inhibitors

Cytochrome P-450 from livers of mice, rats, cattle, and sheep was inhibited by SKF-525A, octylamine, naphthylamine, acetone, DPEA, quinuclidine, and sodium deoxycholate (Gyurik et al., 1981). The N-hydroxylation of 2-N-fluorenylacetamide was inhibited by 3-methylcholanthrene, 7,8-benzoflavone, benzo(a)pyrene, miconazole, harman, and paraoxon, while metyrapone was not (Razzouk and Roberfroid, 1982). In guinea pig microsomes, SKF-525A inhibited N-dealkylation of methadone isomers, while dithiothreiol inhibited N-oxidation (Beckett et al., 1971). Cytochrome P-450 imine N-hydroxylase from rabbits, rats, and guinea pigs was inhibited by DPEA, SKF-525A, N-octylamine, α-naphthoflavone, quinolidine, MMI, aniline, and β-naphthoflavone, but 1-naphthylthiourea, bromazepam, and acetone were ineffective (Gorrod and Christou, 1982). N-Oxidase activity in rabbit hepatic microsomes is reversibly inhibited by diethylpyrocarbonate (Hlavica and Hehl, 1976). Piperonyl butoxide inhibits hamster N-hydroxylase (Hinson et al., 1975). Carbon monoxide, cyanide, and 2,4-dichloro-6-phenylphenoxyethylamine inhibit rat hepatic N-hydroxylase activity (Sum and Cho, 1977). Hamster microsomal cytochrome P-448 N-hydroxylase is inhibited by Triton X-100, desoxycholate, and cholate (Lotlikar and Dwyer, 1976). The 4-hydroxylation of aniline by rabbit microsomal preparations is inhibited by $CuCl_2$, triparnol, SKF-525A, iproniazid, and β-hydroxyquinoline (Kampffmeyer and Kiese, 1964). The multiple forms of aniline p-hydroxylase in rat hepatic microsomes are inhibited by 4-nitroanisole (Bidlack and Lowery, 1982). The conversion of N,N-dimethylaniline to an N-oxide by rat microsomal preparations was inhibited by light and rose bengal (Hlavica and Hehl, 1976). Hepatic microsomes from various species that metabolized heteroaromatic amines to N-oxides are inhibited by carbon monoxide, SKF-525A, OPEA, N-octylamine, and other aliphatic and aromatic amines (Gorrod and Damini, 1979; Gorrod, 1978). The N-oxidation of N-ethylaniline decreased rapidly with increased pH (Uehleke, 1973). The instability of aliphatic primary and secondary hydroxylamines results in autooxidation, and as the pH increases they are converted into nitroso compounds or nitrones. The reaction increases in the presence of Cu^{2+} and Mn^{2+} ions but not in the presence of Fe^{2+}, Ag^{+} or Mg^{2+} ions (Beckett and Gibson, 1977; Johnsson et al., 1978; Beckett et al., 1977).

Enzyme Inducers

Numerous xenobiotics increase the amount of cytochrome P-450 monooxygenases in the liver and also the NADPH-cytochrome c reductase and in some instances the activity of UDP-glucuronyltransferase. This results in increased biotransformation of xenobiotics. Pretreatment of rabbits and guinea pigs with the enzyme inducer phenobarbital results in increased P-450 cytochrome monooxygenase activity in the former but not in the latter. In contrast, neither species responded to 3-methylcholanthrene (Gyurik et al., 1981). Aroclor 1254 produced enzyme induction in the mouse, rat, and guinea pig but not in the hamster and rabbit; phenobarbital was an inducer in the guinea pig and rabbit and 3-methylcholanthrene in the rat and guinea pig (McMahon et al., 1980). The N-hydroxylase of hepatic microsomes of mice, rats, hamsters, and rabbits was induced by pretreatment with 3-methylcholanthrene (Lotlikar and Hong, 1981). Similar results were obtained in the N-hydroxylation of 4-chloroacetanilide, with pretreatment of hamster with 3-methylcholanthrene but not phenobarbital and sodium fluoride increased the yield of the N-hydroxy metabolite (Hinson et al., 1975). Pretreatment of mice with TCDD increased their hepatic mixed-function oxidase N-hydroxylation and O-dealkylation of phenacetin and its analogs (Kapetanovic et al., 1979). Rat colon P-450 mixed-function oxidases were induced by β-naphthoflavone and Aroclor 1254 but not by phenobarbital/hydrocortisone (Fang and Strobel, 1978). Pretreatment of rats with β-naphthoquinone increased the cytochrome P-448 content of rat colon eightfold (Strobel et al., 1980). Rats fed N-2-fluorenylacetamide had increased N-hydroxylase activity in their hepatic microsomes (Sato et al., 1981). A 13-fold increase in rat hepatic N-hydroxylase activity occurred after 3-methylcholanthrene treatment, whereas phenobarbital treatment only doubled activity (Takahashi and Omori, 1975). Treatment of rabbits with β,β-dimethylcysteine resulted in enhanced 4-hydroxylation of aniline by mixed-function oxidases (Kampffmeyer and Kiese, 1964). Pretreatment of male and female rats with phenobarbital or 3-methylcholanthrene increased microsomal 4-hydroxylation of aniline, and the additions of spermine or spermidine enhanced the reaction (Chapman, 1976). C-Hydroxylation of 1-nitro-[9-^{14}C]-(3-dimethylamino-N-propylamino)acridine by cytochrome P-450 was increased by induction with phenobarbital, whereas P-448 activity was increased with 3-methylcholanthrene in subcellular fractions from rat liver and HeLa cells (Pawlak and Konopa, 1979). Enzyme induction in rat microsomes, the 10,000 × g supernatant and purified cytochrome P-450 by 3-methylcholanthrene, phenobarbital, β-naphthoflavone and pregnenolone-16 α-carbonitrile increased the ring hydroxylation of N,N-dimethyl-4-aminoazobenzene (Levine and Lu, 1982). Increased N-oxidation of N,N-dimethylaniline occurred when rabbit hepatic cytochrome P-450 and NADPH-cytochrome c (P-450) reductase were induced by pregnolone-16 α-carbonitrile (Lu et al., 1972) or glucocorticoids (Leakey and Fouts, 1979; Arrhenius, 1968; Devereux and Fouts, 1975). A flavoprotein mixed-function oxidase distinct from NADPH-cytochrome c reductase isolated from porcine and rabbit liver can be induced by N-octylamine, DPEA, and some guanidine derivatives (Hlavica and Hulsmann, 1979; Pettit et al., 1964; Ziegler et al., 1969; Ziegler and Mitchell, 1972; Masters and Ziegler, 1972). Pretreatment of rats with DDT or phenobarbital enhances N-oxidation by hepatic microsomes (Mattlocks and White, 1971). Many xenobiotics can enhance mixed-function oxidases in hepatic and other tissues, but the problem is the lack of standardization of methodology plus pronounced species differences in response. This should be corrected in future investigations.

Physiological Factors Affecting Biotransformation

Age In young animals a poorly developed hepatic monooxygenase system results in decreased metabolism of xenobiotics. There is also a lack of conjugation reaction, causing a retention of the toxicant. With increasing age, there is a decline in the ability of the organism to biotransform many compounds, and adverse reactions can result.

Sex Biotransformation of xenobiotics by females occurs at a lesser rate than by males because the transforming enzymes are inhibited by estradiol. Androgens in males appears to stimulate the cytochrome P-450 monooxygenase, thus converting toxicants to less toxic substances, but not in every instance. The organophosphate pesticides naled and GC6506 were more toxic to females while fospirate was more toxic to males (Haley et al., 1975b). Similar results were obtained with organothiophosphate pesticides (Haley et al., 1975a). The carbamate pesticides—formetanate, mexacarbate, and C-8353—also were more toxic to females (Haley et al., 1974a). Subchronic exposure of mice to N-2-fluorenylacetamide showed that males developed pericardial fibrosis and mineralization at twice the rate of females (Haley et al., 1974b).

Species Biotransformations of foreign compounds show many species differences. The metabolic response to disulfiram differs significantly between humans and rats (Haley, 1979a). Comparative studies of N-demethylase activity with various species gave the following results: rat liver > guinea pig liver > pigeon liver $\geq$ bull frog liver $\geq$ edible frog liver > adult cockroach fat body > carp liver > adult honey bee abdomen > whole rice stem borer (Usui and Fukami, 1978).

Strain There are numerous reports of strain differences in the biotransformation of xenobiotics in the literature. Toxicity from 2,4,5-T differed between CD-1 mice and (C57VL/6 × A/JAX)F_1 and (C3H/He × BALV/c)F_2 hybrid strains

(Highman et al., 1976). Analysis of control animal data indicates a wide difference between rat strains in the development of a wide variety of tumors (Haley, 1978).

Genetics Pharmacogenetics play a large part in xenobiotic metabolism by animals but particularly by humans. The main difference in inbred mouse strains is the choice of inducible and noninducible monooxygenases resides in the nature of the cytosolic receptor protein. The system also operates in human lymphocytes. Constituted enzymes show interindividual variation due to allelism in structural or regulatory genes. In humans, variation in cholinesterase results in prolongation of succinylcholine paralysis of respiratory muscles. Caucasians have a high incidence of atypical esterase, while Alaskan Eskimos have a nonfunctional esterase (Kalow, 1983). Human metabolism of pentobarbital gives N-hydroxypentobarbital, representing 11–15% of the administered dose (Tang et al., 1977a). In humans, amobarbital and phenobarbital are metabolized by N-hydroxylation, accounting for 24–30% of the administered dose. It was also found, based on female twins, that there was a genetically linked lack of N-hydroxylation of amobarbital. This deficiency is a recessive trait controlled by a single pair of allelic autosomal genes (Tang et al., 1977a). Sulfa drugs are acetylated by rabbits, and this characteristic is inherited autosomally, with rapid acetylators dominating slow acetylators. Acetylation of sulfonamides is polymorphic in humans, and human liver homogenates demonstrated that this trait resides in the enzyme acetyltransferase, which transfers acetyl groups from acetylcoenzyme A to the acceptor drug molecule. Two human studies have shown a bimodal pattern, with 61% fast acetylators to 39% slow acetylators (Haley, 1983).

Body Temperature Xenobiotics have decreased metabolism at low temperatures and increased at high temperatures. Such effects are coupled to the rate of body distribution, protein binding, and excretion.

Nutritional Status Nutritional status markedly affects both the enzyme systems and the enzyme activity. There is decreased enzyme activity to metabolism of xenobiotics in mineral, vitamin, and protein deficiencies, as in the lack of required cofactors.

Pathological States Hepatoma, jaundice, and hepatic carcinoma all reduce hepatic enzyme activity.

Drug Interactions Of great importance in modifying the biotransformation process in the multiplicity of xenobiotics to which the human is exposed, such as cigarette smoking, dietary items, and various combinations of chemicals taken for therapeutic purposes. This is illustrated in Table 1 (Thienes and Haley, 1972).

SPECIFIC BIOTRANSFORMATION REACTIONS

N-Dealkylation

N-Dealkylation is a major biotransformation pathway for aliphatic alkyl and dialkyl amines, heterocyclic compounds, carbamates, aliphatic tricyclics, 1-aryltriazenes,

Table 1 Drug Interactions[a]

Drugs	Combined with	Interaction
Alcohol	Amphetamines	Increases biotransformation
	Warfarin	Decreases effect
Barbiturates	Warfarin	Decreases effect
Diazepine derivatives and meprobamate	Alcohol	Additive effect
	Anticoagulants	Decreased effect
	Barbiturates	Additive effect
	MAO inhibitor	Enhanced sedation
	Phenothiazines	Additive effect
	Tricyclic antidepressants	Additive effect
Phenothiazines	Alcohol	Enhanced sedation
	Antihistamines	Additive effect
	Antihypertensives	Increased antihypertensive effect
	Barbiturates	Enhanced sedation
	MAO inhibitor	Decreased MAO inhibition
	Meperidine	Enhanced sedation
	Morphine	Enhanced sedation
	Reserpine	Increased reserpine action
	Thiazide diuretics	Shock
	Tricyclic antidepressants	Additive effect
Antihistamine	Alcohol	CNS depression
	Alkaloids	CNS depression
	Barbiturates	Inhibit each other
	Hydrocortisone	Inhibits hydrocortisone
	Hyposensitization therapy	Inhibits therapy
	MAO inhibitor	Enhances antihistamine
	Parasympathomimetics	Increases parasympathetic activity
	Phenothiazines	Additive effect
	Reserpine	CNS depression
Aspirin	Anticoagulants	Enhances anticoagulant
	para-Aminosalicylic acid (PAS)	PAS toxicity
	Phenobarbital	May decrease analgesia
Meperidine	Atropine	Additive effect
	MAO inhibitor	MAO inhibition decreased Mepiridine action increased
	Phenothiazines	Enhanced sedation
Phenybutazone	Anticoagulants	Potentiates anticoagulant, later decreases
Phenyramidol	Biohydroxycoumarin	Enhances effect
	Diphenylhydantoin	Increased action

[a]From Theines and Haley (1972).

triazines, and many miscellaneous compounds. Derivatives of phenylethyldimethy-lamine are demethylated to various degrees by microsomal preparations from mice, rats, and guinea pigs (McMahon, 1961). Dealkylation studies of aniline derivatives have shown that dealkylation is optimal with ethyl and decreases as the alkyl chain length increases, and with *sec*-butyl and *tert*-butyl the process stops. Substitution with diethyl, di-*n*-propyl, and di-*n*-butyl gives partial dealkylation, while diisobutyl and di-*tert*-butyl do not (Gorrod et al., 1979). *N*-Dealkylation of 4-aminoantipyrine deriva-tives decreases and chain length increases from methyl to *n*-butyl, and dialkyl analogs are less dealkylated than are their monoalkyl analogs (LaDu et al., 1955). Variation in the alkyl moiety of amphetamine from monomethyl to mono-*sec*-butyl and dimethyl to di-*n*-butyl shows the least *N*-dealkylation with the monomethyl analog and the greatest with the methylpropyl analog. These results indicate the effect of chain length, steric hindrance, and lipophilicity on the *N*-dealkylation process (Donike et al., 1974; Testa and Salvesen, 1980). *N*-Dealkylation of meperidine derivatives is greatest with C_2 and then decreases, with C_5 to C_9 being essentially constant (Abdel-Monem and Portoghese, 1971). Where the methyl moiety was attached to the carba-mate nitrogen, only two out of 40 were not *N*-demethylated (Hodgson and Casida, 1961). Substitution of alkyl chains for hydrogen on the third carbon atom of a series of morphine analogs showed an increased rate of demethylation up to C_4, then a decreased rate until C_{10} and C_{12} where no demethylation occurred (Duquette et al., 1980). The mechanism for *N*-dealkylation of the foregoing compounds proceeds via the formation of the carbinolamine derivative (Hucker, 1973).

N-Hydroxylation

N-Hydroxylation is a minor biotransformation pathway for the metabolism of aliphatic primary and secondary amines and amides, and of aromatic primary and secondary amines, amides, and imines (Hlavica, 1982). The addition of an *ortho-, meta-,* or *para*-chloro substituent into the benzene moiety of aniline increases its *N*-hydroxylation (Hlavica, 1982), and *N*-substitution of aniline increases *N*-hydroxylation four to fivefold, but with aromatic secondary amines the rate of *N*-hydroxylation decreases as the chain length of the substituent group increases (Kiese and Uehleke, 1961). It has been shown that a rat microsomal preparation *N*-hydroxylated *N*-methyl-, *N*-ethyl, *N*-butyl, 4-chloro-, and 4-ethoxyaniline more rap-idly than aniline (Kiese and Uehleke, 1961). Metabolic studies with the phenacetin analogs 4-methoxy-, 4-ethoxy-, and 4-(*n*-butyl)acetanilide showed they were *N*-hydroxylated and *O*-dealkylated to acetaminophen. *N*-Hydroxylation rates gave the following order: 4-methoxy < 4-ethoxy < 4-(*n*-butoxy). *N*-Hydroxylative activity but not *O*-dealkylating activity was markedly increased by increasing the alkyl chain length (Kapetanovic et al., 1979). Hamster microsomal preparations convert *trans*-4-acetamide-stilbene and its 4-fluoro, 4-chloro, and 4-bromo derivatives into *N*-hydroxylated compounds. The rate of reaction was greatest with the parent compound (Gammans et al., 1977). Studies of the metabolic effect of 4-CN, 4-CH_3, 4-$C(CH_3)$ and 4-CF_3 analogs of 4-*trans*-acetamidostilbene showed that such substituents mark-edly decreased *N*-hydroxylation. This was attributed to the physicochemical properties of the substituents and their susceptibility to metabolic oxidation (Hanna et al., 1980).

N-Oxide Formation

N-Oxide formation is the biotransformation pathway utilized in the metabolism of aliphatic, aromatic, alicyclic, and heteroaromatic tertiary amines, tertiary amides, imines, and hydrazines. N,N-Dimethylaniline is converted to an N-oxide by purified cytochrome P-450LM$_4$, NADPH-cytochrome c (P-450) reductase, and lipid factor (Hlavica and Hulsman, 1979). Porcine hepatic microsomal preparations contain a flavoprotein mixed-function oxidase distinct from NADPH cytochrome c reductase, and it N-oxidizes N,N-dimethylaniline (Pettit et al., 1964; Ziegler et al., 1969, 1973; Ziegler and Mitchell, 1972; Masters and Ziegler, 1972). This amine oxidase converts 2-naphthylamine, methylhydrazine, 1,1-dimethylhydrazine, and 1,2-dimethylhydrazine into N-oxides (Prough, 1973; Ziegler et al., 1971, 1973; Prough et al., 1977). Hepatic microsomal cytochrome P-450 of various species metabolized heteroaromatic amines, such as 3-substituted pyridines, to N-oxides (Gorrod and Damini, 1979). Metyrapone is converted into 2-N-oxides by rat hepatic microsomes (DeGraeve et al., 1979). The pyrrolizidine alkaloid retrosine, an alicyclic tertiary amine, is converted into an N-oxide by rat liver microsomes (Mattlocks and White, 1971).

C-Hydroxylation

C-Hydroxylation is a minor biotransformation pathway for converting aromatic primary, secondary, and tertiary amines and amides, making them more polar for urinary excretion. Moreover, occupation of the 4-position of the aromatic nucleus—4-chloroaniline, 4-chloromercuribenzoate, or 4-aminopropiophenone—prevents 4-hydroxylation. 4-C-Hydroxylation of aniline is affected by the size of the alkyl group attached to the nitrogen, with butyl more effective than methyl in increasing the rate of hydroxylation. Rabbit microsomal preparations 4-hydroxylate aniline maximally at pH 7.0–7.5 (Kampffmeyer and Kiese, 1964). The effect of pH on 4-hydroxylation of aniline and acetanilide in a THAM-phosphate buffer has been shown to be most active at pH 8.2 (Mitoma et al., 1956). Guinea pig and rabbit microsomal preparations biotransform N,N-dimethyl-4-aminophenol, N-methyl-2-aminophenol, N-methyl-4-aminophenol, 2-aminophenol, and 4-aminophenol (Gorrod and Gooderham, 1981). Induced rat hepatic microsomes convert 5-nitroacenaphthene into 1-hydroxy-5-nitroacenaphthene, 1-hydroxy-5-amino-acenaphthene, cis-1,2-dihydroxy-5-nitroacenaphthene, 2-hydroxy-5-nitroacenaphthene, and several oxo compounds (El-Gayoumy and Hecht, 1982). Hepatic microsomes from mice, rats, and hamsters ring-hydroxylate N-2-fluorenylacetamide in positions C-3, C-5, and C-7, while guinea pigs hydroxylate only C-5 and C-7 and rabbits only position C-7 (Lotlikar and Hong, 1981). Ring-hydroxylation of N-2-fluorenylacetamide in positions C-1, C-3, C-5, and C-7 were produced by rat and hamster microsomal preparations (Razzouk et al., 1980). Ring-hydroxylation of methylaminoazobenzene was produced by hepatic cytochrome P-450 (Vasder et al., 1982). Human hepatic microsomal preparations ring-hydroxylate N-2-fluorenylacetamide in positions C-1, C-3, C-5, C-7, and C-9 (Dybling et al., 1979).

Arene Oxide Formation

Aromatic compounds are converted to phenols by hepatic monooxygenases via highly reactive arene oxides in which the formal aromatic double bond is epoxidized by epoxide hydrase. It is this enzyme that converts arene oxides to *trans*-dihydrodiols. Although benzene undergoes this reaction, its intermediate is too unstable to be isolated; however, naphthylene is converted to a stable naphthylene 1,2-oxide, which has been isolated. In vitro, this intermediate is converted to 1-naphthol, 2-naphthol, and *trans*-1,2-dihydroxy-1,2-dihydronaphthylene. Catechol metabolites of xenobiotic aromatic compounds are produced via dehydrogenation of *trans*-dihydrodiols rather than by sequential hydroxylations of the aromatic ring. Intermediates in toluene metabolism are arene oxides, which isomerize to *ortho*- and *para*-cresols while the methyl group is hydroxylated to form benzyl alcohol. It has also been shown that electron-withdrawing substituents stabilize arene oxides, while electron-donating substitutents have a destablizing effect. The latter type compounds, such as anisoles, alkylbenzenes, or acetanilides, form phenols, while the former type compounds (i.e., halobenzenes or nitrobenzene) form phenols, dihydrodiols, and permercapturic acid. Hepatic microsomal hydrases biotransform benzene oxide, naphthalene, 1,2-oxide, and phenanthrone 9,10-oxide and hydrate benzo(a)anthracene 5,6-oxide, benzo(a)pyrene 7,8-oxide, benzo(a)pyrene, 9,10-oxide, 7,12-dimethylbenz(a)anthracene 5,6 oxide, benz(a)anthracene 8,9-oxide, dibenz(a,c)anthracene 10,11 oxide, and 7-hydroxymethylbenz(a)anthracenes 5,6-oxide. It has also been shown that halobenzenes are metabolized to arene oxides, which produce hepatic necrosis, while polycyclic hydrocarbon oxides are mediators of carcinogenicity; in both cases the reactive intermediates interact with tissue nucleophiles and macromolecules (Jerina and Daly, 1974; Schreiber, 1974).

Olefin Oxidation

Olefinic compounds are converted into dihydrodiols via epoxides (i.e., aldrin into dieldrin). Epoxides of styrene, indene, and cyclohexene are intermediates in their conversion to glycols. Rat liver microsomes convert trichloroethylene into chloral hydrate. In the presence of 1,2-epox-n-octane, an epoxide hydrase inhibitor, seconbarbital is biotransformed into a tetrahydrofuropyrimide via nucleophilic attack of the oxirane ring (Hucker, 1973). Vinyl chloride is metabolized into an epoxide, chloroethylene oxide, and then into chloroacetaldehyde (Haley, 1975b). Vinylidene chloride also follows the epoxide pathway (Haley, 1975c).

The "NIH" Shift

This reaction involved hydroxylation-induced migration of substituents on the aromatic nucleus. When 4-substituted phenylalanines are hydroxylated, halogen or methyl groups migrate from the 4- to the 3-position. Arene oxides produced by epioxidation of aromatic compounds undergo ready isomerization to phenols, with a concomitant migration and retention of substituents (i.e., isotopes of hydrogen, halogens, and alkyl groups) (Jerina and Daly, 1974; Schreiber, 1974).

Azo and Nitro Reduction

Two enzyme systems are involved in reduction of azo and nitro compounds. NADPH-cytochrome c reductase acts on some xenobiotics, while others require a complete cytochrome P-450 monooxygenase system. These types of compounds can also be reduced by enteric bacteria in the gut (Gillette, 1969).

Transferase Reactions

Acetyl Transferases   These acetylate aromatic primary amines, hydrazines, sulfonamides, and a few aliphatic amines and they require acetylcoenzyme A as a cofactor. Acetylation of isoniazid illustrates a situation where there are rapid and slow acetylators in humans, and the reaction is controlled by hepatic acetylase, which is under genetic control (Evans et al., 1960; Sunahara et al., 1961). Sulfonamide acetylation in humans is polymorphic, and this effect resides in hepatic acetyltransferase (Haley, 1982).

Methyl Transferases   These methylate aliphatic and aromatic amines, N-heterocyclics, mono- and polyhydric phenols, and sulfhydryl-containing compounds, and they require the coenzyme S-adenosylmethionine for activation. The enzyme catechol-O-methyltransferase (COMT) catalyses the ring O-methylation of catechols and catecholamines (i.e., L-DOPA and α-methylDOPA). Family studies indicate that erythrocyte COMT activity is an inherited monogenic trait with the low and high methylators, and these variations are common and due to the effects of two alleles at a single locus. Similar genetic characteristics have been found with thiopurine methyltransferase, which S-methylated 6-mercaptopurine, 6-thioguanine, and azothiopurine (Weinshilboum, 1983).

Sulfotransferases   These are found in the tissue cytosol fraction, and they transfer sulfate to the aliphatic alcohols, phenols, and aromatic amines, utilizing the cofactor 3'-phosphoadenosine 5'-phosphosulfate. In the case of alcohols and phenols, this gives rise to ethereal sulfates, which are more water-soluble and more easily excreted.

Glutathione S-Transferases   These are found in the hepatic cytosol of the rat. They catalyze the formation of mercapturic acid derivatives using glutathione as the cofactor (Jakoby et al., 1976). Substrates for this enzyme are various electrophilic xenobiotics. Glutathione derivatives are enzymatically cleaved; gluthathionase removes the glutamic acid moiety; a peptidase removes the glycine moiety; and finally N-acetylase acetylates the product to a mercapturic acid. A related reaction, thioether conjugation, utilized glutathione, cysteine, and N-acetylcysteine in xenobiotic biotransformations. Methylthioethers have been obtained in the metabolism of naphthalene, bromobenzene, tetrachlorobiphenyl, mecloqualone, clozapine, biphenyl, acetaminophen, phenacetin, and bromazepam. Several mechanisms are involved in the cleavage of glutathione or cysteine conjugates to thiols and their subsequent methylation to methylthiol ethers (Stillwell, 1983).

Glucuronyl Transferases These are found in the microsomal endoplasmic reticulum, and the coenzyme for this reaction is uridine 5'-diphospho-α-D—gluronic acid. The substrates for this conjugation reaction include aliphatic and aromatic alcohols, some carboxyl groups, sulfhydryl groups, and primary and secondary aromatic and aliphatic amines. Both ester and ether types of glucuronides are formed and can serve as substrates for the tissue enzyme β-glucuronidase (Testa and Jenner, 1976). Hepatic glucuronidation has a high capacity for making xenobiotics more excretable via the bile or urine (Ingelmann-Sundberg, 1983).

Alcohol and Aldehyde Dehydrogenases These catalyze a wide variety of aliphatic alcohols to aldehydes and ketones, using NAD^+ as a cofactor, and reduce aldehydes and ketones to their corresponding alcohols using NADH as a cofactor. Aldehyde dehydrogenases oxidize aldehydes to acids using NAD^+ as a cofactor.

Esterases and Amidases These are found in mammalian tissues and hydrolyze ester and amide linkages in xenobiotics. Varieties of esterases use different substrates: arylesterases hydrolyze aromatic esters; carboxylesterases hydrolyze aliphatic esters; cholinesterases hydrolyze esters containing choline; and acetylesterases hydrolyze those esters containing the acetyl moiety (Testa and Jenner, 1976). Amidases are less specific in their substrates and hydrolyze xenobiotics more slowly.

ROUTES OF EXCRETION

Urinary

The kidney is the most important organ for removal of xenobiotics and their metabolites and conjugates from the body. Polar compounds are readily excreted in the urine. The amount of drug filtered through the glomerulus into the tubular lumen depends on the filtration rate, protein binding, and pH. The proximal renal tubule adds strong organic acids and bases to the glomerular filtrate by active, carrier-mediated tubular secretion. In the proximal and distal renal tubules, nonionized weak acids and bases are resorbed or excreted by passive diffusion, a bidirectional mechanism in which xenobiotics diffuse in either direction depending on their concentration and the pH on the two sides of the tubular cells. When the pH gradient in the distal tubule favors diffusion into the urine, resorption can occur because strong electrolyte and water creates a concentration gradient of the nonionized form favoring diffusion from urine to blood. Passive resorption of the ionized form can also occur. When tubular urine is more alkaline than plasma, weak acids are excreted more rapidly due to a decrease in net passive resorption. The reverse is true when the urine is more acidic than plasma. With weak bases, the acidification or alkalinization of the urine causes excretion opposite that of weak acids (Orloff and Berliner, 1961; Mudge and Weiner, 1963).

Hepatic and Fecal

Metabolites of xenobiotics can be excreted into the intestinal tract via the bile and subsequently can be resorbed and excreted in the urine or excreted in the feces. Strong organic acids and bases are actively transported into the bile by processes similar to those seen in renal tubule secretion. The liver also has a transport system for handling metals (e.g., lead) (Klaassen, 1976). The toxicity of some xenobiotics is directly related to the amount excreted via the bile, i.e., indomethacin (Duggan et al., 1975). In newborn animals, the administration of microsomal enzyme inducers increases the development of hepatic excretory mechanisms (Klaassen, 1974).

Pulmonary

Both gases and volatile liquids are principally excreted by the lungs. Elimination is accomplished by simple diffusion. With highly lipid soluble agents, excretion is prolonged because they must diffuse from adipose tissue.

Minor Routes

Sweat and saliva are very minor routes of excretion of xenobiotics. With the former, excretion is dependent on the nonionized lipid-soluble form of the xenobiotic. With the latter, the saliva containing the chemical can be swallowed, absorbed, and metabolized in the liver.

Many xenobiotics are excreted in the milk of humans and animals and can give rise to symptoms of toxicity, particularly in the young. Basic compounds concentrate in milk because it is more acidic than plasma, while acidic compounds are lower in milk than plasma. Lipid-soluble xenobiotics, such as cyclodiene pesticides, tend to concentrate in milk (Klemmer et al., 1977).

REFERENCES

Abdel-Monem, M. M., and Portoghese, P. S. 1971. Correlation of analgesic potencies of N-substituted normepheridines and in vitro N-dealkylation. *J. Pharm. Pharmacol.* 23:875–876.

Arrhenius, A. 1968. Effects on hepatic microsomal N- and C-oxidation of aromatic amines by in vivo corticosteroid, aminofluorene treatment, diet or stress. *Cancer Res.* 28:264.

Autor, A. P. 1977. *Biochemical Mechanisms of Paraquat Toxicity,* p. 240. New York: Academic.

Axelrod, J. 1983. The discovery of the microsomal drug-metabolizing enzymes. In *Drug Metabolism and Distribution, Current Revues in Biomedicine,* ed. J. W. Lamble, pp. 1–6. New York: Elsevier Biomedical.

Baker, J., and Chaykin, S. 1960. The biosynthesis of trimethylamine-*N*-oxide. *Biochim. Biophys. Acta* 41:548-550.

Barnett, R. J. 1959. The demonstration with the electron microscope of the end-products of histochemical reactions in relation to the fine structure of cells. *Exp. Cell Res. Suppl.* 7:65-89.

Beckett, A. H., and Gibson, G. G. 1977. Identification of the in vitro *N*-oxidized metabolites of (+)- and (−)-benzylamphetamine. *J. Pharm. Phamacol.* 29:756.

Beckett, A. H., Mitchard, M., and Shinab, A. A. 1971. The influence of methyl substitution on the *N*-demethylation and *N*-oxidation of normethadone in animal species. *J. Pharm. Pharmacol.* 23:941-946.

Beckett, A. H., Purkaystha, A. R., and Morgan, P. H. 1977. Oxidation of aliphatic hydroxylamines in aqueous solutions. *J. Pharm. Pharmacol.* 25:15.

Benjamin, S. A., Hahn, F. F., Chiffelle, T. L., Boecker, B. B., Hobbs, C. H., Jones, R. K., McClellan, R. O., and Snipes, M. B. 1975. Occurrence of hemangiosarcomas in beagles with internally deposited radionuclides. *Cancer Res.* 35:1745-1755.

Bidlack, W. R., and Lowery, G. L. 1982. Multiple drug metabolism: *p*-Nitroanisole reversal of acetone enhanced aniline hydroxylation. *Biochem. Pharmacol.* 31:311-317.

Blume, H., and Oelschalager, H. 1981. Biotransformation des lokalanasthetikums fomocain durch ratten leber-mitrochondrein. *Arzneim-Forsch.* 31:1731-1735.

Chapman, S. L. 1976. Polyamines and drug oxidations. *Drug Metab. Dispos.* 4:417-422.

Cohn, V. H. 1971. Transmembrane movement of drug molecules. In *Fundamentals of Drug Metabolism and Drug Disposition,* eds. B. N. LaDu, H. G. Mandel, and E. L. Way, pp. 3-21. Baltimore: Williams & Wilkins.

DeGraeve, J., Gielen, J. E., Kahl, G. F., Tuttenberg, K. H., Kahl, P., and Maume, B. 1979. Formation of two metyrapone *N*-oxides by rat liver microsomes. *Drug Metab. Dispos.* 7:166.

Devereaux, T. R., and Fouts, J. R. 1975. Effect of pregnancy on treatment with certain steroids on *N,N*-dimethylaniline demethylation and *N*-oxidation by rabbit liver or lung microsomes. *Drug Metab. Dispos.* 3:254.

Donike, M., Iffland, R., and Jaenicke, L. 1974. Der einfluss der *N*-alkylgruppe auf die *N*-dealkylierungsgeschwindig keit bei *N*-Alkyl und *N,N*-dialkylamphetamiderivaten. In vivo. Arzneim-Forsch. 24:556-560.

Duggan, D. E., Hooke, K. F., Moll, R. M., and Kwan, K. C. 1975. Enterohepatic circulation of indomethacine and its role in intestinal irritation. *Biochem. Pharmacol.* 24:1749-1754.

Duquette, P. H., Erickson, R. R., and Holtzman, J. L. 1980. Effect of substrate lipophilicity on the *N*-dealkylation of 3-*O*-alkyl-morphine analogs. In *Microsomes, Drug Oxidations and Chemical Caricinogenesis.* New York: Academic.

Dybling, E., vonBahr, C., Aune, T., Glaumann, H., Levitt, D. S., and Thorgeirsson, S. S. 1979. In vitro metabolism and activation of carcinogenic aromatic amines by subcellular fractions of human liver. *Cancer Res.* 39:4206-4211.

El-Gayoumy, K., and Hecht, S. S. 1982. Identification of mutagenic metabolites formed by *C*-hydroxylation and nitroreduction of 5-nitroacenaphthene by rat liver. *Cancer Res.* 42:1243-1248.

Evans, D. A. P., Manley, K. A., and McKusick, V. A. 1960. Genetic control of isoniazid metabolism in man. *Br. Med. J.* 2:485-491.

Fang, W. F., and Strobel, H. W. 1978. Activation of carcinogens and mutagens by rat colon mucosa. *Cancer Res.* 38:2939-2944.

Finkel, M. P. 1956. Internal emitters and tumor induction. *Proc. Int. Conf. Peaceful Uses of Atomic Energy, Aug. 8-20, 1955, Geneva, Biological Effects of Radiation,* pp. 160-164. New York: United Nations.

Friberg, L. 1978. The toxicology of cadmium. In *Cadmium 77, Proc. 1st Int. Cadmium Conf.,
San Francisco, Calif., Metal Bulletin,* New York, pp. 167–175.

Gammans, R. E., Sehon, R. D., Anders, M. W., and Hanna, P. E. 1977. Microsomal *N*-hydroxylation of *trans*-4'-halo-4-acetamido-stilbenes. *Drug Metab. Dispos.* 5:226–231.

Gillette, J. R. 1969. Significance of mixed oxygenases and nitroreductase in drug metabolism. *Ann. NY Acad. Sci.* 160:558–570.

Gorrod, J. W. 1978. On the multiplicity of microsomal *N*-oxidase systems. In *Mechanisms of Oxidizing Enzymes,* eds. T. P. Singer and R. N. Ondarze, p. 189. Amsterdam: Elsevier.

Garrod, J. W., and Christou, M. 1982. Enzyme characteristics of imine *N*-hydroxylation. *Adv. Exp. Med. Biol.* 136B:1133–1142.

Garrod, J. W., and Damini, L. W. 1979. The effects of various potential inhibitors, activators and inducers on the *N*-oxidation of 3-substituted pyridines in vitro. *Xenobiotica* 9:219.

Gorrod, J. W., and Gooderham, N. J. 1981. The in vitro metabolism of *N,N*-dimethylaniline by guinea pig and rabbit tissue preparations. *Eur. J. Metab. Pharmacokinet.* 6:195–206.

Gorrod, J. W., Temple, D. J., and Beckett, A. H. 1979. The *N*- and *C*-oxidation of *N,N*-dialkylanilines by rabbit liver microsomes in vitro. *Xenobiotica* 9:17–25.

Gyurik, R. J., Chow, A. W., Zaber, B., Brunner, E. L., Miller, J. A., Villani, A. J., Petka, L. A., and Parrish, R. C. 1981. Metabolism of albendazole in cattle, sheep, rats and mice. *Drug Metab. Dispos.* 9:503–508.

Haley, T. J. 1975a. Asbestosis: A reassessment of the overall problem. *J. Pharm. Sci.* 64:1435–1449.

Haley, T. J. 1975b. Vinyl chloride: How many unknown problems? *J. Toxicol. Environ. Hlth.* 1:47–73.

Haley, T. J. 1975c. Vinylidene chloride: A review of the literature. *Clin. Toxicol.* 8:633–643.

Haley, T. J. 1977a. Evaluation of the health effects of benzene inhalation. *Clin. Toxicol.* 11:531–548.

Haley, T. J. 1977b. Pediatric plumbism sources, symptoms and therapy. In *Clinical Chemical Toxicology,* ed. S. S. Brown, pp. 179–182. Amsterdam: Elsevier.

Haley, T. J. 1978. Retrospective analysis of control animal data—The rat. *Clin. Toxicol.* 12:249–253.

Haley, T. J. 1979a. Disulfiram (tetraethylthioperoxydicarbonic diamide): A reappraisal of its toxicity and therapeutic application. *Drug Metab. Rev.* 9:319–335.

Haley, T. J. 1979b. A review of the toxicology of paraquat. *Clin. Toxicol.* 14:1–46.

Haley, T. J. 1982. Sulfanilamide. *Dangerous Properties Ind. Mater. Rep.* 2:13–17.

Haley, T. J. 1983. Sulfathiazole. *Dangerous Properties Ind. Mater. Rep.* 3:9–13.

Haley, T. J. 1984. Arsenic. *Dangerous Properties Ind. Mater. Rep.* 4:9–17.

Haley, T. J., Farmer, J. H., Dooley, K. L., Harmon, J. R., and Peoples, A. 1974a. Determination of the LD_{01} and extrapolation of the LD_{001} for five methylcarbamate pesticides. *Eur. J. Toxicol.* 7:152–158.

Haley, T. J., Schieferstein, G., Jaques, W. E., Farmer, J., Frith, C., and Sprawls, R. W. 1974b. Dose-response predictability of urinary bladder hyperplasia by *N*-2-fluorenylacetamide feeding in mice: Its modification by sex. *J. Pharm. Sci.* 63:1946–1947.

Haley, T. J., Farmer, J. H., Harmon, J. R., and Dooley, K. L. 1975a. Estimation of the LD_1 and extrapolation of the $LD_{0.1}$ for five organothiophosphate pesticides. *Eur. J. Toxicol.* 8:229–235.

Haley, T. J., Farmer, J. H., Harmon, J. R., and Dooley, K. L. 1975b. Estimation of the LD_1 and extrapolation of the $LD_{0.1}$ for five organophosphate pesticides. *Arch. Toxicol.* 34:103–109.

Hanna, P. E., Gammans, R. E., Sehon, R. D., and Lee, M-K. 1980. Metabolic N-hydroxylation. Use of substituent variation to modulate the in vitro bioactivation of 4-acetamido-stilbene. *J. Med. Chem.* 23:1038–1044.

Highman, B., Gaines, T. B., Schumacher, H. J., and Haley, T. J. 1976. Strain differences in histopathologic, hematologic, and blood chemistry changes induced in mice by a technical and a purified preparation of 2,4,5-trichlorophenoxyacetic acid. *J. Toxicol. Environ. Health* 1:1041–1054.

Hinson, J. A., Mitchell, J. R., and Jollow, D. J. 1975. Microsomal N-hydroxylation of p-chloroacetanilide in hamsters. *Biochem. Pharmacol.* 25:599–601.

Hlavica, P. 1982. Biological oxidation in organic compounds and disposition of N-oxidized products. *CRC Crit. Rev. Biochem.* 12:39–101.

Hlavica, P., and Hehl, M. 1976. Comparative studies on the N-oxidation of aniline and N,N-dimethylaniline by rabbit liver microsomes. *Xenobiotica* 6:679–689.

Hlavica, P., and Hulsman, S. 1979. Studies on the mechanisms of hepatic N-oxide formation. N-Oxidation of N,N-dimethylaniline by a reconstituted rabbit microsomal cytochrome P-448 enzyme system. *Biochem. J.* 182:109.

Hodgson, E., and Casida, J. E. 1961. Metabolism of N,N-dialkyl carbamates and related compounds by rat liver. *Biochem. Pharmacol.* 8:179–191.

Hucker, H. B. 1973. Intermediates in drug metabolism reactions. *Drug Metab. Rev.* 2:33–56.

Ingelmann-Sundberg, M. 1983. Bioactivation or inactivation of toxic compounds? In *Drug Metabolism and Distribution, Current Revues in Biomedicine 3*, ed. J. W. Lambe, pp. 22–29. New York: Elsevier Biomedical.

Jakoby, W. B., Habig, W. H., Keen, J. H., Ketley, J. N., and Pabst, M. J. 1976. Glutathione S-transferases: Catalytic aspects. In *Glutathione: Metabolism and Function*, eds. I. M. Arias and W. B. Jakoby, pp. 189–211. New York: Raven.

Jerina, D. M., and Daly, J. W. 1974. Arene oxides: A new aspect of drug metabolism. *Science* 185:573–582.

Johnsson, U., Lundquist, G., Bergstrand, B., Eriksson, S. O., and Lindeke, B. 1978. Autoxidation of N-hydroxy-phenylalkylamines. In *Biological Oxidation of Nitrogen*, ed. J. W. Gorrod, p. 275. Amsterdam: Elsevier.

Kalow, W. 1983. Pharmacogenetics of drug metabolism. In *Drug Metabolism and Distribution. Current Revues in Biomedicine 3*, ed. J. W. Lambe, pp. 110–114. New York: Elsevier Biomedical.

Kampffmeyer, H., and Kiese, M. 1964. Further factors affecting the hydroxylation of aniline, and some of its derivatives by liver microsomes. *Naunyn-Schmiedebergs Arch. Exp. Pathol. Pharmakol.* 241:397–412.

Kapetanovic, I. M., Strong, J. M., and Mieyal, J. J. 1979. Metabolic structure-activity relationship for a homologous series of phenacetin analogs. *J. Pharmacol. Exp. Ther.* 209:117–129.

Kiese, M., and Uehleke, H. 1961. Der Ort der N-Oxidation der Anilins im Loheren Tier. *Naunyn-Schmeideberg's Arch. Exp. Path. Pharmakol.* 242:117–129.

Klaassen, C. D. 1974. Stimulation of the development of hepatic excretory mechanism for ouabain in newborn rats with microsomal enzyme inducers. *J. Pharmacol. Exp. Ther.* 191:212–218.

Klaassen, C. D. 1976. Biliary excretion of metals. *Drug Metab. Rev.* 5:165–196.

Klaassen, C. D., and Shoeman, D. W. 1972. Biliary excretion of lead. *Proc. 5th Int. Cong. Pharmacology*, p. 757.

Klemmer, H. W., Budy, A. M., Takahashi, W., and Haley, T. J. 1977. Human tissue distribution of cyclodiene pesticides—Hawaii, 1964–1973. *Clin. Toxicol.* 11:71–82.

LaDu, B. N., Gaudette, L., Trousof, N., and Brodie, B. B. 1955. Enzymatic dealkylation of aminopyrine (Pyramidon) and other alkylamines. *J. Biol. Chem.* 214:741–752.

Leakey, J. E. A., and Fouts, J. R. 1979. Precocious development of cytochrome P-450 in neonatal rat liver after glucocorticoid treatment. *Biochem. J.* 182:233.

Levine, W. G., and Lu, A. Y. H. 1982. Role of isozymes of cytochrome P-450 in the metabolism of N,N-dimethyl-4-aminoazobenzene in the rat. *Drug Metab. Dispos.* 10:102–109.

Lotlikar, P. D., and Dwyer, E. N. 1976. Effect of detergents on the N- and ring-hydroxylation of 2-acetamidofluorene by hamster liver microsomal preparations. *Biochem. J.* 160:821–824.

Lotlikar, P. D., and Hong, Y. S. 1981. Microsomal N- and C-oxidations of carcinogenic aromatic amines and amides. *Natl. Cancer Inst. Monogr.* 58:101–107.

Lu, A. Y. H., Somogyi, A., West, S., Kuntzman, R., and Conney, A. H. 1972. Pregnenolone-16-α-carbonitrile: A new type of inducer of drug metabolizing enzymes. *Arch. Biochem. Biophys.* 152:457.

Martland, H. S., and Humphries, R. E. 1929. Osteogenic sarcoma in dial painters using luminous paint. *Arch. Pathol.* 7:406–417.

Masters, B. S. S., and Ziegler, D. M. 1972. The distinct nature and function of NADPH-cytochrome *c* reductase and the NADPH-dependent mixed-function amine oxidase from porcine liver microsomes. *Arch. Biochem. Biophys.* 145:358.

Mattlocks, A. R., and White, I. N. H. 1971. The conversion of pyrrolizidine alkaloids to N-oxides and to dihydropyrrolizine derivatives by rat-liver microsomes in vitro. *Chem. Biol. Interact.* 3:383.

McMahon, R. E. 1961. Demethylation studies. I. The effect of chemical structure and lipid solubility. *J. Med. Pharm. Chem.* 4:67–68.

McMahon, R. F., Turner, J. C., and Whitaker, G. W. 1980. The N-hydroxylation and ring-hydroxylation of 4-aminobiphenyl in vitro by hepatic mono-oxygenases from rat, mouse, hamster, rabbit and guinea pig. *Xenobiotica* 10:469–481.

Mitoma, C., Posner, H. S., Reitz, H. C., and Underfriend, S. 1956. Enzymatic hydroxylation of aromatic compounds. *Arch. Biochem.* 61:431.

Mudge, G. H., and Weiner, I. M. 1963. Renal excretion of weak organic acids and bases. In *Proc. 1st Int. Pharmacol. Meeting, Mode of Action of Drugs. Drugs and Membranes,* ed. C. A. M. Hogben, vol. 4, pp. 157–164. Oxford: Pergamon.

Nenot, J. C., and Stather, J. W. 1979. *The Toxicity of Plutonium, Americium and Curium,* p. 225. New York: CBC Publication, Pergamon.

Noack, E. 1983. The interaction of drugs with mitochondrial functions: A possible mechanism for certain pharmacological effects. In *Drug Metabolism and Distribution,* ed. J. W. Lambe, pp. 49–54. New York: Elsevier Biomedical.

Orloff, J., and Berliner, R. W. 1961. Renal pharmacology. *Annu. Rev. Pharmacol.* 1:287–314.

Pawlak, J. W., and Konopa, J. 1979. In vitro binding of metabolically activated (^{14}C)-ledakrin or 1-nitro-9-^{14}C-(3'-dimethyl-n-propylamino)acridine, a new antitumor and DNA cross-linking agent, to macromolecules from subcellular fractions isolated from rat liver and HeLa cells. *Biochem. Pharmacol.* 28:3391–3402.

Pettit, F. H., Orme-Johnson, W., and Ziegler, D. M. 1964. The requirements for flavine adenine dinucleotide by liver microsomal oxygenase catalysing the oxidation of alkylaryl amines. *Biochem. Biophys. Res. Commun.* 16:444–448.

Prough, R. A. 1973. The N-oxidation of alkylhydrazines catalyzed by the microsomal mixed-function amine oxidase. *Arch. Biochem. Biophys.* 158:442–444.

Prough, R. A., Coomes, M. L., and Dunn, D. I. 1977. The microsomal metabolism of carcinogens and/or therapeutic hydrazines. In *Microsomes and Drug Oxidations,* ed. V. Ullrich, p. 500. Oxford: Pergamon.

Razzouk, C., and Roberfroid, M. B. 1982. Species differences in the biochemical properties of liver microsomal arylamine and arylamide N-hydroxylases. *Chem. Biol. Interact.* 41:251–264.

Razzouk, C., Mercier, M., and Roberfroid, M. 1980. Induction, activation and inhibition of hamster and rat liver microsomal arylamide and arylamine N-hydroxylase. *Cancer Res.* 40:3540–3546.

Reichart, E. R., Klemmer, H. N., and Haley, T. J. 1978. A note on dermal poisoning from mevinphos and parathion. *Clin. Toxicol.* 12:33–35.

Sanders, E., and Ashworth, C. T. 1961. A study of particulate intestinal absorption of hepatocellular uptake. Use of polystyrene latex particles. *Exp. Cell Res.* 22:137–145.

Sato, M., Yoshida, T., Suzuki, Y., Degawa, M., and Hashimoto, Y. 1981. Selective induction of microsomal 2-acetylamino-fluorene N-hydroxylation by dietary 2-acetylamino fluorene in rats. *Carcinogenesis* 2:571–574.

Schreiber, E. C. 1974. Metabolically oxygenated compounds: Formation, conjugation and possible biological implications. *J. Pharm. Sci.* 63:1177–1190.

Singh, A., Jolly, S. S., Bansal, B. C., and Mathur, C. C. 1963. Endemic fluorosis: Epidemiological, clinical and biochemical study of chronic fluorine intoxication in Punjab (India). *Medicine* 42:229.

Stillwell, N. G. 1983. Methylthiolation: A new pathway of drug metabolism. In *Drug Metabolism and Distribution, Current Revues in Biomedicine 3,* ed. J. W. Lambe, pp. 99–103. New York: Elsevier Biomedical.

Strobel, H. W., Fang, W-F, and Oshinsky, R. J. 1980. Role of colonic cytochrome P-450 in large bowel carcinogenesis. *Cancer* 45:1060–1065.

Sum, C. Y., and Cho, A. K. 1977. The N-hydroxylation of phenteramine by rat liver microsomes. *Drug Metab. Dispos.* 5:464–468.

Sunahara, S., Urano, M., and Ogawa, M. 1961. Genetical and geographic studies on isoniazid metabolism. *Science* 134:1530.

Takahashi, A., and Omori, Y. 1975. Species differences of N-hydroxylation of aminoazo dyes. I. *Jpn. J. Pharmacol.* 25(Suppl.):123P–124P.

Tang, B. K., Inaba, T., and Kalow, W. 1977a. N-Hydroxylation of pentobarbital in man. *Drug Metab. Dispos.* 5:71–74.

Tang, B. K., Inaba, T., and Kalow, W. 1977b. N-Hydroxylation of barbiturates. In *Biological Oxidation of Nitrogen,* ed. J. W. Gorrod, pp. 151–156. Amsterdam: Elsevier.

Testa, B., and Jenner, P. 1976. *Drug Metabolism: Chemical and Biochemical Aspects.* New York: Dekker.

Testa, B., and Salvesen, B. 1980. Quantitative structure-activity relationship in drug metabolism and disposition: Pharmacokinetics of N-substituted amphetamines in humans. *J. Pharm. Sci.* 69:497–501.

Thienes, C. H., and Haley, T. J. 1972. *Clinical Toxicology,* 5th ed., p. 273. Philadelphia: Lea and Febiger.

Uehleke, H. 1973. The role of cytochrome P-450 in the N-oxidation of individual amines. *Drug Metab. Dispos.* 1:299–313.

Usui, T., and Fukami, J. 1978. Comparative study of microsomal mixed-function oxidases in several animals, with special references to contents of cytochrome P-450 and oxidase activity. *Nippon Noyaky Sakkaishe* 3:149–154.

Vasder, S., Tsuruta, Y., and O'Brien, P. J. 1982. A free radical mechanism for arylamine induced carcinogenesis involving peroxides. *Biochem. Pharmacol.* 31:607–608.

Weinshilboum, R. M. 1983. "Methylator status" and assessment of variation in drug metabolism. In *Drug Metabolism and Distribution, Current Revues in Biomedicine 3,* ed. J. W. Lambe, pp. 104–109. New York: Elsevier Biomedical.

Williams, R. T. 1959. *Detoxication Mechanisms,* 2d ed. New York: Wiley.

Williams, R. M., and Beck, F. 1969. A histochemical study of gut maturation. *J. Anat.* 105:487–501.

Ziegler, D. M., and Mitchell, C. H. 1972. Microsomal oxidase IV: Properties of a mixed function oxidase isolated from pig liver microsomes. *Arch. Biochem. Biophys.* 150:116–125.

Ziegler, D. M., McKee, E. M., and Poulsen, L. L. 1973. Microsomal flavoprotein-catalyzed *N*-oxidation of arylamines. *Drug Metab. Dispos.* 1:314–321.

Ziegler, D. M., Mitchell, C. H., and Jollow, D. 1969. Properties of a purified hepatic microsomal mixed function oxidase. In *Microsomes and Drug Oxidations,* eds. J. R. Gillette, A. H. Conney, G. J. Cosmides, R. W. Estabrook, J. R. Fouts, and G. Mannering, p. 173. New York: Academic.

Ziegler, D. A., Poulsen, L. L., and McKee, E. M. 1971. Interaction of primary amines with a mixed-function amine oxidase isolated from pig liver microsomes. *Xenobiotica* 1:523–531.

Chapter 3

Biochemical and Pharmacological Aspects of Neurotoxicity from and Tolerance to Organophosphorus Cholinesterase Inhibitors

I. K. Ho

Beth Hoskins

INTRODUCTION

Organophosphorus agents produce diverse effects on both the central and peripheral nervous systems in animals and humans. Prior to World War II, only the "reversible" anticholinesterase agents, such as physostigmine (Eserine), were generally known. Prior to and during World War II, potential chemical warfare agents, such as the "nerve gases" soman, sarin, and tabun, were developed in Germany by Schrader's group (Taylor, 1980). Later on, organophosphorus compounds that were less toxic to humans were developed and widely used as pest control agents (e.g., malathion, parathion, mipafox) (Murphy, 1980). Their toxic properties apparently are related to their actions to inhibit esterases throughout the nervous system (Holmstedt, 1959; Davies et al., 1960; Johnson, 1975, 1976; Ecobichon, 1983). Diisopropyl fluoro-phosphate (DFP), synthesized by McCombie and Saunders (1946), has been one of the most extensively studied organophosphorus cholinesterase inhibitors (OP-ChE-Is) (Taylor, 1980).

According to their mechanisms of action, most of the organophosphorus agents can be classified into three main categories. The most extensively studied group is

This chapter was supported by a contract from the U.S. Army Medical Research and Development Command (contract DAMD17-81-C-1238). Thanks are due to Jewel Harper for her secretarial assistance.

composed of many organophosphorus agents [e.g., diisopropyl fluorophosphate (DFP), soman, sarin, tabun, and organophosphorus insecticides] known to inhibit acetylcholinesterase (AChE) (O'Brien, 1960, 1967; Heath, 1961; Koelle, 1963). Symptoms of acute toxicity in animals and humans exposed to these compounds are mainly cholinergic, including involuntary defecation, urination, lacrimation, muscular twitching, weakness, tremors, and convulsions (Davis and Richardson, 1980; Ecobichon, 1983). Usually these agents inhibit AChE by changing it into an inactive form that can no longer be reactivated either spontaneously or by oximes (Davies and Green, 1956; Hobbiger, 1956). This irreversible inhibition is termed "aging." The rate of aging caused by some of the potent OP-ChE-Is is fairly rapid. Harris et al. (1971) have reported that the time required for aging caused by soman is 2.4 min in guinea pigs.

A second group of organophosphorus compounds, comprising certain 4-alkyl derivatives of 1-phospha-2,6,7-trioxabicyclo[2,2,2]-octane 1-oxide, produces convulsions and death within a few minutes in mice (Bellet and Casida, 1973; Gordon et al., 1983). It has been demonstrated that brain AChE is not inhibited by these compounds. While the mechanism of their action is still unknown, it has been suggested that γ-aminobutyric acid (GABA) (Bowery et al., 1976) or cyclic guanosine monophosphate (GMP) (Mattsson et al., 1977) may be involved.

Third, many organophosphorus agents (e.g., tri-2-cresyl phosphate and DFP), after a single dose, can produce a delayed polyneuropathy, including a symmetrical distal axonal degeneration occurring in the peripheral nervous system and in selected tracts of the central nervous system (Spencer and Schaumburg, 1976). The initiation of this effect does not involve the inhibition of AChE, but rather the inhibition of another esteratic enzyme, termed "neurotoxic esterase" by Johnson (1975, 1976).

This chapter deals mainly with the aspects of OP-ChE-I-induced neurotoxicity and the phenomenon of tolerance development to compounds on multiple exposures to these agents. Names and structures of the OP-ChE-Is that are mentioned in the text are given in Table 1.

MECHANISMS OF ACUTE EFFECTS OF OP-ChE-Is

Cholinergic Mechanism

The extreme toxicity of OP-ChE-Is was found to be due to their irreversible inactivation of acetylcholinesterase (AChE), thereby exerting long-lasting inhibitory activity. DFP has been shown by Adrian et al. (1947) and others [details in the following reviews: Holmstedt (1959), Usdin (1970), Davis and Richardson (1980), Ecobichon (1983)] to inhibit AChE irreversibly. It was first demonstrated that the administration of this compound to humans resulted in specific effects attributable to the depression of AChE activity in tissues (Grob et al., 1947a,b,c; Harvey et al., 1947). This agent produced symptoms of acute poisoning such as anxiety, restlessness, insomnia, confusion, slurred speech, tremor, ataxia, and convulsions. However, it is not well established whether all of the toxic symptoms are due to the derangement of cholinergic function or if other neurochemical changes might be, in part, responsible.

Table 1. Organophosphorus Cholinesterase Inhibitors Included in the Text

Structural formula	Trade, common, or other name	Chemical name
Leptophos structure: CH_3O, $P{=}S$, $-O-$ (4-Bromo-2,5-dichlorophenyl with Br_2, Cl, Cl), phenyl	Leptophos; VCS-506; Phosvel; Abar; Lepton	O-(4-Bromo-2,5-dichlorophenyl)O-methylphenyl phosphonothioate
$\begin{array}{c}CH_3O\\CH_3O\end{array} P{=}S\!-\!S\!-\!CH(COOC_2H_5)\!-\!CH_2\!-\!COOC_2H_5$	Malathion; Cython; insecticide no. 4049; Phosphothion; Malathon; Malathiozol; Malathiozoo; Malaspray; Chemathion	S-[1,2-Dicarbethoxyethyl]-O,O-dimethyldithio phosphate
$\begin{array}{c}C_2H_5O\\C_2H_5O\end{array} P{=}S\!-\!S\!-\!CH_2CH_2N(C_2H_5)_2$	Tetram; systox (mixture of isomers)	O,O-Diethyl S-(β-diethylamino) ethyl phosphorothiolate
(i) P=S Isomer $\begin{array}{c}C_2H_5O\\C_2H_5O\end{array} P{=}S,\ P\!-\!O\!-\!CH_2\!-\!CH_2\!-\!S\!-\!C_2H_5$	Demeton O; Bayer 1C756; E-1059	O,O-Diethyl-O-[2-(ethylthio)ethyl] phosphorothioate
(ii) P=O Isomer $\begin{array}{c}C_2H_5O\\C_2H_5O\end{array} P{=}O,\ P\!-\!S\!-\!CH_2\!-\!CH_2\!-\!S\!-\!C_2H_5$	Demeton S	O,O-Diethyl-S-[2-(ethylthio)ethyl] phosphorothioate
$\begin{array}{c}C_2H_5O\\C_2H_5O\end{array} P{=}S,\ P\!-\!S\!-\!CH_2\!-\!CH_2\!-\!S\!-\!C_2H_5$	Di-syston; disulfoton; Bayer 19639; S276; Dithio-Systox; Thiodemeton; Dithiodemeton	O,O-Diethyl S-2-ethyl-2-mercaptoethyl phosphorodithioate

Structure	Common names	Chemical name
C_2H_5O, C_2H_5O — P(=S) — O — (4-nitrophenyl)	Parathion; E605; Alkron; Aphamite; DNTP; Etilon; Niran; Paraphos; Ethel parathion; Folidol; Orthophos; ACC; 3422; SNP; Thiophos; Fosferno; Bladan	Diethyl O-(4-nitrophenyl) phenylphosphonothioate
C_2H_5O, C_2H_5O — P(=O) — O — (4-nitrophenyl)	Paraoxon; mintacol; E600	Diethyl 4-nitrophenylphosphate
i-C_3H_7O, i-C_3H_7O — P(=O) — F	DFP; isoflurophate	Diisopropyl fluorophosphate
i-C_3H_7NH, i-C_3H_7NH — P(=O) — F	Mipafox	N,N'-Diisopropylphosphorodiamidic fluoride
CH_3O, CH_3O — P(=O) — O — CH=CCl₂	Dichlorvos Bayer 19149; Dichlorovos, Dedevap; Nerkol; Vapona; Herkol; DDVF; Nogos; Nuvan; Oko; Mafu	Dimethyl-2,2-dichlorovinyl phosphate
CH_3O, CH_3O — P(=O) — O — (nitro-tolyl, NO_2, CH_3)	Fenitrothion; Accothion; Folithion; Bay 41831; Sumithion; Cytel; Cyfen	O,O-Dimethyl O-(4-nitro-m-tolyl) phosphorothioate
dioxane ring with S—P(=S)(OC_2H_5)₂ substituents	Delnav; dioxathion, Hercules 528; Navadel	2,3-p-Dioxane S-bio-(O,O-diethyl dithiophosphate)

Table 1. Organophosphorus Cholinesterase Inhibitors Included in the Text (*Continued*)

Structural formula	Trade, common, or other name	Chemical name
C_2H_5O—$P(=O)(CH_3)$—$SCH_2CH_2N(i\text{-}C_3H_7)(i\text{-}C_3H_7)$	VX	Ethyl *S*-diisopropylaminoethyl methylphosphonothiolate
$(CH_3)_2N$—$P(=O)(C_2H_5O)$—CN	Tabun (GA)	Ethyl *N*-dimethylphosphoramidocyanidate
C_2H_5O—$P(=S)(C_6H_5)$—O—C_6H_4—NO_3	EPN	*O*-Ethyl *O*-(4-nitrophenyl) phenylphosphonothioate
$i\text{-}C_3H_7O$—$P(=O)(CH_3)$—F	Sarin (GB)	Isopropyl methylphosphonofluoridate
$(CH_3)_2N$—$P(=O)$—O—$P(=O)$—$N(CH_3)_2$ with $N(CH_3)_2$	OMPA; schradan	Octamethyl pyrophosphoramide
$(CH_3)_3C$—$CHO(CH_3)$—$P(=O)(CH_3)$—F	Soman (GD)	Pinacolyl methylphosphonofluoridate

It has been suggested that various cholinergically mediated behaviors would be disrupted only if the AChE activity in brain fell below some critical level, such as 40% of normal (Glow and Rose, 1965; Glow et al., 1966a,b; Russell, 1964; Russell et al., 1961). However, some of the behavioral changes induced by DFP do not entirely correlate with the degree of AChE inhibition. Kozar et al. (1976) have demonstrated that significant recovery of AChE after DFP administration preceded the return of the relevant behaviors to baseline levels. They showed that AChE in the lateral hypothalamus and the anterior preoptic area showed significant recovery by 16 h, while the corresponding behaviors did not recover to normal until 48 and 20 h, respectively. They further showed that there was no significant recovery of AChE in the caudate nucleus until 48 h after DFP, while the measures of alternation performance had still not returned to baseline levels by 71 h.

Wecker et al. (1977) have shown that atropine in high doses blocked the increase in ACh levels in the brain induced by OP-ChE-Is, but it did not significantly alter the convulsions and lethality produced by these compounds. Furthermore, it has been reported that no relation has been demonstrated between protection by atropine-like drugs against poisoning by OP-ChE-Is and their central or peripheral antimuscarinic activity (Faff et al., 1976; Green et al., 1977). Jovic (1974) also showed that after a single injection of soman, a close relationship existed between the severity of the symptoms of poisoning and the level of cholinesterase (ChE) inhibition only during the first 30–120 min in the acute phase. However, 2–48 h after the injection, the toxic symptoms, hyperglycemia and depression of spontaneous motor activity, disappeared despite continued ChE inhibition in blood, brain, and diaphragm. Meeter and Wolthuis (1968) showed that only 2% of ChE activity in brain was sufficient to preserve spontaneous respiration in rats after anticholinesterase poisoning. It is possible that only certain sites have to be inhibited in the brain to cause death, and the determinations of AChE inhibition carried out on whole brain may be inadequate to demonstrate the inhibition of these sites if certain compounds attack them selectively.

Duffy et al. (1979) have reported long-term electroencephalogram (EEG) changes in workers who have been exposed to sarin. The abnormality reported in this study was found in subjects with normal red-blood-cell ChE values at the time they were studied and who were exposure-free for more than 1 year. Burchfiel et al. (1976) and Burchfiel and Duffy (1982) also reported that monkeys exposed to sarin showed EEG abnormalities 1 year after exposure. If symptoms and signs of acute toxicity of OP-ChE-Is are produced mainly via inhibition in ChE activity, the recovery should be completed 3–4 months after exposure. This is based on reports that tissue ChE activity returns to normal at an approximate rate of 1% per day after acute exposure to sarin and other OP-ChE-Is (Grob and Harvey, 1958; Milby, 1971). Therefore, it has been suggested that sarin exposure can produce long-term changes in brain function (Duffy et al., 1979).

Other Neuronal Mechanisms that May Be Involved in Acute Toxicity of OP-ChE-Is

Studies of interactions between phenothiazine neuroleptics and anticholinesterase agents have been carried out; however, the results are somewhat contradictory, varying with the neuroleptic agent and animal used. A protective effect by phenothiazine against poisoning by several OP-ChE-Is has been reported in guinea pigs and in rabbits (Dahlbom et al., 1953; Fradá and Gucciardi, 1957; Wills, 1961). In contrast, potentiation of the toxic effects of organophosphorous insecticides by promazine or chlorpromazine also has been reported in humans (Arterberry et al., 1962) and in rats (Gaines, 1962; Michalek and Stavinoha, 1978). Studies of how phenothiazines affect OP-ChE-I-induced toxicity have not been well carried out. Although effects of the combination of chlorpromazine and OP-ChE-I (e.g., dichlorvos) on both ChE and butyrylcholinesterase (BuChE) activity in the brain have not been measured, Michalek and Stavinoha (1978) have measured potentiation of physostigmine effects by chlorpromazine in discrete brain regions (cerebellum, medulla oblongata plus pons, hypothalamus, striatum, midbrain, hippocampus, and cerebral cortex) and showed a quantitative similarity of effects on enzyme activities in various regions. Potentiation of BuChE inhibition, however, was slightly more pronounced than that of the total ChE activity. Potentiation did not depend on possible anticholinesterase effects of chlorpromazine in vivo, since the drug alone did not produce any inhibition of total ChE either in whole brain or in discrete brain regions (Michalek and Gatti, 1976), and it only produced a slight inhibition of BuChE. Therefore, whether potentiation by chlorpromazine of OP-ChE-I-induced toxicity is produced mainly via some cholinergic mechanism or not remains to be elucidated. Since the main mechanism of action of phenothiazine-type neuroleptics is blockade of postsynaptic dopamine (DA) receptors (Snyder, 1981; Seeman, 1981), studies of the involvement of the dopaminergic system in OP-ChE-I-induced toxicity have been warranted.

Glisson et al. (1972, 1974) have shown that acute administration of DFP significantly increased the brain level of DA in rabbits. They also showed that DFP-induced elevation of ACh levels in the thalamus and hypothalamus was lowered by pretreatment with the monoamine oxidase inhibitor, JB-835, and dihydroxyphenylalanine (DOPA) (Glisson et al., 1974). When rabbits were pretreated with atropine methylnitrate prior to DFP, the increase in DA induced by DFP was prevented. In chronic experiments, Freed et al. (1976) showed that mipafox administered to rats daily for 35 days produced ataxia and a reduction of DA levels in the corpus striatum. Treatment with leptophos for the same period of time produced slight motor dysfunction and a small but significant decrease in striatal DA levels. Fenitrothion neither induced motor dysfunction nor changed striatal DA levels. All three compounds inhibited ChE activity in the corpus striatum. These results led to the suggestion of an involvement of striatal DA in the delayed neurotoxic effects of certain OP-ChE-Is. In a histological study, Dasheiff et al. (1977) demonstrated that increased catecholamine stores were found in the locus ceruleus and the zona compacta of the substantia nigra in rats following a 0.33 LD50 dose of sarin. These increases returned to normal after 10 days. In a case report of possible organophosphorus insecticide-induced parkinsonism, there was the suggestion that chronic exposure of organophosphorus agents altered the cholinergic and dopaminergic activity in the striatum (Davis et al., 1978).

It has also been suggested that GABA may play an important role in organophosphorus insecticide-induced convulsions (Kar and Matin, 1972; Matin and Kar, 1973). Compounds (e.g., benzodiazepines) acting via GABAergic mechanisms (Costa et al.,

1975, 1976; Haefely et al., 1975) are potent inhibitors of organophosphorus compound-induced seizure activity (Lipp, 1973; Rump et al., 1973). Cyclic GMP levels appear to reflect the GABAergic inhibitory activity in the cerebellum (Mao et al., 1974a,b), and it has been shown that soman elevated cyclic GMP levels in rat cerebellum (Lundy and Magor, 1978). Benzodiazepines that block soman-induced convulsions also block the increase in cyclic GMP at the onset of convulsions (Lundy and Magor, 1978). Lundy et al. (1978) further showed that diazepam and two GABA-transaminase inhibitors, aminooxyacetic acid and n-dipropyl acetic acid, greatly reduced soman convulsions. Other organophosphorus agents that cause convulsions and death but do not inhibit AChE (Bellet and Casida, 1973) are also believed to exert their effects by altering GABAergic function (Bowery et al., 1976). Thus, evidence suggests that organophosphorus-induced convulsions appear to be abolished by altering GABA/ACh (acetylcholine) balance in an unknown manner, possibly via neuronal depression.

More recently, Sevaljevic et al. (1981) reported that inhibition of AChE in soman and VX (ethyl S-diisopropylaminoethyl methylphosphonothiolate) poisoning coincides with a significant increase in plasma cyclic adenosine monophosphate (AMP) levels. They further showed that administration of 1-(2-hydroxyiminomethyl-1-pyridino-3-(4-carbamoyl-1-pyridinio)-2-oxapropane dichloride (HI-6), an oxime, provided a full protection in poisoning by lethal doses of soman and VX; however, its effects on restoration of plasma cyclic AMP levels and red-blood-cell (RBC) AChE activity were dependent on the agent used. In VX intoxication, HI-6 reactivated RBC AChE and remarkably reduced the level of cyclic AMP in plasma, whereas in soman poisoning, HI-6 administration caused neither RBC AChE reactivation nor decreased cyclic AMP. The authors suggest that even though HI-6 failed to reactivate RBC AChE, it may reactivate AChE at some other vital site(s) in the body. They therefore speculated that cyclic AMP generation via catecholamine activation of adenylate cyclase may participate in the VX-induced increase of plasma cyclic AMP. This is based on the proposal that induction of catecholamine release may be involved in soman intoxication (Stitcher et al., 1977). Pharmacologically, Stitcher et al. (1977) showed the combination of theophylline and N^6,O^2-dibutyryl cyclic AMP significantly enhanced the toxicity of soman in mice. Therefore, it has been suggested that cyclic AMP participates in OP-ChE-I poisoning, possibly by enhancing the levels of ACh in the brain (Askew and Ho, 1975) or enhancing the release of ACh at neuromuscular junctions (Breckenridge et al., 1967; Goldberg and Singer, 1969).

Lundy and Shaw (1983) have demonstrated elevated cyclic GMP levels in the cerebella of rats that received one or two times the LD50 of soman. These increases in cyclic GMP occurred before the onset of cholinergic symptoms and prior to convulsions. Pretreatment of animals with an antimuscarinic or antinicotinic agent plus an oxime (HI-6) that attenuated soman-induced lethality had little effect on soman-induced convulsion or cyclic GMP levels. However, pretreatment with clonazepam, which reduced the convulsive activity of soman, also attenuated the increased cyclic GMP in the cerebellum. Their results also showed that soman-induced convulsion and the resulting increase in cerebellar cyclic GMP concentrations could not be related mainly to increased cholinergic activity or to muscarinic effects, since pretreatment of poisoned animals with antimuscarinic or antinicotinic compounds or with atropine plus an oxime had little effect on severity of convulsions or on cyclic GMP levels. Therefore they suggested that cyclic GMP may play a role in the initiation and continuation of soman-induced convulsions that were not related to specific cholinergic receptors but to general neuronal excitation.

DEVELOPMENT OF TOLERANCE
TO ORGANOPHOSPHORUS
CHOLINESTERASE INHIBITORS

General Aspects of Tolerance Development to OP-ChE-Is

Along with studies of acute toxicity of OP-ChE-Is, tolerance to these agents has aroused interest since the phenomenon was first reported by Barnes and Denz (1951). Their studies revealed that rats fed diets containing 50 ppm of E.605 (parathion) showed reduced signs of toxicity after 2 months on the diet. The amount of parathion used was demonstrated to be the threshold dose, in that above this level animals could not survive and below 20 ppm no symptoms were detected. Consequently, Rider et al. (1952) reported the phenomenon of tolerance to octamethyl pyrophosphoramide (OMPA) by gradually increasing the daily dose or by treating rats daily with a sublethal dose for a prolonged period of time. In 1953, Sumerford et al. also reported a phenomenon of tolerance to organophosphorus insecticides in residents living near orchards in Wenatchee, Washington. They reported that some workers had erythrocyte and plasma ChE values as low as 15% of the normal level without complaining of any symptoms throughout the spray season. Barnes and Denz (1954) confirmed the tolerance phenomenon in rats that had been chronically fed with the organophosphorus insecticides OMPA and Systox (mixture of isomers, see Tetram, Table 1). They observed that ChE activity in brains from Systox-treated rats was inhibited more than 85% at the time when toxic signs were not apparent. Hodge et al. (1954) showed that in male and female rats that were maintained on ethyl p-nitrophenyl thionobenzene phosphonate (EPN) (up to 150 and 75 ppm, respectively) for 2 years, the agent had no effect on growth. Similar phenomena were also demonstrated in dogs. Since these early reports, there have been other reports of tolerance to OP-ChE-Is. Bombinski and Dubois (1958) demonstrated that rats can tolerate about 50% of the LD50 of Di-Syston (see Table 1 for structure) given repeatedly at daily intervals for a period of 60 days. Oliver and Funnell (1961) showed that chronic parathion poisoning produced complete inhibition of erythrocyte ChE without concurrent skeletal-muscle paralysis in swine. Cooper (1962) reported that in guinea pigs that were dosed orally with Delnav [2,3-p-dioxane S-bis-(O,O-diethyl dithiophosphate)] at 25 mg/kg for 6 times at weekly intervals, weight losses occurred for up to 3 weeks. However, the body weights recovered to normal despite continued treatment.

DFP has been widely studied in terms of tolerance development to OP-ChE-Is (Glow et al., 1966a,b; Russell et al., 1969, 1971a,b,c, 1975, 1979; Overstreet, 1973, 1974). Russell, Overstreet and associates have reported on studies of chronic administration of DFP and the resulting behavioral tolerance to low-dose administration of DFP. In their studies of tolerance to DFP, an initial dose of DFP of 1.0 mg/kg to rats was followed at 3-day intervals by 0.5-mg/kg doses. Animals were housed in 24-h lighted quarters, and the 1-h consummatory behavioral responses such as drinking, lapping, and eating were measured after 23 h of food and water deprivation. Results of their studies showed not only that behavioral tolerance does develop to chronic maintenance of ChE at lwo levels of activity, but they also provided evidence indicating that the time characteristics of development of tolerance to DFP were different for the different consummatory behaviors. Development of tolerance was reported to be significantly faster as evidenced by eating behavior than by drinking behavior, the latter behavior requiring about twice as long to become normal as did eating behavior. Our recent studies using DFP injections (Lim et al., 1983) agree, in part, with those of Russell et al. (1969, 1971b), in that we have found that tolerance develops to DFP in terms of both eating and drinking behaviors. However, we found that chronic DFP treatment yielded similar effects on both of these behaviors.

Tolerance development to other OP-ChE-Is such as nerve-gas agents and other organophosphorus insecticides has also been reported. Sterri et al. (1980) showed that when rats were exposed daily to one-half LD50 doses of soman, some of the animals did not show symptoms of soman poisoning and survived a total exposure of four to seven times the acute LD50 dose of soman. During this period, brain and diaphragm AChE activities declined steadily during the chronic soman exposure. They later reproduced the phenomenon of tolerance to soman in both guinea pigs and mice (Sterri et al., 1981). Costa and Murphy (1982) have also demonstrated that mice develop tolerance to disulfoton during daily administration of 10 mg/kg for 14 days. They showed that signs of poisoning disappeared after 5–8 days of treatment, indicating that the animals had developed tolerance to disulfoton. At the end of 14 days of treatment, AChE activity was inhibited 75–93% in hippocampus, cerebral cortex, striatum, and cerebellum of disulfoton-tolerant mice.

The literature also reveals that chronic administration of an OP-ChE-I is accompanied by the development of cross-tolerance to the cholinomimetic effects of other cholinergic agents. Brodeur and DuBois (1964) have shown that rats made tolerant to Di-Syston are also less sensitive to the lethal effects of carbachol. McPhillips (1969) showed that rats that had developed tolerance to Di-Syston were found to be less susceptible to the subacute lethal action of OMPA than were control rats. They also showed that the sensitivity of Di-Syston-tolerant rats to the acute lethal action of oxotremorine was also reduced. Schwab and Murphy (1981) demonstrated that rats fed 7.5 ppm disulfoton that were without cholinergic toxicity were significantly more resistant to the lethal effects of carbachol than were rats given carbachol after 58 and 62 days on a control diet. In addition, rats fed 20 ppm disulfoton in the diet initially showed signs of toxicity that gradually disappeared with time on the diet. Rats fed at this level were more resistant to the lethal effects of carbachol than were control rats on all challenge dates and were more resistant than were those animals fed 7.5 ppm. Thus, it appears that the cross-tolerance between disulfoton and carbachol is dose-dependent.

Biochemical and Pharmacological Aspects
of Tolerance to OP-ChE-Is

The development of tolerance to OP-ChE-Is has since been well established as being a consequence of repeated administration of these agents. The exact biochemical mechanisms involved in tolerance processes have been difficult to pinpoint. During the past two decades, an increase in the number of studies pertaining to OP-ChE-Is has resulted in some understanding of how alterations of cholinergic functional states might be involved in the tolerance phenomenon induced by these agents (Costa et al., 1982a). Dispositional tolerance and other neurochemical changes may also contribute to the phenomenon of tolerance development to OP-ChE-Is. Therefore, the following sections highlight attempts to relate metabolic dispositions, cholinergic functions, and other neurochemical changes to OP-ChE-I-induced tolerance.

Metabolic Dispositional Tolerance As for barbiturates and other drugs (Remmer, 1964; Conney, 1967; Conney and Burns, 1962), the phenomenon of induction of drug-metabolizing enzymes by Op-ChE-Is has been reported (Neal, 1967; DuBois, 1969; Stevens et al., 1972). Therefore, chronic administration of Op-ChE-Is might enhance their own metabolism, consequently leading to decreased toxicity. Although OP-ChE-Is have been demonstrated to inhibit microsomal mixed-function oxidase activity when given acutely (Rosenberg and Coon, 1958; Stevens et al., 1972; Hodgson et al., 1980), they also have been shown to induce cytochrome P-450 and microsomal enzymes when animals were repeatedly administered organophosphorus insecticides (Stevens et al., 1972). Furthermore, pretreatment with phenobarbital, which induces cytochrome P-450 and drug-metabolizing enzymes, has been shown to decrease the acute toxicity of several organophosphorus insecticides (DuBois, 1969). Therefore, the evidence suggests that Op-ChE-Is that induce higher activity of microsomal mixed-function oxidase activity may enhance their own metabolism and consequently lead to the development of tolerance upon repeated administration. While this hypothesis seems to be plausible, numerous studies do not support the contention that the dispositional aspect plays a major role in the tolerance phenomenon. It has been consistently demonstrated that AChE activities are persistently inhibited during the repeated administration of OP-ChE-Is (Barnes and Denz, 1954; Russell et al., 1971a,b,c, 1975; Overstreet et al., 1972; Sivam et al., 1983).

Some specific enzymes that are present in other tissues have also been considered to contribute to the development of tolerance to OP-ChE-Is. An enzyme or enzyme complex capable of hydrolyzing DFP or soman has been identified in the squid giant axon (Hoskin et al., 1966; Hoskin, 1971; Hoskin and Long, 1972; Garden et al., 1975; Hoskin and Rousch, 1982). The enzyme has been termed squid-DFPase. The discovery of this type of enzyme has raised the possibility that during the development of tolerance to OP-ChE-Is, this enzyme will be induced and consequently lead to the acceleration of hydrolysis of organophosphorus compounds.

Sterri et al. (1980) have linked tolerance to soman to the storage of lipid-soluble compounds in adipose tissue or binding of soman to plasma or liver proteins. They suggested that "storage depot(s)" for soman may be the enzymes, plasma ChE and especially plasma aliesterase (Sterri et al., 1981). Their suggestion was based on finding that the plasma ChE activity was more than 90% inhibited 1 h after the administration of soman and was returned to 40–50% of the control within 24 h, and the plasma aliesterase activity was about 70% inhibited after 1 h and was fully recovered within 24 h.

Another enzyme system that is distinctively different from ChE and can be phosphorylated by organophosphorus esters has been termed neurotoxic esterase (Johnson, 1975, 1976). Neurotoxic agents such as phosphates, phosphonates, or phosphoramidates have been shown to inhibit neurotoxic esterase. Therefore, this enzyme system could also play a role in the development of tolerance to OP-ChE-Is. It is clear that more studies on the metabolism of organophosphorus esters in tolerant animals are necessary.

Alteration in the Cholinergic Functional State in Op-ChE-I-Induced Tolerance Brodeur and DuBois (1964) were the first to suggest that tolerance to the Op-ChE-Is is due to the development of subsensitivity of cholinergic receptors to acetylcholine. To support this contention, they demonstrated that cholinergic receptors become less sensitive, since the LD50 of carbachol was significantly higher in Di-Syston-tolerant rats than that in control rats. Subsequently, McPhillips (1969) showed that rats that had developed tolerance to Di-Syston were less sensitive to the sublethal dose of OMPA than were control rats. They also showed that Di-Syston-tolerant rats were found to be more resistant to an acute lethal dose of oxotremorine. Costa et al. (1981) showed that mice that developed tolerance to disulfoton also became less sensitive to a lethal dose of carbachol. Schwab and Murphy (1981) showed that animals fed 20 ppm disulfoton daily were also more resistant to the lethal effects of carbachol than control animals. Overstreet et al. (1972) showed that pilocarpine, a cholinomimetic agent, reduced the food intake of DFP-tolerant rats to a much lesser extent than that of controls. Overstreet (1973) further demonstrated that pilocarpine-suppressed water intake in normal rats was not evident in DFP-tolerant animals. Overstreet (1974) also demonstrated that the behavior depressant effects of pilocarpine were reduced in DFP-tolerant animals. Overstreet et al. (1974), by using anticholinesterase agents as well as muscarinic and nicotinic agonists and antagonists, demonstrated that the sensitivity of both muscarinic and nicotinic receptors to AChE may be reduced during chronic treatment with DFP, but that nicotinic receptors may be more resistant to change than are muscarinic receptors. Russell et al. (1975) also showed that pilocarpine was less effective in suppressing the response of rats tolerant to DFP than in suppressing that of control animals. Furthermore, rats tolerant to DFP were resistant to the hypothermic actions of pilocarpine and carbachol (Overstreet et al., 1973), and disulfoton-tolerant mice were resistant to the hypothermic and antinociceptive actions of oxotremorine (Costa et al., 1982b). The evidence above has thus consistently revealed that a decreased sensitivity of cholinergic receptors may be one the mechanisms underlying the development of tolerance to OP-ChE-Is.

These pharmacological and behavioral studies have been further substantiated by biochemical studies on the characteristics of both muscarinic and nicotinic receptors after tolerance development to OP-ChE-Is.

Muscarinic Receptors in Op-ChE-I-Tolerance   Since the availability of specific radioligands for cholinergic receptors (Yamamura and Synder, 1974; Birdsall et al., 1978; Hulme et al., 1978; Ehlert et al., 1980a), direct quantification and characterization of alterations in cholinergic receptors in Op-Che-I-induced tolerance have been possible. By using the specific muscarinic antagonist [³H]quinuclidinyl benzilate ([³H]QNB), Ehlert and Kokka (1977) first demonstrated a decreased binding of [³H]QNB in the ilium of rats that had been repeatedly treated with DFP. Ehlert and Kokka (1978) further reported decreases in [³H]QNB binding levels in rat brain following chronic administration of DFP. Immediately afterward, Schiller (1979) showed that following constant reduction of AChE activity by repeated administration of DFP, there is a decrease in the number of muscarinic acetylcholine receptors as evidenced by the reduction in [³H]QNB binding sites in cholinergic-rich areas of the brain such as striatum, cortex, and hippocampus. Gazit et al. (1979) also demonstrated that chronic administration of Tetram [O,O-diethyl S-(β-diethylamino) ethyl phosphorothiolate] leads to a marked reduction in the level of muscarinic receptors in cortex, hippocampus, hypothalamus, thalamus, caudate, striatum, and brainstem of rat brains. Uchida et al. (1979) also demonstrated that chronic administration of DFP to mice induces decreases in the numbers of muscarinic receptors. However, the binding affinity of muscarinic receptors for [³H]QNB was not altered by chronic administration of DFP. Although detailed studies reported by Ehlert et al. (1980b) supported their previous findings that chronic administration also caused a decrease in the density of [³H]QNB binding sites in homogenates of the striatum, they further reported that an increase in the K_i for inhibition of [³H]QNB by different cholinergic agents was noted in rats treated chronically with DFP. Therefore they reported that chronic administration of DFP significantly decreased affinity of muscarinic receptors in the striatum. Smit et al. (1980) also reported that chronic administration of paraoxon significantly reduced the number of muscarinic binding sites and caused a small decrease in the affinity of the receptors in rats. Reduction of [³H]QNB binding to muscarinic receptors in forebrain and hindbrain in disulfoton-tolerant rats (Schwab et al., 1981) and mice (Costa et al., 1981) has also been demonstrated. In both studies, no significant changes in affinity of muscarinic receptor bindings were found in the brain. Costa et al. (1982b) further differentiated the alterations of cholinergic muscarinic receptors during chronic and acute tolerance to disulfoton. Furthermore, Costa and Murphy (1982) demonstrated that in mice tolerant to disulfoton, the number of muscarinic receptor binding sites was significantly reduced in hippocampus, cortex, striatum, and cerebellum. However, the affinity constants of the muscarinic receptors were not altered in any of the areas studied. We have also demonstrated that subacute administration of DFP to rats for either 4 or 14 days reduced the number of muscarinic sites without affecting their affinity (Sivam et al., 1983). The evidence available therefore suggests that subsensitivity or down-regulation of the muscarinic cholinergic receptors takes place when development of tolerance to OP-ChE-Is occurs.

Nicotinic Receptors in OP-ChE-I-Tolerance   Since Brodeur and DuBois (1964) and Russell et al. (1975) hypothesized that a change in cholinergic receptor sensitivity might be a likely mechanism underlying the development of tolerance to Op-ChE-Is, the involvement of muscarinic cholinergic receptors has been the focus of extensive studies for the past few years, as discussed earlier. However, the possible involvement of nicotinic cholinergic receptors in OP-ChE-I-tolerance has not been as extensively explored. Russell et al. (1975) reported that DFP-treated animals failed to develop cross-tolerance to the reversible anticholinesterase inhibitors physostigmine and neostigmine. Therefore, they suggested that this lack of cross-tolerance may have occurred because of differential involvement of muscarinic and nicotinic receptors in tolerance development to Op-ChE-Is. This hypothesis was based on results of their studies showing that when ChE activity levels were at 46% and 30% of the normal level during chronic treatment with DFP, subsensitivity developed to pilocarpine and carbachol and supersensitivity developed to atropine (Overstreet et al., 1974). However, the sensitivity of nicotinic receptors was altered only when ChE activity was at 30% of the normal level (i.e., not at 45%). Based on these data, they hypothesized that subsensitivity of both muscarinic and nicotinic receptors to acetylcholine may be developed during chronic treatment with DFP, but that muscarinic receptors may be more labile than nicotinic receptors. The nature of an involvement of nicotinic receptors in OP-ChE-I-induced tolerance remains to be elucidated.

Acetylcholine Metabolism in Op-ChE-I-Induced Tolerance It has been demonstrated that the synthetic enzyme for acetylcholine, choline acetyltransferase (CAT), is not affected by either acute or chronic administration of disulfoton (Stavinoha et al., 1969), DFP (Russell et al., 1975), paraoxon (Wecker et al., 1977), soman, sarin, or tabun (Ho et al., 1983). Russell et al. (1975, 1981) further demonstrated that AChE activity was depressed at constantly low levels (below 30%), while acetylcholine content in whole brain was elevated and remained at 140% of the control level during chronic DFP treatment. Wecker et al. (1977) showed that in rats treated chronically with low doses of paraoxon, total acetylcholine levels reached a maximum of 50% over control levels and AChE activity was 55% inhibited. While free acetylcholine levels increased in both acutely and chronically treated animals, bound acetylcholine levels only increased significantly in the acutely treated rats. Russell et al. (1979) also demonstrated that there were no statistically significant differences in the synthesis of acetylcholine or the high-affinity transport of choline into synaptosomal fractions when rats treated chronically with DFP were compared with control rats. Recently, Lundy and Shih (1983) also demonstrated that neither acetylcholine nor choline levels are good parameters to predict the outcome of soman poisoning. In light of the evidence, therefore, it appears unlikely that end-product inhibition of presynaptic acetylcholine metabolism would be involved in OP-ChE-I-induced tolerance.

Since these agents irreversibly inactivate AChE, the dynamic state of this enzyme during chronic administration of these agents should be investigated. The reappearance of AChE activity after irreversible inhibition of the enzyme by OP-ChE-Is may be correlated with de novo synthesis rather than reactivation of inhibited enzyme. Reactivation of DFP- or soman-inhibited ChE has been investigated in mammalian tissue both in vitro (Coult et al., 1966) and in vivo (Fleisher and Harris, 1965; Harris et al., 1971); no evidence for a significant reactivation of DFP-inhibited enzyme has been provided. Therefore, the only means for recovery of AChE has been demonstrated to be a heterogeneous pool of several molecular forms whose profile in mammalian nervous systems can vary considerably (Hall, 1973; Wilson and Walker, 1974; Rieger and Vigny, 1976; Bisso et al., 1980; Gruvic et al., 1981; Michalek et al., 1981). Therefore, it has been suggested that metabolic differences among various forms could be at least partly responsible for differences in neurobehavioral recovery after organophosphorus-induced intoxication (Bignami et al., 1975; Michalek et al., 1979). Three main molecular forms (slow-, medium-, and fast-migrating forms) of AChE have been separated by polyacrylamide gel electrophoresis. Of soluble brain AChE in rats treated acutely with DFP, Michalek et al. (1981) have shown that 80% of the activity was reduced in DFP-treated rats. Of the remaining 20% of AChE activity, the relative contribution of slow-migrating forms to the residual enzymatic activity was decreased, while that of medium-migrating forms was significantly increased. At 4 days after the DFP treatment, these changes became more apparent, while AChE activity had recovered to about 50% of the control level. The partial recovery in the distribution of molecular forms in this period was mainly due to an increase in the medium-migrating forms. Based on these results, they have suggested that the medium-migrating forms may be precursors in the biosynthesis of slow-migrating forms and/or there may be functional specificity of the different forms (Michalek et al., 1981). Gruvic et al. (1981), using cytochemical techniques, studied the recovery of AChE in the diaphragm, brain, and plasma of rats after acute administration of soman. The cytochemical evidence indicated that recovery of AChE was slow during the first 2 days, and only 4-S and 10-S molecular forms of the enzyme activity were present in the endplate regions. However, the synaptic AChE activity had already started to accumulate, and this indicated that the synthesis of AChE in muscle and Schwann cells might even have been enhanced. Furthermore, they demonstrated AChE activity in brain recovered in a similar way as in muscle. Although newly synthesized AChE has not been studied in animal models of OP-ChE-I-induced tolerance, it is tempting to speculate that chronic administration of OP-ChE-Is may alter the rate of synthesis of AChE. By histochemical and biochemical techniques, Chippendale et al. (1974) have demonstrated that AChE activity in both septum and hippocampus after DFP administration in rats exhibited an initially rapid phase of recovery and a slower recovery. Analysis of AChE synthesis in the septum preceded that in the hippocampus. Based on the results, they have suggested that AChE in the hippocampus may be transported from the septum.

Although OP-ChE-Is exert their toxicity mainly through the inhibition of AChE, it has been shown that only 2% of ChE activity in brain is sufficient to preserve spontaneous respiration in rat (Meeter and Wolthuis, 1968). In the literature, reports have consistently shown that when animals had developed tolerance to OP-ChE-Is, the cholinesterase activity still remained at 10–30% of the normal AChE activities (Glow et al., 1966a,b; Russell et al., 1969, 1971a,b, 1975; Overstreet, 1973; Sivam et al., 1983). Therefore, in OP-ChE-I-tolerant animals, the newly synthesized AChE may be accounting for the tolerance to maintenance doses of OP-ChE-I. Consequently, the enzyme activity would remain at a steady-state level without further inhibition. The role of newly synthetized AChE in OP-ChE-I-induced tolerance deserves extensive study.

Evidence reported also shows that various organophosphorus anticholinesterase agents have been reported to stimulate protein synthesis (Clouet and Walsch, 1963; Domschke et al., 1970; Welsch and Dettbarn, 1971; Cehovic et al., 1972). This could lead to increase in synthesis of AChE after chronic administration of OP-ChE-Is. ACh has also been shown to increase the rate of RNA synthesis in vitro (Prives and Quastel, 1969); consequently, the accumulation of ACh after OP-ChE-I administration could lead to increased AChE synthesis, a type of positive feedback.

Other Mechanisms Involved
in OP-AChE-I-Induced Tolerance

Other nonspecific metabolic changes, such as adenosine triphosphatase, alkaline phosphatase, and cytochrome oxidase, have been studied during chronic administration with DFP (Russell et al., 1975). Results showed that neither cytochrome oxidase nor alkaline phosphatase was altered during the treatment. ATPase activity was inhibited by about 20%, but this inhibition did not quite correlate with the behavioral changes during the development of tolerance. They suggested that inhibition of ATPase by DFP could be indirect, since the fluoride ion that is released from DFP upon hydrolysis could be the cause of this inhibition (Lahiri and Wilson, 1971).

Although susceptibility of cholinergic receptors may play a major role in OP-ChE-I-tolerance, other neuronal activities that interact with cholinergic pathways cannot be overlooked. Russell et al. (1975) demonstrated that control and DFP-tolerant animals when treated with methyl p-tyrosine, which depletes both dopamine and norepinephrine content in the brain, affected the behavior of animals to a comparable degree in both control and DFP-tolerant animals. Even though norepinephrine has not been demonstrated to be involved in the development of tolerance to OP-ChE-Is, more extensive studies should be carried out.

The discovery of the variety of neurotransmitters, especially dopamine and γ-aminobutyric acid (GABA), and their participation in the number of neurological and behavioral disorders (Hornykiewicz, 1975; Seeman, 1981; Enna, 1981) suggest that these systems, in addition to the cholinergic system, also may be involved in OP-ChE-I-tolerance. It has been demonstrated that an imbalance of dopaminergic and cholinergic systems in the basal ganglia is associated with motor dysfunction, particularly parkinsonism (Hornykiewicz, 1966, 1975). The basal ganglia are rich in AChE (Quastel, 1962; Dawson and Jarrott, 1981). On the other hand, GABA is an inhibitory neurotransmitter in the mammalian central nervous system (Roberts et al., 1976; McBurney and Baker, 1978; Lal et al., 1980). Evidence suggests that the drugs that increase GABAergic activity in the brain decrease striatal dopamine turnover (Lahti and Losey, 1974). It also has been suggested that acetylcholine may regulate GABA synthesis (Roberts and Hammerschlag, 1972). Based on these reasons, other neuronal systems that may be involved in OP-ChE-I-induced tolerance warrant extensive study. We have demonstrated that acute administration of DFP increases the number of dopamine and GABA receptors without affecting the muscarinic receptor characteristics (Sivam et al., 1983). Whereas chronic administration of DFP for either 4 or 14 days reduced the number of muscarinic sites without affecting the affinity, the DFP treatment caused an increase in the number of dopamine and GABA receptors only after 14 days of treatment; however, the increase was considerably lower than that observed after the acute treatment. The in vitro addition of DFP to striatal membranes did not affect dopamine, GABA, or muscarinic receptors. These data indicate a possible involvement of GABAergic and dopaminergic systems in development of tolerance to DFP. It may be that the GABA and DA systems, singularly or in combination, counteract the enhanced cholinergic activity induced by OP-ChE-Is.

PROBLEMS ENCOUNTERED IN THIS AREA
OF RESEARCH

While most of the OP-ChE-Is are very toxic to all species of animals, there are differences in susceptibility to these agents among species. It has been reported that the LD50 of DFP by oral administration varied widely, for example, 36.8 ± 0.98 and 9.78 ± 0.65 mg/kg for mice and rabbits, respectively (Horton et al., 1946). The intravenous LD50 values were 0.34 ± 0.01, 3.43 ± 0.62, and 1.63 ± 0.03 mg/kg for rabbits, dogs, and cats, respectively (Horton et al., 1946). Frawley et al. (1957) further observed a sex difference in DFP-induced lethality. The LD50 values for oral administration of DFP are 7.7 and 13.5 mg/kg for female and male rats, respectively. Domschke et al. (1970) and Stitcher et al. (1977) have shown that the regeneration of ChE in rats poisoned with DFP is slower than those poisoned with soman. However, the rate of return of blood ChE activity is similar for both soman and DFP in mice (Stitcher et al., 1977).

While species or sex differences could be the reason for different mortality, the variations in potency of different lots of DFP cannot be overlooked. We have studied the variation of three DFP lots obtained from two sources (Ho and Hoskins, 1983). The effects of different lots of DFP on body weights, mortality, and brain AChE activity in rats varied significantly. The in vitro effects of these DFP preparations on brain AChE activity also were markedly different. Since it is apparent that different commercial preparations of DFP do possess different potencies, one can expect that the same dose of different preparations would not produce the same effects on any physiological systems under study. Therefore, the differences in the literature might be due not only to different potencies but also to different protocols for treating the animals, perhaps even to a different procedure for handling DFP in terms of the vehicle and the route of administration, etc.

Different treatment schedules used in different studies may also contribute to the discrepancies. Russell et al. (1969, 1971a) reported significant decreases in both water and food intake, beginning 23 h after a single injection of DFP at 1 mg/kg, with short-term recovery taking place between subsequent injections of 0.5 mg/kg at 3-day intervals. The brain AChE activity 24 h after a single injection of DFP was approximately 30% that of the normal rats (Russell et al., 1969, 1971a,b, 1975; Glow et al., 1966a,b; Overstreet, 1973). Although Glow et al. (1966a) reported no evidence of toxic effects, with brain ChE activity being 20–40% of control, they did report body weight to be significantly depressed from normal body weight during chronic admin- istration of DFP. They also reported a reduction in food consumption only at day 1 and day 4 (following the first and second injections of DFP, respectively), with decreased water consumption throughout the experimental period. Their data showed that tolerance to DFP in terms of water consumption was not obvious. Russell et al. (1969, 1971b) reported tolerance to DFP-induced decreased water consumption and food consumption. As mentioned earlier, Russell et al. (1969, 1971b) reported that the time to develop tolerance was shorter in terms of food intake than drinking behavior, and furthermore that a suprabaseline drinking behavior was found follow- ing withdrawal of DFP and after 25 days of normal drinking. In contrast to the above reports on DFP-induced toxicity and tolerance, we found no acute effect of a single dose of DFP at 1 mg/kg, or of twice this dose, to decrease significantly either eating or drinking behavior (Lim et al., 1983). However, after 4 daily doses of DFP at 2 mg/kg sc, we did observe significant depression in both food and water consumption as well as significant depression in body weight. Our results showed that chronic DFP treatment yielded similar effects on both of these behaviors. In fact, maximum de- creases in both consummatory behaviors occurred at the same time. Therefore, it appears that the differences between our data and those of others are due to different dosing schedules and to the previously mentioned different potencies of DFP prepara- tions.

Even among the same species, different strains of animals show significant varia- tions in their responses to the OP-AChE-Is. Stavinoha et al. (1969) found high levels of acetylcholine in the brains of Charles River but not of Holtzman rats rendered

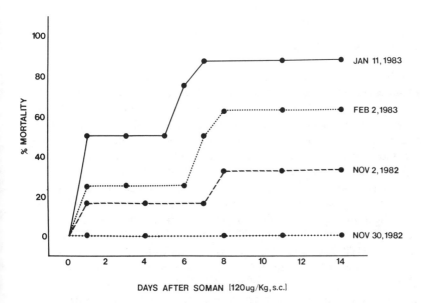

Figure 1 Percent mortality of Sprague-Dawley rats over a 2-week period following a single subcutaneous injection of soman (120 μg/kg). Dates are dates of injections and were generally 5 days after receipt of each animal shipment.

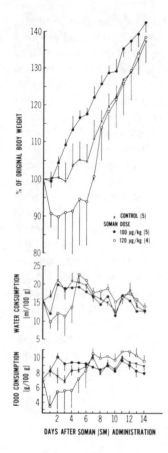

Figure 2 Growth rates (as percent of initial body weights) and consummatory behaviors of rats (initial body weights 209.6 ± 3.4 g) over a 14-day period after a single subcutaneous dose of soman (100 or 120 μg/kg). Data are presented as means ± SEM. Numbers in parentheses represent number of animals per treatment group.

tolerant to disulfoton, although AChE activity was inhibited to the same extent in both strains. Overstreet and Russell (1982) also found that Slinders S-line rats, which were more sensitive than were randomly bred rats to DFP, also showed more sensitivity to the depressive effect of the agonists pilocarpine and physostigmine on locomotive activities, water intake, and operant responding maintained by water reward. On the other hand, the locomotive stimulant effects of scopolamine, a muscarinic antagonist, were less effective in the S-line rats, while depressants of atropine and scopolamine on water intake and operant responding maintained by water reward were comparable in the randomly bred line and S-line. They further showed that S-line rats were more sensitive to the hyperthermic effects of pilocarpine and oxotremorine. Even though two lines of rats show differences in sensitivity to DFP, the brain AChE activity in two lines following DFP treatment were not significantly different (Overstreet et al., 1979). These studies suggest that selection of a particular strain of animals also plays an important role in studying the mechanisms of OP-AChE-I-induced tolerance.

Finally, recent studies in our laboratory have demonstrated variations in response to OP-AChE-Is within the same strain of rats obtained from the same vendor. Figure 1 shows how the same dose of soman caused different mortalities in Sprague-Dawley rats obtained from Charles River Breeding Laboratories. Body weights of the animals were approximately the same for all shipments. Mortality appeared to be higher during cold temperatures (January and February). However, climate does not explain the higher mortality in early November than in late November. Figure 2 summarizes growth rates (as percent of initial body weights) and consummatory behaviors of rats over a period of 2 weeks following a single injection of soman (100 or 120 μg/kg). These studies were carried out in early November when the climate was quite mild, temperatures being in the 60s and 70s (degrees Fahrenheit). Identical experiments were performed in February when the climate was quite cold (10–30 °F) using younger (Fig. 3) and older (Fig. 4) rats. The differences in growth rates and consummatory behaviors between the two age groups are striking. Additionally, when one particular shipment of rats died immediately upon receiving a nonlethal dose of soman, we were able to learn that these rats had been treated for viral infections prior to our receiving them. These results clearly indicate that one must not overlook the many variables (e.g., seasonal, age, vendor, pretreatment, etc.) that may singly or in combination affect the outcome of studies of toxicity and tolerance to organophosphorus compounds.

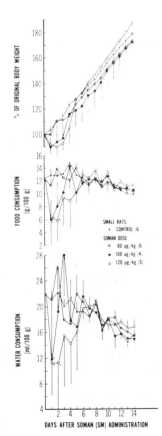

Figure 3 Growth rates (as percent of initial body weights) and consummatory behaviors of rats (initial body weights 136.5 ± 2.1 g) over a 14-day period after a single subcutaneous dose of soman (80, 100, or 120 μg/kg). Asterisks indicate significant ($p < 0.05$) difference from control group. Data are presented as means ± SEM. Numbers in parentheses represent number of animals per treatment group.

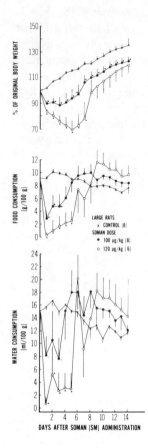

Figure 4 Growth rates (as percent of initial body weights) and consummatory behaviors of rats (initial body weights 241 ± 2.3 g) over a 14-day period after a single subcutaneous dose of soman (100 or 120 μg/kg). Asterisks indicate significant ($p < 0.05$) difference from control group. Data are presented as means ± SEM. Numbers in parentheses represent number of animals per treatment group.

REFERENCES

Adrian, E. E., Feldberg, W., and Kilby, B. A. 1947. The cholinesterase inhibiting action of fluorophosphonates. *Br. J. Pharmacol. Chemother.* 2:56–58.

Arterberry, J. D., Bonifaci, R. W., Nash, E. W., and Quinby, G. E. 1962. Potentiation of phosphorus insecticides by phenothiazine derivatives. Possible hazard, with report of a fatal case. *J. Am. Med. Assoc.* 182:848–850.

Askew, W. E., and Ho, B. T. 1975. Effects of intraventricular injections of N^6,O^2-dibutyryl adenosine $3',5'$-monophosphate on the rat brain cholinergic system. *Can. J. Biochem.* 53:634–635.

Barnes, J. M., and Denz, F. A. 1951. The chronic toxicity of *p*-nitrophenyl diethyl thiophosphate (E. 605); a long term feeding experiment with rats. *J. Hyg.* 49:430–441.

Barnes, J. M., and Denz, F. A. 1954. The reaction of rats to diets containing octamethyl pyrophosphoramide (Schraden) and *O,O*-diethyl-*S*-ethylmercaptoethanol thiophosphate ("Systox"). *Br. J. Ind. Med.* 11:11–19.

Bellet, E. M., and Casida, J. E. 1973. Bicyclic phosphorus esters: High toxicity without cholinesterase inhibition. *Science* 182:1135–1136.

Bignami, G., Rosic, N., Michalek, H., Milósević, M., and Gatti, G. L. 1975. Behavioral toxicity of anticholinesterase agents: Methodological neurochemical and neuropsychological aspects. In *Behavioral Toxicology*, eds. B. Weiss and V. G. Laties, pp. 155–215. New York: Plenum.

Birdsall, N. J. M., Burgen, A. S. V., and Hulme, E. C. 1978. The binding of agonists to brain muscarinic receptors. *Mol. Pharmacol.* 14:723–736.

Bisso, G. M., Nemesio, R., and Michalek, H. 1980. Early post-natal changes in the pattern of molecular forms of acetylcholinesterase in the rat brain. In *Multidisciplinary Approach to Brain Development*, eds. C. Di Benedetta, R. Balázs, G. Gombos, and G. Porcellati, pp. 235–236. Amsterdam: Elsevier/North Holland.

Bombinski, T. J., and DuBois, K. P. 1958. Toxicity and mechanism of action of Di-Syston. *AMA Arch. Ind. Health* 17:192–199.

Bowery, N. G., Collins, J. F., and Hill, R. G. 1976. Bicyclic phosphorus esters that are potent convulsants and GABA antagonists. *Nature (Lond.)* 261:601–603.

Breckenridge, B., Burn, J. H., and Matschinsky, F. M. 1967. Theophylline, epinephrine and neostigmine facilitation of neuromuscular transmission. *Proc. Natl. Acad. Sci. USA* 57:1893–1897.

Brodeur, J., and DuBois, K. P. 1964. Studies on the mechanism of acquired tolerance by rats O,O-diethyl S-2-(ethylthio)ethyl phosphorodithioate (Di-Syston). *Arch. Int. Pharmacodyn. Ther.* 149:560–570.

Burchfiel, J. L., and Duffy, F. H. 1982. Organophosphate neurotoxicity: Chronic effects of sarin on the electroencephalogram of monkey and man. *Neurobehav. Toxicol. Teratol.* 4:767–778.

Burchfiel, J. L., Duffy, F. H., and Sim, V. M. 1976. Persistent effects of sarin and dieldrin upon the primate electroencephalogram. *Toxicol. Appl. Pharmacol.* 35:365–379.

Cehovic, G., Dettbarn, W. D., and Welsch, F. 1972. Paraoxon: Effects on rat brain cholinesterase and on growth hormone and prolactin of pituitary. *Science* 175:1256–1258.

Chippendale, T. J., Cotman, C. W., Kozar, M. D., and Lynch, G. S. 1974. Analysis of acetylcholinesterase synthesis and transport in the rat hippocampus: Recovery of acetylcholinesterase activity in the septum and hippocampus after administration of diisopropylfluorophosphate. *Brain Res.* 81:485–496.

Clouet, D., and Waelsch, H. 1963. Amino acid and protein metabolism of the brain—IX. The effect of an organophosphorus inhibition on the incorporation of [^{14}C]-lysine into the proteins of rat brain. *J. Neurochem.* 10:51–63.

Conney, A. H. 1967. Pharmacological implications of microsomal enzyme induction. *Pharmacol. Rev.* 19:317–366.

Conney, A. H., and Burns, J. J. 1962. Factors influencing drug metabolism. *Adv. Pharmacol.* 1:31–58.

Cooper, F. A. 1962. Delnav [2:3-p-dioxane S-bis-(O,O-diethyl dithiophosphate)] as an ixodicide. *Vet. Rec.* 74:103–112.

Costa, E., Guidotti, A., and Mao, C. C. 1975. Evidence for involvement of GABA in the action of benzodiazepines: Studies on rat cerebellum. In *Advances in Biochemical Psychopharmacology*, eds. E. Costa and P. Greengard, vol. 14, pp. 113–130. New York: Raven.

Costa, E., Guidotti, A., and Mao, C. C. 1976. A GABA hypothesis for the action of benzodiazepines. In *GABA in Nervous System Function*, eds. E. Roberts, T. N. Chase, and D. B. Tower, pp. 413–426. New York: Raven.

Costa, L. G., and Murphy, S. D. 1982. Passive avoidance retention in mice tolerant to the organophosphorus insecticide disulfoton. *Toxicol. Appl. Pharmacol.* 65:451–458.

Costa, L. G., Schwab, B. W., Hand, H., and Murphy, S. D. 1981. Reduced [^{3}H]quinuclidinyl benzilate binding to muscarinic receptors in disulfoton-tolerant mice. *Toxicol. Appl. Pharmacol.* 60:441–450.

Costa, L. G., Schwab, B. W., and Murphy, S. D. 1982a. Tolerance to anticholinesterase compounds in mammals. *Toxicology* 25:79–97.

Costa, L. G., Schwab, B.W., and Murphy, S. D. 1982b. Differential alterations of cholinergic muscarinic receptors during chronic and acute tolerance to organophosphorus insecticides. *Biochem. Pharmacol.* 31:3407–3413.

Coult, D. B., Marsh, D. J., and Read, G. 1966. Dealkylation studies on inhibited acetylcholinesterase. *Biochem. J.* 98:869–873.

Dahlbom, R., Diamant, H., Edlund, T., Ekstrand, T., and Holmstedt, B. 1953. Protective effect of phenothiazine derivatives against poisoning by the irreversible cholinesterase inhibitor dimethylamidoethoxy phosphoryl cyanide (Tabun). *Acta Pharmacol. Toxicol.* 9:163–167.

Dasheiff, R. M., Einberg, E., and Grenell, R. G. 1977. Sarin and adrenergic-cholinergic interaction in rat brain. *Exp. Neurol.* 57:549–560.

Davies, D. R., and Green, A. L. 1956. The kinetics of reactivation by oximes of cholinesterase inhibited by organophosphorus compounds. *Biochem. J.* 63:529–535.

Davies, D. R., Holland, P., and Rumens, M. J. 1960. The relationship between the chemical structure and neurotoxicity of alkyl organophosphorus compounds. *Br. J. Pharmacol.* 15:271–278.

Davis, C. S., and Richardson, R. J. 1980. Organophosphorus compounds. In *Experimental and Clinical Neurotoxicology,* eds. P. S. Spencer and H. H. Schaunburg, pp. 527–544. Baltimore: Williams & Wilkins.

Davis, K. L., Yesavage, J. A., and Berger, P. A. 1978. Possible organophosphate-induced Parkinsonism. *N. Nerv. Ment. Dis.* 166:222–225.

Dawson, R. M., and Jarrott, B. 1981. Response of muscarinic cholinoceptors of guinea pig brain and ileum to chronic administration of carbamate or organophosphate cholinesterase inhibitors. *Biochem. Pharmacol.* 30:2365–2368.

Domschke, W., Domagk, G. F., Domschke, S., and Erdmann, W. D. 1970. Über die wirkung von soman unter diisopropylfluorophosphat auf die enzymbiosynthese in der rattenleber. *Arch. Toxikol.* 26:76–83.

DuBois, K. P. 1969. Combined effects of pesticides. *Can. Med. Assoc. J.* 100:173–179.

Duffy, F. H., Burchfiel, J. L., Bartels, P. H., Gaon, M., and Sim, V. M. 1979. Long-term effects of an organophosphate upon the human electroencephalogram. *Toxicol. Appl. Pharmacol.* 47:161–176.

Ecobichon, D. J. 1983. Organophosphorus ester insecticides. In *Pesticides and Neurological Diseases,* eds. D. J. Ecobichon and R. M. Joy, pp. 151–203. Boca Raton, Fla.: CRC.

Ehlert, F. J., and Nokka, N. 1977. Decrease in [^{3}H]-quinuclidinyl benzilate binding to the muscarinic cholinergic receptor in the longitudinal muscle of the rat ileum following chronic administration of diisopropylfluorophosphate. *Proc. West Pharmacol. Soc.* 20:1–7.

Ehlert, F. J., and Kokka, N. 1978. Decrease in [^{3}H]-quinuclidinyl benzilate binding to the striatum of rats following chronic administration of diisopropylfluorophosphate. *Fed. Proc.* 37:609.

Ehlert, F. J., Dumont, Y., Roeske, W. R., and Yamamura, H. I. 1980a. Muscarinic receptor binding in rat brain using the agonist [^{3}H] *cis* methyldioxolane. *Life Sci.* 26:961–967.

Ehlert, F. J., Kokka, N., and Fairhurst, A. S. 1980b. Altered [^{3}H]-quinuclidinyl benzilate binding in the striatum of rats following chronic cholinesterase inhibition with diisopropylfluorophosphate. *Mol. Pharmacol.* 17:24–30.

Enna, S. J. 1981. GABA receptor pharmacology. Functional considerations. *Biochem. Pharmacol.* 30:907–913.

Faff, J., Borkoruska, E., and Bak, W. 1976. Therapeutic effects of some cholinolytics in organophosphate intoxications. *Arch. Toxicol.* 36:139–146.

Fleischer, J. H., and Harris, L. W. 1965. Dealkylation as a mechanism for aging of cholinesterase after poisoning with pinacolyl methylphosphonofluoridate. *Biochem. Pharmacol.* 14:641–650.

Fradá, G., and Gucciardi, G. 1957. Influenza della cloropromazine sull'intossicazione da esteri fosforici (Effect of chlorpromazine on phosphoric ester poisoning). *Med. Lav.* 48:301–306.

Frawley, J. P., Fuyat, H. N., Hagan, Z. C., Blake, J. R., and Fitzhugh, O. G. 1957. Marked potentiation in mammalian toxicity from simultaneous administration of two anticholinesterase compounds. *J. Pharmacol. Exp. Ther.* 121:96–106.

Freed, V. H., Matin, M. A., Fang, S. C., and Kar, P. P. 1976. Role of striatal dopamine in delayed neurotoxic effects of organophosphorus compounds. *Eur. J. Pharmacol.* 35:229–232.

Gaines, T. B. 1962. Poisoning by organic phosphorus pesticides potentiated by phenothiazine derivatives. *Science* 138:1260–1261.

Garden, J. M., Hause, S. K., Hoskin, F. C. G., and Rousch, A. H. 1975. Comparison of DFP-hydrolyzing enzyme purified from head ganglion and hepatopancreas of squid (*Loligo pealei*) by means of isoelectric focusing. *Comp. Biochem. Physiol.* 52C:95–98.

Gazit, H., Silman, I., and Dudai, Y. 1979. Administration of an organophosphate causes a decrease in muscariniic receptor level in rat brain. *Brain. Res.* 174:351–356.

Glisson, S. N., Karczmar, A. G., and Barnes, L. 1972. Cholinergic effects on adrenergic neurotransmitters in rabbit brain parts. *Neuropharmacology* 11:465–477.

Glisson, S. N., Karczmar, A. G., and Barnes, L. 1974. Effects of diisopropyl phosphorofluoridate on acetylcholine, cholinesterase and catecholamines of several parts of rabbit brain. *Neuropharmacology* 13:623–631.

Glow, P. H., and Rose, S. 1965. The effects of reduced acetylcholinesterase levels on the extinction of a conditioned response. *Nature (Lond.)* 206:475–477.

Glow, P. H., Richardson, A., and Rose, S. 1966a. Effects of acute and chronic inhibition of cholinesterase upon body weight, food intake, and water intake in the rat. *J. Comp. Physiol. Psychol.* 61:295–299.

Glow, P. H., Richardson, A., and Rose, S. 1966b. The effect of acute and chronic treatment with diisopropylfluorophosphate on cholinesterase activities of some tissues of the rats. *Aust. J. Exp. Biol. Med.* 44:73–86.

Goldberg, A. L., and Singer, J. J. 1969. Evidence for a role of cyclic AMP on neuromuscular transmission. *Proc. Natl. Acad. Sci. USA* 64:134–141.

Gordon, J. J., Inns, R. H., Johnson, M. K., Leadbeater, L., Maidment, M. P., Upshall, D. G., Cooper, G. H., and Rickard, R. L. 1983. The delayed neuropathic effects of nerve agents and some other organophosphorus compounds. *Arch. Toxicol.* 52:71–82.

Green, D. M., Muir, A. W., Stratton, J. A., and Inch, T. D. 1977. Dual mechanism of the antidotal action of atropine-like drugs in poisoning by organophosphorus anticholinesterases. *J. Pharm. Pharmacol.* 29:62–64.

Grob, D., and Harvey, T. C. 1958. Effects in man of the anticholinesterase compound sarin (isopropyl methylphosphorofluoridate). *J. Clin. Invest.* 37:350–368.

Grob, D., Lilienthal, J. L., Jr., Harvey, A. M., and Jones, B. F. 1947a. The administration of diisopropylfluorophosphate (DFP). I. Effect on plasma and erythrocyte cholinesterase; general systemic effects; use in study of hepatic function and erythropoiesis; and some properties of plasma cholinesterase. *Bull. Johns Hopkins Hosp.* 81:217–244.

Grob, D., Lilienthal, J. L., Jr., and Harvey, A. M. 1947b. The administration of di-isopropyl fluorophosphate (DFP) to man. II. Effect of internal motility and use in the treatment of abdominal distention. *Bull. Johns Hopkins Hosp.* 81:245–257.

Grob, D., Harvey, A. M., Langworthy, D. R., and Lilienthal, J. L., Jr. 1947c. The administration of di-isopropyl fluorophosphate (DFP) to man. III. Effect on the central nervous system with special reference to the electrical activity of the brain. *Bull. Johns Hopkins Hosp.* 81:257–266.

Gruvic, Z., Sketelj, J., Klinar, B., and Brzin, M. 1981. Recovery of acetylcholinesterase in the diaphragm, brain, and plasma of the rat after irreversible inhibition by soman: A study of cytochemical localization and molecular forms of the enzyme in the motor end plate. *J. Neurochem.* 37:909–916.

Haefely, W., Kulcsar, A., Mohler, H., Pierei, L., Polc, P., and Schaffner, R. 1975. Possible involvement of GABA in the central actions of benzodiazepines. In *Advances in Biochemical Psychopharmacology*, eds. E. Costa and P. Greengard, vol. 14, pp. 131–151. New York: Raven.

Hall, Z. W. 1973. Multiple forms of acetylcholinesterase and their distribution in end plate and non plate regions of rat diaphragm muscle. *J. neurobiol.* 4:343–361.

Harris, L. W., Yamamura, H. I., and Fleisher, Y. H. 1971. De nova synthesis of acetylcholinesterase in guinea pig retina after inhibition of pinacolyl methylphosphonofluoridate. *Biochem. Pharmacol.* 20:2927–2930.

Harvey, A. M., Lilienthal, J. L., Jr., Grob, D., Jones, B. F., and Talbot, S. A. 1947. The administration of di-isopropyl fluorophosphate in man. IV. The effects on neuromuscular function in normal subjects and in myasthenia gravis. *Bull. Johns Hopkins Hosp.* 81:267–292.

Heath, D. F. 1961. *Organophosphorus Poisons.* New York: Pergamon.

Ho, I. K., and Hoskins, B. 1983. Variation of commercial diisopropyl fluorophosphate preparation in toxicological studies. *Drug Chem. Toxicol.* 6:421–427.

Ho, I. K., Sivam, S. P., and Hoskins, B. 1983. Acute toxicity of diisopropylfluorophosphate, Tabun, Sarin and Soman in rats: Lethality in relation to cholinergic and GABAergic enzyme activities. *Fed. Proc.* 42:656 (abst.).

Hobbiger, F. 1956. Chemical reactivation of phosphorylated human and bovine true cholinesterases. *Br. J. Pharmacol.* 11:295–303.

Hodge, H. C., Maynard, E. A., Hurwitz, L., DiStefano, V., Downs, W. L., Jones, C. K., and Blanchet, H. J., Jr. 1954. Studies of the toxicity and of the enzyme kinetics of ethyl p-nitrophenyl thionobenzene phosphonate (EPN). *J. Pharmacol. Exp. Ther.* 112:29–39.

Hodgson, E., Kulkarni, A. P., Fabacher, D. L., and Robacker, K. M. 1980. Induction of hepatic drug metabolizing enzymes in mammals by pesticides: A review. *J. Environ. Sci. Health B* 15:723–754.

Holmstedt, B. 1959. Pharmacology of organophosphorus cholinesterase inhibitors. *Pharmacol. Rev.* 11:567–688.

Hornykiewicz, O. 1966. Dopamine (3-hydroxytyramine) and brain function. *Pharmacol. Rev.* 18:925–975.

Hornykiewicz, O. 1975. Parkinson's disease and its chemotherapy. *Biochem. Pharmacol.* 24:1061–1065.

Horton, R. G., Koelle, G. B., McNamara, B. P., and Pratt, H. J. 1946. The acute toxicity of di-isopropyl fluorophosphate. *J. Pharmacol. Exp. Ther.* 87:415–420.

Hoskin, F. C. G. 1971. Diisopropylphosphorfluoridate and tabun enzymatic hydrolysis and nerve function. *Science* 172:1243–1245.

Hoskin, F. C. G., and Long, R. J. 1972. Purification of a DFP-hydrolyzing enzyme from squid head ganglion. *Arch. Biochem. Biophys.* 150:548–555.

Hoskin, F. C. G., and Rousch, A. H. 1982. Hydrolysis of nerve gas by squid-type diisopropylphosphorofluoridate hydrolyzing enzyme on agarose resin. *Science* 215:1255–1257.

Hoskin, F. C. G., Rosenberg, P., and Brzin, M. 1966. Re-examination of the effect of DFP on electrical and cholinesterase activity of squid giant axon. *Proc. Natl. Acad. Sci. USA* 55:1231-1234.

Hulme, E. C., Birdsall, N. J. M., Burgen, A. S. V., and Metha, P. 1978. The binding of antagonists to brain muscarinic receptors. *Mol. Pharmacol.* 14:737–750.

Johnson, M. K. 1975. Organophosphorus esters causing delayed neurotoxic effects. Mechanism of action and structure/activity studies. *Arch. Toxicol.* 34:259–288.

Johnson, M. K. 1976. Mechanism of protection against the delayed neurotoxic effect of organophosphorus esters. *Fed. Proc.* 35:73–74.

Jovic, R. C. 1974. Correlation between signs of toxicity and some biochemical changes in rats poisoned by soman. *Eur. J. Pharmacol.* 25:159–164.

Kar, P. P., and Matin, M. A. 1972. Possible role of γ-aminobutyric acid in paraoxon-induced convulsions. *J. Pharm. Pharmacol.* 24:996–997.

Koelle, G. B. 1963. Cytological distributions and physiological functions of cholinesterases. In *Handbuch der Experimentellen Pharmakologie,* eds. O. Eichler and A. Farah, vol. 15, pp. 187–298. Berlin: Springer-Verlag.

Kozar, M. D., Overstreet, D. H., Chippendale, T. C., and Russell, R. W. 1976. Changes of acetylcholinesterase activity in three major brain areas and related changes in behaviour following acute treatment with diisopropyl fluorophosphates. *Neuropharmacology* 15:291-298.

Lahiri, A. K., and Wilson, I. B. 1971. On the inhibition of (Na^+-K^+)-activated adenosine triphosphatase by diisopropyl fluorophosphate. *Mol. Pharmacol.* 7:46–51.

Lahti, R. A., and Losey, E. G. 1974. Antagonism of the effects of chlorpromazine and morphine on dopamine metabolism by GABA. *Res. Commun. Chem. Pathol. Pharmacol.* 7:31–40.

Lal, H., Fielding, S., Malick, J., Roberts, E., Shah, N., and Usdin, E. 1980. GABA neurotransmission: Current developments in physiology and neurochemistry. *Brain Res. Bull.* 5(Suppl. 2):1–946.

Lim, D. K., Hoskins, B., and Ho, I. K. 1983. Assessment of diisopropylfluorophosphate (DFP) toxicity and tolerance in rats. *Res. Commun. Chem. Pathol. Pharmacol.* 39:399–418.

Lipp, J. A. 1973. Effect of benzodiazepine derivatives on soman-induced seizure activity and convulsions in the monkey. *Arch. Int. Pharmacodyn.* 202:244–251.

Lundy, P. M., and Magor, G. 1978. Cyclic GMP concentrations in cerebellum following organophosphate administration. *J. Pharm. Pharmacol.* 30:251–252.

Lundy, P. M., and Shaw, R. K. 1983. Modification of cholinergically induced convulsive activity and cyclic GMP levels in the CNS. *Neuropharmacology* 22:55–63.

Lundy, P. M., and Shih, T. M. 1983. Examination of the role of central cholinergic mechanisms in the therapeutic effects of HI-6 in organophosphate poisoning. *J. Neurochem.* 40:1321–1328.

Lundy, P. M., Magor, G., and Shaw, R. K. 1978. Gamma-aminobutyric acid metabolism in different areas of rat brain at the onset of soman-induced convulsions. *Arch. Int. Pharma-codyn. Therap.* 234:64–73.

Mao, C. C., Guidotti, A., and Costa, E. 1974a. The regulation of cyclic guanosine monophos-phate in rat cerebellum: Possible involvement of putative amino acid neurotransmitters. *Brain Res.* 75:510–514.

Mao, C. C., Guidotti, A., and Costa, E. 1974b. Interactions between γ-aminobutyric acid and guanosine cyclic 3′,5′-monophosphate in rat cerebellum. *Mol. Pharmacol.* 10:736–745.

Matin, M. A., and Kar, P. P. 1973. Further studies on the role of γ-aminobutyric acid in paraoxon-induced convulsions. *Eur. J. Pharmacol.* 21:217–221.

Mattsson, H., Brandt, K., and Heilbronn, E. 1977. Bicyclic phosphorus esters increase the cyclic GMP level in rat cerebellum. *Nature (Lond.)* 268:52–53.

McBurney, R. N., and Baker, J. L. 1978. GABA-induced conductance fluctuations in cultured spinal neurons. *Nature (Lond.)* 274:596–597.

McCombie, H., and Saunders, B. C. 1946. Alkyl fluorophosphonates: Preparation and physio-logical properties. *Nature (Lond.)* 157:287–289.

McPhillips, J. J. 1969. Altered sensitivity to drugs following repeated injections of a cholines-terase inhibitor to rats. *Toxicol. Appl. Pharmacol.* 14:67–73.

Meeter, E., and Wolthuis, O. L. 1968. The spontaneous recovery of respiration and neuromuscu-lar transmission in the rat after anticholinesterase poisoning. *Eur. J. Pharmacol.* 2:377–386.

Michalek, H., and Gatti, G. L. 1976. Anticholinesterase properties of phenothiazine neurolep-tics. In *Proceedings of European Society of Toxicology,* eds. W. A. M. Ducan, B. J. Leonard, and M. Brunard, vol. XVII, pp. 372–379. Amsterdam: Excerpta Medica.

Michalek, H., and Stavinoha, W. B. 1978. Effect of chlorpromazine pre-treatment on the inhibition of total cholinesterases and butylcholinesterase in brain of rats poisoned by physostigmine or dichlorvos. *Toxicology* 9:205–218.

Michalek, H., Meneguz, A., Bisso, G. M., Carro-Ciampi, G., Gatti, G. L., and Bignami, G. 1979. Neurochemical changes associated with the behavioural toxicity of organophos-phate compounds. In *Advances in Pharmacology and Therapeutics,* vol. 9, *Toxicology,* ed. Y. Cohen, pp. 187–201. Oxford: Pergamon.

Michalek, H., Meneguz, A., and Bisso, G. M. 1981. Molecular forms of rat brain acetylcho-linesterase in DFP intoxication and subsequent recovery. *Neurobehav. Toxicol. Teratol.* 3:303–312.

Milby, T. H. 1971. Prevention and management of organophosphate poisoning. *J. Am. Med. Assoc.* 216:2131–2133.

Murphy, S. D. 1980. Pesticides. In *Casarett and Doull's Toxicology: The Basic Science of Poisons,* 2d ed., eds. J. Doull, C. D. Klaassen, and M. O. Amdur, pp. 357–408. New York: Macmillan.

Neal, R. A. 1967. Studies on the metabolism of diethyl 4-nitrophenyl phosphorothionate (parathion) *in vitro. Biochem. J.* 103:183–191.

O'Brien, R. D. 1960. *Toxic Phosphorus Esters.* New York: Academic.

O'Brien, R. D. 1967. *Insecticides, Action and Metabolism.* New York: Academic.

Oliver, W. T., and Funnell, H. S. 1961. Correlation of the effects of parathion on erythrocyte cholinesterase with sympatomatology in pigs. *Am. J. Vet. Res.* 22:80–84.

Overstreet, D. H. 1973. The effects of pilocarpine on the drinking behavior of rats following acute and chronic treatment with diisopropylfluorophosphate and during withdrawal. *Be-hav. Biol.* 9:257–263.

Overstreet, D. H. 1974. Reduced behavioral effects of pilocarpine during chronic treatment with DFP. *Behav. Biol.* 11:49–58.

Overstreet, D. H., and Russell, R. W. 1982. Selective breeding for diisopropyl fluorophosphate-sensitivity: Behavioral effects of cholinergic agonists and antagonists. *Psychopharmacology* 78:150–155.

Overstreet, D. H., Hadick, D. G., and Russell, R. W. 1972. Effects of amphetamine and pilocarpine on eating behavior in rats with chronically low acetylcholinesterase levels. *Behav. Biol.* 7:217–226.

Overstreet, D. H., Kozar, M. D., and Lynch, G. S. 1973. Reduced hypothermic effects of cholinomimetic agents following chronic anticholinesterase treatment. *Neuropharmacology* 12:1017–1032.

Overstreet, D. H., Russell, R. W., Vasquez, B. J., and Dalglish, A. W. 1974. Involvement of muscarinic and nicotinic receptors in behavioral tolerance to DFP. *Pharmacol. Biochem. Behav.* 2:45–54.

Overstreet, D. H., Russell, R. W., Helps, S. C., and Messenger, M. 1979. Selective breeding for sensitivity to the anticholinesterase, DFP. *Psychopharmacology* 65:15–20.

Prives, C., and Quastel, J. H. 1969. Effect of cerebral stimulation on biosynthesis of nucleotides and RNA in brain slices *in vitro*. *Biochim. Biophys. Acta* 182:285–294.

Quastel, J. H. 1962. Acetylcholine distribution and synthesis in the central nervous system. In *Neurochemistry,* eds. K. A. C. Elliot, I. H. Page, and J. H. Quastel, p. 431. Springfield, Ill.: Thomas.

Remmer, H. 1964. Gewöhnung an hexobarbital durch beschleunigten abbau. *Arch. Int. Pharmacodyn. Therap.* 152:346–359.

Rider, J. A., Ellinwood, L. Z., and Coon, J. M. 1952. Production of tolerance in the rat to octanethyl pyrophosphoramide (OMPA). *Proc. Soc. Exp. Biol. Med.* 81:455–459.

Rieger, F., and Vigny, M. 1976. Solubilization and physicochemical characterization of rat brain acetylcholinesterase: Development and maturation of its molecular forms. *J. Neurochem.* 27:121–129.

Roberts, E., and Hammerschiag, R. 1972: Amino acid transmitters. In *Basic Neurochemistry,* eds. R. W. Albers, G. J. Siegel, R. Katzman, and B. W. Agranoff, pp. 218–245. Boston: Little, Brown.

Roberts, E., Chase, T. N., and Tower, D. B. 1976. GABA in *Nervous System Function.* New York: Raven.

Rosenberg, P., and Coon, J. M. 1958. Increase of hexobarbital sleeping time by certain anticholinesterases OMPA, ZPN, malathion, chlorothion phostex. *Proc. Soc. Exp. Biol. Med.* 98:650–652.

Rump, S., Grudzinska, E., and Edelwejn, Z. 1973. Effects of diazepam on epileptiform patterns of bioelectrical activity of the rabbit's brain induced by fluostigmine. *Neuropharmacology* 12:813–817.

Russell, R. W. 1964. Neurophysiological and biochemical correlates of effects of drugs on behaviour: The acetylcholine system. In *CIBA Foundation Symposium: Animal Behavior and Drug Action,* ed. H. Steinberg, pp. 144–159. Boston: Little, Brown.

Russell, R. W., Watson, R. H. J., and Trankenhaeuser, M. 1961. Effects of chronic reductions in brain cholinesterase activity on acquisition and extinction of a conditioned avoidance response. *Scand. J. Physiol.* 2:21–29.

Russell, R. W., Warburton, D. M., and Segal, D. S. 1969. Behavioral tolerance during chronic changes in the cholinergic system. *Commun. Behav. Biol.* 4:121–128.

Russell, R. W., Vasquez, B. J., Overstreet, D. H., and Dalglish, F. W. 1971a. Effects of cholinolytic agents on behavior following development of tolerance to low cholinesterase activity. *Pscyhopharmacologia* 20:32–41.

Russell, R. W., Vasquez, B. J., Overstreet, D. H., and Dalglish, F. W. 1971b. Consummatory behavior during tolerance to and withdrawal from chronic depression of cholinesterase activity. *Physiol. Behav.* 7:523–528.

Russell, R. W., Warburton, D. M., Vasquez, B. J., Overstreet, D. H., and Dalglish, F. W. 1971c. Acquisition of new responses by rats during chronic depression of acetylcholinesterase activity. *J. Comp. Physiol. Psychol.* 77:228–233.

Russell, R. W., Overstreet, D. H., Cotman, C. W., Carson, V. G., Churchill, L., Dalglish, F. W., and Vasquez, B. J. 1975. Experimental tests of hypotheses about neurochemical mechanisms underlying behavioral tolerance to the anticholinesterase diisopropyl fluorophosphate. *J. Pharmacol. Exp. Ther.* 192:73–85.

Russell, R. W., Carson, V. G., Jope, R. S., Booth, R. A., and Macri, J. 1979. Development of behavioral tolerance: A search for subcellular mechanisms. *Psychopharmacology* 66:155–158.

Russell, R. W., Carson, V. G., Booth, R. A., and Jenden, D. J. 1981. Mechanisms of tolerance to the anticholinesterase, DFP: Acetylcholine levels and dynamics in the rat brain. *Neuropharmacology* 20:1197–1201.

Schiller, G. D. 1979. Reduced binding of [³H]-quinuclidinyl benzilate associated with chronically low acetylcholinesterase activity. *Life Sci.* 24:1159–1164.

Schwab, B. W., and Murphy, S. D. 1981. Induction of anticholinesterase tolerance in rats with doses of disulfoton that produce no cholinergic signs. *J. Toxicol. Environ. Health* 8:199–204.

Schwab, B. W., Hand, H., Costa, L. G., and Murphy, S. D. 1981. Reduced muscarinic receptor binding in tissues of rats tolerant to the insecticide disulfoton. *Neurotoxicology* 2:635–647.

Seeman, P. 1981. Brain dopamine receptors. *Pharmacol. Rev.* 32:229–313.

Sevaljevic, L., Krtolica, K., Poznanovic, G., Boskovic, B., and Maksimovic, M. 1981. The effect of organophosphate poisoning on plasma cyclic AMP in rats. *Biochem. Pharmacol.* 30:2725–2727.

Sivam, S. P., Norris, J. C., Lim, D. K., Hoskins, B., and Ho, I. K. 1983. Effect of acute and chronic cholinesterase inhibition with diisopropyl fluorophosphate on muscarinic, dopamine, and GABA receptors of the rat striatum. *J. Neurochem.* 40:1414–1422.

Smit, M. H., Ehlert, F. J., Yamamura, S., Rose, W. R., and Yamamura, H. I. 1980. Differential regulation of muscarinic agonist binding sites following chronic cholinesterase inhibition. *Eur. J. Pharmacol.* 66:379–380.

Snyder, S. H. 1981. Dopamine receptors, neuroleptics and schizophrenia. *Am. J. Psychiatr.* 138:460–464.

Spencer, P. S., and Schaumberg, H. H. 1976. Central and peripheral distal asonopathy—The pathology of dying-back polyneuropathies. In *Progress in Neuropathology,* ed. H.Zimmerman, vol. III, pp. 253–295. New York: Grune and Stratton.

Stavinoha, W. B., Ryan, L. C., and Smith, P. W. 1969. Biochemical effects of an organophosphorus cholinesterase inhibitor on the rat brain. *Ann. NY Acad. Sci.* 160:378–382.

Sterri, S. H., Lyngaas, S., and Fonnum, F. 1980. Toxicity of soman after repetitive injection of sublethal doses in rat. *Acta Pharmacol. Toxicol.* 46:1–7.

Sterri, S. H., Lyngaas, S., and Fonnum, F. 1981. Toxicity of soman after repetitive injection of sublethal doses in guinea-pig. *Acta Pharmacol. Toxicol.* 49:8–13.

Stevens, J. T., Stitzel, R. E., and McPhillips, J. J. 1972. Effects of anticholinesterase insecticides on hepatic microsomal metabolism. *J. Pharmacol. Exp. Ther.* 181:576–583.

Stitcher, D. L., Harris, L. W., Moore, R. D., and Heyl, W. C. 1977. Synthesis of cholinesterase following poisoning with irreversible anticholinesterases: Effects of theophylline and N^6,O^2-dibutyryl adenosine $3',5'$-monophosphate on synthesis and survival. *Toxicol. Appl. Pharmacol.* 41:79–90.

Sumerford, W. T., Hayes, W. J., Johnston, J. M., Walker, K., and Spillane, J. 1953. Cholinesterase response and symptomatology from exposure to organic phosphorus insecticides. *AMA Arch. Ind. Hyg. Occup. Med.* 7:383–398.

Taylor, P. 1980. Anticholinesterase agents. In *Goodman and Gilman's The Pharmacological Basis of Therapeutics,* 6th ed., eds. A. G. Gilman, L. S. Goodman, and A. Gilman, pp. 100–119. New York: Macmillan.

Uchida, S., Takeyasu, K., Matsuda, T., and Yoshida, H. 1979. Changes in muscarinic acetylcholine receptors of mice by chronic administration of diisopropylfluorophosphate and papaverine. *Life Sci.* 24:1805–1812.

Usdin, E. 1970. Reactions of cholinesterases with substrates inhibitors and reactivators. In *Anticholinesterase Agents. International Encyclopedia of Pharmacology and Therapeutics, Section 3,* ed. A. G. Karczmar, vol. 1, pp. 47–354. Oxford: Pergamon.

Wecker, L., Mobley, P. L., and Dettbarn, W. D. 1977. Central cholinergic mechanisms underlying adaptation to reduced cholinesterase activity. *Biochem. Pharmacol.* 26:633–637.

Welsch, F., and Dettbarn, W. D. 1971. Protein synthesis in lobster walking leg nerves. *Comp. Biochem. Physiol.* 38B:393–403.

Wills, H. H. 1961. Anticholinergic compounds as adjuncts to atropine in preventing lethality by sarin in the rabbit. *J. Med. Pharm. Chem.* 3:353–359.

Wilson, B. W., and Walker, C. R. 1974. Regulation of newly synthesized acetylcholinesterase in muscle cultures treated with diisopropylfluorophosphate. *Proc. Natl. Acad. Sci. USA* 71:3194–3198.

Yamamura, H. I., and Snyder, S. H. 1974. Muscarinic cholinergic binding in rat brain. *Proc. Natl. Acad. Sci. USA* 71:1725–1729.

Chapter 4

Hepatotoxicity

Harihara M. Mehendale

INTRODUCTION

Simply stated, hepatotoxicity may be defined as the effect of any agent on the liver that results in a deviation from the normal function and morphology of this organ. Hepatic toxicity inflicted by foreign or natural chemicals has been recognized for slightly over a century. During the latter part of the 19th century, attempts to understand the toxicology of yellow phosphorus and the haloalkane anesthetic chloroform resulted in an appreciation of the hepatotoxic potential of chemicals (Zimmerman, 1978). Interest in the chemically inflicted hepatic toxicity has steadily grown since then and has led to the remarkable progress in our understanding of the mechanisms governing many toxicological manifestations induced by toxic chemicals. From a practical point of view, it has become necessary to classify hepatic toxicity into several categories. One such categorization is based on the type of toxic hepatic response. Thus, chemicals may lead to fatty changes, necrosis, cirrhosis, or carcinoma. Accompanying these types of toxicities are changes in physiological or biochemical functions of the liver. Thus, secretion of bile may be increased or decreased and, at least intuitively, the latter response is of greater concern than the former. Similarly, intermediary metabolism of carbohydrates, lipids, and protein synthesis and turnover may be altered as a consequence of many toxicological phenomena.

Associated with these subcellular changes, morphological and functional changes may also be seen at the cellular level.

The susceptibility of the liver to injury by chemical agents appears to be a consequence of the anatomical position of this organ and the central role it plays in the metabolism and disposition of foreign chemicals. Liver contains by far the highest level of enzymatic systems capable of biotransforming foreign chemicals. Often, the intermediate biotransformation products are more reactive and undergo toxicological interactions with tissue macromolecules. Many chemicals are eliminated from the liver via the biliary route. Bile acids, which play a very important role in the formation of bile fluid itself and in the solubilization of lipids in the intestine, are conserved by reabsorption and enterohepatic recirculation. Foreign chemicals, excreted by the biliary route, often enter into the enterohepatic recirculation cycle, enabling them to repeatedly enter the liver tissue. Depending on the physicochemical properties of the foreign chemical, the parent compound or its biotransformation products may accumulate in the liver. Many chemicals are biotransformed further beyond the biologically activated intermediates to less reactive polar metabolites, and may be eliminated either by the liver via bile or by the kidney via urine after entering the systemic circulation. It is apparent that the central role played by the liver in the removal of the chemicals from the portal circulation and subsequent metabolism and disposition makes this organ especially susceptible to first and often persistent attack by these offending chemicals, culminating in toxic injury.

Recent developments have established that hepatotoxicity may be inflicted by thousands of synthetic chemicals, drugs, and naturally occurring chemicals such as bacterial, fungal, plant, and animal toxins. Some toxicological responses of the liver may be exacerbated by combinations of these chemicals. One of the most challenging current problems in toxicology is to devise ways by which such potentially exacerbating toxicological interactions may be discerned, so that we may be able to predict potentially hazardous situations after exposure to combinations of chemicals. Other toxic responses may be related to the individuality of the host giving rise to idiosynchratic reactions. It is the responsibility of experimental toxicologist to study the mechanisms of toxicity governing these toxicological manifestations in an attempt to protect the host from the deleterious toxic effects of these chemicals.

Liver Morphology and Anatomical Considerations

The functional unit of the liver is a lobule (Fig. 1) described in relation to the vascular architecture. The terms classic lobule, portal lobule, and liver acinus (Fig. 2) represent a central vascular vantage point used to describe the lobular structure (Jones and Mills, 1973). Thus, *classic lobule* represents the lobular structure around the central vein, while the lobular pattern centered around portal zones is referred to as *portal lobule* or *liver acinus*. The classic lobule is arranged around the central vein and is composed of a continuous system of communicating parenchymal cells, which lie in one-cell-thick sheets arranged roughly perpendicular to the central vein. Throughout the entire lobule, the parenchymal cells are interconnected and subdivided by sinusoids or lacunae. Each sinusoidal space opens into the central vein. The perisinusoidal

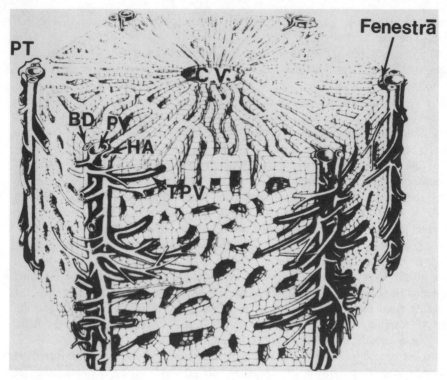

Figure 1 A diagrammatic representation of the current concepts of the liver lobule: BD, bile duct; PV, portal vein; HA, hepatic artery; TPV, terminal portal venule; CV, central vein; S, sinusoid; PT, portal triad; F, fenstrae. *[Reproduced with permission from Jones and Schmuckler (1977).]*

space occupying the periphery of each lacuna is referred to as the space of Disse. The portal triad consists of the portal vein, hepatic artery, and bile duct. In the terminal branches the hepatic artery, portal vein, and bile duct traverse the parenchyma through the fenestrae in the limiting plate that circumscribes the portal triad.

The liver is a highly vascularized organ and receives one quarter of the cardiac output (Jones and Schmuckler, 1977). The total venous system drains the intestinal blood flow, and the hepatic artery brings the arterial flow from the celiac trunk of the aorta. The main arterial and the venous afferent trunks enter the organ at the hilum and branch repeatedly, distributing via the portal zones throughout the organ in company with each other and the biliary system, forming the portal triad of the classic lobule (Fig. 1). The larger branches of the arterial and venous vessels traverse the organ, giving rise to vessels of smaller caliber that branch further into thin-walled vessels, which penetrate the outer limiting plate of hepatocytes in the lobule to empty into the sinusoidal bed, permeating the curving and splitting plates and bridging the sheets of hepatocytes. Most of the arterial and portal blood enters the periphery of the lobule, with the resultant mixture containing both the portal contribution of material absorbed from the intestinal lumen and the oxygenated arterial blood containing sys-

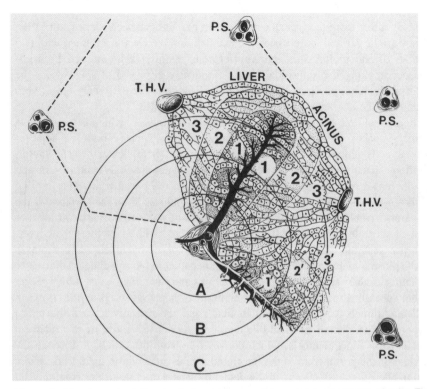

Figure 2 Blood supply of the simple liver acinus and the zonal arrangement of cells. The acinus occupies adjacent sectors of neighboring hexagonal fields. Zones 1, 2, and 3, respectively, represent areas supplied with blood of first, second, and third quality with regard to oxygen and nutrients. These zones center about the terminal afferent vascular branches, terminal bile ductules, lymph vessels, and nerves, and extend into the triangular portal field from which these branches crop out. Zones 1', 2', and 3' designate corresponding areas in a portion of an adjacent acinar unit. In Zones 1 and 1' the afferent vascular twigs empty into the sinusoids. Circles B and C indicate peripheral circulatory areas as commonly described around a "periportal" area, A; P.S., portal space; T.H.V., terminal hepatic venules ("central veins"). *[Reproduced with permission from Rappaport (1975).]*

temic constituents. Sinusoids can be looked on as specialized vessels that lack the basal lamina or a muscular cell layer reinforcing the endothelium. The contents of the vascular space therefore apparently pass freely to and from the space of Disse. Thus the surfaces of hepatocytes and both sides of the cells forming the walls of the vessels bathe in the pools of both vascular and perivascular space. The centrilobular veins, which receive sinusoidal flow, in turn empty into the vessels of larger caliber that, although they traverse the lobule, do not directly receive sinusoidal outflow. In addition to the drainage of the space of Disse via the sinusoidal outflow to the efferent hepatic flow, there is lymphatic drainage by portal lymphatic vessels abutting the space surrounding the arterial and portal venous branches penetrating the lobule. In some areas of the lobule, the space of Disse may receive direct outflow from the lymphatic vessels.

Sinusoids differ from the typical capillaries in two basic aspects (Jones and Mills, 1973). They are larger and more variable in caliber, and their walls are lined with two distinct types of endothelial cells and Kupffer cells. Kupffer cells are active phagocytes and occur along the sinusoidal walls, frequently observed at sites where the sinusoids branch, functioning as luminal guards. The cells are extremely large, with an irregular surface characterized by folds, ruffles, and villi.

The functional unit of the biliary system is bile canaliculus, which is the smallest of the biliary spaces (1–2 μm) and is usually centrally located between adjacent parenchymal cells (Jones and Mills, 1973; Jones and Schmuckler, 1977; Taylor, 1975). Biliary space is smallest between the hepatocytes near the central vein and gradually increases in volume along a gradient toward the portal triad. The limiting walls of the canaliculi are composed of localized specialization on the surfaces of the adjacent parenchymal cells. Microvilli bearing cores of microfilaments protrude into the lumen of the bile canaliculus from the canalicular surfaces of the hepatocytes. Canaliculi are separated from adjacent intracellular spaces by junctional complexes between the plasma membranes of the adjoining hepatocytes. Immediately adjacent to the canalicular luminar space are the tight junctions and junctional gaps, which represent another specialization of the plasma membrane of hepatocytes. Bile fluid flows in the canalicular lumen from the central lobular zone centripetally toward the portal triads, where it enters small terminal bile ductules. At this level, one or two fusiform ductule cells form short channels, which convey bile from the canaliculi through the limiting plate of the portal triad to the interlobular bile ducts within the portal canals. Interlobular bile ducts (30–40 μm in diameter) transport the bile to the continuously anastomosing network of ducts, which form larger conduits as they approach the hepatic portal and finally exit through the hilum as the common bile duct.

The classic lobule, along with its various morphologically and functionally specialized cells, the interconnecting biliary system, and the vasculature, is demarcated by connective tissue to form not only a functional, but a morphologically distinct unit of the hepatic architecture. The unit is most obvious in those species whose livers contain thick bands of connective tissue that practically encapsulate each lobule. Thus, such a lobular structure is dramatically demarcated in pig and racoon, while in the human it appears incomplete and poorly defined (Jones and Schmuckler, 1973). However, expert morphologists and pathologists can identify the transit lobule by locating the central vein and following the regularly placed portal triads that encircle the periphery of the classic lobule.

Physiology and Functional Considerations

Although toxicologists often refer to the liver as if it were built entirely on one type of cell—namely, the liver parenchymal cell (commonly also referred to as hepatocytes)—there are in fact many other types of cell present in the liver that are vital for its overall function. These include endothelial cells that line the blood vessels, bile ductular cells, collagenous connective-tissue cells, nerve cells, Kupffer cells, and the parenchymal cells or hepatocytes. Generally, however, the normal liver is dominated by the parenchymal or hepatocyte cells. In addition to the heterogeneity of the liver in terms of cell types, there is a marked heterogenous distribution of functional characteristics within the liver lobule. Pathologists have based their description of the hepatic acinus (Fig. 2) on the liver tissue primarily supplied by the terminal branches of the hepatic artery and portal vein (Rappaport, 1975). The parenchymal cells are grouped into concentric zones, those surrounding the terminal afferent vessels being zone 1, or the first to receive blood and nutrients, the last to undergo most necrosis, and the first to regenerate. Those liver cells in the region more distal to the afferent blood supply—namely, zones 2 and 3—receive blood of considerably less nutritive value and are less resistant to potential hepatotoxins and other vectors of possible hepatotoxicity. Consequently, these factors may influence the regiospecific action of hepatotoxins. For instance, centrilobular necrosis, characteristic of carbon tetrachloride toxicity, is an example of regiospecific hepatic lesion.

The liver, an essential organ for maintenance of life in many higher forms of vertebrates, has an extraordinary reserve capacity and potential, as well as regenerative capabilities. In addition to bile secretion, which is required for the emulsification of dietary fats before digestion, the liver takes up digested and absorbed nutrients from the systemic circulation and stores carbohydrates in the form of glycogen, while proteins and lipids are synthesized and used for various synthetic and other metabolic activities. These and other stored substances may be utilized by the hepatocyte or released into the blood circulation, either unbound or in association with carrier lipoproteins. Certain substances are synthesized by the liver in response to the demands of the body, such as albumin and plasma proteins, glucose, fatty acids, cholesterol, and phospholipids, representing a functional response of this organ to bodily demands. The liver is also an important hemopoietic site during early embryogenesis, and the large hepatic vascular capacity in adult livers serve as a storehouse for blood. Finally, the abundance of sinusoidal Kupffer cells makes the liver one of the principal filters for foreign particulate matter and intruding bacteria entering the enterohepatic blood circulation.

Much is known about the biology of the liver cells and organelle structure and function in normal health and disease (Arias et al., 1980). In recent years much attention has been directed toward the hepatic capacity to metabolize, activate, and detoxify exogenous compounds such as drugs, insecticides, any other foreign chemicals, and endogenous agents such as bile acids, fatty acids, steroids, and other hormones and nonhormonal substances. Hepatic parenchymal cells are relatively large polyhedral units and contain one or more spherical nuclei. Each hepatocyte is in direct contact with adjacent parenchymal cell, the biliary space, and the space of Disse. Hepatocytes carry on a multitude of functions and accordingly contain a well-developed system of organelles. Mitochondria are abundantly numerous in the liver cells. In addition to housing the energy-producing enzyme systems, mitochondria also serve other functions. For instance, mitochondria play a key role in regulating cytosolic Ca^{2+} levels. Lysosomes are common to the hepatocytes and are usually more abundant in the peribiliary regions. Microbodies like lysosomes are surrounded by a single membrane and occupy approximately 2–3% of the total cell volume. Unlike cells in most other tissues, both the rough-surfaced and the smooth-surfaced varieties of endoplasmic reticulum are well developed in the hepatocytes. The amounts of these two categories of membranes, their intracellular distribution, and particular arrangement vary from cell to cell and depend on the location of the cell within the hepatic lobule, the physiological state of the animals, and the experimental conditions and exposure to chemical inducers. In recent years, the endoplasmic reticulum or microsomal fractions of homogenized hepatocytes have been the subject of intensive study. This organelle participates in the synthesis of albumin, fibrinogen, and other plasma proteins; the synthesis of cholesterol and bile acids; the conjugation of bilirubin, drugs, and steroids prior to biliary excretion; the oxidative metabolism of drugs and steroids; the esterification of fatty acids to triglycerides; the breakdown of glycogen; and the deiodination of tetraiodothyronine to triiodothyronine. Smooth endoplasmic reticulum also contains necessary Ca^{2+}-sequestering mechanisms, and this undoubtedly plays a role in regulating cytosolic Ca^{2+} levels. Although some of the evidence remains conjectural, most of the hepatic drug-metabolizing enzyme activity is confined to the smooth endoplasmic reticulum. This membrane system has an enormous surface area. It is generally recognized that there are localized areas with specific functional capacities within this extensive band of membranes (Jones and Mills, 1973). This concept is supported by the fact that drug-induced hypertrophy of this membrane system does not always necessarily result in the uniform increase in all of its functional aspects. The presence of more smooth endoplasmic reticulum in the centrolobular hepatocytes may explain why certain compounds such as carbon tetrachloride (CCl_4) when metabolized to hepatotoxic agents by the smooth-endoplasmic-reticulum enzymes primarily affect the liver cells in this zone (Slater, 1978). Such observations also serve to reemphasize the functional heterogeneity of hepatocytes within the liver tissue.

The processes involved in the formation of bile fluid are incompletely understood (Jones and Myers, 1979; Klaassen, 1978). It has been proposed that the primary event in the formation of bile is the active transport of bile-acid anions from parenchymal cells into the bile canaliculi. Recent morphological evidence has suggested a close participation of the Golgi apparatus with the formation of bile fluid. Bile-acid clearance from the portal blood is extremely efficient, and parenchymal cells closest to the portal area also represent Golgi-rich areas in the periportal zone. In any event, excretion of bile acids is closely tied in with the formation of bile fluid in the bile canaliculi. Various studies have revealed the formation of two distinct pools of bile fluid. One pool appears to be directly related to the excretion of bile acids and is referred to as *bile-acid-dependent flow*. The second pool of bile fluid appears not to be related to bile acids and is referred to as *bile-acid-independent flow*. In general, exposure to enzyme-inducing agents results in increased secretion of the bile-acid-independent flow. The mechanism of formation of bile fluid and the factors governing the control of these events are rather important considerations for toxicology, since many foreign chemicals are excreted in the bile fluid (Levine, 1978). Biliary excretion of foreign chemicals may take place with or without biotransformation catalyzed by the enzymes contained in the endoplasmic reticulum or other enzymes contained in the cytoplasm of the hepatocytes.

Spectrum of Hepatic Toxicity

The diverse variety of toxic chemicals that are capable of inflicting hepatotoxicity may be categorized based on the circumstances of exposure (Zimmerman, 1978). Occupational exposure represents a situation where either routine or accidental exposures may be encountered. In this connection, although one readily thinks of industrial environment, occupational exposure may not be restricted to these situations alone. Anesthesiologists may be exposed to halogenated anesthetics, and farmers may be exposed to pesticide sprays. Domestic situations allowing exposure to hepatotoxins are accidental, suicidal, ingestion of contaminated food, and abuse of drugs as exemplified by the use of euphorogenic chemicals. Certain toxins may be synthesized enterically, either via chemical reactions or mediated by bacterial growth and activity. Ethionine and nitrosamines are biosynthesized by the bacterial flora in the gastrointestinal (GI) tract. Environmental pollutants represent yet another type of exposure situation where either synthetic chemicals or natural toxins may be encountered. Iatrogenic responses represent hepatoxicities encountered in therapeutic applications of a variety of drugs.

Hepatotoxins may also be classified based on the property of the toxin or the host characteristics (Zimmerman, 1978). The mechanism of liver toxicity is considered to be either due to the toxic property of the chemical or due to the unusual host vulnerability. Agents that are capable of producing hepatic toxicity in a wide variety of species may be referred to as *intrinsic hepatotoxins*. When the toxic action of chemicals depends on the unusual susceptibility of the host, these are referred to as *hepatotoxins,* the toxic interaction being referred to as *idiosyncrasy.* However, such a classification is an oversimplification, since within the the class of intrinsic toxins the toxic reactions depend on the idiosyncratic state of the host. Toxicity is modified by a number of variables and involves several different mechanisms. Idiosyncratic state and the intrinsic toxicity may either complement to accentuate a toxic response or counteract to reduce toxicity. For example, CCl_4- or bromobenzene-induced hepatic necrosis may be modified depending on the prior exposure to particular enzyme-inducing agents. Similarly, necrotic response to a given dose of acetaminophen may depend on the hepatic levels of reduced glutathione (GSH).

A variety of morphological and biochemical lesions are produced in the liver by chemicals or biological agents. The extent of hepatic toxicity depends on any number of factors that relate to the types of toxic chemicals, exposure situation, and host. Thus, the hepatic toxicity can be acute, subchronic, or chronic, depending on these various factors. In toxicology, the term *acute* may be used to indicate exposure to a single dose. Often, however, it is also used to indicate the severity of hepatotoxicity. Similarly, the term *chronic* is used to indicate either repeated exposure over an extended period of time or the presence of a hepatotoxic response over an extended period of time. While acute toxicity may result in necrosis of the liver, continued exposure may lead to additional cell death, and withdrawal may lead to a partial or complete recovery. Repeated and prolonged exposure results in subchronic expression of toxicity such as necrosis. Continuous and repeated exposure may lead to cirrhosis. Although these expressions of toxicity appear to be stepwise and progressive, one may see the stepwise progression of a lesion only upon careful manipulation of dose and other exposure situations. Conversely, one may escape observation of such a progression with some toxic chemicals. We are only now experiencing a rapid progress in our understanding of the mechanisms of chemically induced carcinogenicity. Carcinogenicity may result from a single exposure to a chemical or after multiple exposures under acute or chronic situations. Some chemicals may require a latent period for carcinogenesis, and may need to be bioactivated, while others may be direct-acting. Effects of some chemicals may include abolishing a latent period of virally or chemically induced cancer. Genotoxic carcinogens act by adduct formation with DNA, RNA, and other macromolecules, while other chemicals may induce cancer by epigenetic mechanisms.

In addition to classifying hepatotoxic substances on the basis of intrinsic capability and host susceptibility as well as the circumstances of exposure, Zimmerman (1978) classified hepatotoxic agents also on the basis of mechanisms. Zimmerman divided intrinsic hepatotoxins into either direct or indirect hepatotoxins. According to this concept, a direct toxin can injure many tissues, including the liver. In the liver, the direct toxin would affect a number of organelles such as the endoplasmic reticulum, the mitochondria, and the lysosomes. An example of this type of agent is CCl_4. Indirect toxins are thought to affect a particular metabolic pathway. This effect should lead to an uncoupling of the metabolic organization of the hepatocytes. Galactosamine is an example of this category. Galactosamine enters the pathway by which galactose is metabolized, with the resultant formation of UDP-galactosamine, thus tying up uridylate nucleotide. This leads to a metabolic "blind alley," which in turn leads to the trapping of metabolically needed uridylate (Zimmerman, 1978). Since the rate of trapping exceeds the capacity of the adult rat liver to generate uridylate, a striking decrease in the concentration of UDP-glucose, UDP-galactose, UTP, UDP, UMP, and UDP-glucuronide is observed. For the cholestatic lesions one would find the examples of α-naphthylisothiocyanate (ANIT) or anabolic steroids. Although the precise mechanism of action of either of these chemicals is not understood, it is recognized that they interfere with the mechanisms of bile formation. From the above discussion, it may be realized that various pathologic processes induced by a multitude of chemicals are involved in hepatotoxicity. Our understanding of how initial or midlevel expressions of hepatotoxicity relate to terminal hepatotoxic responses such as cirrhosis and hepatocarcinoma is at a stage of infancy. First, we do not fully understand the precise progression of toxic responses leading to hepatocarcinoma. Second, our understanding of whether there is a threshold in terms of the progression of hepatocellular responses to injury leading to hepatocellular cancer is at a primitive stage.

Since hepatic toxicity can be induced by a wide spectrum of toxic chemicals (Plaa, 1980) and drugs (Ishak, 1982), several attempts have been made to classify the toxic responses of the liver. Popper and Schaffner (1959) described five groups of reactions. The first group includes zonal hepatocellular alterations without inflammatory reaction. This group is represented by a wide variety of compounds causing either necrosis or fat accumulation in the hepatocytes. The second group is called intrahepatic cholestasis. This category contained many chemicals of dissimilar chemical structure, producing jaundice closely resembling that produced by extrahepatic biliary obstruction. These two groups differ from each other with respect to dose dependency, predictability, and demonstrability in animal models, extrahepatic cholestasis being in obedience to these principles. The third group of reactions includes hepatic necrosis with inflammatory reaction. The dominant feature here is the progression to a massive necrosis characteristic of viral hepatitis. The fourth group is called the unclassified group and contains a number of hepatotoxic responses that did not appear to fit into any other scheme. The fifth group contains hepatocarcinogens. Although at the time of original classification none were included in this category, at the present time a number of toxic chemicals are recognized as being hepatocarcinogens.

Finally, there are a multitude of factors that can affect hepatocellular responses to a challenge by toxic chemicals. Allergic and hypersensitivity reactions present special considerations. Interactions of several chemicals upon simultaneous exposure or upon exposure to individual chemicals separately present a problem of an additional dimension in interpreting experimental data. Zimmerman's classification of intrinsic and idiosyncratic agents would appear not to accommodate the hepatotoxic responses as a result of chemical interactions in the liver tissue. In addition, the present classifications of hepatotoxic chemicals do not take into account reversible and irreversible hepatotoxic reactions. The action of genotoxic carcinogenic compounds would seem to be irreversible, while the actions of anabolic steroids in bringing about cholestatic reaction would appear to be reversible. Modulating action of inducing agents in certain toxic responses, synergistic action of several nontoxic chemicals acting to potentiate the toxic responses of chemicals, promoters in the case of liver cancer, and the unique host susceptibility present certain special cases in point. The present classifications of toxic responses or toxic agents should only be used as guides to assist in conceptualizing and consolidating the presently available knowledge while continuously modifying these concepts as additional knowledge accrues.

Subcellular Sites of Liver Toxicity

In recent years the availability of electron-microscopy techniques has enabled a closer scrutiny of the ultrastructural changes taking place within liver cells after injury by a variety of hepatotoxins (Arias et al., 1980). Although in many cases ultrastructural changes at the cellular or subcellular level cannot be correlated with biochemical or functional parameters of toxicity, the advent of transmission and scanning electron microscopy techniques has contributed greatly to our understanding of many subcellular manifestations of toxic reactions. Certain specific subcellular sites of injury will be considered in the following discussion as examples of toxic responses of the liver.

Hepatocellular permeability may be altered by many toxic chemicals and represents a toxicant-induced perturbation of membrane function. Elevated blood levels of many proteins and other endogenous substances have been associated with the changes in the membrane permeability of hepatocytes. Necrosis leads to high levels of certain enzymes in the blood released from the damaged liver. In most clinical circumstances, this is demonstrated by elevated levels of serum transaminases (glutamate–oxalate transaminase and glutamate–pyruvate transaminase), which may be increased to 10- to 100-fold, depending on the degree of damage. Similarly, many other enzymes are released from the hepatocytes as a result of a variety of hepatocellular injury. These enzymes include alkaline and acid phosphatases, lactic dehydrogenase isozymes, isocitric dehydrogenase, sorbitol dehydrogenase, and many others. In many instances of hepatocellular necrosis induced by a variety of toxic chemicals and in the cholestatic injury resembling extrahepatic obstructive jaundice, a complement of serum enzymes is measured as an indication of the degree of hepatocellular damage. In CCl_4-induced hepatocellular necrosis, accumulation of Ca^{2+} has also been demonstrated, indicating a change in cellular permeability. Nitrosamines and phalloidins (*Amanita phalloides*) are two other specific agents known to modify membrane permeability of the hepatocytes.

In response to many toxic chemicals, a conspicuous increase of smooth endoplasmic reticulum has been observed. While the proliferation of smooth endoplasmic reticulum on exposure to a variety of inducing agents appears to be an adaptive and potentially useful phenomenon, it may become counterproductive as the challenge by the offending chemical continues (Conney, 1967). Thus, prolonged exposure to some inducing agents may lead to an ultimately decreased metabolic activity of smooth endoplasmic reticulum, despite persistent increase in the amount. Accompanying the proliferation of smooth endoplasmic reticulum are a number of chemical and enzymatic changes that indicate the adaptive nature of this change. Since smooth endoplasmic reticulum houses many of the important biotransformation enzymes, such an adaptive response by the liver has important implications in terms of both the expression of hepatic injury and the susceptibility of the liver to subsequent challenges by other offending chemicals. The phenomenon of hyperplastic, hypoactive endoplasmic reticulum described above is perhaps an early manifestation of toxicity. The ability to induce mixed-function monooxygenases of the endoplasmic reticulum has been demonstrated for virtually hundreds of foreign chemicals. A few examples include the insecticides DDT and mirex, the barbiturate phenobarbital, the antiepileptic drug diphenylhydantoin, and many other foreign chemicals. The ability to alter quantitatively the smooth endoplasmic reticulum is not restricted to foreign compounds alone. Steroids are some of the important inducers of smooth endoplasmic reticulum.

Specific damage to endoplasmic reticulum by toxic chemicals has also been noted. Such chemicals include CCl_4, thioacetamide, dimethylnitrosamine (DMN), phosphorus, ethionine, dimethylaminoazobenzene (DMAB), pyrrolizidine alkaloids, and galactosamine. In CCl_4-induced hepatic toxicity, the formation of trichlorocarbon free radical ($\cdot CCl_3$) and subsequent lipid peroxidative reactions result in the destruction of endoplasmic reticulum. Such damage can be measured both by decreased incorporation of amino acids into proteins and by the destruction of cytochrome P-450. ANIT, which induces intrahepatic cholestasis, is metabolically activated before causing damage to the smooth endoplasmic reticulum. Since the drug-metabolizing enzyme activity is situated in the smooth endoplasmic reticulum, such interactions are known to greatly influence the toxicity of other chemicals to the liver tissue.

The mitochondrial changes include increase in size, alteration in the density of matrices, loss of cristae, and decrease in number. In chronic alcoholic disease, enlarged mitochondria (megamitochondria), pleomorphism, and damaged cristae are readily observed. Mitochondrial membrane becomes more permeable to Ca^{2+}, which accumulates to form large granules in CCl_4 toxicity. Many chemicals cause mitochondrial changes as indicated above. Pyrrolizidine alkaloids, ethionine, allyl formate, many chlorinated solvents, phosphorus, and DMN are known to cause similar changes in mitochondria. While there is no doubt that mitochondrial distortion and fragmentation are caused by chemical injury, the specificity of these changes remains in doubt, since other physiological changes such as anoxia can cause similar changes in mitochondria.

Disintegration of lysosomes and leakage of hydrolytic enzymes into the cell have been noted following experimental injury. Lysosomes are cell scavengers providing the means of ridding the cell of debris. Cellular autophagy results in secondary lysosomal structures, which also contain digestive enzymes. The number of the secondary lysosomes appears to increase in many types of sublethal hepatic toxicities. Damage to lysosomal structure has been recorded after the administration of CCl_4, pyrrolizidine alkaloids, beryllium, thymidine, and phosphorus to experimental animals.

The most prominent changes in the nucleus are those produced by hepatotoxic agents that are also hepatocarcinogens. The nuclei increase in size and there may be striking anisonucleosis. Changes in the nucleoplasm include the production of increased amounts of interchromatin and of satellite granules, as has been shown to occur with toxic effects of aflatoxins, DMN, pyrrolizidine alkaloids, tannic acid, and thioacetamide. These changes are now believed to be due to the formation of highly reactive electrophiles, generated in the cells, that react covalently within many of the major components of the hepatocytes, including the cell nucleus and nucleolus, plasma membrane, smooth and rough endoplasmic reticulum, and ribosomes. Many other changes have been noted in other subcellular organelles after challenge by many toxic chemicals. These include abnormalities in peroxysomes, the microfilamental structure and organization, the Golgi apparati, and many cytosolic components. Changes in the bile canaliculi are characteristic of intrahepatic cholestasis. Chloestasis induced by chlorpromazine, anabolic contraceptives, and many drugs have similar features as any other cholestasis. Bile secretion ceases because of an obstruction in the extrahepatic ducts or because of interference with cholate excretion. Many bile canaliculi loose their microvilli and dilate, more so in the centrilobular zone. Canaliculi rupture when the cell death occurs, but very seldom in early cholestatic response. Often, changes in bile canalicular membranes are also accompanied by changes in smooth endoplasmic reticulum discussed earlier.

From the above discussion, it is clear that many toxic chemicals are capable of altering a whole spectrum of ultrastructural and morphological features of the hepatocytes. Most often, it is very difficult to associate a particular morphological change with a particular toxin. This is, and will continue to be, a challenging area of toxicology. One way the multisensitive changes in the subcellular structure elicited by foreign chemicals may be rationalized is by assuming that changes brought about by the toxic chemical in specific organelles give rise to self-propagating organoleptic changes in other organelles. Despite the lack of specificity in cellular actions of many chemicals, morphological observations have indeed aided the understanding of cellular sites and mechanisms of action of many chemicals by providing morphological and cytochemical correlation of biochemical and physiological parameters of toxicity.

EXPERIMENTAL MODELS OF HEPATOTOXICITY

Liposes

Accumulation of lipid in the liver tissue has been variously referred to as fatty infiltration, fatty degeneration, and liposis (Dianzan, 1979). *Liposis* refers to excessive accumulation of fat or lipid material predominantly consisting of triglycerides and fatty acids. Normal liver may contain as much as 5% of its weight as fat. Lipidotic liver may contain as much as 50% of its weight as fat, most of it being triglycerides. Under conditions of hepatic triglyceride accumulation, lipid droplets appear surrounded by membranes to form liposomes. Hepatic triglycerides seem to be contained in two separate pools, which mix poorly. Only one of these pools is involved actively in secreting triglycerides into the plasma.

Many models of drug-induced lipidosis have been described. These include CCl_4, ethionine, orotic acid, ethanol, tetracycline antibiotics, corticosteroids, and yellow phosphorus. Lipidotic liver is also observed in hepatic resection and in disease states such as diabetes. Choline-deficient diet has also been used to produce fatty liver, and this model has been studied extensively.

The plasma concentration of triglycerides can be reduced to half the normal value within $1/2$ h after CCl_4 administration in fasted animals. Abnormal accumulation of triglycerides in the hepatic cells has been demonstrated as early as 2 h after the administration of this hepatotoxic compound. Such accumulation of fat has been documented by following the incorporation of labeled fatty acids, measuring freshly secreted triglycerides, by morphometric analysis of appropriately stained liver sections, and trapping with the use of detergents in intact animals as well as in perfused liver preparations. There is also evidence for the blocked release of triglycerides from the liver. Hepatic accumulation of fat after ingesting alcohol has been well documented (Zimmerman, 1978). This can be attributed to the introduction of physiological lesions at multiple sites of lipid metabolism. No only can individual factors be evoked to explain the abnormal accumulation of fat in alcoholic liver—the problem may be compounded by indirect effects mediated via nutritional imbalances such as choline deficiency. Moreover, such effects may also be mediated via hormonal mechanisms such as the effects of catecholamines on mobilization of body fat.

Ethionine-induced and orotic acid-induced accumulation of fat in the liver is a result of striking reduction in the transport of lipid from the liver. Depressed plasma levels of very-low-density lipoprotein (VLDL) have been attributed either to defective glycosylation or to impaired synthesis of the phospholipid component of VLDL. The initial biochemical event triggering the accumulation of fat in the liver tissue in response to orotic acid appears to be related to deficiency of ATP consequent to the acceleration of uridine synthesis (Zimmerman, 1978). Ethionine also causes a decrease in ATP, which leads to accumulation of fat in the liver. The complex biochemical manifestations of ethionine include depressed serum triglycerides, phospholipids, cholesterol, cholesterol esters, lipoproteins, and glucose. Changes in hepatic function include impaired excretion of sulfobromophthalein (BSP) and mild elevation of serum bilirubin. Several other experimental models of fatty liver have been studied extensively (Zimmerman, 1978).

Administration of large intravenous doses of tetracycline and its derivatives is associated with the fine fatty vacuolization of the liver. Corticosteroid administration also results in fatty infiltration of the liver. Injection of a large dose of yellow phosphorus, a component of many rat poisons, results in fatty infiltration of the liver. Hepatic lipid increases twofold within 10 h after partial hepatectomy in experimental animals. The majority of the lipid accumulating after this surgical practical removal of the liver is in the form of triglycerides. After the resection recovers to normal size, the triglycerides fall to normal levels, indicating that the elevation of liver fat is a specific response to partial hepatectomy.

Necrotic Reactions

Hepatic necrosis or cell death can be produced by a variety of chemicals. Some examples of these include CCl_4, bromobenzene, thioacetamide, dimethylnitrosamine, pyrrolizidine alkaloids, aflatoxin B_1, toxins of *Amanita phalloides,* galactosamine, allyl formate, and endotoxins. For relative ease in associating the lesion with a class of necrogenic agents or at least with the extent of exposure to necrogenic agents, morphologically hepatic necrosis has been classified in various ways (Zimmerman, 1978). Hepatic necrosis may be zonal, massive, or diffuse. Zonal necrosis may be in the central, midzone, or peripheral area of the classical lobule, depending on the necrogenic agent (Fig. 2). Galactosamine produces diffuse necrosis. Precise location of necrosis may depend on the agent causing hepatocellular necrosis. CCl_4 and bromobenzene produce centrilobular necrosis. CCl_4 and bromobenzene cause centrilobular necrosis because these chemicals require bioactivation and the enzyme systems mediating the biotransformation are present in the centrilobular zone. The type of necrosis produced by toxic agents may depend on a number of factors, such as prior or simultaneous exposure to other chemicals, age, species, intrinsic toxicity of the chemical in question, duration, and concentration of the chemical. Combination of toxic chemicals may accentuate the necrogenic response of the liver subsequent to challenge by a necrotic agent. There are also species differences in necrosis produced by certain toxic agents. Aflatoxins, for example, produce centrilobular necrosis in the rat and midzonal and peripheral necroses in the pigs.

Despite the large number of experimental models available for the production of hepatocellular necrosis and the voluminous descriptive information available, the precise mechanism leading to cell death is still unclear. Generally speaking, two schools of thought have prevailed in the literature. The first one holds that unavailability of cellular energy and the impairment of energy-production mechanisms result in cellular bankruptcy, leading to deterioration of organelles and cellular structure, leading to cell death. Certain changes such as excessive accumulation of Ca^{2+} within the cells and in mitochondria may be associated with the events leading to cellular death. The second school of thought holds that cell death represents an active process and reflects a free-radical reaction of the cells (Farber and Fisher, 1980). Inhibitors of protein synthesis are known to protect against the necrogenic effect of CCl_4. In support of the proposal that cell death reflects an active process in response to toxic chemicals, protective action of protein-synthesis inhibitors against CCl_4-induced necrosis may be cited. This and other observations have been produced as evidence of the active suicidal response of the hepatic cells to toxic chemicals. Better understanding of the underlying mechanisms will undoubtedly come from future investigations in this area.

Hepatobiliary Dysfunction

A variety of toxic chemicals may modify hepatic function by induction of microsomal enzyme systems. Liver plays an important role in the metabolism of toxic chemicals to reactive or inactive intermediates or their final products. Liver also plays a central role in the elimination of these chemicals via the bile or in returning these to the systemic circulation. Alteration of hepatobiliary function represents an important measurable response of the liver to toxic chemicals. Such a consideration does not take into account the precise mechanisms or consequences of the toxic injury to the liver tissue but can be used to assess the impact on the hepatobiliary function. Two principal aspects of hepatobiliary function include excretory and secretory functions of the liver. Under certain circumstances, each of these functions may be jointly or independently affected to partially or completely impair these functions (Klaassen, 1978; Levine, 1978). An examination of the events that lead to biliary excretion indicates that a number of factors individually or in any combination may affect biliary excretion (Popper and Schaffner, 1959). These include (a) hepatic blood flow, (b) binding to plasma proteins, (c) permeability of sinusoidal membrane, (d) interaction with cytoplasmic binding proteins, (e) rate and extent of biotransformation, (f) permeability of the bile canalicular membranes, and (g) bile flow and transport of the excreted substances in the biliary tree. Some of these processes are active, carrier-mediated, while others may include simple diffusion or facilitated diffusion. Additional factors such as the substrate concentration, presence of inhibitors, and adequate energy supply, the molecular weight of the chemical in question, polarity, and lipid solubility may also become important.

Several chemicals that are known to be inducers of the mixed-function oxidase system of the liver modify biliary excretion of a number of model compounds (Klaassen, 1978; Levine, 1978). Phenobarbital, spironolactone, DDT, and other agents have been used to demonstrate these effects. The overall effect of these inducers is to increase the biliary excretion of model compounds such as sulfobromophthalein (BSP), indocyanine green (ICG), and a variety of other drugs. On the other hand, toxic chemicals such as the pesticides hexachlorobenzene, toxaphene, chlordecone, and mirex have been shown to cause impaired biliary excretion of model compounds such as BSP, phenolphthalein glucuronide, and polar metabolites of polychlorinated biphenyls and imipramine (Mehendale, 1979). While the biliary excretion of these chemicals was impaired by prior exposure to the above pesticidal compounds, bile secretion was increased in these models of impaired hepatobiliary function. Since these chemicals that impair the biliary excretion of model compounds are also potent inducers of drug-metabolizing enzyme systems, the effect of enzyme-inducing agents on hepatobiliary function cannot be predictably generalized as being favorable or unfavorable to biliary excretion of other chemicals and to bile secretion itself.

Hepatic cholestasis can be induced in experimental animals by administration of certain steroids and ANIT, and clinically this has been observed with chlorpromazine and certain tricyclic antidepressant drugs. Studies with these model cholestatic agents have provided important contributions to the understanding of the etiology of cholestasis. Cholestasis can also be induced by naturally occurring bile-acid conjugates, taurolithocholic acid, and chenodeoxycholic acid. Cholestatic reaction has also been associated with the antibiotics and contraceptive steroids. Intravenous administration of manganese, inorganic substances such as sulfate produces cholestatic response in experimental animals. Studies with these and various other models of intrahepatic cholestasis have aided in gaining some insight into and understanding of the mechanisms underlying intrahepatic cholestasis.

Cirrhosis

Cirrhosis can be defined as a chronic disease condition presenting morphological alterations of the lobular structure characterized by destruction and regeneration of parenchymal cells and increased connective tissue (Zimmerman, 1978). Major morphological changes include granular or nodular appearance and are characterized by the presence of septae of collagen throughout the liver. The aggregated liver cells circumscribed by sheath-like fibrous growth of collagenized connective tissue give the appearance of nodules of hepatic cirrhosis. Portal cirrhosis is characterized by small nodules, granular appearance, and pale-yellow coloration, although the color may depend a great deal on fatty infiltration, iron deposition, necrosis, and the degree and duration of jaundice. In postnecrotic cirrhosis, the liver is acute yellow, atrophied, and coarsely nodular with broad and dense bands of connective tissue dividing the liver into nodules of varying size. In portal cirrhosis, heavy involvement of parenchymal tissue surrounding the portal blood supply may be seen. Biliary cirrhosis is characterized by dark-green coloration and firm, granular, and nodular appearance of the liver. In primary biliary cirrhosis there is a reduction in the interlobular bile ducts, while in the cirrhosis secondary to obstruction jaundice there is an increase in the interlobular ducts. In most cases, single-cell necrosis appears to be the major cause of pathogenesis that is associated with deficiency in the repair mechanism of the residual cells. This deficiency leads to accumulation of fibrotic tissue, giving rise to scar formation. The precise mechanism of pathogenesis of cirrhosis is not clearly understood, and several other factors may play a role in the causation of cirrhosis.

Several models of drug-induced cirrhosis are available. These include the chronic administration of CCl_4, aflatoxins, DMN, and several other carcinogens. Drug-induced cirrhosis is known to occur as in the case of methotrexate, a folic-acid antagonist used in the treatment of leukemia, lymphoma, and psoriasis. The single foremost cause of cirrhosis in humans is, however, the consumption of alcoholic beverages. In experimental animals, production of alcoholic cirrhosis has not been completely successful. There has been a great deal of controversy concerning the causation of cirrhosis by ethanol. Two hypotheses have prevailed in regard to the cause of alcoholic cirrhosis. One hypothesis holds that ethanol produces nutritional deficiency and that cirrhosis is a secondary effect related to this nutritional imbalance. Evidence in support of this hypothesis comes from studies in which adequate supplemental nutrition administered along with ethanol fails to produce classical alcoholic cirrhosis. Not supplementing these nutritional factors such as proteins, vitamin B_{12}, folic acid, methionine, and choline promotes the incidence of cirrhosis. An alternative hypothesis has held that ethanol is capable of directly inflicting cirrhosis and that inability to demonstrate cirrhosis in experimental animals is because of the inappropriate experimental animal models for alcohol-induced cirrhosis. Evidence for such a proposal comes from studies where preconditions of cirrhosis such as increased collagen synthesis have been observed after chronic administration of ethanol even when nutritional supplementation was administered. One group of investigators has been able to demonstrate cirrhosis of the liver in the baboon even after adequate supplementation of nutritional requirements. In any case, interest in alcoholic cirrhosis will continue in view of the worldwide alcohol consumption and the close relationship with the incidence of cirrhosis of the liver.

Carcinogenesis

The liver is susceptible to cancer induction by a variety of different humanmade and naturally occurring chemical substances. Naturally occurring substances known to cause liver cancer in experimental animals include aflatoxin B_1, pyrrolizidine alkaloids, cycasin, and safrole (Fig. 3). Among humanmade substances one finds dimethyl- or diethylnitrosamine, DDT, polychlorinated biphenyls, CCl_4, chloroform, vinyl chloride, dimethylaminoazobenzene, acetylaminofluorine, thioacetamide, urethane, ethionine, dimethylbenzanthracene, several other polycyclic hydrocarbons, and galactosamine (Fig. 4). Angiosarcoma, a rare form of liver cancer caused by vinyl chloride in some industrial workers employed in the plastics industry, provides an excellent example of human liver cancer caused by humanmade chemicals. Induction of liver cancer in experimental animals was one of the first experimental models of hepatic response to carcinogens that has been studied extensively. The success in early development of animal models for liver cancer has resulted in detailed characterization of various responses to experimental carcinogens.

Studies in experimental animals indicate quite clearly that development of cancer of the liver is associated with a number of obvious nonmalignant lesions appearing prior to the occurrence of neoplastic malignancy (Farber and Fisher, 1980). Induction of liver cancer requires several weeks of exposure to most liver carcinogens. In rats and mice, a single injection of carcinogens such as urethane, dimethylbenzanthracene, dimethyl- or diethylnitrosamine, methyl nitrosonitroguanidine, and nitrosomethyl urea produces cancer. A necrogenic dose of CCl_4 also produces cancer. Partial hepatectomy in conjunction with the administration of these carcinogens enhances the production of cancer. In the degenerative and regenerative changes that follow, two populations of hepatocytes become evident: the original population, and the new proliferative population of cells, which enlarges to become hyperplastic nodules, which are believed to be the precursors for the subsequent development of neoplasia

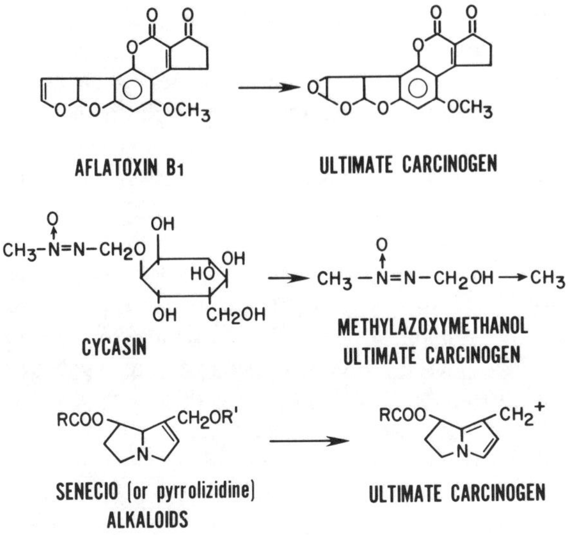

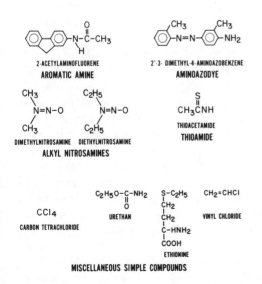

Figure 3 Natural agents causing hepatic cancer with major forms of ultimate carcinogens.

and cancer. Hyperplastic nodules show distinct biochemical, morphological, and functional changes in comparison to normal hepatocytes. Although the initiating event may be mutation, misguided cell differentiation also may play a role in the proliferation of the hyperplastic nodules. Acute inhibition of normal mitotic activity has been suggested to be the triggering factor leading to the proliferation of a new population of cells that can grow in a new cytotoxic environment containing the challenging

Figure 4 Structures of some chemical carcinogens.

chemical. Most of the hepatocellular carcinomas differ in cellular organization from normal adult livers and assume a configuration resembling that of the fetal liver. Such a pseudofetal organization is also evident from biochemical markers such as α-fetoprotein, complement of fetoisozymes, and fetoantigens. Hyperplastic nodules may undergo maturation and revert back to normal-appearing liver, and when this does not happen the persisting nodules give rise to cancerous tissue. After the initiation, a long latent period is required, however, ranging from 6 months to 2 years in the laboratory rat, for the final expression of liver cancer to occur.

There is considerable evidence to believe that many carcinogens are inactive per se as carcinogens but need to biotransform to electrophilic reactants that are ultimate carcinogens. These ultimate forms of carcinogens interact with tissue constituents such as DNA, RNA, protein, and other macromolecules. Hepatocytes are capable of most of the enzymatic activation of procarcinogens to ultimate carcinogens, and the mixed-function monooxygenase plays a major role in this activation process.

Carcinogens have been classified depending on origin, on chemical structure, or on the basis of the mechanism by which they cause cancer. Mechanistic classification of carcinogens separates all the known carcinogens into two major classes (Weisburger and Williams, 1980). *Genotoxic carcinogens* are agents that function as electrophilic reactants, either directly or after bioactivation to ultimate carcinogens. The second class is referred to as *epigenetic carcinogens* and includes those agents for which there is no evidence of direct interaction with genetic material. This category includes hormones, solid-state carcinogens, immunosuppressors, cocarcinogens, and promotor substances.

In order to facilitate future direction and investigation in the area of mechanisms of carcinogenesis, Farber (Farber and Fisher, 1980) has suggested the use of sequential analysis of neoplastic tissue in experimental carcinogenesis. Such an approach embodies the advantages of a unifying hypothesis, ability to control the process at each step, synchronization, and quantitation of new cell populations; molecular and possibly genetic markers for different cell populations allow the collection of sufficiently large cell populations for identification and further work. There are four models in the sequential analysis approach suggested by Farber. Model A involves the use of a single exposure to diethylnitrosamine or other carcinogens such as DMN, 2-acetylaminofluorine, dimethylaminoazobenzene, aflatoxin B_1, or ethionine to intact or partially hepatectomized female rats 20–24 h after the surgical procedure. The number, size, and behavior patterns of islands of new hepatocytes histochemically deficient in enzyme markers are studied. Model B utilizes young weanling rats in which proliferating hepatocytes are quite numerous. Animals are exposed to 2-acetylaminofluorine in the diet for 18 days and following a short recovery period of 1 week are fed a diet containing 0.05% phenobarbital for several months. Nodules are much more numerous under these conditions than without the phenobarbital, and there also occurs an increase in number of hepatocellular carcinomas. The young animals receiving only 2-acetylaminofluorine also develop nodules and liver cancer but to a considerably lesser degree. Model C utilizes rats that are subjected to partial hepatectomy and within 24 h are exposed to a single dose of diethylnitrosamine or other carcinogens. After 2 months on a normal diet, the animals are fed a diet containing 0.05% phenobarbital and examined at the end of 6–8 months. Under such conditions the number of enzyme-altered islands is about seven times higher in animals exposed to phenobarbital than in controls. Also, some animals develop hepatocellular carcinoma under this regimen. Model D is based on a functional analysis of the properties of the presumed precursor hepatocyte populations for cancer. Animals are exposed to a single dose or several doses of a carcinogen. Only after recovery from any necrosis or other acute degenerative–regenerative processes in the bulk of the original hepatocytes, the animals are exposed to 2-acetylaminofluorine in the diet for 7 days in order to create a mitoinhibitory effect and are then subjected to a strong stimulus for self-proliferation, by partial hepatectomy. Under these conditions, the bulk of the hepatocytes show no self-proliferation. However, the isolated hepatocytes widely scattered throughout the liver now rapidly proliferate to form foci and visible tiny nodules within 10 days after partial hepatectomy. The number of foci and their size can be determined and related to the dose and type of carcinogen administered. These models meet the prerequisites for a satisfactory sequential model of carcinogenesis and allow stepwise analysis of chemically induced liver cancer.

MECHANISMS OF HEPATIC TOXICITY

Liposes

As pointed out earlier, most of the lipid that accumulates in the tissue in response to a toxic agent is composed primarily of triglycerides, followed by fatty acids. Six general mechanisms can account for the accumulation of lipid material in the liver tissue (Zimmerman, 1978; Alpers and Isselbacher, 1975): (a) increased triglycerides synthesis, (b) decreased release of triglycerides from the liver into the blood stream, (c) triglyceride synthesis may be shunted to nonsecretory or slow-secreting pools, (d) combination of increased rate of synthesis and decreased release of triglycerides and fatty acids, (e) increased supply of fatty acids, and (f) decreased synthesis of glycoproteins.

Clearly, some effects that lead to liposes are mediated via changes in transport, synthetic, or catabolic mechanisms. Some of these effects could be indirectly mediated via alterations in hormonal regulating mechanisms. Catecholamine regulation of body-fat mobilization can be altered by toxic chemicals to result in increased availability of fatty acids. Increased hepatic triglyceride synthesis could occur because of the increased availability of fatty acids and glycerol phosphate. The triglyceride synthesis can directly cause increased accumulation of triglycerides in the liver. Increased synthesis of fatty acids has been demonstrated after ethanol in a variety of in vitro and in vivo models. This may be related to the increased NADPH/NAD ratios as a result of alcohol metabolism. Alcohol metabolism by alcohol and aldehyde dehydrogenases results in increased generation of NADPH, and acetyl fragments which facilitate the availability of fatty acids. Increased supply of fatty acids to the liver can also result from alcohol-evoked mobilization of peripheral fat. Increased production of reducing equivalents may also produce a block in the utilization of acetyl fragments that can be shunted to elongation of fatty acids. Thus, ingestion of alcohol can result in a dual effect of decreased oxidation of fatty acids and increased synthesis, as well contributing to the elevation of fatty acids.

Decreased release of triglycerides from the liver into the bloodstream has been associated with CCl_4-, ethionine-, and phosphorus-induced hepatic steatosis. Hepatic triglyceride is released from the liver in the form of lipoproteins. In general, agents that cause liposes, cause one or another metabolic aberration that results in impaired synthesis of normal lipoproteins. CCl_4 and ethionine cause a fall in the circulating levels of VLDL, the fraction that is predominently involved in the transport of hepatic triglycerides to the extrahepatic tissues. With ethionine and yellow phosphorus, the principal mechanism whereby lipids accumulate in the liver appears to be related to a defect in the synthesis of lipoproteins. With CCl_4 and ethionine, synthesis of the protein part of the VLDL appears to be defective. In choline deficiency, which results in fatty liver, the phospholipid synthesis is impaired. Secretion of VLDL has been reported to be impaired by orotic acid, as well as by choline deficiency. Ethionine-induced fatty liver results from a deficient synthesis of apoprotein of VLDL, required for the movement of triglycerides from the liver. Deficiency of ATP induced by both orotic acid and ethionine results in trapping of adenosyl moieties as S-adenosyl ethionine, since the turnover of this molecule is much slower than that of the normal metabolite S-adenosyl methionine.

Regenerating livers represent a unique instance of abnormal accumulation of fat in the liver tissue. After a two-thirds hepatectomy in experimental animal, high levels of lipids accumulate in the liver, ranging up to 10 times the normal levels. The triglyceride levels fall to normal range after the regeneration of the liver. In CCl_4-induced lipidosis, protective agents can prevent appearance of hepatic necrosis but do not seem to affect fat accumulation in the liver. These examples serve to illustrate that mere accumulation of fat in the tissue does not necessarily represent a toxic response of the liver tissue to injury inflicted by toxic chemicals. In most cases, high accumulation of fat in the liver tissue should be taken to mean that many metabolic pathways have been altered from the norm by the toxic chemical. This would signal the high-risk status of the liver for hepatotoxic mechanisms to operate, for instance, the free-radical mechanisms that may result in lipid peroxidation, as exemplified by CCl_4 hepatotoxicity. Accumulation of a high level of fat in the liver must add to the lipid peroxidative damage that ensues. Thus, in most instances it is clear that accumulation of fat by itself may not represent a toxic response but may in fact represent a high-risk status of the liver tissue for damage by other agents.

Lipid Peroxidation

One of the most clearly defined hypotheses relating to the action of hepatotoxic agents is the lipid peroxidative damage of cellular membranes. Lipid peroxidation may be looked upon as occurring in two steps (Fig. 5). Some toxic event initiates lipid peroxidation, and organic free radicals generated by the initiation process serve to propogate the reactions. The concept of lipid peroxidative damage was advanced by Slater (1975) as the principal mechanism of CCl_4-induced liver injury and has found ample experimental support (Recknagel and Glende, 1978). This theory holds that

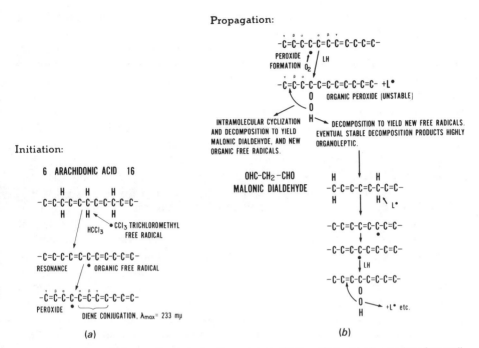

Figure 5 Lipid peroxidation of a typical polyunsaturated fatty acid by trichlorocarbon free radical. The scheme illustrates the initiation (a) of lipid peroxidation by CCl₃ and self-propagating reactions (b) involved in the lipid peroxidative damage of membranes; γ, wavelength. [Adapted from Recknagel and Glende (1973).]

CCl₄ is homolytically cleaved by a cytochrome P-450 monooxygenase system to produce the ˙CCl₃ free radical. In the aerobic environment, the CCl₃ free radical enters a hydrogen abstraction reaction (Fig. 5) to form an organic free radical of the fatty acid chloroform. The cytochrome P-450 system is encased in a phospholipid membrane rich in polyenoic fatty acids. Hence these polyenoic fatty acid are the most likely immediate targets for the initial lipid peroxidative attack to occur. In the aerobic environment of the hepatocyte, the organic fatty acid radical rearranges, yielding organic peroxy and hydroperoxy radicals. These radicals destroy the cytochrome P-450 hemoprotein, thus compromising the mixed-function oxygenase activity. The rapid decomposition of the endoplasmic reticulum and its function is a direct result of this lipid peroxidative process. The lipid peroxides and hydroperoxides attack the lipids and possibly the proteins, especially the functional groups such as sulfhydryl groups, compromising their function. Generation of organic radicals by the ˙CCl₃ free radical causes another chain of reactions. The organic radicals themselves interact with other lipids, either in the same membrane or in other membranes after being diffused from the original site of formation. This interaction results in the formation of other organic free radicals and peroxy and hydroperoxy radicals (Fig. 5). The entire process is propagated to continue the autocatalytic reactions until the membranes are destroyed and many cell functions are disrupted, culminating in the demise of the hepatocyte.

Destruction of cytochrome P-450 has been demonstrated in animals treated with CCl_4 and in vitro incubations containing CCl_4. Two hypotheses have been put forward concerning the mechanisms by which cytochrome P-450 system is destroyed (Dianzani, 1979). One holds that the $\cdot CCl_3$ free radical formed at the cytochrome P-450 catalytic site directly attacks the phospholipid casing of the membrane-bound P-450 complex. An alternative hypothesis holds that the $\cdot CCl_3$ free radical is liberated from the catalytic site of cytochrome P-450 and interacts with cellular membranes to initiate lipid peroxidation. Resultant organic fatty acid radicals and peroxy and hydroperoxy radicals attack and destroy the cytochrome P-450 complex. In any case, destruction of cytochrome P-450 hemoproteins does occur in CCl_4-induced liver injury. This is in fact the basis for autoprotection afforded in experimental animals by prior exposure to a small dose of CCl_4, against a subsequently administered larger dose of CCl_4. Actual decrease in cytochrome P-450 levels in the liver tissue of animals treated with CCl_4 as well as in vitro microsomal incubations with CCl_4 have been demonstrated by a number of investigators. Loss of glucose 6-phosphatase activity and representative monooxygenase activities, of protein synthesis, and of capacity to form and secrete low-density lipoproteins are some of the other consequences of CCl_4-induced liver injury on the function of endoplasmic reticulum.

Several lines of evidence are available in support of the bioactivation of CCl_4 being central to the mechanism of CCl_4-induced liver injury. Phenobarbital treatment, which enhances the hepatic cytochrome P-450-catalyzed monooxygenase activity, increases and SKF-525A diminishes the lipid peroxidation and CCl_4-induced hepatic necrosis. Irreversible binding of CCl_4 to microsomal incubations is also accordingly altered by phenobarbital and SKF-525A, in support of the bioactivation mechanism. Recent evidence has indicated that CCl_4 toxicity may not correspond to the total cytochrome P-450 in the liver tissue (Plaa, 1980). Newborn animals contain less cytochrome P-450 in the liver, and yet CCl_4 is equally toxic to these animals. Exposure to very low amounts of the pesticide chlordecone results in greatly potentiated CCl_4 hepatotoxicity (Curtis et al., 1979) in the absence of elevated total cytochrome P-450 levels. On a molar basis, potentiation of CCl_4 by chlordecone is much greater than by phenobarbital and lethality is also greatly amplified by chlordecane in comparison to much higher levels of phenobarbital (Mehendale, 1984). Although these findings are not inconsistent with the bioactivation of CCl_4 to $\cdot CCl_3$ free radical, these findings are indicative of the flaws in directly relating bioactivation potential as measured by biochemical parameters such as total cytochrome P-450, to the haloalkane hepatotoxicity. Other lines of evidence are available in support of the central role played by $\cdot CCl_3$ in the hepatotoxicity of CCl_4. The brominated analog $BrCCl_3$ is more toxic than the fully chlorinated analog CCl_4. Since the energy required for the homolytic cleavage of C—Br bond (49 kcal/mol) is less than that required for C—Cl bond (69 kcal/mol), $BrCCl_3$ would be expected to be more toxic if the toxicity by either compound is related to the formation of $\cdot CCl_3$ free-radical. Experimentally, this has been found to be the case. Furthermore, toxicity of $BrCCl_3$ is also enhanced by phenobarbital and chlordecone, although the latter is much more potent in this regard.

Lipid peroxidation is also reported to occur after the administration of tetrachloroethane to mice. Iodoform produces a hepatocellular lesion similar to that produced by CCl_4. Phosphorus poisoning also produces lipid peroxidation in the liver. Several other hepatotoxic substances cause hepatic necrosis in the absence of lipid peroxidation. These include 1,1-dichloroethylene, DMN, ethylene dibromide, thioacetamide, and acetaminophen. Whether lipid peroxidation is involved in the ethanol-induced fatty liver is still debated.

It may be that many free radicals initiate the lipid peroxidation process. For instance, many autooxidations, certain oxidases, and leakage of electrons from normal electron-transport chains result in the generation of superoxide anions (O_2^-). These anions may give rise to other radical forms of oxygen, such as singlet oxygen, $OH^{\cdot}$ radical, and H_2O_2, which may initiate autocatalytic lipid peroxidative processes. Evidence for the involvement of O_2^- radical in the initiation of lipid peroxidation comes largely from the inhibition of such processes in the presence of superoxide dismutase, an enzyme responsible for removing the O_2^-. Antidotes for lipid peroxidative damage are not available. Antioxidant compounds can protect against lipid peroxidation, but prior presence is required for their protective action. These include vitamin E, ascorbic acid, and GSH, which stop the propagation of the lipid peroxidative process. CCl_4-induced lipid peroxidation can be obtunded by antioxidants such as pyrogallol and other polyols and sulfhydryl compounds such as cysteamine. However, these agents have to be administered prior to, simultaneously with, or immediately after the administration of CCl_4 in order for their protective action to be manifested.

Protein Synthesis

Many hepatotoxic compounds have been reported to interfere with the hepatocellular protein synthesis. These include galactosamine, 2-acetylaminofluorene, CCl_4, 3,4-dimethylaminoazobenzene, diethylnitrosamine, DMN, thioacetamide, and ethionine, all of which have been shown to inhibit incorporation of amino acids into hepatic proteins. These findings have led a number of investigators to believe that inhibition of protein synthesis is the cause of hepatic necrosis. However, such conclusions may not be entirely accurate. For example, proper doses of ethionine can result in inhibition of protein synthesis without the appearance of liver necrosis. Cycloheximide also inhibits protein synthesis without inducing liver necrosis. Administration of cycloheximide has been shown to protect rats against hepatotoxic effects of CCl_4 and against the acute biliary epithelial necrosis observed following the administration of ANIT. Thus, the precise role of protein synthesis in the manifestation of hepatotoxic responses to administration of toxic chemicals is not entirely clear. Extensive work has been carried out to determine the mechanism by which protein synthesis is altered by hepatotoxic agents. Representative agents used in such studies include galactosamine, DMN, and CCl_4. Administration of galactosamine reduces synthesis of RNA and plasma proteins such as the coagulation factors. The depression of protein synthetic activity appears to be as a result of the deficiency in UTP, since the administration of uridine reverses the inhibition. The galactosamine 1-phosphate formed in the liver leads to the accumulation of UDP-galactosamine and other related derivatives. This results in a depletion of hepatic UTP and other UDP-hexoses, since most of the uridine would be tied up by galactosamine or its derivatives. This leads to a depression of uracil nucleotide-dependent biosynthesis of macromolecules. Ethionine inhibits amino acid incorporation into microsomal proteins as a result of the replacement of methionine in S-adenosyl methionine, which leads to a trapping of cellular adenine, which in turn leads to the decreased rate of ATP synthesis. Ethionine-induced fatty liver characterized by the accumulation of triglycerides is a consequence of the interference with protein metabolism. Decreased or abnormal VLDL leads to excessive accumulation of triglycerides in the liver. DMN-induced decrease in protein synthesis is especially noted in the microsomes. The effect is apparently mediated by a loss of messenger RNA from polyribosomes. It is likely that methylation of RNA is the underlying mechanism for disrupting the messenger RNA of the polyribosomes. CCl_4 causes a marked reduction in the incorporation of amino acids into lipoproteins relatively soon after the administration of the toxic agent. Decreased amino acid incorporation into hepatic proteins, albumin, and plasma clotting factors has been noted. CCl_4-induced damage to protein synthesis appears to be an irreversible effect that leads to cellular death.

The precise role played by alterations in protein synthesis caused by the administration of toxic chemicals in the toxic responses of the liver has not been fully understood. While many secondary effects can be visualized to be operative as a result of hindered protein synthesis, whether these events have any direct toxicological significance has not been fully investigated.

Activation of Toxic Agents

Activation of toxic substances in the liver is now a well-established phenomenon for several classes of hepatotoxins. These include haloalkanes, aromatic compounds, halogenated aromatics and aliphatics, nitrosamines, aromatic amines, polycyclic hydrocarbons, mycotoxins, plant toxins such as pyrrolizidine alkaloids, and others. Toxins for which bioactivation is not required are also known to cause hepatotoxicity. Examples of such compounds include all of the direct-acting hepatocarcinogens, such as bis-chloromethyl ether, and other hepatotoxic agents such as chlordecone and mirex. Most activation reactions are catalyzed by enzymes, although some spontaneous chemical rearrangement reactions have been invoked to explain certain activation processes. Before the implication of these biotransformation reactions was fully recognized, these reactions were referred to variously as biodegradation, biotransformation, intoxication, and detoxication reactions. Modern advances in analytical methodology and the availability of stable and radiolabeled isotopes have aided immensely in the identification of intermediate steps in a series of biotransformation reactions. Subsequent chemical synthesis of many of these intermediate biotransformation products has allowed the recognition of toxicity characteristics of these activated biotransformation products and structure-activity relationships.

There is considerable evidence in support of bioactivation of haloalkanes such as CCl_4 and chloroform. CCl_4 is bioactivated to the $\cdot CCl_3$ free radical by the cleavage of the C—Cl bond. This occurs in the endoplasmic reticulum, is catalyzed by the cyto-

chrome P-450 monooxygenase system, and requires NADPH. This product of homolytic cleavage becomes incorporated into the endoplasmic reticulum and can be measured as covalently bound $^{14}CCl_4$-derived radiolabel. Free-radical scavengers such as
pyrogallol and cysteamine and lipid antioxidants such as α-tocopherol can reduce
such irreversible tissue binding and protect against liver injury. Two $\cdot CCl_3$ can con-
dense to form hexachloroethane, which has been demonstrated in animal experiments. The $\cdot CCl_3$ undergoes a hydrogen abstraction reaction with polyenoic fatty
acids to form chloroform and to generate the organic fatty-acid free radical (Fig. 5).
Recent evidence suggests that complete oxidation of CCl_4 may involve the formation
of phosgene intermediate. Both hepatotoxicity and metabolism of CCl_4 to various
products are augmented by exposure to inducing agents such as phenobarbital. Recent
evidence suggests, however, that the inducing property of the inducer may not be the
only determinant in potentiated hepatotoxicity of CCl_4 (Mehendale, 1984).

Chloroform is known to be metabolized by the mixed-function monooxygenase
system. Activation is catalyzed by the cytochrome P-450 system, and covalent binding of the $H^{14}CCl_3$-derived radiolabel to microsomal proteins also occurs as in the
case of CCl_4. Metabolism, covalent binding, and toxicity of chloroform are increased
by prior exposure to phenobarbital. GSH is depleted in the phenobarbital-treated
animals receiving $CHCl_3$, indicating enhanced formation and interaction of activated
products with this protective ligand. Recent evidence suggests the formation of free-
radical intermediate phosgene in the complete oxidation of $CHCl_3$. This activation
proceeds through hydroxylation of $CHCl_3$ to trichloromethanol, which spontaneously
dehydrochlorinates to form phosgene. Vinyl chloride is another haloalkane that is
known for angiosarcoma, a rare form of liver cancer in some industrial workers. It is
believed to be bioactivated by the cytochrome P-450 monooxygenase system via
epoxidation, since its bioactivation can be completely blocked by inhibitors of cytochrome P-450. After bioactivation, metabolism of vinyl chloride proceeds via conjugation with GSH to form urinary mercapturic acid metabolites.

Acetaminophen-induced hepatic necrosis is also mediated via chemically reactive
intermediate, formation of which is catalyzed by cytochrome P-450 monooxygenase
system (Gillette, 1978). Bioactivation can be followed by irreversible binding of
acetaminophen-derived radiolabel to tissue macromolecules. The association between
hepatotoxicity and irreversible tissue binding has been supported by several lines of
experimental evidence. Little irreversible tissue binding occurs after therapeutic
doses of acetaminophen. After toxic doses, greater tissue binding occurs. Normally,
active intermediate(s) combine with GSH, and mercapturic acid conjugates appear in
the urine. After toxic doses, hepatic GSH levels are depleted and toxic intermediates
of acetaminophen accumulate in the liver tissue, giving rise to elevated tissue binding
and increase in hepatic necrosis. Induction by phenobarbital potentiates the toxicity,
and cytochrome P-450 inhibitors decrease the toxicity. The generation of active intermediates that bind to tissue protein irreversibly to cause tissue injury has been demonstrated for other substances such as furosemide and N-acetylisoniazid. Studies with
these hepatotoxic agents have aided not only in the understanding of the underlying
mechanisms of hepatotoxicity but also in the appreciation of the importance of normally minor activation pathways in the causation of tissue toxicity. Thus, although

acetaminophen activation normally proceeds, the deactivation mechanisms by way of conjugation with GSH can protect the tissue from injury. At toxic doses, the tissue level of activated acetaminophen becomes excessive, protective mechanisms are overwhelmed, and tissue toxicity ensues.

Another example of bioactivation mechanism for hepatotoxicity is that of bromobenzene-induced centrilobular necrosis. Bromobenzene is activated to the 3,4-arene oxide intermediate by cytochrome P-450 monooxygenase system. This active intermediate covalently binds to tissue macromolecules to cause necrosis. The presence of adequate levels of cysteine and GSH results in the formation of innocuous mercapturic acid conjugates, and injury does not occur. Toxicity can be enhanced by depleting cysteine or tissue GSH levels, or by prior exposure to inducing agents. Conversely, inhibitors of cytochrome P-450 decrease bromobenzene-induced hepatotoxicity.

Bioactivation of procarcinogens has been demonstrated to be important in the expression of this type of toxicity. Since liver is the organ with greatest capacity for metabolizing chemical carcinogens, this has important implications for carcinogenicity of other organs and tissues as well. 2-Acetylaminofluorine causes hepatic and urinary-bladder carcinomas in experimental animals. This carcinogen requires a series of bioactivation steps. It first undergoes *N*-hydroxylation, and this product has been demonstrated to be a more active carcinogen than the parent compound in animal models. However, the *N*-hydroxy metabolite by itself is not highly reactive and requires additional activation, which is provided by the esterification of the *N*-hydroxy group with sulfate or acetate, or it may undergo a peroxidating reaction giving rise to arylamidating products such as the ring-hydroxy products (Fig. 6). These products can undergo electrophilic reactions with DNA, RNA, proteins, and other tissue macromolecules. Thus, in the case of 2-acetylaminofluorine, bioactivation involves a number of enzyme systems acting in concert to produce highly electro-

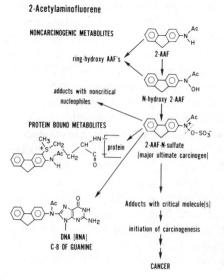

Figure 6 Interaction of ultimate carcinogens with guanine bases of nucleic acids. Simplified pathways for metabolism of activated forms of 2-AAF and adduct formation are illustrated.

philic reactants. *N*-Hydroxylation of 2-acetylaminofluorine is a cytochrome P-450-mediated reaction. *N*-Acetylation and sulfation are conjugation reactions catalyzed by soluble enzymes in the liver cytosol. DMN is also bioactivated by the cytochrome P-450 monooxygenase system to the highly reactive electrophilic methyl carbonium radicals, which interact with nucleic acids and tissue proteins in a manner analogous to the arylamidating reactions of 2-acetylaminofluorene (Fig. 6).

Bioactivation of the mycotoxin aflatoxin B_1 has been recognized as being important in the carcinogenesis of this naturally occurring fungal toxin. The lactone ring of the aflatoxin molecule is expoxidized by a cytochrome P-450 monooxygenase system, and this expoxide metabolite reacts with DNA, RNA, and proteins to form various adducts. The bioactivation, adduct formation, and hepatotoxicity are all increased by inducers of cytochrome P-450 and decreased by the inhibitors of this enzyme system.

Much interest has been generated in the interaction of electrophilic carcinogens or ultimate carcinogens (Weisburger and Williams, 1980) with nucleic acids. Current effort is devoted to the characterization of the resultant adducts. 2-Acetylaminofluorine metabolites interact with the C-8 position of the guanine base of RNA or DNA. Methyl carbonium ions generated from the bioactivation of DMN alkylate the guanylic acid of DNA at the O-6 or N-7 position. Although greater amounts of adduct may be formed at the N-7 position, adduct formation at the O-6 position may be more closely related to the carcinogenicity of DMN. Aflatoxin B_1 epoxide also reacts with the N-7 position of guanine. Similarly, the epoxide product of vinyl chloride interacts with nucleic acid bases. Thus, considerable knowledge has accumulated concerning the interaction of electrophilic active intermediates with nucleic acids. Further effort will undoubtedly be devoted to determining the relationship between these reactions to form various adducts with nuclear materials and carcinogenicity produced by these compounds.

Several other examples exist where bioactivation mechanisms have been known to be involved in the toxic responses of the liver. Hepatotoxic reactive metabolites have been proposed for thioacetamide to account for the acute necrogenic effects. Hepatotoxicity of the anesthetic agent halothane has been related to the biotransformation of this chemical, and necrotic lesions can be enhanced in animals pretreated with inducers of the hepatic cytochrome P-450 monooxygenase system. The pyrrolizidine alkaloids of *Crotolaria* have been known to cause veno-occlusive hepatic disease. These compounds are also activated to toxic metabolites in the liver tissue. Finally, the cholestatic response of ANIT is known to be enhanced by prior administration of inducing agents. Although the active intermediates have not been identified and characterized, all of these examples are widely believed to represent bioactivation mechanisms.

Depletion of Endogenous Protective Ligands

Recent developments in toxicology have resulted in a better appreciation of the important role played by protective ligands present in the tissue in the manifestation of the hepatic responses to the administration of toxic agents. Examples of such endogenous ligands include GSH, cysteine, sulfate, glucuronic acid, methyl groups, vitamin E, and others.

It was noted that irreversible binding of acetaminophen- and bromobenzene-derived active intermediates to tissue macromolecules was increased, with concomitant decrease in tissue levels of GSH. As the GSH level decreased, increased irreversible binding and tissue necrosis were observed. Higher toxicity of the compounds could be demonstrated by depleting GSH levels by administering agents such as diethylmaleate or iodomethane. GSH is known to undergo conjugation reactions with electrophilic reactants, either via enzymatically catalyzed reactions by a family of GSH transferases or via nonenzymatic reactions. Increased toxicities associated with depleted GSH levels were explained on the basis of diversion of the biotransformation pathway via the increased accumulation of active intermediates, which interacted with tissue macromolecules to cause toxicity. With the advent of the discovery that acetaminophen- and bromobenzene-induced hepatic necrosis could be related to the hepatic content of GSH came the realization that toxic responses of the liver may not be only a function of the bioactivation steps. GSH levels can be elevated by administration of glutathione precursors such as cysteine or methionine to provide protection against bromobenzene- and acetaminophen-induced hepatic necrosis. Experimental manipulation of GSH levels has become a standard experimental protocol in attempts to explain the toxicity of a variety of toxic chemicals. It is important to realize that although depletion of protective agents such as GSH can result in a diversion of the biotransformation pathway to a more toxic route, quantitatively such alteration only becomes important when depletion is more severe and when it falls below a certain critical level.

Similarly, it is possible that the availability of sulfate and glucuronic acid, two important ligands in the detoxication of a variety of foreign chemicals, may be important in the expression of toxicity. We have increasingly come to realize that the threshold levels of toxic intermediates can be regulated not only by the rate of formation of the activated intermediates but also by the manipulation of conjugative reactions that serve to remove reactive intermediates. Sulfate and glucuronide conjugation reactions are important in deactivation pathways, and the availability of these ligands may become limiting under certain circumstances. For example, in galactosamine toxicity, the availability of activated glucuronic acid will become limiting since galactosamine ties up the majority of uridilate and galactosamine interferes with the availability of cellular energy. In general, the availability of sulfur is limited in the mammalian species, and depletion of available sulfur via sulfate conjugation results in a drain on sulfur-containing amino acids, as well as additional expenditure of cellular energy required for the sulfate conjugation pathway. This in part explains the predominance of the glucuronic acid pathway for elimination of foreign chemicals in mammalian species, with the possible exception of the cat. Further work to determine the precise role of these ligands in altering toxicity of foreign chemicals will undoubtedly be stimulated after the role played by GSH in such toxicities has been appreciated and well understood.

Finally, there are other ligands, such as vitamin E and ascorbic acid, that can protect against bioactivation-mediated cellular toxicities such as the free-radical mechanisms. These ligands can protect against radical-initiated tissue injury, as has been demonstrated for vitamin E and ascorbic acid. The protection afforded by vitamin E in terminating lipid peroxidation reactions is a result of the trapping of an electron from the free radical by this compound. Vitamin E in turn does not reduce oxygen, and hence propagation of peroxidation is interrupted. The precise role of such endogenously occurring ligands in protecting against toxic reactions by radical-generating foreign chemicals will be further investigated with greater interest in the future.

Arrested Hepatocellular Repair

Liver tissue is capable of regeneration, and this ability is particularly noticeable after partial hepatectomy (Farber and Fisher, 1980) or after limited injury by any number of toxic chemicals. It follows then that any event that might interfere with the ability of the liver to regenerate might increase the toxic response of the liver to a chemical. Such a mechanism might be operative in the chlordecone potentiation of CCl_4 hepatotoxicity (Fig. 7).

An earlier study of histomorphological changes associated with chlordecone plus CCl_4 toxicity was not very revealing at 24 h of CCl_4 administration. Hence, at time-course study was undertaken (Lockard et al., 1983a,b). This study showed that either CCl_4 or a combination of chlordecone and CCl_4 produced the same basic morphologic alterations in hepatocytes, that is, dilatation of rough endoplasmic reticulum, lipid accumulation, and necrosis. The differences in the two experimental groups were seen in the pattern of lobular distribution and of the degree of severity of the hepatic alterations. While a low dose of CCl_4 alone resulted in temporary, minimal alterations of pericentral hepatocytes, a massive dose of CCl_4 alone resulted in classic pericentral and midzonal necrosis. The combination of chlordecone and a small dose of CCl_4 caused progressively severe alterations in hepatocytes throughout the entire lobule over the time course of the experiment, without any particular localization to a specific zone. These observations suggest that although the chlordecone plus CCl_4 combination resembles intoxication with a massive dose of CCl_4, the histological findings indicate some differences in the progression and distribution of hepatocellular damage in the lobular architecture of the liver.

Morphometric analyses (Lockard et al., 1983b) were revealing in several biochemical and physiological aspects of hepatocellular repair and renovation that takes place at an accelerated rate after the initial injury. After the administration of CCl_4 alone, hepatic injury peaked around 12 h; recovery was apparent as seen by restoration of hepatocellular glycogen, arrested lipid accumulation, repair and restoration of endoplasmic reticulum, and restoration of hepatocytes with healthy nuclei. Indeed, soon after the initial injury became evident, cellular repair and regeneration accelerated, as evidenced by increased mitotic index (Fig. 8). CCl_4 at a dose of 0.1 ml/kg does not cause any significance alterations in functional, biochemical, or histological indices of hepatic injury measured 24 h after CCl_4, indicating lack of any tissue injury. However, tissue injury was evident as early as 4 h after CCl_4, and it was clear from histomorphometric studies (Lockard et al., 1983a,b) that liver tissue is able to

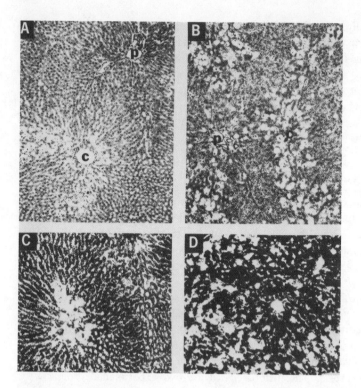

Figure 7 All fields show livers (at ×45) of rats killed 24 h after single injection of 100 μl/kg CCl₄. Fields A and B were stained by the PAS method without diastase hydrolysis. Fields C and D are frozen sections stained with Sudan black to show lipid. Key: c, central vein; p, portal vein. Field A: CCl₄ alone. Limited centrilobular necrosis characterized by greatly swollen cells with agranular cytoplasm. In the nonnecrotic cells, the dark-staining cytoplasmic material is glycogen. Another portal vein is at upper left. Field B: chlordecone feeding (10 ppm in diet) for 15 days followed by CCl₄ (100 μl/kg). Necrosis (areas of swollen, almost unstained cells) involves portions of all zones in a diffuse and irregular fashion. Shrunken hyperbasophilic nuclei can be recognized in some of the necrotic cells. Note decreased PAS positivity (compare with field A), which demonstrates loss of glycogen from nonnecrotic cells. Field C: same liver as in field A. Very dark midzonal staining demonstrates liposis. The lighter staining of periportal parenchyma demonstrates a smaller amount of lipid in these cells. A portal vein is at lower right. Field D: same liver as in field B. Abundant liposis in middle and periportal zones. Another central vein is at upper right. In fields C and D, the cells that show little if any sudanophilia are necrotic hepatocytes. *[Reproduced with permission from Curtis et al. (1979).]*

recover from this injury. Soon after the initial injury was evident, repair and renovation of injured tissue began to occur. Hepatocellular regeneration continued until complete recovery at 36 h after this dose of CCl₄.

In contrast, a combination of chlordecone and CCl₄ resulted in hepatic changes that became progressively severe with time. There were progressive and greater loss of glycogen, greater and progressive lipid accumulation, and increased numbers of swollen hepatocytes (Lockard et al., 1983b). In animals receiving the chlordecone and CCl₄ combination, approximately 37% necrosis indicated by pyknotic nuclei was present at 36 h, and this was progressive and there was no evidence of hepatic regeneration. The extensive liver necrosis observed morphologically was consistent with extremely high levels of serum enzymes that progressively increased during the time course of the experiment. Particularly noteworthy in this regard are the observations on hepatocellular mitotic index, which remained suppressed (Fig. 8), thus preventing the liver tissue from repair and renovation of damaged tissue. The level of hepatocellular injury far exceeds the capacity for repair. The hepatocellular regeneration which should have been stimulated is arrested, and consequently a progressive hepatic injury is observed in animals treated with the chlordecone plus CCl₄ combination.

This time-course study of histopathological alterations (Lockard et al., 1983a) and morphometric analysis of morphological changes associated with chlordecone sensitization of CCl₄ hepatotoxicity suggest that two dynamic aspects of cellular physiology need to be examined: first, the reason for the initial greater injury associated with chlordecone pretreatment; and second, the events leading to the arrest or prevention of mechanisms responsible for cellular multiplication and tissue renovation after the initial injury. These findings are consistent with greater initial CCl₄ damage seen after chlordecone treatment. Although the mechanism for the prevention of cellular repair and renovation is not understood, recent studies (Mehendale, 1984) have indicated that starting 3 h after CCl₄ administration, cytosolic Ca^{2+} increases progressively in animals preexposed to chlordecone (Fig. 9), while no changes were observed after treatment with CCl₄ alone to animals maintained on normal diet. This is followed by a progressive increase (Mehendale, 1984) in initially mitochondrial but later microsomal sequestration of cytosolic calcium progressively. Whether the disrepair of hepatocellular renovation and restoration can be explained by greatly perturbed calcium homeostasis, or whether other mechanisms might be involved, re-

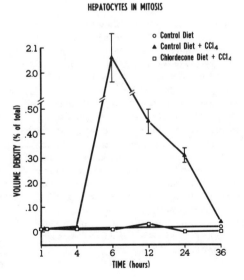

HEPATOCYTES IN MITOSIS

o Control Diet
▲ Control Diet + CCl₄
□ Chlordecone Diet + CCl₄

VOLUME DENSITY (% of total)

TIME (hours)

Figure 8 Volume density of hepatocytes with mitotic figures is shown for control, CCl₄, and chlordecone plus CCl₄ groups at various time intervals. Chlordecone (10 ppm in the diet for 15 days) and CCl₄ (100 μl/kg) treatments were as described earlier. Mitotic index was measured at various times after CCl₄ administration. *[Reproduced with permission from Lockard et al. (1983b).]*

mains to be experimentally tested. Recent studies with cytotoxic menadione (Mehendale et al., 1985) have indicated that hepatocellular accumulation of extracellular CA^{2+} precedes any appearance of hepatotoxicity. Such findings are indicative of the critical role played by the influx of extracellular Ca^{2+} in vital cellular processes.

Hepatobiliary Function

Modification of biliary excretory function may be mediated via a number of mechanisms. Increased biotransformation results in enhanced biliary excretion of some chemicals. This is especially true for chemicals that need biotransformation to polar metabolites prior to biliary excretion. Evidence in favor of such a mechanism comes from experiments in which biliary excretion of model compounds was enhanced by agents that stimulate drug-metabolizing enzyme systems and was decreased by agents that inhibit these enzymes. Phenobarbital-induced enhancement of BSP excretion is thought to be associated with increased bile flow. A good correlation was found between bile flow and excretion of the chemical in the bile for several compounds whether or not they required prior metabolism. For example, increased bile flow and increased biliary excretion of drugs that require no metabolism to appear in the bile correlated well (ouabain, amaranth, and dibromoanalog of BSP), as for those that were metabolized before excretion (BSP, bilirubin, thyroxin, probenecid, and procainamide ethobromide). Other mechanisms may play a role in modified biliary excretory function. Transport of substances from blood to the liver and from the liver to the bile may be considered important mechanisms. Competitive inhibition by toxic chemicals for the transport of normally excreted substances into the bile canaliculi may be considered a possibility. Evidence for reabsorption of substances along the canalicular duct has been reported, and an enhancement of this mechanism by agents that modify biliary excretory function would be expected to result in decreased biliary excretion. Toxic chemicals may stimulate the synthesis and excretion of bile salts,

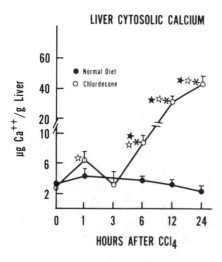

Figure 9   Male Sprague-Dawley rats were maintained on a diet containing 0 or 10 ppm chlordecone for 15 days. On day 15, they received a single ip injection for 100 μl CCl_4/kg in corn-oil vehicle (1 ml/kg). Total cytosolic Ca^{2+} was determined at various time points after the administration of CCl_4. Asterisk denotes the values are significantly different from zero time point of normal diet plus corn oil group of rats. Open star denotes that the values are significantly different from the zero time point of chlordecone plus corn oil group of rats. Solid star is an indication of the value being significantly different from the respective time point of normal-diet group of rats. The values were considered to be significant at $p \le 0.05$.

which in turn are known to alter bile secretion and the excretion of other chemicals. Chlordecone- and mirex-induced impairment of biliary excretory function has been attributed to the aberration of transport of model compounds across the bile canalicular membrane (Mehendale, 1979). This may be related to impaired energy production and utilization in the hepatic cells. The enhancement of bile flow by prior exposure to inducing agents has been demonstrated to be due to the increased bile-acid-independent bile flow.

There is considerable evidence to indicate that cholestatic response of the liver to the administration of ANIT may be mediated by a metabolite. Marked species variation, the potentiation of cholestatic response to ANIT by enzyme inducers, and diminished cholestatic response by enzyme inhibitors are some of the observations that support the view that cholestatic response is mediated by a metabolite of ANIT. The cholestatic reaction associated with anabolic steroids may be mediated by the effect on permeability of the biliary tree, by a reduced bile-salt-independent bile flow, and by decreased clearance of bile salts. These alterations are consistent with the observations that a number of contraceptive steroids decrease bile flow and decrease the excretory maximum for bilirubin. Manganese sulfate elicits a widespread dilatation of bile canaliculi with the microvilli, which is observed within a day after the treatment. This may be related to impaired hepatobiliary function seen after the administration of manganese sulfate. There is considerable controversy as to whether chlorpromazine causes cholestasis in humans because of a direct toxic effect or because of a hypersensitivity reaction. Since there is wide variation in the response in experimental animals, the experimental confirmation of the mechanism by which chlorpromazine causes intrahepatic cholestasis has not been scrutinized. The morphologic features of chlorpromazine-induced cholestasis have not been produced in experimental animals. A number of mechanisms leading to cholestasis have been put forth based on a variety of experimental evidence. These include decreased bile-salt-independent canalicular bile flow for chlorpromazine, canalicular membrane dysfunction for ANIT, altered ductular-cell permeability for ANIT, hypotoxic hypoactive smooth endoplasmic reticulum for ANIT, and intracanalicular mycellar precipitation for chlorpromazine. However, none of these mechanisms have been definitively validated. It is also possible to conceptualize that a combination of these mechanisms may operate to precipitate a cholestatic response.

FACTORS AFFECTING HEPATIC TOXICITY

Biotransformation-Enzyme Induction

Many factors can influence the responses of the liver to toxic chemicals. These include such factors as species, age, sex and hormonal status, exposure to other chemicals, nutritional and dietary deficiency, genetic factors, and site and route of exposure to toxic chemicals. In most cases, the underlying principal mechanism appears to be altered biotransformation of the chemical in question. For those chemicals that undergo biotransformation reactions, it is apparent that the qualitative and quantitative considerations of biotransformations would directly affect the toxic responses of the liver. How altered biotransformation affects hepatotoxicity depends on the chemicals involved and on whether the toxic chemical requires bioactivation in order to exert its toxic effect.

Prior or simultaneous exposure to enzyme-inducing or -inhibiting agents can have a profound effect on the response of the liver to the hepatotoxic chemicals. Whether the toxicity is increased or decreased depends on which of the various steps involved in the metabolism of the toxic chemical are altered and on the extent to which each step is altered relative to the other. When more than one enzyme is altered in the biotransformation pathway, the net effect is dependent on the influence that each of the steps has in the bioactivation and detoxication reactions.

Potentiation of CCl_4 hepatotoxicity has been reported after prior exposure to inducing agents such as phenobarbital and DDT. Subsequently, it was shown that several aliphatic alcohols such as methanol, ethanol, isopropanol, and butanol exert similarly potentiating effects on acute inhalation toxicity of CCL_4. Recently it has been shown that dietary exposure to a small level of chlordecone results in greatly potentiated CCl_4 hepatotoxicity (Fig. 7). This property was not shared by mirex or photomirex, two close structural analogs of chlordecone. Furthermore, the potentiating property of chlordecone on CCl_4 toxicity is approximately 100-fold higher than that of phenobarbital. Hepatotoxicity of chloroform has also been shown to be similarly potentiated by chlordecone but not by mirex (Plaa, 1980). Whatever the underlying mechanism for potentiation of toxicity, it is apparent that simultaneous exposure to a number of chemicals results in an altered expression of hepatotoxicity by chemicals. There are many examples of hepatotoxins whose toxic actions have been reported to be modified by prior, simultaneous, or subsequent exposure to other chemicals. In fact, such experimental manipulations have become important tools in experimental toxicology.

Many factors that affect the metabolism and distribution of toxic chemicals also affect chemical carcinogenesis (Williams, 1984). A decrease of dietary proteins, for instance, decreases cytochrome P-450, which converts DMN to its toxic metabolite, and hence the hepatocarcinogenesis is decreased. This results in increased nephrocarcinogenicity, however, presumably due to greater accumulation of DMN in that tissue, where it is bioactivated to exert the carcinogenic effect. Some carcinogens such as aflatoxin B_1 require only a single administration for their effect to be manifested, while others require repeated administration. Carcinogens in general require a latent period for the final expression of carcinogenicity to occur.

Promoters are agents that increase the tumorigenic response of a genotoxic carcinogen when applied after the carcinogen. Certain inducers of hepatic drug-metabolizing enzymes, such as phenobarbital, DDT, and butylated hydroxytoluene, are capable of exerting a very powerful promoting effect when administered after minimal doses of procarcinogens. Much experimental evidence has accumulated to believe that the enhanced bioactivation of procarcinogens to ultimate carcinogens is the underlying mechanism. When these promoters are administered with procarcinogens, often the effect may be reversed, mostly by increasing the detoxication reactions or interfering with activation reactions. Thus, promoters appear to exert their effects via epigenetic mechanisms and are believed to be important in the causation of human cancer. Consideration and quantitation of the precise role played by the promoters in human cancer is a challenge for the toxicologist in evaluating the genotoxic potential of carcinogens.

Physiological Considerations: Hepatic Blood Flow

Among the many physiological factors that effect the hepatic toxicity, one important factor might be the rate and degree of delivery of the toxin to the liver. The rate of delivery and quantity of toxic agent delivered to the liver will undoubtedly affect the metabolism, interaction with liver cells, and elimination of the chemical in question. Many chemical hepatotoxic agents are nonpolar compounds, and when they are not transformed to polar metabolites these tend to accumulate in adipose tissue, from which they may be released into the circulation for long periods of time. Chemicals that rapidly undergo activation or inactivation transformation processes in the liver are almost entirely removed by the liver in one pass. Generally speaking, many hepatotoxins undergo this "first-pass" phenomenon. When the chemical dose is overwhelming, the removal and metabolism processes are dependent on hepatic blood flow. After removal by the liver, depending on the end products of biotransformation, these may be eliminated via biliary excretion, stored in the liver, or dumped into the systemic circulation for excretion via the kidney. Hepatic blood flow may affect all of these processes and hence the toxic response of the liver.

Upon administration of a hepatotoxic agent, it can be demonstrated that hepatic blood flow is affected as an initial or continuous response to the toxic injury. Blood supply to the liver may be affected, as in the case of phenobarbital, which can double the blood flow through the liver. Blood flow within the liver may be diverted preferentially between different lobes of the liver. In addition, within the liver lobes, hepatic microcirculation can be altered by many hepatotoxic agents. These include CCl_4, bromobenzene, thioacetamide, allyl formate, DMN, acetaminophen, pyrrolizidine alkaloids, phalloidins, chronic alcohol consumption, and attendant malnutrition. Within hours after administration of hepatotoxins such as CCl_4 and bromobenzene, changes in sinusoidal organization and intregrity can be observed. Sinusoidal flow becomes discontinuous, and clumping erythrocytes, edema, congestion, and hemorrhagic spots may be seen in the centrilobular area. These changes spread to other zones within the lobular structure. The severity of the injury increases in response to the exposure situation. Such changes in microcirculation result in quicker deterioration of the tissue in the affected areas. Consideration of the role played by physiological factors such as hepatic blood flow and microcirculation must bear an even greater importance in connection with the toxic responses of the liver to combinations of hepatotoxins. In many experimental protocols, inducing agents, enzyme inhibitors, or GSH-depleting agents are used to pretreat the animals. The precise role of alteration in hepatic blood flow and microcirculation in the liver on hepatic responses after the toxic agent is administered is poorly understood. This lack of understanding may often result in erroneous conclusions from such experimental protocols involving combinations of treatment.

REFERENCES

Alpers, D. H., and Isselbacher, K. J. 1975. Fatty liver: Biochemical and clinical aspects. In *Diseases of the Liver,* ed. L. Schiff, pp. 815–832. Philadelphia: Lippincott.

Arias, I. M., Popper, H., Sehachter, D., and Shafritz, D. A. 1980. *The Liver: Biology and Pathobiology.* New York: Raven.

Conney, A. H. 1967. Pharmacological implications of microsomal enzyme induction. *Pharmacol. Rev.* 19:317–366.

Curtis, L. R., Williams, L. W., and Mehendale, H. M. 1979. Potentiation of the hepatotoxicity of carbon tetrachloride following preexposure to chlordecone (Kepone) in the male rat. *Toxicol. Appl. Pharmacol.* 51:283–293.

Dianzani, M. U. 1979. Reactions of the injury: Fatty liver. In *Toxic Injury of the Liver,* eds. E. Farber and M. M. Fisher, pp. 281–331. New York: Marcel Dekker.

Farber, E., and Fisher, M. M. 1980. *Toxic Injury of the Liver,* part A and B. New York: Dekker.

Gillette, J. R. 1978. Formation of reactive metabolites of foreign compounds and their covalent binding to cellular constituents. In *Handbook of Physiology, section 9, Reactions to Environmental Agents,* eds. D. H. K. Lee, H. L. Falk, and S. D. Murphy, pp. 577–590. Washington, D.C.: American Physiological Society.

Ishak, K. G. 1982. The liver. In *Pathology of Drug-Induced and Toxic Diseases.* New York: Churchill Livingstone.

Jones, A. L., and Mills, E. S. 1973. The liver and gallbladder. In *Histology,* 3rd ed., eds. R. O. Greep and L. Weiss, pp. 599–644. New York: McGraw-Hill.

Jones, S. R., and Myers, W. C. 1979. Regulation of hepatic biliary secretion. *Annu. Rev. Physiol.* 41:62–87.

Jones, A. L., and Schmuckler, D. L. 1977. Current concepts of liver structure as related to function. *Gastroenterology* 73:833–851.

Klaassen, C. D. 1978. Biliary excretion. In *Handbook of Physiology, section 9, Reactions to Environmental Agents,* eds. D. H. K. Lee, H. L. Falk, and S. D. Murphy, pp. 537–554. Washington, D.C.: American Psychological Society.

Levine, W. G. 1978. Biliary excretion of drugs and other xenobiotics. *Annu. Rev. Pharmacol. Toxicol.* 18:81–96.

Lockard, V. G., Mehendale, H. M., and O'Neal, R. M. 1983a. Chlordecone-induced potentiation of carbon tetrachloride hepatotoxicity: A light and electron microscopic study. *Exp. Mol. Pathol.* 30:230–245.

Lockard, V. G., Mehendale, H. M., and O'Neal, R. M. 1983b. Chlordecone-induced potentiation of carbon tetrachloride hepatotoxicity: A morphometric and biochemical study. *Exp. Mol. Pathol.* 39:246–256.

Mehendale, H. M. 1979. Modification of hepatobiliary function by toxic chemicals. *Fed. Proc.* 38:2240–2245.

Mehendale, H. M. 1984. Potentiation of halomethane hepatotoxicity. *Fundam. Appl. Toxicol.* 4:295–308.

Mehendale, H. M., Svensson, S.-Å., Baldi, C., and Orrenius, S. 1985. Accumulation of Ca^{2+} induced by cytotoxic levels of menadione in the isolated perfused liver. *Eur. J. Biochem.* 149:201–206.

Plaa, G. L. 1980. Toxic responses of the liver. In *Toxicology, The Basic Science of Poisons,* eds. J. Doull, C. D. Klaassen, and M. O. Amdur, pp. 206–231. New York: Macmillan.

Popper, H., and Schaffner, F. 1959. Drug-induced hepatic injury. *Ann. Intern. Med.* 51:1230–1252.

Rappaport, A. M. 1975. Anatomic considerations. In *Diseases of the Liver*, 4th ed., ed. L. Schiff, pp. 1-49. Philadelphia: J. B. Lippincott.

Recknagel, R. O., and Glende, E. A., Jr. 1978. Lipid peroxidation: A specific form of cellular injury. In *Handbook of Physiology, Section 9, Reactions to Environmental Agents*, eds. D. H. K. Lee, H. L. Falk, and S. D. Murphy, pp. 591-602. Washington, D.C.: American Physiological Society.

Slater, T. F. 1978. Biochemical studies on liver injury. In *Biochemical Mechanisms of Liver Injury*, ed. T. F. Slater, pp. 1-95. New York: Associated.

Taylor, W. 1975. *The Hepatobiliary System. Fundamental and Pathological Mechanisms*. New York: Plenum.

Weisburger, J. H., and Williams, G. M. 1980. Chemical carcinogens. In *Toxicology: The Basic Science of Poisons*, eds. J. Doull, C. D. Klaassen, and M. O. Amdur, pp. 84-138. New York: Macmillan.

Williams, G. M. Modulation of chemical carcinogenesis by xenobiotics. *Fundam. Appl. Toxicol.* 4:325-344.

Zimmerman, H. J. 1978. *Hepatotoxicity*. New York: Appleton-Century-Crofts.

Chapter 5

Pulmonary Toxicology

Hanspeter Witschi

Jerold A. Last

INTRODUCTION

Lung injury caused by chemicals is a major health problem. Chronic obstructive lung disease is widespread in the general population; it is a crippling and eventually killing condition whose direct and indirect economic costs in the United States have been estimated to exceed 12 billion dollars per year. Inhaled airborne chemicals, such as found in tobacco smoke or present in polluted ambient air and originating from motor vehicles or fossil-fuel-burning power plants, have been identified as causative agents. Industrial exposure to toxic agents, as in certain mining operations and manufacturing processes, is often accompanied or followed by pulmonary disease; examples are silicosis, asbestosis, or coal miners' lung. Another form of lung damage caused by toxic agents is lung cancer; death from this cause has increased dramatically during the last few decades. Chemicals inhaled in tobacco smoke are primarily responsible for the increased incidence of lung cancer. Finally, it is known that quite a few bloodborne agents may cause acute or chronic lung damage, such as the antineoplastic agents bleomycin or busulfan, nitrofurantoin (a drug used to treat urinary-tract infections), or the weedkiller paraquat.

Research sponsored by the Office of Health and Environmental Research, U.S. Department of Energy under contract DE-AC05-840R21400 with the Martin Marietta Energy Systems, Inc.

A great many chemicals thus have the potential to cause toxic lung damage, whether they reach their target organ by inhalation or in the bloodstream. Some chemicals cause acute discomfort within minutes following exposure, and signs of impaired pulmonary function, sometimes leading to death, may develop rapidly. However, more often than not, signs of acute lung injury may go unnoticed, and it takes months or even years until it becomes apparent that a chemical agent has compromised the structural and functional integrity of the conducting airways and of the alveolar zone. Industrial diseases such as silicosis or asbestosis or lung diseases caused by common air pollutants or by tobacco smoke may take years to develop fully. Yet it is known that practically all chemicals implicated in the etiology of chronic lung disease may cause lung damage after one single episode of exposure. It is one of the challenges in pulmonary toxicology to link early damage in a meaningful way to late manifestations of toxic lung injury. However, regardless of whether toxic lung damage progresses rapidly or more slowly, the most important physiological functions of the lung will be diminished or even crippled: the uptake of oxygen from the air and the elimination of CO_2 from the venous blood. Inadequate pulmonary ventilation and reduced gas exchange will affect the entire organism, enhancing disease and eventually causing death.

STRUCTURE AND FUNCTION OF THE LUNG

Anatomy

Air is brought into the lung through the upper airways and the conducting airways. Most of the upper airways, which include the nasal passages, nasal turbinates, oropharynx, and larynx, are covered by a ciliated epithelium, beneath which lie mucus-secreting glands; only the nasal entrance, oropharynx, and larynx are covered by a squamous, nonciliated epithelium (Swift and Proctor, 1977).

The nasal turbinates increase the surface with which inspired air comes into first contact with the interior of the body, warm inhaled air to body temperature, and saturate it with water. Turbulence created in the air flow by the turbinates causes larger particles (those larger than about 5–10 μm) to become impacted and trapped in the mucosa. The upper airways thus serve also as a first filter and prevent larger particles from reaching the deeper regions of the lung.

Past the larynx, air enters the conducting airways, which consist of the trachea and bronchial tree. The trachea is lined by a ciliated epithelium, containing mucus-producing goblet cells; the submucosa also contains numerous mucosal glands. The trachea divides at the carina into two main bronchi that ventilate the left and right lungs. Once each main bronchus enters the pulmonary parenchyma, it subdivides into two daughter airways of different diameter, which then become parent branches themselves and undergo further division (irregular dichotomy). In humans, the average number of generations from the trachea (generation 0) down to the last conducting airways, the terminal bronchioles, numbers about 16.

The conducting airways are lined by a complex epithelium consisting of ciliated cells, mucus-producing goblet cells, brush cells, Clara cells, and a few rare cell types. Beneath the epithelium lie numerous mucus-producing glands; their secretions form a continuous blanket, which covers the luminal surface of the bronchial tree.

The smallest purely conducting airways, the terminal bronchioles, open into alveolar ducts, which contain a few alveoli in their walls. Alveolar ducts undergo further dichotomic divisions until they end in a final blind airway. This is the alveolar sac, a dome-shaped space whose walls are lined with wide-open air chambers, the alveoli (Gil, 1982) (Fig. 1)

Gas exchange takes place in the alveoli. Air and blood remain separated from each other at all times by the alveolar septum or the so-called air–blood barrier. The alveolar septum consists of three layers: the alveolar epithelium, a narrow interstitial space, and the capillary endothelium. Capillary endothelial cells are squamous cells with an organelle-poor cytoplasm. A characteristic feature of endothelial cells are small vesicles, which are capable of engulfing bloodborne molecules through pinocytosis and transporting them across the endothelial cells. The interstitial space is in most places extremely thin, often consisting only of the fused basement membranes of the endothelial and epithelial cells. In other places the interstitial space contains elastic fibers and small bundles of collagen fibrils, fibroblasts, and other less well characterized cell types (Fig. 2).

The alveolar epithelium consists of essentially two cell types. Type I alveolar cells or membraneous pneumonocytes are thin sheets whose organelle-poor cytoplasm may extend to 50 μm from the nucleus. Type II alveolar cells or granular pneumonocytes are of cuboidal shape and often lie in the corners of the alveoli. Their surface is covered with microvilli, and the cytoplasm is rich in organelles. Most prominent in type II alveolar cells are the so-called lamellar bodies, the intracellular storage sites of surfactants. A third cell type, type III alveolar cells, is extremely rare (Weibel, 1973).

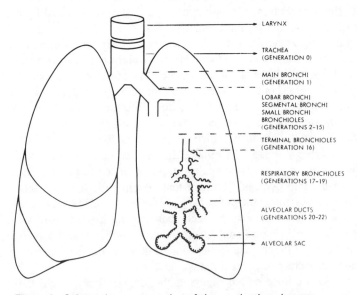

Figure 1 Schematic representation of the conducting airways.

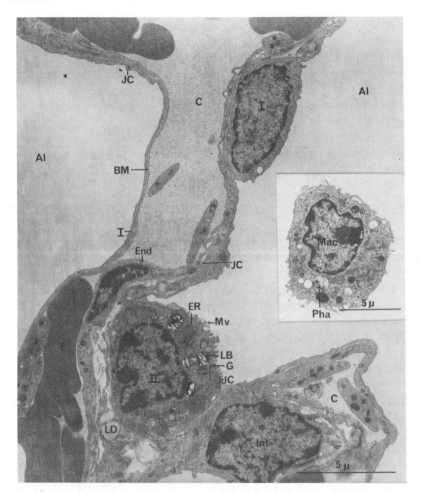

Figure 2 Alveolar septum from a normal mouse lung. Type I and type II cells cover the alveolar surface. The cells are joined together by junctional complexes. Endothelial cells, interstitial cells, and a macrophage (inset) are of normal appearance. Abbreviations: Al, alveolus; BM, basement membrane; C, capillary lumen; E, erythrocyte; End, capillary endothelium; ER, endoplasmic reticulum; G, Golgi apparatus; Int, interstitial cell; JC, junctional complex; LB, lamellar body; LD, lipid droplet; M, mitochondrion; Mac, macrophage; Mv, microvilli; Pha, phagocyte; I, type I cell; II, type II cell. [*From Hirai et al. (1977)*.]

Morphometric data show the following relative number of the 4 main cell types in population in the alveolar zone of rat lung: type I alveolar cells, 8.3%; type II alveolar cells, 14.1%; capillary endothelial cells, 39%; and interstitial cells, 38.6%. More than 90% of the alveolar surface is covered by the type I alveolar cells (Weibel et al., 1976).

An important nonsessile cell population found in the lung is the alveolar macrophages (Brain et al., 1977). Alveolar macrophages are originally formed in the bone marrow and carried via the bloodstream into the lung, where they migrate into the alveolar interstitium. There they may lie dormant until the presence of foreign materials within the alveoli, such as bacteria or inhaled particles, produces some activating stimulus. The cells move then from the interstitium into the alveolar space and begin to ingest the foreign particles by phagocytosis. Alveolar macrophages contain numerous lysosomes, small organelles filled with digestive enzymes, particularly acid hydrolases. Degradable foreign particles such as bacteria are readily digested by the lysosomal enzymes. However, other particles such as inorganic dusts may resist digestion and can remain within the macrophages. Eventually, macrophages may leave the alveolar zone via the airways, through the pulmonary lymphatics or through pulmonary blood vessels.

Physiology

Ventilation   Ventilation consists of moving air through the upper respiratory tract and the tracheobronchial tree into the terminal respiratory units. After gases are exchanged in the alveolar zone, air enriched in CO_2 is expelled from the lung. During inspiration, the thoracic cage is enlarged and the diaphragm moves downward; the lung passively follows this expansion. During expiration, the chest wall and diaphragm relax or, in forced expiration, become compressed, and air is expelled from the lung. Efficient ventilation requires proper expansion and recoil of the lung parenchyma and of the tracheobronchial tree; pathologic processes that alter the elastic properties of lung tissue will adversely affect proper ventilation (Murray, 1976).

The volume of air that can be moved in and out of the lung with a maximum inspiratory and expiratory movement is called *vital capacity* (VC). In humans, vital capacity is approximately 4500 cm^3. However, even after the most vigorous expiration the lung never collapses totally but retains approximately 1200 cm^3 air. This air volume, which cannot be expelled from the lung, is called *residual volume* (RV). The sum of vital capacity (VC) and of residual volume (RV) gives the total volume of air a lung can contain and is called *total lung capacity* (TLC). In humans, total lung capacity is approximately 5700 cm^3.

Under resting conditions, the amount of air moved with each breath in and out of the lung is only a fraction of the vital capacity. It is called *tidal volume* (TV) and, in humans, measures approximately 500 cm^3. If an increased delivery of fresh air to the terminal respiratory units is required, as for example in heavy exercise, both the tidal volume and the respiratory rate can be increased. The amount of air moved in and out of the lung may, in humans, vary from 20 l/min up to 180 l/min. Accordingly, the delivery of airborne toxicants to the lung will vary. In areas where there is heavy air pollution it is often recommended not to exercise during episodes of particularly severe smog conditions, in order to keep delivery of toxic agents to the lung as low as possible.

The total lung capacity as well as the ratio between vital capacity and residual volume may change if the lung is diseased. Under certain pathologic conditions, the alveoli become overdistended and air is trapped. While total lung capacity would remain unchanged or might even increase, the amount of air that can effectively be moved in and out of the alveoli would diminish. This condition would result in a decreased vital capacity and an increased residual volume. On the other hand, should part of the lung collapse or should the alveoli become filled with liquid, both total lung capacity and vital capacity would decrease.

Perfusion With each beat, the heart pumps blood into two large vessels, the aorta and the pulmonary artery; the left ventricle ejects approximately 70–80 cm^3 blood into the aorta, and the right ventricle delivers an equal amount into the pulmonary artery. The blood pumped into the aorta and from there into the systemic circulation is fully oxygenated and will be distributed to all organs in the body. In the different organs, blood passes through capillary networks and becomes depleted of oxygen. It then returns via the venous system back to the right ventricle, from where it is pumped into the pulmonary artery. The blood ejected from the right ventricle perfuses only the pulmonary capillary bed; the lung is thus the only organ to receive, at any given time, the entire cardiac output (i.e., the volume of blood leaving one heart chamber). The lung may thus be exposed to substantial amounts of bloodborne agents. Moreover, any agent injected into a peripheral vein will reach the pulmonary capillary bed before it comes into contact with the capillaries of any other organ. In humans, cardiac output pumped into the lung under resting conditions is 6–8 l/min and, during heavy exercise when the heart rate increases, may increase to 20–30 l/min.

The blood pressure in the pulmonary circulation is much lower than it is in the systemic circulation. Gravitational forces therefore favor in humans a better perfusion of the lower parts of the lung than of the upper ones. Uneven distribution of blood flow is probably less pronounced in nonsupine animals, particularly small animals (Murray, 1976).

Diffusion In the pulmonary capillary bed, the blood comes in intimate contact with the alveolar air, although air and blood remain separated from each other at all times by the alveolar septum. It has been estimated that 80–95% of the alveolar surface in humans (80 m^2) contains capillaries. Air and blood are thus in close proximity over an approximately 70-m^2 area. Contact with airborne toxic agents thus occurs on a surface that is approximately 40 times larger than skin, another body area exposed directly to environmental agents.

Gas exchange takes place along the entire alveolar surface. Oxygen moves by diffusion from the alveolar air into the blood, and CO_2 diffuses from the blood into the alveoli; the venous blood becomes oxygenated. Oxygen has to diffuse across the pulmonary epithelial cells and their basement membranes, the interstitial space, the basement membrane, and the body of the capillary endothelial cells, through a thin film of plasma, and finally across the wall of the erythrocyte, before it can react with hemoglobin to form oxyhemoglobin. Resistance to diffusion of oxygen may be increased by pathologic alterations in any of these successive layers; a thickening of the interstitial space, as for example in fibrosis, or in replacement of the usually flat and thin alveolar epithelial cells by more cuboidal-shaped cells, such as follows acute epithelial damage, will compromise the diffusion of oxygen across the air–blood barrier.

CO$_2$ is an end product of cell metabolism in all body tissues. It diffuses into the plasma of the capillary blood and enters the erythrocytes, where it is mainly transformed into H$_2$CO$_3$, a reaction accelerated by a Zn-containing enzyme, carbonic anhydrase. A concentration gradient exists in the pulmonary capillaries from blood toward the CO$_2$-poor inspired alveolar air; CO$_2$ thus diffuses across the air–blood barrier into the alveolar air and is expired.

A quantitative index of the amount of gas traveling across the air–blood barrier is the diffusion capacity. It is expressed as cubic centimeters of gas transferred per minute per unit pressure difference across the air–blood barrier. Since CO$_2$ is much more soluble in water than is O$_2$, CO$_2$ diffuses about 20 times faster across the alveolar septum than does oxygen. If the structure of the air–blood barrier is altered by pathologic processes, it is the diffusion capacity for oxygen that may become the limiting factor; the result is inadequate oxygenation of the venous blood. A possible way to correct for this is to increase the partial pressure of O$_2$ in the alveolar air by increasing the oxygen concentration in the inspired air (however, there are possible problems of oxygen toxicity in this approach, as will be discussed below).

Nonventilatory Functions of the Lung

Lungs have several functions other than gas exchange. They include removal of vasoactive agents from the circulating blood, production and release of hormones and mediators, and biotransformation of foreign chemicals. For example, the polypeptide angiotensin I is converted during one single pulmonary passage into the vasoactive angiotensin II; the converting enzyme is located in part in the pulmonary capillary cells. The major site for inactivation of 5-hydroxytryptamine in the body is the lung. Prostaglandins E and F (but not prostaglandin A) are also inactivated or removed from the circulation in the lung, as are adenine nucleotides. However, other vasoactive agents such as histamine, epinephrine, or vasopressin are not affected in the pulmonary circulation (Bakhle and Vane, 1977).

It is also established that lungs have the capability to metabolize foreign chemicals. Many basic amines such as imipramine, methandone, and chlorcylizine accumulate in the lung; metabolites may subsequently be released into the circulation. A pulmonary mixed-function oxidase system has been identified in the lungs of many species, probably including humans; the enzymes have been shown to transform numerous substrates, including aromatic polycyclic hydrocarbons, through hydroxylation, epoxidation, and N-demethylation. The lung mixed-function oxidase system is located in the microsomal fraction and is in many respects similar to the hepatic mixed-function oxidase system; however, an entire lung probably contains only about 3% of the total amount of drug-metabolizing enzymes present in liver. It is now generally thought that, as compared to other organs, particularly the liver, the lung plays only a small role in the overall biotransformation of drugs and toxicants. However, selective uptake of certain compounds into the lungs or metabolic activation of certain substrates into highly reactive alkylating agents may play a substantial role in producing lung toxicity; examples are the herbicide paraquat and the lung toxic furans, discussed below. Selective uptake and biotransformation of chemicals by the lung may thus be important factors in pulmonary toxicity (Philpot et al., 1977).

INHALATION TOXICOLOGY

Exposure Techniques

To study the effects of toxic agents on the respiratory tract, animals are allowed to inhale gases or aerosols. Proper exposure to airborne toxic agents requires the use of sophisticated and specialized equipment. In principle, experimental animals (or under certain conditions even human volunteers) are put into an enclosed space, a so-called inhalation chamber. Within this chamber an atmosphere is created that contains the test agent at the desired concentrations. The generation of gas mixtures usually poses no major problems other than accurate monitoring of concentrations, whereas generation of well-characterized aerosols containing particles of respirable size is technically more demanding. Suitable analytical procedures must be used to determine the concentration of the agent within the chamber during the entire experiment. The most commonly used procedures can be described as follows (MacFarland, 1976) (Fig. 3).

    Whole-Body Chambers The most widely used technique for exposure is to place a suitable number of animals into an airtight chamber. Such chambers may range in size from a few liters up to several cubic meters. The size of the chamber is largely determined by the number and size of the animals one wants to expose. Experience has shown that to maintain animals comfortable within a closed chamber, without having to deal with excessive build-up of heat and humidity, their total body volume should not exceed 5% of the total chamber volume (chamber loading rule). A 1-m^3 chamber (1000 l) could thus theoretically contain maximally 50 kg of animals,

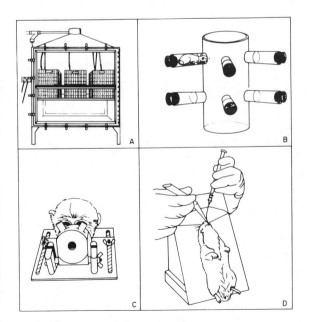

Figure 3 Exposure techniques: (A) whole-body exposure chamber; (B) nose-only chamber; (C) face mask; (D) intratracheal instillation.

corresponding to approximately 200 young rats or if necessary 2000 mice; however, space has to be allowed for cages and their manipulation and eventual analytical equipment. Ideally, within the chamber animals should be housed in individual cages. Animals have a tendency to huddle together and to bury their nose into each other's fur if they are exposed to toxic materials; this may produce a filter effect and reduce the amount of material actually inhaled. When designing inhalation chambers and loading them with animals, it is preferable to err on the side of having a larger chamber volume than was calculated from the chamber loading rule. Most inhalation chambers range in size between 1 and 2 m^3 total capacity. One advantage of whole-body exposure is that the animals are kept in relative comfort. One hypothetical disadvantage is that the location of the animals within the chamber, at least in the case of exposure to particles and aerosols, may to some extent determine what concentrations of the test agent the animals are exposed to (if the agent is fed into the chamber at its top, animals in the bottom cages may receive less of the test agent). This problem is usually circumvented by appropriate chamber design and rapid airflow through the chamber to maintain constant concentrations of inhaled agents. Good chamber design and fast flows (30 changes/h of chamber atmosphere is appropriate) also prevents inappropriate buildup of CO_2 and NH_3 (from animal excreta) in the exposure chamber. As a general rule, fewer animals per chamber is preferable for the above reasons and to minimize spontaneous outbreaks of disease, especially viral, that are prone to occur under crowded conditions. In whole-body exposures, material may become deposited in the fur of the animals, from which it is removed during grooming; it may then become absorbed by the gastrointestinal tract rather than by the lung. The amount of test material needed to achieve the desired chamber concentration is usually quite large, and this may limit exposures to materials in short supply.

Modes of Operation of Chambers Inhalation chambers may be operated in two modes: static or dynamic. In a statically operated chamber, a desired amount of test agent is introduced into or released within an already closed chamber and uniformly distributed by mixing the test agent thoroughly with the air. The animals are then kept in this atmosphere for the desired length of the experiment. This method is only used if comparatively small amounts of test agent are available. The disadvantages of static exposure conditions are that heat and humidity may build up rather rapidly in a totally enclosed system. The chamber concentration of the test agent will of course decrease during exposure time, since some of the agent will be taken up by the animals internally or externally; oxygen depletion and CO_2 and NH_3 accumulation may be another problem.

In a dynamically operated system, the inhalation chamber is ventilated throughout the experiment with a constant flow of air, preferably at a flow rate of at least one-half of the total chamber volume per minute. The test agent is added to the air delivered into the chamber at the desired concentration. This system guarantees a constant concentration of the test agent in the chamber and prevents CO_2 accumulation and oxygen depletion. However, to operate a chamber in a dynamic way uses considerable amounts of test materials, as well as a constant or at least periodic monitoring of the chamber atmosphere; this is necessary to ascertain that the test agent is present at the desired concentrations at all times. A second point to consider is the velocity at which a test agent will equilibrate with the air present in the chamber at the beginning of the experiment. The equation that describes the time it takes until an agent reaches equilibrium within a chamber is

$$C = (W/b)[1 - \exp(bt/a)]$$

where C is the concentration in the chamber after time t, W is the weight of agent introduced per minute, a is the volume of the chamber, and b is flow rate through the chamber. The equation can be used to calculate the time it takes to reach 99% of a desired concentration in the chamber and can be rewritten

$$t = k \left(\frac{a}{b}\right)$$

where a equals chamber volume and b equals flow rate. Note that the second equation does not contain the concentration of the test agent as a factor: the time it takes to obtain any desired percentage of a desired concentration depends only on the volume of the chamber and the flow of air through the chamber. The constant k to reach 99% equilibrium is 4.605. If, for example, one has a 1000-l chamber in which one wants to obtain a concentration of 100% oxygen, it would take approximately 10 min if oxygen is delivered into the chamber at the rate of 500 l/min; if oxygen flow were reduced to only 5 l/min, equilibrium would be reached only after about 15 h. Therefore, it may often be necessary at the beginning of an experiment to operate a dynamic chamber at higher air inflow, in order to reach rapid equilibration. Once the desired concentration has been reached, the airflow may then be reduced.

Nose-Only Exposure Chambers have been designed in which only the head or the nose of an animal is exposed to a toxic inhalant. The test atmosphere is introduced into a cylinder or a rectangular chamber fitted with holes in the wall. Into these holes are inserted conical tubes designed to hold the animals; the nose or head of the animals alone protrudes through the end of the holder into the chamber proper. Advantages of this exposure technique are that the volume of the exposure chamber can be held quite small and therefore less test material is required, and that only a small part of the animal's body will come in direct contact with the test agent. The overall dimensions of nose-only exposure chambers are usually smaller than those of whole body chambers. This allows them to be placed, if necessary, into a large second chamber. This is an advantage when animals are exposed to radioactive aerosols or to carcinogens, which need to be entirely contained. A disadvantage of nose-only exposure is that the animals have to be put into their holders at the beginning of the experiment and removed at the end; the procedure is labor-intensive. A more serious drawback is the stress placed on animals restrained in a tube, with consequent morbidity and even mortality; this requires a shortening of the maximum daily length of exposure. Finally, it is necessary during lifetime exposures to increase gradually the size of the animal holders as the animals grow.

Face Masks   It is possible to fit animals with a tight face mask and to deliver the test atmosphere directly into the mask. Suitable valves at the inlet and outlet of the mask prevent rebreathing of carbon dioxide and of the toxic agent. With this technique, animals must be restrained and the procedure is labor-intensive, making it impractical for large-scale experiments.

Other Methods   Occasionally, quite satisfactory results may be obtained by injecting a test agent directly into the airways; this can be done in anesthetized animals either through a tracheostomy or by inserting a blunt needle under visual control through the mouth and past the vocal chords into the trachea. In larger animals such as dogs, a tracheal cannula can be inserted via tracheostomy and left in place for repeated exposures. The major advantage of intratracheal injections is that they are easy to perform; the main disadvantage is that instilled material may be regurgitated or unevenly distributed within the lung. On the other hand, the intratracheal method offers the unique advantage that, with the help of specialized equipment, circumscribed segments only of the trachea might be exposed to a particular agent (Nettesheim and Marchok, 1983).

Deposition and Clearance

Toxic materials in the inhaled air may be either gases or aerosols; an aerosol consists of droplets of liquid or particles suspended in a gas. Insoluble gases will reach all regions of the lung upon inhalation, unless they are highly irritant and produce voluntary or involuntary cessations of respiratory movements or extensive bronchoconstriction. For highly soluble gases such as SO_2 that are efficiently absorbed by the nasopharynx, penetration into the deeper lung regions may not occur, especially under conditions of nose-only breathing such as is obligatory for laboratory rodents. Inhaled particles, be they droplets of liquid or solid material, may be removed from the lung with the next expiration or, more likely, may become deposited in various regions of the upper respiratory tract, of the tracheobronchial tree, or even in the alveolar zone. Once they have been deposited, particles may be removed from the respiratory tract or they may persist for varying lengths of time within the lung; occasionally they remain there for years. In inhalation toxicology, the term *deposition* is used to denote the initial accumulation of inhaled particles within the nose, the conducting airways, and the functional respiratory units of the alveolar zone. Removal of inhaled and deposited particles from the respiratory tract is called *clearance*; occasionally the term clearance is also used to describe elimination of particles from the entire body if they have been translocated to other organs following original deposition in the lung. *Retention* denotes the fraction of deposited material that is not removed but remains within the body; it may refer to both lung burden or to total body burden of an originally inhaled material. Both deposition and clearance of inhaled particles are of prime importance in determining the toxic potential of inhaled agents (Stuart, 1976; Raabe, 1982).

Mechanisms of Deposition   The initial site of deposition of inhaled particles in the lung depends on the anatomy of the respiratory tract, the air flow and turbulence in the various segments of the conducting airways, and the aerodynamic properties of the inhaled particles. As a general rule, larger particles (5 μm or larger or an equivalent) are deposited in the nasopharynx or in the tracheobronchial tree. For smaller particles (0.1–2 μm diameter), deposition in the conductive airways is usually negligible compared to deposition in the alveolar zone, and total deposition may be roughly equated with alveolar deposition alone. However, these general rules are not absolute. For example, asbestos fibers as large as 50 μm in length (rods 0.4–1 μm in diameter) can penetrate to the alveolar zone. Deposition of particles occurs by three mechanisms: inertial impaction, sedimentation, and diffusion. Particles with an aerodynamic diameter from a few micrometers to more than 100 μm will impact against the walls of upper respiratory passages and of the bronchial tree when the airstream in which they are carried is abruptly deflected by the nasal turbinates or by branching of the airways. The greater the velocity of the airstream and the larger the particle, or the smaller the airway radius is, the greater will be the probability of deposition by inertial impaction of the airway walls.

A second mechanism of deposition is sedimentation by gravity. Particles suspended in air tend to fall; this leads to deposition. Sedimentation is of primary importance in the deposition of particles in the smaller bronchi, the bronchioles, and the alveolar spaces where the airways are small and airflow velocity is low.

Diffusion is the third mode of deposition and applies to particles only with a diameter of 0.5 μm or less. Such small particles, suspended in a gas, are in Brownian motion. This eventually produces contact between particles and surrounding walls of the respiratory tract. Brownian motion increases with decreasing particle size. Diffusional deposition is important in small airways and bronchioles and at airway bifurcations. However, particles of molecular size, as for example radioactive radon and thorium daughters, may also be deposited to a considerable extent by diffusion in the nasal passageways and large airways such as the trachea.

Deposition by inertial impaction occurs mostly in the upper regions of the respiratory tract, where air flow is greatest and where nasal turbinates and bronchial bifurcation cause abrupt changes in air flow. Deposition by sedimentation takes place mainly in small bronchi and bronchioli, and deposition by diffusion occurs mostly in the smallest airways and the alveoli and their associated ducts.

Clearance   The term clearance refers to all mechanisms by which deposition particles are removed from the airways and from the alveolar zone. Highly water-soluble particles and gases are absorbed directly through the epithelial layer of the respiratory tract and reach the bloodstream near their site of original deposition. Insoluble particles behave differently. If deposited in the upper airways and the tracheobronchial tree, structures lined by a ciliated epithelium covered by a mucus blanket, insoluble particles are transported upward by the mucociliary escalator past the larynx into the pharynx; they are either swallowed or removed from the body altogether by coughing. Swallowed material may subsequently be absorbed from the gastrointestinal tract into the general circulation and produce secondary toxic effects.

In the alveoli, no ciliated epithelium or mucus-producing cells are found; rather, the surface of the alveoli is covered with a continuous layer of extracellular material. It consists mainly of phospholipids and is called surfactant; its low surface tension prevents the alveoli from collapsing when the lung volume decreases during expiration. The defense of the alveolar region against foreign materials rests mainly with mobile cells, the alveolar macrophages, which are able to engulf and to destroy microorganisms. They then may migrate upward through the tracheobronchial tree or leave the alveolar zone through the lymphatic vessels; occasionally, macrophages will tend to aggregate beneath the pleura or accumulate around small airways, intraalveolar septa, or small blood vessels. Macropahges may also engulf particles other than microorganisms. However, such materials are not always successfully digested by the macrophages and may even kill and destroy the phagocytic cells. Dead macrophages may be removed by tracheobronchial clearance or retained in granulomas. Many insoluble agents that are deposited in the terminal respiratory units thus have a tendency to remain in this region and elicit abnormal tissue responses such as development of fibrotic changes, rarefaction of pulmonary tissue as in emphysema, or even malignant transformation of pulmonary cells. Insoluble particles smaller than 0.01 μm may become directly embedded in the alveolar interstitial space and eventually diffuse directly into the bloodstream. Removal of foreign particles from the alveolar zone may also occur via the pulmonary lymphatic vessels. On occasion, materials deposited in the alveolar zone may eventually be removed by dissolution and diffusion into the capillary blood.

Dosimetry

The effective dose of a toxic agent may be defined as the amount of a chemical that reaches and interacts with the target site where it produces its untoward effect. This number can only rarely be obtained in toxicity studies. More often, doses are expressed as grams or milligrams of material administered to the test species per kilogram of body weight or per square meter of body surface area.

To express the dose to an organism in an inhalation experiment presents additional problems. If a toxic agent were inhaled in one breath only, then dose might be calculated from the concentration in the inspired single breath and the concentration in the immediately expired air. Calculations of dose would require introduction of a factor that takes into account the partial retention of the agent in the respiratory tract. Theoretically, this factor might vary from 0 to 100%. If the duration of exposure is longer than the time it takes for a complete breath, the dosimetric formula could be written as

$$\text{Dose} = \alpha C t (\text{MV})$$

where α is the retention factor, C is the concentration of test agent in inspired air, t is the time of exposure, and MV is the minute volume.

This formula is an oversimplification, but may be used to yield estimates of dose, provided α, C, t, and MV (under conditions of exposure) are known. The most difficult parameter to estimate is the retention factor α; it depends on the solubility of the agent and, for aerosols, also on particle size. If α is assumed to be 1, the absolute amount of effectively retained agent needed to produce a response will in most instances be overestimated. Experimentally determined values of α are generally closer to 0.1–0.2.

It is customary in inhalation toxicology to express data not in terms of absolute dose, but to make use of the so-called Ct product; C denotes concentration of the agent in the test atmosphere, and t indicates time of exposure. A rule, generally known as Haber's rule, states that for a fixed response, the Ct product is constant; for example, if C_1t_1 produces death of half the animals, then the same will be true for C_2t_2, provided C_1t_1 equals C_2t_2. The rule has two important hypothetical deviations. At extremely high values of C_1, the time to produce a response may no longer become shortened (i.e., the biological response takes a minimum time to develop regardless of how much test agent is absorbed). On the other hand, at extremely low values of C_1, exposure can go indefinitely without the development of a toxic lesion, because of threshold limits (i.e., actual doses absorbed are too small to produce a biological response). Haber's rule is an oversimplification, albeit a useful one; for example, relatively brief transient exposures to high concentrations of ozone result in toxicity related to the maximal level of ozone encountered, not to total concentration × time experience.

For practical purposes, two values may be determined in inhalation studies that give some indication about the toxicity of a test agent. One is called the LC50, or lethal concentration at which 50% of the animals will die within a predetermined test period. The alternative is to expose animals for various lengths of time to a fixed concentration of test agent in air and to calculate the LT50, or lethal time, the time it takes for half of the animals to die in this particular atmosphere.

RESPONSE OF THE LUNG TO INJURY

The effects of toxic inhaled materials on the respiratory tract can be assessed in several ways. A great many foreign agents with widely differing chemical structures can gain access to the respiratory tract. However, the conducting airways and the terminal respiratory units of the lung generally respond in almost sterotypical ways only to acute or chronic insult. The primary damage produced by the initial interaction of a toxic substance with the pulmonary tissue is usually followed by repair processes (Witschi and Côté, 1977). Whether the initial damage to the cells of the lung results in cell death without recovery, is successfully repaired, or will elicit a chronic, sometimes worsening, condition depends on the nature of the toxic material and on the quantities deposited in the lung. Whether the agent can be successfully removed from the lung or whether it will persist, and whether exposure is a single episode or repeated several times over a lifetime, are other important factors in determining ultimate toxicity.

Airways

In the conducting airways, noxious inhalants such as sulfur dioxide (SO_2) may affect the functions of the ciliated and secretory cells. Inhibition of ciliary movement may slow down the flow of mucus and thus removal of particles through the mucociliary escalator. Acute and, more importantly, chronic damage to the secretory cells lining the airways can also diminish proper formation of mucus and produce changes in its chemical composition (Reid, 1978). Secretory cells undergo changes in appearance and may increase in number (metaplasia, hyperplasia). This produces a shift in the overall cell population lining the conducting airways. Excessive mucus produced both by cell dysfunction and by increased numbers of mucus-producing cells can eventually plug the conducting airways. The cells lining the conducting airways, after prolonged exposure to chemicals, can also undergo metaplasia and eventually malignant transformation and give origin to bronchogenic carcinoma (Harris, 1978).

In the smallest airways, the terminal bronchioles, a common event is acute cell death followed by tissue recovery. The walls of the terminal bronchioles are lined essentially by two cell types, the so-called Clara cells and the ciliated cells. Ciliated cells are readily damaged by several agents, particularly nitrogen dioxide (NO_2) and ozone, two components of photochemical smog. Irreversibly damaged ciliated cells may be replaced by division and proliferation of the nonciliated or Clara cells; acutely damaged ciliated cells can therefore be effectively replaced, but we do not yet understand the function of consequences of such cellular changes (Evans et al., 1976b). However, Clara cells themselves are vulnerable; newer experiments document that they are particularly rich in drug-metabolizing enzymes and have the capability to activate foreign compounds into highly reactive and toxic metabolites (Boyd, 1980). This can cause widespread destruction and death of Clara cells, precluding successful recovery of the bronchiolar epithelium. Sustained chemical insults to the bronchiolar epithelium may decrease the number of Clara cells while increasing the number of goblet cells and stimulating mucus production. These changes may be accompanied by proliferation of the smooth muscle cells and fibroblasts and by infiltration of migratory inflammatory cells. Chronic alterations of this kind in the small airways is thought to be the fundamental mechanism underlying chronic obstructive lung disease (Niewoehner and Cosio, 1978).

Alveolar Zone

Agents that reach the terminal respiratory units may cause acute death of the alveolar epithelial cells and of the capillary endothelial cells. There seems to be no general rule that the route of access to the alveoli determines the initial site of damage. Inhalants may cause necrosis of either first the epithelial cells, as does for example NO_2 or ozone, or first the endothelial cells, as does oxygen; on the other hand, certain bloodborne agents may cause initial damage to the endothelium (bleomycin), whereas others first damage the epithelium (paraquat). Damage to the cells of the air–blood barrier is followed by sloughing off of the dead cells into the alveolar spaces, by formation of hyaline membranes, by leakage of fluid into the alveoli (edema), and by leakage and migration of inflammatory cells into the airspaces (Witschi and Côté, 1977).

Alveolar type I cells appear to be more susceptible to toxic agents than are type II cells; it is thought that the type I cells with their organelle-poor cytoplasm are less able to resist chemical insult. Type I cell necrosis is a common feature in many forms of toxic lung damage. To replace the damaged epithelium, type II cells begin to proliferate, to divide, and to transform eventually into type I cells, thus restoring again a normal air–blood barrier (Adamson and Bowden, 1974). Necrotic capillary endothelial cells are replaced by proliferation and division of undamaged endothelium. In many instances, particularly following a single episode of insult to the lung parenchyma, a morphologically and functionally normal air–blood barrier is restored by this process within a few days.

Two of the most frequent chronic lesions in the alveolar region are fibrosis and emphysema. Repeated chemical insults to the cells of the alveoli may interfere with efficient recovery, and alveoli may become lined with a thickened epithelium, consisting of cuboidally shaped cells, instead of with a thin epithelial layer. Type II alveolar and capillary endothelial cells are not the only cells that proliferate following toxic lung injury. Fibroblasts lying within the alveolar septa may begin to divide, presumably under the influence of factors produced by the accompanying influx of inflammatory and phagocytic cells into the alveoli. The result is a profound change in the cell population forming the alveolar zone, characterized by a decrease in type I epithelial cells, an increase in cells resembling type II epithelial cells, accumulation of macrophages, and an increase in the interstitial cells, particularly fibroblasts and smooth muscle cells. The process may be accompanied by an increase in the amount of collagen present in the alveolar zone with a progressive thickening of the air–blood barrier and impairment of gas exchange (Rennard et al., 1982). This condition, if it persists, may develop into pulmonary fibrosis. The term fibrosis denotes only the morphologic and functional aspects of the disease and does not necessarily give an indication as to its etiology; while numerous toxic agents have the potential to cause pulmonary fibrosis, such as paraquat, bleomycin, or even radiation damage to the lung, most pulmonary fibrosis seen in humans remains of unknown origin.

Emphysema denotes another form of chronic lung damage. In this disease there is a decrease and restructuring of the connective-tissue elements supporting the alveolar structures, and a subsequent remodeling of the alveolar space. The end result is an abnormal dilation of the air spaces with accompanying destruction of the walls of many alveoli, of alveolar ducts, and of terminal respiratory bronchioles. In emphysema, gas exchange is severely compromised, mainly because air can no longer be moved efficiently into and out of the enlarged air spaces (Kuhn et al., 1982).

Cancer originating from the cells of the alveolar walls or from the cells lining the surface of the lung, the pleural cells, is much rarer than cancer originating from the bronchial epithelium. In certain mouse strains, both benign (adenoma) and malignant (adenocarcinoma) tumors arising from type II alveolar cells are readily induced by a great many carcinogens, regardless of route of exposure (inhalation or injection) (Shimkin and Stoner, 1975).

Initial responses of the cells of the lung to toxic insults include acute cell proliferation as an attempt to repair the damage. Cell death is often accompanied by leakage of fluid or blood into the air space, infiltration by inflammatory cells, and altered biochemical functions, such as abnormal production of mucus. If the insult is repeated, the cell population in the lung may change, and this can cause narrowing of the small airways, thickening of the air–blood barrier, or rarefication of the alveolar septum, with resulting increases in air space. All of these processes are likely to decrease the efficiency of the lung by inhibiting gas exchange.

ANALYSIS OF TOXIC LUNG DAMAGE

Morphological Methods

Examination of the tissues of the respiratory tract by gross inspection and under the microscope allows detection and identification of acute lung damage, chronic degenerative changes, and development of cancerous lesions. Any morphologic evaluation not only should focus on the lung parenchyma proper, but should also involve an inspection of the nasal turbinates, the larynx, and the large conducting airways. Occasionally it is of advantage to clear the lungs with appropriate procedures and to inspect them under a dissection microscope. This is particularly important if one wishes to detect the presence of tumors in the conducting airways or in the alveolar zone (Dungworth et al., 1976).

Preparation of tissue for histological analysis needs careful consideration of methods of fixation, selection of tissue blocks, and sectioning. Proper fixation may be accomplished either by perfusion of the lungs with fixative through the pulmonary artery or by installation through the trachea into the airways: proper head pressure of fixative must be used in order to avoid creation of artifacts. Ordinary paraffin sections will give a general impression of tissue lesions; however, such sections are usually too thick to allow identification of individual cell types in the lung. Tissue embedded in epon or glycol methacrylate can be cut in section of 1 μm or less. Individual cell types can then be identified with certainty.

Fine-structural alterations in the lung parenchyma, such as degenerative changes and necrosis of type I pneumonocytes, are usually only detected with certainty by using transmission electron microscopy. Scanning electron microscopy allows one to visualize the surface of interior lung structures, permits identification of alterations of the tissue surface, and will detect rearrangement of cells in the overall cell population. An advantage of this technique is that it allows comparative examination of large areas of the lung and detection of structural changes such as emphysema. Histochemical methods are used to attempt to correlate biochemical findings with morphology; however, histochemistry of the lung requires that sections be cut at considerable thickness, and this makes identification of individual cell types difficult.

Autoradiography has proved to be a particularly valuable tool to study acute lung damage. If animals are injected with radioactive thymidine, those lung cells that actively synthesize DNA will become selectively labeled. It has been documented that an excellent correlation exists between the extent of damage to type I alveolar cells, produced by inhalation of a toxic agent, and the subsequent proliferation of type II cells; measurement of DNA synthesis in lung may be used under certain conditions as an approach to detect and quantitate initial toxic damage (Evans et al., 1978). Cell kinetic studies done by autoradiography have established the important role the type II alveolar cells and bronchiolar Clara cells play in the renewal of damaged epithelium. Autoradiographic studies may also be used to examine the fate of toxic inhaled materials and to identify those cell types that preferentially metabolize certain compounds.

Morphometric techniques allow one to quantitate the number of cells in a given lung area or a given lung volume and to measure the volume of cells, the thickness of the air–blood barrier, the volume and number of intracellular organelles, and the size of air spaces (Weibel, 1973). While extremely useful for obtaining quantitative information, morphometric techniques tend to be time-consuming and to require that careful consideration be given to adequate sampling procedures and to adequate techniques. Their use in routine toxicological evaluation of toxic lung damage has therefore been somewhat limited, although ultimately quantitation morphometric techniques must be used to define subtle damage occurring at low levels of toxic exposure (Barry and Crapo, 1985).

Respiratory-Function Tests

Respiratory-function tests were originally developed in humans and are used clinically to detect and quantitate pathologic changes in the structure of the respiratory system. Most human tests have been adapted for use in laboratory animals and allow one to measure the performance of the lung after exposure to toxic agents. Many tests require an active cooperation of the subject, as for example tests involving breath holding, forced inspiration, or forced expiration. In animals it is obviously impossible to obtain such cooperation. Methods have therefore been developed that allow one to measure certain parameters by forcing the animals to perform the desired maneuvers. This can be accomplished by placing the entire animal into a body plethysmograph. By variation of the pressure on the entire body in an airtight chamber, the thorax will compress or expand and the lungs will be ventilated in a passive way. Similar results may be obtained by cannulating the trachea and producing changes in lung volume with air flowing through the cannula into the lung or by mimicking expiration by air withdrawal. Some measurements, such as pressure–volume curves, may also be done on excised lungs after the animals have been killed.

An overview of currently used pulmonary function tests is given below; for more detailed analysis and reference, the review by Wilson et al. (1976) should be consulted (Table 1).

Ventilation Respiratory rate and tidal volume can easily be measured in both humans and experimental animals with conventional spirometric techniques. The total volume of breathing in 1 min (minute ventilation) can be obtained by multiplying the frequency of breaths by the volume of air inspired with each breath.

Static Lung Volumes Total lung capacity, vital capacity, and residual volume are determined by inhalation of an inert gas such as helium; the gas will eventually equilibrate throughout the lung, and total lung volume can be measured from its distribution. To measure vital capacity, a maximal inspiratory and expiratory effort is needed in humans; in animals, vital capacity can be measured by applying external

Table 1 Respiratory-Function Parameters[a]

Parameters	Definition
Respiratory rate	Frequency of breathing per minute
Tidal volume	Volume of air exchanged per normal breath
Minute ventilation	Volume of air exchanged in 1 min
Total lung capacity (TLC)	Air volume in entire lung
Vital capacity (VC)	Air volume exhaled by maximum expiration following maximum inspiration
Residual volume (RV)	Air remaining in lung after a normal expiration
Compliance	Index of stiffness of the respiratory system; decreased compliance indicates increased stiffness
Forced expired volume versus time	Overall mechanical lung function
Closing volume	Closure of small airways
Pulmonary blood flow	
Diffusion capacity	Gas exchange across air–blood barrier in the alveolus
Blood-gas analysis	Efficiency of gas exchange and index of total alveolar ventilation

[a]Compiled from Murray (1976), MacFarland (1976), and Wilson et al. (1976).

distending and withdrawing pressures to the lung. Additional static lung volumes are expiratory reserve volume (defined as the amount of air that can be expired after a normal expiration by additional effort), functional residual capacity (lung volume at the end of a normal expiration), and inspiratory capacity (additional maximal air intake after a normal inspiration).

Respiratory Mechanics Lung expands during inspiration by expansion of the thoracic cage and a downward movement of the diaphragm. The lung closely follows the movement of the chest wall because it is tightly coupled to it by a thin film of liquid lying between the outer surface of the lung and the inner chest wall. During expiration the elastic tissue within the lung retracts and exhalation occurs passively. Even after the deepest forced expiration, the lung tissue is still partially expanded, and an excised lung (or if air is introduced into the pleural space) will recoil further and assume a much smaller volume than it actually occupies within the thoracic cavity. The lung must therefore comply with normal movements of the chest wall. Many disease processes affect the elastic properties of the lung tissue, and the lung may no longer follow expansion of the thorax wall with ease. An index of the functional stiffness of the respiratory system is the so-called compliance. It reflects the distention of the elastic respiratory system and may be defined as the rate of change in volume with change in pressure. Compliance is determined by plotting changes in lung volume during inspiration and expiration against pleural pressure; pleural pressure can be measured with comparative ease in the esophagus. Compliance may also be determined by measuring static volume–pressure curves on excised lungs. Pathologic processes that diminish the elastic properties of the lung—for example, fibrosis or other infiltrative diseases—will usually produce a decrease in compliance, whereas other conditions, such as loss of lung tissue as in emphysema, may increase pulmonary compliance. When air-filled lungs are studied, content and quality of surfactant have a predominant effect on the pressure–volume curves. Hence, lung compliance is best determined with saline-filled lungs, where pressure–volume curves accurately reflect distensibility of tissue.

The overall mechanical function of the lungs and of the thoracic wall can also be evaluated by measurement of the volume of forced expired air versus time. Often the volume of air exhaled during the first second of forced expiration is taken as an index of airflow (FEV_1); more refined techniques determine flow rate at various lung volumes. The test can be done in both animals and humans. Resistance to airflow is mainly determined by the first generation of major airways and is not greatly affected by more peripheral changes in the lung parenchyma. Increased resistance to airflow may be caused by changes in the muscular tone of the airways (bronchospasm), swelling of the mucosa by edema, or increased amounts of mucus in the bronchial lumen. Early literature on pulmonary-function testing in animals often failed to make proper allowances for resistance to airflow in cannulas or tubing, thereby generating artifacts in these determinations. Obviously, resistance to flow must be a property of the lungs and not of the plumbing for these results to be valid.

Distribution of Ventilation Pathologic changes in the conducting airways may produce uneven distribution of pulmonary ventilation; techniques have been developed in humans and in larger animals to detect this condition. A commonly used technique is to replace inhaled air by 100% oxygen; upon repeated expiration, nitrogen is washed out from the lung and the so-called single-breath N_2-washout curve may provide evidence for uneven distribution of ventilation.

During maximum expiration, the small airways with a diameter less than 1 mm in the lower lung portions are believed to close, leaving trapped air behind in the alveoli. In a forced expiratory maneuver, the fraction of the vital capacity not yet expired at the moment the small airways collapse can be determined and is referred to as *closing volume*. It can be measured in humans and in experimental animals. Diseases of the small airways may cause them to collapse earlier than normal, and this may produce an increase in closing volume. The closing volume has been advocated by some as representing a sensitive test to detect early pathologic changes in the small airways.

Pulmonary Circulation Pulmonary blood flow, blood volume, and pressure may be studied by cardiac catheterization in both animals and humans. Toxic agents will often produce abnormal leakage of fluid out of the vascular bed into the alveoli and the pulmonary interstitial tissue. Leakage of large molecules can be measured by the use of radiolabeled serum proteins. A convenient and simple, but sensitive, method to detect the presence of pulmonary edema is to determine the wet weight/dry weight ratio in lung; this can only be done on the excised tissue of freshly killed animals.

Diffusion An abnormal thickening of the air–blood barrier may inhibit proper gas diffusion between alveolar air and blood. The term diffusion capacity for any gas denotes the amount of gas that crosses the air–blood barrier per unit time for a given mean pressure difference of the gas in the alveolar air and the pulmonary capillary blood. Most inert gases diffuse rapidly and quickly establish equilibrium in pressure between air and blood. Oxygen and CO combine chemically with the hemoglobin (Hb) of the red blood cells. In order to saturate the blood hemoglobin, O_2 or CO must diffuse in such large quantities across the alveolar–capillary membrane that it may not be possible to reach complete equilibrium, and a detectable alveolar end–capillary pressure difference may be detected. Both gases may therefore be used to measure diffusion capacity. CO is most frequently used; if CO is inhaled in small amounts, it will immediately combine with red-cell Hb, and its partial pressure in the blood will remain practically zero. Diffusion capacity can thus be expressed as the quantity of CO crossing the air–blood barrier per unit time in response to its mean pressure in the alveolar air. As an alternative to physiological measurements of diffusion capacity, the use of morphometric techniques has been suggested (Weibel, 1973).

Blood-Gas Analysis Pulmonary-function tests can be complemented by determining the tensions or pressures of oxygen and CO_2 in arterial or venous blood. Reduced arterial oxygen tension may indicate impaired ventilation, uneven blood flow to the different regions of the lung, or a decrease in diffusion capacity. Impaired pulmonary function may also produce an increase in arterial CO_2 pressure and a decrease in blood pH; however, metabolic factors and renal function may also affect the same parameters, and the data must thus be interpreted taking all these possibilities into account.

Biochemical Parameters of Toxic Lung Damage

Many biochemical processes in the lung are affected and profoundly altered by toxic agents (Witschi and Côté, 1977; Mustafa and Tierney, 1978) (Table 2). Ideally, it should thus be possible to measure and to quantitate pathologic changes with biochemical techniques. However, it has not been possible to establish causal relationships between biochemical alterations and cell degeneration and cell death in lung. In view of the considerable cellular heterogeneity of lung tissue, it is often not possible to detect biochemical changes that occur only in highly selected or comparatively small cell populations. The problem is compounded by the observation that a reduction in food intake may considerably change the activity of several enzymes and metabolic pathways in the lung; biochemical changes in the lung originally attributed directly to a toxic agent may merely reflect altered food intake. Many workers have shown that several oxidant gases will depress lung mitochondrial respiration, inhibit or destroy microsomal enzymes, influence pulmonary synthesis of protein and other macromolecules, reduce pulmonary surfactant levels, or initiate lipid peroxidation of

Table 2   Selected Biochemical Parameters of Toxic Lung Damage[a]

Indicator	Damage indicated
Wet weight/dry weight ratio	Increased in most forms of pulmonary edema
Total lung wet weight	Increased in all forms of pulmonary edema
Incorporation of thymidine into pulmonary DNA	Cell proliferation following injury; inflammatory changes
Lipid metabolism, particularly quantity and biosynthesis of surfactant	Status of metabolic integrity of type II alveolar cells
Collagen biosynthesis	Fibrotic changes
Glucose-6-phosphate dehydrogenase (G6PDH)	Increased activity of pentose shunt or changes in lung cell populations
Ethane and pentane production	Lipid peroxidation that may lead to tissue damage; however, tissue of origin is uncertain and gut microflora may be an important source
Sulfhydryl metabolism; glutathione levels and nonprotein SH-group	Defense mechanisms against oxidant damage or changes in lung cell populations
Superoxide dismutase (SOD)	Oxidant tolerance or lung cell changes
Glutathione peroxidase	Oxidant tolerance or lung cell changes
Catalase	Oxidant tolerance or lung cell changes, presence of blood in lung

[a]Compiled from Witschi and Côté (1977) and Mustafa and Tierney (1978).

biological membranes (Mustafa and Tierney, 1978). However, these studies have been of rather limited value in quantifying pulmonary injury. Since many pulmonary toxins cause pulmonary edema soon after administration, an increase in lung weight or an increase in the ratio of pulmonary wet to dry weight is one of the earliest reliable indices of acute toxic lung damage. With certain compounds undergoing metabolic activation in the lung, it has also been possible to correlate lung toxicity with the amount of toxic agent covalently bound to pulmonary macromolecules.

In many forms of toxic lung injury, the initial damage to the tissue is followed within a few days by a period of reparative processes. Toxic agents may initiate, as a secondary response, cell proliferation, formation of increased amounts of tissue constituents such as collagen and elastin, and changes in the activities of several enzymes related to the inflammatory influx of cells to sites of injury. Cell proliferation in lung, if it is substantial following necrosis of alveolar epithelial cells, may be quantitated by measurement of pulmonary DNA synthesis. Although the biochemical approach does not allow identification of which cell types proliferate, the technique provides quantitative information with ease and speed. Formation of excessive amounts of collagen and evaluation of the rate of collagen synthesis can be another reliable indicator of a reaction to a toxic injury (Last et al., 1979). Enzymes involved in the pentose phos-

phate pathway, particularly G6PDH,* are often measured as an indicator of pulmonary injury and/or repair, and the activity of SOD,[†] is often measured to assess the
influence of exposure to oxidants, particularly oxygen. Overall changes in the pulmonary amounts of nucleic acids, proteins, and phospholipids indicate changes in the
pulmonary cell population. Altered biosynthesis of mucus in tracheal explants may
reflect changes in the number and activity of mucus-secreting cells and thus complement histopathological analysis (Last et al., 1977). Induction of mixed-function oxidases, particularly AHH,[‡] often occurs within hours after insult to pulmonary parenchyma and may be used as a biochemical parameter for monitoring exposure to toxic
inhalants.

In summary, evaluation of the effects of toxic agents on airways and lung parenchyma has in the past relied mainly on qualitative pathological evaluation of the lung,
complemented by pulmonary-function tests. By a combination of both approaches,
specific information as to nature and extent of lesions in the respiratory apparatus
becomes available. Biochemical studies to assess toxic lung damage are feasible,
although specificity and sensitivity are not as satisfactory, especially in acutely damaged lung, as for histopathological analyses.

LUNG INJURY CAUSED BY CHEMICALS

General

Lung tissue may become damaged by a wide variety of chemical agents. For the
purpose of the following discussion, we may arbitrarily divide chemicals into three
large classes. In one group we place agents to which a comparatively large segment
of the population is exposed at one time or another. Among them are the so-called air
pollutants, most notably ozone, nitrogen oxides, and sulfur oxides. However, it must
be realized that these gases are not the only components of polluted air; other chemicals present include formaldehyde, acrolein, peroxyacetyl nitrate (PAN), a vast variety of hydrocarbons emitted in the exhaust of gasoline and diesel-powered internal
combustion engines, particulate matter, and other agents produced by burning of
fossil fuels, particularly coal. A special form of "voluntary" (or involuntary with
respect to sidestream smoke) air pollution is cigarette smoking: tobacco smoke is a
complex mixture of over 1500 or more identified compounds.

Much research has been done during the last decade on the toxicology of air
pollutants. Ozone, nitrogen oxides, and sulfur dioxide will be discussed in this section
in more detail because of their overall presence in polluted air and also because their
mechanism of action has been elucidated to a great extent. This will be followed by a
discussion of oxygen toxicity. Oxygen toxicity may be a problem in medicine. Recently, much progress has been made toward understanding its mechanism of action
from the cellular to the molecular level.

*G6PDH, glucose 6-phosphate dehydrogenase.
[†]SOD, superoxide dismutase.
[‡]AHH, aryl hydrocarbon hydroxylase.

For a second class of agents, exposure occurs mostly in industrial settings. Chronic lung disease caused by mineral dusts such as silica, asbestos, or coal dust has been known for a long time. Metals such as aluminum, antimony, beryllium, tin, and several others, if inhaled, damage the respiratory tract. Other agents may sensitize particularly susceptible individuals and cause occupational asthma; grain dust, enzymatic detergents, and certain solvents such as toluene diisocyanate are known to produce this kind of lung damage. Allergic alveolitis can be caused by inhalation of organic dust, among them bacteria, yeasts, molds, pollen, and organic fibers. Examples of such disease are farmer's lung, produced by spores of certain thermophilic actinomycetes growing on moldy hay, and bagassosis, caused by exposure to moldy bagasse (sugar cane). Byssinosis is a lung disease caused by inhalation of cotton bracts (fine cotton dust). Of all these possible etiological agents, silica, asbestos, and the metals beryllium, cadmium, and nickel will be discussed in more detail; additional information can be found in textbooks of toxicology, lung pathology, or occupational lung disease.

Lung damage may also be caused by agents that are carried into the lung via the bloodstream. One of the best-known examples is the herbicide paraquat, which, if swallowed, will cause extensive and often fatal lung damage in humans and experimental animals within a few days. Among other agents, there are several drugs such as the anticancer agents busulfan, cyclophosphamide, and bleomycin, the antibacterial agent nitrofurantoin, naturally occurring agents such as 4-ipomeanol, perilla ketone, and pyrrolizidine alkaloids, the antioxidant butylated hydroxytoluene, and many others. A recent review on drug-induced lung disease (Gillett and Ford, 1978) lists nearly 100 drugs known to damage the lung. The morphologic and biochemical events caused by many bloodborne toxicants have been summarized (Witschi and Côté, 1977). In this section, the agents paraquat, bleomycin, 4-ipomeanol, and 3-methylfuran will be reviewed in some detail in order to provide an overview of possible mechanisms of action for agents causing lung damage when administered systemically.

Air Pollutants

Ozone
Human Toxicity Ozone is naturally present in the higher atmosphere. In the human environment it is produced in photochemical smog. It may also be represent in the cabins of high-flying aircraft and in the gas produced by arc welding. In a polluted atmosphere, considerable amounts of ozone may be formed if ultraviolet (UV) light interacts with NO_2. This sets in motion a series of photochemical reactions that eventually produce ozone. Ozone is a respiratory irritant. Exposure usually causes acute signs of discomfort such as chest pain and irritation of the upper airways; if inhaled in sufficient concentrations, ozone may produce fatal acute pulmonary edema. Controlled studies in humans have detected impaired pulmonary function following inhalation of ozone, such as a reduced forced expiratory volume, increase in airway resistance, decrease in vital capacity, and decreased diffusion capacity. Effects have

been observed during exposure to as low an ozone concentration as 0.2 ppm for 2 h. Concentrations above 0.6 ppm are usually not well tolerated. Vigorous exercise may increase the undesirable effects of inhaled ozone, since more ozone reaches the deep regions of the lung if ventilation is increased (National Research Council, 1977b).

Animal Toxicity Exposure of rodents to ozone concentrations of 4.5–5.0 ppm for 3 h causes death (drowning) from pulmonary edema. Common values encountered in the Southern California Air Basin in summer months are as high as 0.5 ppm peak concentration, and about 0.2 ppm average concentration. Exposure to concentrations as low as 1–3 ppm for a few hours or 0.4–5.0 ppm for a few days are sufficient to produce pathologic changes in the deep regions of the lung. These changes are similar to those found with other oxidants. Death of alveolar and bronchiolar epithelial cells is preceded by abnormal swelling of the mitochondria, blebbing, and eventual disruption of the cell membrane, followed by leakage of serum and formed blood elements into the air spaces. The initial phase of tissue destruction is followed by tissue repair (Evans et al., 1976a; Schwartz et al., 1976). Changes in pulmonary function measured in animals include increase in respiratory frequency and increase in airway flow resistance. Chronic exposure of animals to ozone over prolonged periods of time produces fibrotic changes in the lung. Early experiments suggesting that chronic exposure to ozone causes emphysema may need to be investigated with healthy animals exposed to pure ozone in air; early workers did not use respiratory-disease-free rodents and usually generated ozone from air (by electric discharge), thereby giving rise to NO_2, a known emphysematous agent, as well.

Mechanism of Action In model systems using artificial membranes, ozone in the presence of water will produce short-chain aldehydes and hydrogen peroxide as major products. The reaction is called ozonolysis and must be clearly distinguished from lipid peroxidation; ozonolysis does not involve formation of free-radical intermediates, lipid peroxides, or conjugation of double bonds. However, an endpoint of both ozonolysis and lipid peroxidation is malonaldehyde. This compound is often measured in studies on the interaction of ozone with membrane systems, and accordingly the terms *ozonization* and *peroxidation* are usually used synonomously. However, it has been stressed that lipid peroxidation in biological systems exposed to ozone is only a secondary event (Mudd and Freeman, 1977). Although ozone increases the permeability of model membrane systems in vivo, actual ozonization of lipid components of membranes may be a secondary event only. It is conceivable that in vivo ozone not only may react preferentially with proteins of the cell membrane but may even penetrate, without harming the cell membrane, into the cell's interior before causing damage. For example, in alveolar macrophages, ozone does not inhibit uptake of bacteria by the cells but inhibits enzymes involved in their subsequent digestion. This suggests that ozone may inhibit enzymes within cells, rather than having a primary deleterious effect on cell membranes. Biochemical investigation on lungs of animals exposed to ozone have shown swelling of mitochondria, decreased mitochondrial respiration, and decreased activity of microsomal enzymes. Ultimately, cell death may result from a combination of the effects of ozone both on cellular membranes and on key enzymes in cellular metabolism.

Modifying Factors Ozone toxicity is thought to be a consequence of its oxidant capacity. Pulmonary damage resulting from ozone exposure can be altered by manipulation of the various host biological antioxidant systems. Vitamin E functions as a chemical antioxidant. Animals fed diets directly deficient in vitamin E exhibit an increased susceptibility to ozone toxicity; however, supplementing the diet with vitamin E does not diminish the toxicity of ozone in animals fed a complete diet. The glutathione peroxidase–glutathione reductase system also appears to be involved in protecting mammalian cells from ozone-induced damage, based on experiments performed with selenium-deficient rats (Se is a cofactor for lung glutathione peroxidase). Exposure of animals to low levels of ozone enables them to withstand a subsequent exposure to normally lethal levels. The basis of this tolerance probably relates to changes in pulmonary and nonpulmonary cells caused by the low-level exposure. Conversely, selenium-deficient animals, which have decreased activity of the selenoenzyme glutathione peroxidase, are more susceptible to ozone-induced damage. There is no cross-tolerance between ozone and oxygen, suggesting different mechanisms of action of these two oxidant gases, even though ozone and NO_2 do exhibit cross-tolerance.

Oxides of Nitrogen

Human Toxicity Oxides of nitrogen (NO_x) originate from many natural and human made processes. The largest amount of NO_x released into the atmosphere comes from the heating of atmosphere N_2 that occurs during the combustion of fossil fuels such as coal, oil, or gasoline; emissions from gasoline-powered automobiles and from oil-burning power plants are the two most important sources of NO_x in the atmosphere. Oxides of nitrogen are a major component of photochemical smog. The compound of most concern for human health is nitrogen dioxide (NO_2), both in its own right and as an immediate precursor of ozone. Large amounts of NO_2 are usually not directly emitted into the atmosphere, but arise from photochemical oxidation of nitric oxide (NO). Chronic exposure to NO_2 has been linked directly to lung diseases in man (National Research Council, 1977a). The impact of NO_2 upon the human respiratory tract has been studied both in controlled exposure studies and by analysis of the health impact of episodes of accidental or occupational accumulation of high NO_2 concentrations in the ambient air. Exposure to NO_2 under controlled conditions has shown that NO_2 may cause narrowing of the airways, accompanied by an increase in flow resistance and a reduction in maximum air expiratory flow rate. In episodes where humans were exposed accidentally to extremely high concentrations of NO_2 (150–200 ppm), severe respiratory distress developed, followed later by obliteration of the small airways through proliferation of connective tissue (bronchiolitis obliterans). This process has resulted in human fatalities (for example, silo filler's disease). Exposure to lower levels of NO_2 produces bronchopneumonia and reversible inflammatory changes in the small airways. It is also believed that exposure to NO_2 may be followed by an increased incidence of respiratory disease caused by infectious agents. Of particular concern is epidemiologic evidence suggesting that children exposed to NO_2 in early life might be susceptible to more frequent development of respiratory illness at a later age. There is, therefore, good evidence to suggest that exposure to NO_2 (as well as to other oxides of nitrogen) is instrumental in producing human lung disease.

Animal Toxicity   Exposure to less than 25 ppm of NO_2 rarely produces acute lethality in experimental animals. However, changes in lung structure and function may be seen in animals exposed to concentrations of NO_2 as low as 0.5–2 ppm after exposure times of only a few hours. In animals exposed continuously to NO_2, lung damage develops within the first 24 h of exposure. Damage is usually first seen in the terminal bronchioles and spreads into the proximal portions of the alveolar ducts. It is characterized by necrosis of the ciliated bronchiolar and alveolar epithelial cells, accompanied by exudation of fibrin and macrophage aggregation. Repair is accomplished by proliferation of the Clara cells and the type II pneumonocytes (Evans et al., 1976b). Newborn and young animals are relatively resistant to NO_2, whereas in older animals pulmonary edema develops more readily. Old animals also show a delay in onset of replacement of injured alveolar cells. Changes in interstitial connective tissue may lead to a thickening of the alveolar walls, and later pathologic changes resembling emphysema develop. Animals exposed acutely to NO_2 increase markedly their respiratory rate and, upon chronic exposure, develop decreased compliance and reduced lung volumes (i.e., fibrosis or restrictive lung disease).

Mechanism of Action NO_2 is relatively insoluble in water, hence penetrating more deeply into the lung than does ozone (which is about seven times more water-soluble than is NO_2). Small amounts of NO_2 are absorbed into the mucous layer covering the epithelium of the nasal cavity, where NO_2 can react with water to form nitric and nitrous acids (HNO_3 and HNO_2), respectively. Once absorbed in the upper airways or in the deeper portions of the lung, NO_2 or its chemical derivatives may be retained in the lung for long periods of time. Two mechanisms to account for the pulmonary toxicity of NO_2 have been postulated: NO_2 may initiate lipid peroxidation, which would subsequently cause cell injury and death, or NO_2 may oxidize proteins and low-molecular-weight substances such as sulfhydryl compounds and pyridine nucleotides (Menzel, 1976). Evidence that lipid peroxidation is a pathogenetic mechanism in NO_2 toxicity is derived chiefly from in vitro experiments that have demonstrated that NO_2 can initiate oxidation of unsaturated fatty acids via a free-radical mechanism. Acute exposure to NO_2 also affects several pulmonary enzymes, such as increased activity of the hexose monophosphate shunt or the citric acid cycle. It is not yet clear, however, to what extent these changes reflect true alterations in pulmonary biochemistry rather than changes in the cellular composition of the lung with accompanying secondary biochemical changes.

Modifying Factors   It has been shown in several species that NO_2 increases the susceptibility of pulmonary tissue to infectious agents. Animals are exposed to NO_2 and, following cessation of exposure, challenged with an aerosol containing infectious microorganisms such as *Klebsiella pneumoniae* or influenza A/PR-8 virus. Mortality in NO_2-exposed animals is usually significantly higher than in controls and increases in proportion to the concentration of NO_2 inhaled or the length of exposure to NO_2 (Ehrlich et al., 1970). It is important to note, however, that inoculum sizes of bacteria or viruses in these experiments are orders of magnitude larger than occur naturally. One important conclusion of these studies is that the concentration of NO_2 to which animal are exposed is more important than the duration of the exposure. In addition, intermittent exposure to NO_2 may have essentially the same effect as continuous exposure, although a longer intermittent exposure time is required to elicit quantitively similar effects as those observed after continuous exposure. The increased susceptibility of the lung to infectious agents after NO_2 inhalation may be due to an impairment of mucociliary transport, or, more likely, may be caused by damage to the alveolar macrophages. Increased susceptibility to NO_2 may also be brought about by environmental stress. In vitro, such antioxidants as butylated hydroxytoluene or butylated hydroxyanisole retard the autooxidation of unsaturated fatty acids induced by NO_2 and it is tempting to speculate that, in vivo, antioxidants might similarly afford protection against free radical reactions (Menzel, 1976).

Sulfur Oxides

Human Toxicity The burning of fossil fuel, particularly of coal, releases sulfur-containing products such as SO_2, sulfuric acid, and organic sulfates into the atmosphere. More than 95% of the total SO_x in urban polluted atmospheres at low relative humidity and relatively low intensity of sunlight (i.e., northeastern and midwestern urban United States, northern Europe) is in the form of SO_2. At concentrations found in heavily polluted community air, SO_2 produces discomfort, irritation of the eyes and of the nasal mucosa, and bronchial constriction. Bronchoconstriction develops in normal people exposed to 1–5 ppm SO_2, although particularly susceptible individuals (e.g., asthmatics) may react at lower concentrations (although controversial, levels as low as 0.1–0.2 ppm have been reported). Decreased flow of nasal mucus after exposure to SO_2 has been observed. If SO_2-containing air is inhaled through the nose, most SO_2, which is very soluble in water, is absorbed in the nasal passages; during mouth breathing, more SO_2 may be expected to reach the conducting airways, and impairment of mucociliary clearance mechanisms might compromise the capability of the respiratory tract to deal effectively with the inhaled toxic or infectious particles. Chronic exposure to SO_2 has been associated in humans and animal studies with increased susceptibility to acute upper respiratory tract infections, chronic bronchitis, bronchial asthma, and chronic degenerative lung disease (Rall, 1974). Death from inhaled SO_2 alone may occur when excessively high amounts are released accidentally into the atmosphere. Extensive necrosis of the mucosa of the upper airways and pulmonary hemorrhage and edema may be seen.

Animal Toxicity Numerous studies on the toxicity of SO_2 have been performed in animals. Animals usually tolerate 30–50 ppm SO_2 without any apparent adverse health effects. Higher concentrations produce discomfort and signs of ocular irritation. In the lung, the effects of SO_2 are almost exclusively limited to the upper respiratory tract down to the level of bronchi, where airway constriction and increased secretion of mucus are produced. Narrowing of the airways occurs within a matter of minutes and is reversible. Lethality was produced in guinea pigs within 20 h after exposure (continuously) to 1000 ppm and within 6–7 days after exposure to 130 ppm. Edema and hemorrhage were the most prominent pathologic findings. Chronic exposure of rats produces a disease similar to chronic bronchitis in the upper airways, with hypertrophy of goblet cells and hypertrophy of mucus glands. The mucus lining the airways may become of abnormal consistency, affecting the mucociliary beat. This may affect the efficient removal of agents from the lung by the mucociliary escalator. The changes may be subtle, however, and exposure of guinea pigs to about 6 ppm of SO_2 for 12 months or of monkeys to 0.14–1.3 ppm for 78 consecutive weeks apparently produced no significant pathological changes.

Sulfuric acid and particulates of sulfate produced changes in the respiratory tract of experimental animals essentially similar to those of SO_2. Guinea pigs are the species most sensitive to sulfuric acid inhalation and develop readily signs of bronchoconstriction and laryngeal spasm upon acute exposure. Sulfuric acid may also cause parenchymal lung damage, characterized by hemorrhage, edema, and congestion. Increased pulmonary flow resistance is easily found. Quantitative comparisons between the effects of SO_2 and of sulfuric acid have shown that, if calculated as milligrams sulfur per cubic meter, sulfuric acid is considerably more irritating under conditions of both acute and chronic exposure than is SO_2 (National Research Council, 1978).

Mechanism of Action Exposure of either the lungs or the upper airways alone to SO_2 produces increased resistance to air flow almost instantaneously. The response may be abolished either by cooling of the cervical vasosympathetic nerves or by atropine. Bronchoconstriction is caused by increased tone of the smooth bronchial musculature and depends on intact parasympathetic pathways.

In the respiratory tract, absorbed SO_2 reacts with water to form bisulfite and then is further metabolized by sulfite oxidase to sulfate; sulfate is ultimately excreted by the kidneys. However, by interacting with biochemical reducing agents such as NADH or NADPH, a free radical, SO_3^- may be formed. This free radical might hypothetically compete for NAD(P)H with many enzymes requiring important macromolecules (Gause et al., 1977).

Modifying Factors The irritant properties of SO_2 are greatly enhanced if the gas is mixed with an aerosol of certain salts. In an atmosphere of more than 70% humidity, aerosols of NaCl or of salts of manganese, vanadium, or iron form droplets and SO_2 becomes dissolved in those droplets. The effects of SO_2 are then aggravated by carrier effects bypassing nasopharyngeal deposition or by transformation of SO_2 into more irritating compounds such as sulfuric acid and sulfate salts. If the aerosol particles are in the submicrometer range, they may gain access to the deeper regions of the lung.

A second concern is that SO_2 enhances morbidity and mortality of people afflicted with chronic lung disorders or other preexisting diseases. In the famous London fog episode in 1952, approximately 4000 persons died within a 2-week period of excessive air pollution, with SO_2 levels reaching 1–2 ppm (Ellison and Waller, 1978). Most victims were older people suffering from preexisting cardiac or respiratory disease. A drop in ambient air temperature, as occurs close to the ground during episodes of temperature inversion, is likely to increase frequency of breathing and at the same time may slow down the movement of the cilia in the nose and upper airways. With increased breathing frequency and diminished efficiency of the mucociliary escalator, particulates and infectious microorganisms could theoretically gain access to the deep lung regions. Partial removal might occur via the lymphatic system; however, increased lymph flow is likely to reduce the filtration efficiency of the regional lymph nodes. A combination of all these factors together with the presence of preexisting disease might have accounted for the increase in morbidity and mortality by respiratory-tract infection. Alternatively, the high humidity (fog) may have carried more SO_2 past the nasal defenses, thereby raising the effective dose to the deeper lung.

Oxygen

Human Toxicity Lung damage caused by oxygen in humans is well documented, although to recognize with certainty its clinical signs and symptoms is not always easy (Deneke and Fanburg, 1980). Administration of oxygen in higher concentrations than found in ambient air may prove to be a life-saving measure in newborn infants suffering from respiratory distress or in adult patients with acute or chronic breathing problems. Unfortunately, too much oxygen damages the cells of the lung. Oxygen pneumonitis is characterized by cytoplasmic edema and necrotic changes in the capillary endothelial cells. Type I alveolar cells degenerate and may slough off the basement membrane, and hyaline membranes are formed. The thin pulmonary epithelium becomes replaced by a cuboidal epithelium. This produces a thickened air–blood barrier with reduced diffusion capacity. In premature infants, oxygen treatment is known to permanently damage the retina and to cause blindness (retrolental fibroplasia). What concentration of oxygen in the inspired air produces lung damage and how long elevated oxygen concentrations may be administered without serious toxicity or without development of persistent untoward effects are still evaluated on a case-by-case basis, rather than by a good understanding of dose–effect and time–effect relationships (Balentine, 1982).

Lung Damage in Animals Placed into 100% oxygen at atmospheric pressure, most experimental animals will die within a few days. Their lungs are congested and edematous, and liquid accumulates in the pleural cavity. Light- and electron-microscopic studies show essentially similar lung damage as observed in humans. Detailed cytodynamic studies have shown extensive proliferation of both epithelial and capillary endothelial cells. If animals are removed from oxygen before they die, cell proliferation will eventually restore a normal lung structure; acute oxygen toxicity can be reversible. However, under conditions of prolonged exposure or intermittent exposures to hyperoxia, pulmonary fibrosis may develop.

Some data are available on dose effects of oxygen in animals. Concentrations of 60% or more oxygen in the inspired air for up to 1 week produce measurable cell damage, whereas concentrations below 60% seem to have less effect (Hackney et al., 1975). While exposure to normobaric oxygen, even up to 100%, usually causes predominantly lung damage, exposure to hyperbaric oxygen (more than 1 atm pressure) produces profound metabolic alterations in the central nervous system, convulsions, and death (Balentine, 1982).

Mechanisms of Oxygen Toxicity   The molecular mechanisms underlying oxygen toxicity are beginning to be understood. Molecular oxygen itself is relatively unreactive. The biologic effects of elevated concentrations of oxygen suggest that hyperoxia enhances the formation of toxic oxygen metabolites. Some enzymes involved in normal oxygen metabolism are capable of reduction of molecular oxygen without the formation of detectable intermediates in free form. Other enzymes produce reactive intermediates, however, that can cause cellular damage. In the presence of elevated concentrations of oxygen, an excess of free radicals is apparently formed that can no longer be efficiently detoxified. Potentially harmful oxygen radicals include superoxide (O_2^-) and peroxide (O_2^{2-}), which are produced by biological systems, as well as singlet oxygen and the highly reactive hydroxyl (HO) radical. The cellular macromolecules with which these highly reactive molecular species interact are not known with certainty. Possible targets include polyunsaturated fatty acids, which are essential components of cell membranes; they could become peroxidatively damaged. Direct evidence for lipid peroxidation following hyperoxia in vivo is not available; however, there are data suggesting that excess oxygen inhibits sulfhydryl enzymes and interferes with mitochondrial function. It is also possible that the various oxygen radicals interact with and damage cellular membrane proteins and lipids without causing measurable lipid peroxidation (Autor, 1982).

Modifying Factors   Since all aerobic cells produce some oxygen radicals under normal conditions, they have developed a variety of enzymatic systems to protect themselves. The enzymes believed to be most important include superoxide dismutase, which converts superoxide radicals to hydrogen peroxide and ground-state oxygen, catalase, and the glutathione peroxidase–glutathione reductase system, which converts hydrogen peroxide to oxygen and water. Changes in all these systems alter the susceptibility to pulmonary oxygen toxicity; these observations further underline the importance of oxygen radicals in the pathogenesis of oxygen-induced lung damage (Ciba Foundation, 1979). Newborn animals are resistant to the toxic effects of oxygen up to the age of 15 days and partially resistant to 30 days. This resistance correlates with their ability to increase the pulmonary activities of superoxide dismutase, catalase, and glutathione peroxidase (Autor and Stevens, 1978). Up to 15 days of age, each of these enzymes is inducible and these animals exhibit no lung damage. In rats 15–30 days of age, only catalase and glutathione peroxidase are inducible, and some lung damage is evident after hyperoxic exposures. Rats older than 30 days succumb to oxygen toxicity within 4 days. Tolerance can be induced, however, by prior exposure of these animals to 85% oxygen for several days, a treatment that increases the pulmonary activity of superoxide dismutase. Guinea pigs, hamsters, and mice, which fail to develop tolerance to oxygen toxicity after pretreatment with 85% oxygen, exhibit little increase in pulmonary superoxide dismutase (Crapo and Tierney, 1974). It is also of interest that adult rats injected with bacterial endotoxin develop resistance to the toxic effects of oxygen. These animals also exhibit elevated lung levels of catalase, glutathione peroxidase, and superoxide dismutase (Frank and Roberts, 1979). Vitamin E may also be important in protecting lung cells from the toxic effects of oxygen, since animals placed on a vitamin E-deficient diet show an increased susceptibility to oxygen toxicity.

Industrial and Environmental Chemicals

Silica

Human Toxicity Inhalation of particles containing crystalline silicon dioxide (silica) causes a chronic, progressive fibrotic disorder in the lung called silicosis. Silica is one of the most abundant constituents of the earth's crust, and silica dust may be created in almost any situation where rocks are mined or ground, such as in tunneling, mining, and quarrying operations. Occupational exposure to silica dust may also occur in masonry or in sand blasting (polishing metal surfaces with a jet of finely ground sand). Silicosis was, and to a certain degree still is, one of the most important occupational diseases. However, with the introduction of stringent dust-control measures, the incidence of silicosis over the last few decades has decreased.

Simple silicosis, once it has developed, often has a tendency to progress further even if exposure to silica dust ceases to exist. Clinical signs and symptoms are those of lung fibrosis and development of cardiorespiratory failure. At one time, one of the most serious complications of silicosis was concomitant infection with tuberculosis; with the advent of effective chemotherapy against tuberculosis, the incidence of so-called silicotuberculosis and its implications for health have been greatly diminished (in the Western World). An acute form of silicosis that may progress rapidly within a short time to death can occur where there is exposure to extremely high concentrations of silica dust (Seaton, 1975a).

Animal Toxicity Silicosis has been produced in experimental animals by exposing them to silica dust or by instilling silica (quartz) directly via the trachea into the lung. The developing lesions usually resemble the changes found in human situations (Heppleston, 1975; Reiser et al., 1982).

Mechanism of Action Respirable-sized quartz particles (2–5 μm) once deposited in the lung parenchyma are subsequently ingested by alveolar macrophages into phagosomes through endocytosis. Lysosomes, as they behave when bacteria are engulfed by macrophages, then fuse with the phagosomes and form phagolysosomes in an attempt to destroy the foreign agents. However, on the surface of quartz particles, silicic acid groups are formed. These groups can act as powerful hydrogen-bonding groups that can interact with secondary amide groups of proteins or of phosphate ester groups of phospholipids. Since biological membranes contain both proteins and phospholipid, the interaction between hydrogen donor and hydrogen acceptor groups may eventually destroy both phagolysosomal and cellular membranes. As a result, digestive enzymes and quartz crystals are released into the alveoli (Allison et al., 1966). The liberated silica particles are reengulfed by other macrophages or by type II alveolar cells, and the process of phagocytosis and subsequent cell damage repeats itself until alveoli are filled with fragments of membranes, proteins, and phospholipids. Cell debris and silica particles may subsequently move through the lymphatic channels. During this journey, silica particles enter connective-tissue histiocytes and kill them in a similar way as they kill alveolar macrophages. Surrounding cells may become stimulated by the products released from damaged cells and begin to proliferate. Areas develop where there are dead or dying macrophages, proliferating mononuclear cells and fibroblasts, and an excessive production of reticulin and collagen fibers. Quartz particles may continue to spread through the lymphatic channels up into the lymph nodes of the lung hilus, or they may reach subpleural lymph nodes. With time, multiple foci of so-called silicotic islets develop throughout the lung, having a diameter of 0.5–5.0 mm. Particles of silica can be demonstrated in the nodules.

Damage of pulmonary macrophages appears therefore to be the key mechanism in the pathogenesis of silicosis. This sets in motion multiple cell–cell interactions. It is possible that, besides the reactions described above, the immune system may also play an important role in producing the full pathologic picture (Reiser and Last, 1979).

Modifying Factors   Much of the evidence supporting such a mechanism of action as described for silica has been found in systems studying isolated pulmonary macrophages. When silica particles are coated with an efficient electron acceptor, poly(2-vinyl pyridine 1-oxide) (PVPNO), and incubated in vitro with macrophages, damage to lysosomal and cellular membranes is prevented. This would appear to be a rational approach, based on knowledge of molecular mechanisms, to prevent and possibly to treat silicosis; however, PVPNO has to date not found use in human therapy. (Scattered anecdotal reports of its use for this purpose occur in the Eastern European literature, but we know of no controlled clinical trials of this agent.)

Asbestos

Human Toxicity   Asbestos is a naturally occurring fibrous material that is highly resistant to destruction by physical and chemical agents. Asbestos is incorporated into insulation and building materials such as tiles and felts, fireproof fabric and paint, and the lining of some furnaces and kilns. Asbestos-containing rock is mined by drilling and blasting, and asbestos is isolated by crushing and milling. Most asbestos is produced in South Africa, Canada, and the Soviet Union, although there are active asbestos mines in the United States, in Vermont and California. Chemically, asbestos consists of mineral silicates. The most commonly produced forms are chrysotile, which tends to form hollow tubes or fiber bundles, and crocidolite, amosite, and tremolite, which tend to form straight needle-like fibers.

Asbestos has been recognized for centuries as an etiologic agent in the pathogenesis of chronic lung disease. Asbestosis is found in the lungs of workers mining the material (although to a surprisingly small extent), as well as in lungs of workers in other occupations such as ship-building, construction, brake-repairing, etc. Four major lung diseases have been associated with exposure to asbestos: parenchymal asbestosis, pleural asbestosis, mesothelioma, and asbestos-associated carcinoma. Diffuse interstitial fibrosis of the lung, similar to many other forms of interstitial fibrosis, is the main characteristic of parenchymal asbestosis. The lesions are usually more developed in the lower portion of the lung. Alveolar spaces may be filled with macrophages and, later, the cellular debris may become organized by deposition of fibrin and of collagen. A pathognomonic feature of asbestosis is the so-called asbestos bodies, yellow–brown structures 20–150 μm long and 2–4 μm wide. At the center of the body one may often find an asbestos fiber coated with proteinacious material, mostly iron-containing ferritin. Asbestos bodies and free asbestos fibers may be detected in the sputum and may help to indicate the presence of the disease; however, their presence does not provide formal proof of asbestosis or provide an index of severity of the disease. The airways are usually not affected in asbestosis. The disease progressively reduces total and vital lung capacity and diminishes diffusion capacity. The changes in pulmonary function are similar to those found in lung fibrosis caused by other toxic agents.

Inhaled asbestos fibers may pierce alveoli that lie directly underneath the visceral pleura and may gain access to the pleural space. This leads to pleural effusions and to the formation of calcified or fibrous plaques on the pleural surface; asbestos fibers are occasionally found within these structures.

Mesothelioma is a comparatively rare malignant tumor originating from the cells lining the outer surface of the lung or the interior of the thoracic cage or from cells lining the peritoneal cavity. The rareness of the tumor helped to identify asbestos exposure as an etiologic cause. Mesothelioma was found predominantly, although not exclusively, in people working with or otherwise exposed to asbestos. Mesothelioma may be found in both the thoracic and the abdominal cavity. One characteristic feature of the tumor is that the latency period between initial exposure and clinical signs of tumor presence may be exceedingly long, sometimes 25–40 years. There seems to be no relationship between severity of exposure and tumor incidence. Epidemiological evidence originally suggested that only crocidolite would produce mesothelioma. It now seems that other forms of asbestos (chrysotile) may have similar action.

Pulmonary carcinoma following exposure to asbestos may develop with or without concomitant asbestosis. Pathological features and clinical course of the disease are not different from other forms of bronchogenic carcinoma (Seaton, 1975b). There is (unlike mesothelioma) a strong synergistic interaction between asbestos exposure and cigarette smoking as risk factors for this disease.

Animal Toxicity Diffuse fibrotic changes, as well as tumors in various sites of the respiratory tract, have been observed in animals exposed over a lifetime to respirable dusts of asbestos fibers. In one study the average daily exposure was 10–13 mg/m^3 and the average incidence of tumors in the respiratory tract was approximately 30%. In the same study it was also found that if asbestos exposure was stopped after 6 months, fibrosis of the lung continued to progress. It is thought that in humans the disease takes a similar course. No increase in tumor incidence in organs other than the lung was found (Selikoff and Lee, 1978).

Mechanism of Action If asbestos fibers are incubated with red blood cells in vitro, they produce hemolysis by damaging the cell membranes. In nucleated cells such as macrophages or lymphocytes, asbestos fibers have marked toxic effects and may kill cells within a few minutes. Delayed toxicity involves the lysosomes of the cells. Damage to the lysosomal membrane with subsequent release of acid hydroxylases might produce fibrosis in a way similar to that postulated to occur in silicosis. As far as carcinogenic effects of asbestos fibers are concerned, it has been speculated that the physical properties of the fibers (such as length or chemical properties of asbestos itself) or that carcinogenic materials absorbed on the fiber surface, such as polycyclic hydrocarbons or metals, might cause malignant transformation of lung cells. It is also possible that asbestos fibers act in the respiratory tract as cocarcinogens by accentuating the carcinogenic action of other inhalants (Selikoff and Lee, 1978).

Modifying Factors   The risk of developing lung cancer from exposure to asbestos is greatly enhanced in cigarette smokers. Asbestos and cigarette smoke appear to act as cocarcinogens, and their effects are probably synergistic rather than only additive (Selikoff and Lee, 1978).

Metal Fumes and Dusts

Human Toxicity   Pulmonary toxicity due to inhalation of dusts and fumes of various metals and their compounds occurs most often in industrial settings. Acute exposure to many metals causes chemical pneumonitis and inflammatory changes in the airways. Chronic exposure is known to produce pulmonary fibrosis, to favor the development of emphysema, or, with certain metals, to cause development of bronchial cancer. Inhalation and deposition of metals in the lung are occasionally followed by absorption into the circulation, and signs and symptoms of systemic toxicity follow.

Metals of particular concern include beryllium (Be) (Stokinger, 1966), cadmium (Friberg et al., 1971), nickel, and chromium. Exposure to even small amounts of beryllium may precipitate a chronic, often progressive form of lung disease characterized by the development of granulomatous lesions. There is no straightforward dose–effect relationship in berylliosis. Some individuals may be exposed to substantial amounts of Be during their lifetimes, and develop only mild forms or no disease at all. In other individuals, exposure to very small amounts of Be precipitates the development of progressive and wasting chronic lung lesions (Tepper, 1972). It is believed that immunologic mechanisms are involved and that only a particularly susceptible segment of the exposed population is likely to develop beryllium disease (Reeves, 1977). Inhaled Be produces toxic systemic effects in other organs than lung. Beryllium is suspected as a human carcinogen, although definite proof is still lacking.

Acute inhalation of cadmium fumes causes severe and acute signs of toxicity and is often fatal. Death may be delayed for several days. Absorption of cadmium from the lung may produce kidney damage; after long-term exposure to cadmium, pulmonary emphysema develops.

Chromium and nickel have been identified as human carcinogens. Exposure to dusts of chromium ores is found essentially in mining and electroplating industries. In exposed workers (especially exposed to chromates), the death rate from lung cancer is increased (as is incidence of nasal tumors). Another known human carcinogen is nickel in its various forms. Workers in nickel mining and nickel-processing industries have a higher risk for the development of cancer in the nasal sinuses and in the lung than has the normal population. For both nickel and chromium, it has not yet been established with certainty whether all metal compounds are carcinogens or whether only some have carcinogenic potential. The problem may be complicated by the fact that workers in industrial settings are rarely exposed to one potentially carcinogenic compound alone. Nickel dusts may be inhaled together with the dust of other metals—for example, chromates—or with other agents suspected to be carcinogens, such as polycyclic aromatic hydrocarbons. Nickel and metals in general may thus not be direct carcinogens, but could conceivably act as promoting agents or cocarcinogens.

While acute and chronic lung disease caused by Ni, Cr, Be, and Cd, as well as other metals, is well documented in humans, it must be emphasized that the incidence of disease has been greatly reduced with the introduction of proper industrial hygiene (primarily dust removal and abatement in milling, crushing, and other industrial processes).

Animal Toxicity   Inhalation of metal aerosols or direct instillation of metal solutions into the trachea has been shown to produce lung damage in several animal species. Some metal compounds—for example, nickel carbonyl or certain organometal compounds—also cause lung damage if injected intravenously (Hackett and Sunderman, 1968). The changes seen after exposure to these agents usually resemble the ones seen with other acutely toxic agents: necrosis of the cells lining the alveoli, followed by proliferation of type II pneumocytes. This effect is accompanied by biochemical changes reflecting tissue damage and repair. Evidence for the carcinogenicity of beryllium, nickel, and chromium, has been obtained in chronic inhalation studies with rodents (Sunderman, 1978).

Mechanisms of Action   Little information is available on how metals and their compounds exert their deleterious effects on lung tissue. In liver, metals such as beryllium or nickel have been found to interfere with the biosynthesis of macromolecules, particularly DNA and RNA; how changes such as these may relate to eventual lung damage remains to be established (Sunderman, 1978).

Modifying Factors   The primary goal in treatment of metal toxicity is to eliminate the toxic agent from the body. For this purpose, chelating agents (EDTA, BAL) are generally used. No evidence is available that documents that such treatment substantially relieves lung burdens. The possibility also exists that metals may be shifted from the lung to other target sites; this has been documented in experimental beryllium disease, where treatment with corticosteroids produces a translocation of the metal from the lung to other organs, particularly the liver. Such shifts in organ distribution are thought to influence the course of Be disease in humans, where it is known that a dormant disease may suddenly flare up in periods of stress and changed overall hormonal status, such as following surgical interventions or in pregnancy (Tepper, 1972).

Paraquat

Human Toxicity   Paraquat is a bipyridylium salt and is widely used as a herbicide. Unfortunately, several episodes of accidental, suicidal, or homicidal poisoning have shown that paraquat is very toxic to humans. Estimates of the oral lethal dose in humans range as low as about 30 mg/kg of body weight, corresponding to a few mililiters of the concentrated paraquat solutions available commercially. Acute clinical signs of paraquat poisoning are vomiting, diarrhea, and decreased kidney function. However, the most serious effect is lung damage. Early after poisoning the lungs are congested and edematous. Later a severe and progressive fibrosis develops for which no effective treatment has as yet been found. Patients who do not recover rapidly usually die within a few weeks from respiratory failure after paraquat ingestion (Pasi, 1978).

Animal Toxicity   Oral or parenteral paraquat administration produces lung toxicity in several species of animals. The initial lesions are degeneration of type I alveolar cells. Contrary to what is seen with many other toxic agents, paraquat also causes extensive type II cell damage. It is thought that this specific action of paraquat on type II cells is one of the key events in paraquat toxicity. Perivascular edema and necrosis of the capillary endothelial cells are seen. Within a few days after paraquat intoxication, small mononuclear cells fill the alveolar spaces and severe pulmonary fibrosis develops (Smith and Heath, 1974). Besides causing lung damage, paraquat also induces lesions in other tissues, particularly the kidney.

For reasons we do not yet fully understand, paraquat has a particular affinity for lung tissue. Incubation of lung slices in vitro in the presence of paraquat shows that it is taken up by an active transport mechanism into the lung, presumably into the type II alveolar cells. Several drugs, among them chlorpromazine, imipramine, spermine, and other amines (and also metabolic energy-generation inhibitors) block paraquat accumulation. In vivo, paraquat reaches high lung concentrations within a few hours after administration (by any mode) and is only slowly lost from the lung. The affinity of lung tissue for the herbicide appears therefore to be a crucial step in the toxic action of paraquat. This discovery suggests that the most important measure to be taken in acute poisoning is to inhibit paraquat accumulation in the lung. In experimental animals and with more limited success in humans, paraquat absorption from the gut can be decreased with administration of Fullers earth, a clay to which paraquat binds. Removal of still-circulating paraquat from the blood by hemodialysis is another feasible approach to reduce lung burden (Rose and Smith, 1977). The importance of paraquat accumulation in the lung in determining its toxicity has been further strengthened by studies with the closely related herbicide diquat. Both in vivo and in vitro, diquat is taken up with about 10 times less affinity by the lung than is paraquat. Accordingly, diquat produces only minimal lung damage.

Mechanism of Action   The herbicidal property of paraquat is thought to be mediated through cyclic oxidation and reduction of the molecule. In plant cells, paraquat is reduced to form the free radical. Oxygen reacts with this radical and removes an electron by forming superoxide and oxidized paraquat. The superoxide anion dismutases further into H_2O_2 or O_2, either spontaneously or enzymatically. The formation of hydrogen peroxide and superoxide anion is presumably accompanied by other reactions in which the highly reactive hydroxyl radical is formed. Continuous cycling of paraquat in the oxidation–reduction cycle would serve as a continuous source of several highly reactive molecule species and cause extensive cell damage. While evidence for this mechanism of action has been obtained in studies with plant cells, it is not yet fully established whether paraquat acts the same way in mammalian cells, particularly lung cells. Generation of superoxide ions, hydrogen peroxide, and hydroxyl radicals could initiate a reaction in which unsaturated lipids of cellular membranes are peroxidized. Self-perpetuating lipid peroxidation would ultimately produce cell death. While circumstantial evidence for this possibility is very good, it has proven difficult to document unequivocally the occurrence of lipid peroxidation in the lungs of paraquat-treated animals, and the possibility that other forms of free radical toxicity are crucial cannot be dismissed. Cyclic reduction and oxidation of paraquat is accompanied by concomitant oxidation of NADPH and NADP, and, eventually, diminution and destruction of cellular pyridine nucleotides occurs. Paraquat also severely inhibits synthesis of pulmonary fatty acids, presumably by depleting type II cells of the necessary cofactor NADPH. Biosynthesis of pulmonary surfactant might become compromised and further contribute to acute paraquat toxicity.

The many studies done with paraquat demonstrate the difficulty of defining biochemical mechanisms of tissue damage in an organ containing as many different cell types as has the lung. Oxidation and loss of pyridine nucleotides after paraquat are not excessive. However, as long as it cannot be determined whether such changes, measured in whole lung tissue, affect all lung cells in a uniform manner or whether they occur only in the apparent target cells of paraquat (the type II pneumocytes, which represent only 8% of all lung cells), it will be difficult to interpret such biochemical changes (Autor, 1978).

Modifying Factors Animals injected with paraquat and placed into an atmosphere containing 60–100% O_2 will develop signs of toxicity much earlier than animals kept in air (Fisher et al., 1973). The mean survival time between paraquat administration and death is considerably shortened. Oxygen treatment also lowers dramatically the LD50 for paraquat. It is believed that an increase in the alveolar oxygen concentration enhances the rate at which free radicals are formed. Interestingly enough, diquat, which also can form free radicals similar to paraquat but causes only minimal lung damage in animals kept in air becomes more toxic in oxygen than is paraquat and causes extensive lung damage (Witschi et al., 1977).

It is possible to increase levels of pulmonary superoxide dismutase, and this will protect animals to some extent against paraquat toxicity. Younger animals are naturally more resistant to oxygen and are also protected to some extent against paraquat. If rats are kept on a selenium-deficient diet and have diminished reduced glutathione peroxidase levels in lung, they will have a shorter survival time if given paraquat than do normal animals. It is not clear whether all these effects on survival are directly related to differences in lung protective agents against oxidant damage. Young animals, for example, excrete more paraquat by the kidneys and thus may simply accumulate less of the toxic agent in the target organ. Young animals also have low levels of drug-metabolizing enzymes and could lack specific uptake systems for paraquat in the lung.

Bleomycin and Other Antineoplastic Agents

Human Toxicity Bleomycin is a polypeptide antibiotic first isolated from *Streptomyces verticillatus*. It is a promising drug for the treatment of certain cancers, particularly squamous cell-carcinoma, multiple lymphoma, and testicular tumors. Compared with other antineoplastic agents, bleomycin produces little toxic damage to the hematopoietic and gastrointestinal tissues. However, it has been noted that patients treated with bleomycin often develop lung fibrosis. Several other antineoplastic agents are also known to produce lung damage as a secondary toxic effect, for example, busulphan, melphalan, cyclophosphamide, and methotrexate. Pathologic changes in the lung include a decrease in type I alveolar cells, increased number of type II pulmonary cells with sometimes bizarre shapes, and extensive interstitial fibrosis. The pulmonary complications during cancer treatment can be fatal. It is believed that they are the consequence of a truly toxic reaction, and their severity usually depends on the total dose of the drug administered (Sostman et al., 1977; Cooper et al., 1986).

Animal Toxicity Bleomycin produces lung toxicity in mice, rats, hamsters, dogs, and birds. The first lesions are seen in the capillary endothelial cells and are accompanied by interstitial edema. The endothelium is thus the primary site of injury in bleomycin toxicity. Necrosis of type I epithelial cells develops later, 4–8 days after a single injection of bleomycin. Later, or during the course of repeated treatment, a fibrinous exudate accumulates in the alveoli, and their lumen eventually becomes filled with fibroblasts. Development of interstitial fibrosis leds to a thickening of the air–blood barrier. Upon repeated treatment, type II alveolar cells assume bizarre forms and shapes, and on occasion ciliated cells are found within the alveoli (Adamson and Bowden, 1977). This observation led to the suggestion that bleomycin not only causes primary cell necrosis but also interferes with subsequent normal tissue repair. Pulmonary fibrosis may be reproduceably induced in animals if bleomycin is injected intravenously, subcutaneously, or directly into the trachea. After intratracheal instillation, as little as 0.5–1 mg bleomycin may cause persistent fibrosis in the lung (Snider et al., 1978).

Mechanism of Action Bleomycin inhibits the growth of tumor cells by producing single-strand scissions in DNA. Consequently, some cells may be inhibited from entering mitosis altogether, whereas others may replicate abnormally. Although inhibition of cell division by bleomycin does not necessarily explain initial necrosis of endothelial and type I alveolar cells, it could explain the subsequent formation of abnormal type II cells observed in several experimental studies. The effect of the drug on DNA may compromise proper cell division and subsequent differentiation of type II epithelial cells into type I cells. It has recently been shown that after a single injection, bleomycin is present for some 10 days in alveolar epithelial cells. Repeated injection leads to accumulation of the drug in the lung. Continuous presence of the drug presumably causes continuing injury. Dividing epithelial cells might be particularly susceptible, normal cell–cell interactions may become disturbed, and excessive growth of fibroblasts presumably leads to fibrosis (Adamson and Bowden, 1979).

Modifying Factors Pulmonary toxicity of several anticancer drugs may be enhanced by concomitant irradiation of the thorax with X-rays. Radiation pneumonitis and fibrosis are well-recognized clinical entities that may follow irradiation of the lung. However, fibrosis usually takes several weeks to several months to develop fully. In combination with drug therapy by bleomycin, doxorubicin, or methotrexate, the onset of progressive and often fatal fibrosis may be accelerated and diffuse fibrosis may develop within weeks rather than within months. The exact mechanism underlying this synergistic interaction is only partially understood (Gross, 1977).

Miscellaneous

During the last few years, attention has been focused on a group of toxic furans that produce acute and severe lung damage in domestic and experimental animals. Although no human toxicity data are known yet, two of these agents deserve to be discussed in more detail. Analysis of their toxicity illustrates particularly well several important aspects of mechanisms of toxic lung damage. The two compounds are 4-ipomeanol and 3-methylfuran (Boyd, 1980). Ipomeanol is produced in sweet potatoes infected with a common mold. Traces of 4-ipomeanol have been found in commercially sold sweet potatoes. Methylfuran has been identified in urban smog. It is believed to be a breakdown product of natural terpenes originating from evergreen trees, especially pine trees.

Animal Toxicity   An outbreak of poisoning in cattle fed moldy sweet potatoes first called attention to the toxic properties of 4-ipomeanol. Cattle dying from ingestion of moldy sweet potatoes show severe hemorrhagic and edematous lesions in the lung. Similar lesions have subsequently been produced with purified 4-ipomeanol in the lungs of mice, rats, rabbits, and guinea pigs. There appear to be some subtle differences between species. In mice, intraalveolar and perivascular edema are prominent, whereas in rats massive pleural effusions develop in addition to intraalveolar and perivascular edema. Lung damage follows oral or parenteral exposure. However, toxic lesions are not restricted to the lung, and necrosis of renal tubular or hepatic parenchymal cells is common in several species. Within the lung, particular target cells for 4-ipomeanol are the Clara cells of the small airways (Boyd, 1980).

Clara-cell necrosis is also observed following inhalation or parenteral administration of 3-methylfuran. This compound, if inhaled, will also produce toxic lesions in liver, kidney, and hemotopoietic system.

Mechanism of Action   Both 4-ipomeanol and 3-methylfuran undergo metabolic activation to highly reactive electrophilic metabolites. Evidence for this has been obtained by in vitro studies with lung-tissue preparations or with lung microsomes. Inhibition of mixed-function oxidase metabolism in vivo or in vitro with suitable agents such as cobaltous chloride or piperonyl butoxide mitigates or abolishes the toxicity of both compounds. Activation of the agents to a reactive metabolite is followed by covalent binding of such metabolites to tissue macromolecules such as proteins and nucleic acids. An excellent correlation has been found between covalent binding to the macromolecules of different tissues, measured in vitro, and target-organ toxicity in vivo. Rat kidney microsomes have little activating activity for 4-ipomeanol, whereas mouse kidney microsomes are much more active. In vivo, rat kidneys are usually not damaged by the compound, but adult mice develop extensive renal lesions. Renal microsomes of young mice do not activate 4-ipomeanol, and no kidney damage develops in young animals. A good correlation was also found between in vivo covalent binding of 4-ipomeanol to lung tissue and overall toxicity. The degree to which different tissues and different species are able to activate the compound through the microsomal cytochrome P-450 system thus ultimately determines toxicity, target-organ specificity, and species differences.

Autoradiographic studies have shown that both 4-ipomeanol and 3-methylfuran bind covalently within the Clara cells of the small airways. The cells appear to be particularly rich in mixed-function oxidases, and activation of the furans to toxic metabolites might cause cell death. Additional evidence comes from studies with CCl₄ and 4-nitroquinoline oxide. Both compounds may be activated to reactive metabolites and produce Clara cell death. On the other hand, bird lungs contain virtually no Clara cells and no lung damage is produced in birds by either 4-ipomeanol or 3-methylfuran, although both compounds produce extensive liver necrosis. Metabolic activation of certain foreign agents by the mixed-function oxidase system of Clara cells may well be key events in the pathogenesis of some forms of acute toxic lung damage and possibly also in the development of more chronic lesions such as cancer.

Modifying Factors Studies with both 4-ipomeanol and 3-methylfuran have shown that important differences exist between species and between young and old animals. It is possible to mitigate or totally abolish toxic effects by inhibition of mixed-function oxidases. On the other hand, pretreatment with inducers of mixed-function oxidases (such as 3-methylcholanthrene) can change the target organ of the toxins. In normal rats, most 4-ipomeanol is covalently bound to pulmonary macromolecules, and lung damage is the most prominent feature. In animals pretreated with 3-methylcholanthrene, most covalently bound material is found in the liver, and this coincides with extensive centrilobular hepatic necrosis. It is therefore possible to shift target-organ toxicity by suitable pretreatment (Boyd, 1980). Moreover, these observations suggest that toxicity to a specific organ is likely to occur by formation of reactive metabolites in situ rather than by formation of the reactive metabolite in one organ and subsequent transport to another.

CONCLUSION

It has been recognized for centuries that inhaled gases and particles can cause acute or chronic lung damage. It is now generally known that many agents may damage the cells of the lung if they are carried in the bloodstream. The presence of lung lesions can be detected and quantitated by many sophisticated methods. Lungs have efficient defense mechanisms and can respond successfully to many episodes of acute damage with a wide repertoire of reparative responses. When these mechanisms fail and become overwhelmed, chronic lesions develop. A key factor to allow us to recognize, to predict, and eventually to prevent lung damage caused by chemicals is to understand pathogenetic mechanisms and principles. Such mechanisms will have to be further studied at all levels of biological organization, from molecular events to the biology of lung cells and their interactions, before we truly understand pathogenesis of lung disease.

REFERENCES

Adamson, I. Y. R., Bowden, D. H. 1974. The type 2 cell as progenitor of alveolar epithelial regeneration. A cytodynamic study in mice after exposure to oxygen. *Lab. Invest.* 30:42–55.

Adamson, I. Y. R., and Bowden, D. H. 1977. Origin of ciliated alveolar epithelial cells in bleomycin-induced lung injury. *Am. J. Pathol.* 87:569–580.

Adamson, I. Y.R., and Bowden, D. H. 1979. Bleomycin-induced injury and metaplasia of alveolar type 2 cells. *Am. J. Pathol.* 96:531–544.

Allison, A. C., Harrington, J. S., and Birbeck, M. 1966. The examination of the cytotoxic effects of silica on macrophages. *J. Exp. Med.* 124:141–154.

Autor, A. P. 1978. *Biochemical Mechanisms of Paraquat Toxicity.* New York: Academic.

Autor, A. P., ed. 1982. *Pathology of Oxygen.* New York: Academic.

Autor, A. P., and Stevens, J. B. 1978. Mechanism of oxygen detoxification in neonatal rat lung tissue. *Photochem. PhotoBiol.* 28:775–780.

Bakhle, Y. S., and Vane, J. R. 1977. *Metabolic Functions of the Lung,* vol. 4. *Lung Biology in Health and Disease.* New York: Dekker.

Balentine, J. D. 1982. *Pathology of Oxygen Toxicity.* New York: Academic.

Barry, B. E., and Crapo, J. D. 1985. Application of morphometric methods to study diffuse and focal injury in the lung caused by toxic agents. CRC Crit. Rev. Toxicol. 14:1–32.

Boyd, M. R. 1980. Biochemical mechanisms in chemical-induced lung injury: Roles of metabolic activation. *CRC Crit. Rev. Toxicol.* 7:103–176.

Brain, J. D., Proctor, D. F., and Reid, L. M. 1977. *Respiratory Defense Mechanisms, part II;* vol. 5, *Lung Biology in Health and Disease.* New York: Dekker.

Ciba Foundation. 1979. *Ciba Foundation Symposium on Oxygen Free Radicals and Tissue Damage.* Ciba Foundation Symposium New Series. London: Ciba Foundation.

Cooper, J. A. D., Jr., White, D. A., and Mathey, R. A. 1986. Drug-induced pulmonary disease. Amer. Rev. Respir. Dis. 133:321–340.

Crapo, J. D., and Tierney, D. F. 1974. Superoxide dismutase and pulmonary oxygen toxicity. *Am. J. Physiol.* 226:1401–1407.

Deneke, S. M., and Fanburg, B. L. 1980. Normobaric oxygen toxicity of the lung. *N. Engl. J. Med.* 303:76–86.

Dungworth, D. L., Phalen, R. F., Schwartz, L. W., and Tyler, W. S. 1976. Morphological methods for evaluation of pulmonary toxicity. *Annu. Rev. Pharmacol. Toxicol.* 16:381–400.

Ehrlich, R., Henry, M. C., and Fentes, J. 1970. Influence of nitrogen dioxide on resistance to respiratory infections. In *Inhalation Carcinogenesis,* eds. M. G. Hanna, P. Nettesheim, and J. R. Gilbert, pp. 243–257. AEC Symposium Series.

Ellison, J., and Waller, R. E. 1978. A review of sulphur oxides and particulates matter as air pollutants with particular reference to effects on health in the United Kingdom. *Environ. Res.* 16:302–325.

Evans, M. J., Cabral, L. J., Stephens, R. J., and Freeman, G. 1973. Renewal of alveolar epithelium in the rat following exposure to NO_2. *Am. J. Pathol.* 70:175–198.

Evans, M. J., Dekker, N. P., Cabral-Anderson, L. J., and Freeman, G. 1978. Quantitation of damage to the alveolar epithelium by means of type 2 cell proliferation. *Am. Rev. Respir. Dis.* 118:787–790.

Evans, M. J., Johnson, L. V., Stephens, R. J., and Freeman, G. 1976a. Cell renewal in the lungs of rats exposed to low levels of ozone. *Exp. Mol. Pathol.* 24:70–83.

Evans, M. J., Johnson, L. V., Stephens, R. J., and Freeman, G. 1976b. Renewal of the terminal bronchiolar epithelium in the rat following exposure to NO_2 or O_3. *Lab. Invest.* 35:246-257.

Fisher, H. K., Clements, J. A., and Wright, R. P. 1973. Enhancement of oxygen toxicity by the herbicide paraquat. *Am. Rev. Respir. Dis.* 107:246-249.

Frank, L., and Roberts, R. J. 1979. Endotoxin protection against oxygen induced acute and chronic lung injury. *J. Appl. Physiol.* 47:577-581.

Friberg, L., Piscator, M., and Nordberg, G. 1971. *Cadmium in the Environment.* Cleveland: CRC.

Gause, E. M., Greene, N. D., Meltz, M. L., and Rowlands, J. R. 1977. *In vivo* and *in vitro* effects of sulfur dioxide upon biochemical and immunological parameters. In *Biochemical Effects of Environmental Pollutants,* ed. S. D. Lee, pp. 273-292. Ann Arbor, Mich.: Ann Arbor Science.

Gil, J. 1982. Comparative morphology and structure of the airways. In *Mechanisms in Respiratory Toxicology,* eds. H. P. Witschi and P. Nettesheim, vol. I, pp. 3-26. Boca Raton, Fla.: CRC.

Gillett, D.G., and Ford, G. T. 1978. Drug induced lung disease. In *The Lung. Structure, Function and Disease,* eds. W. M. Thurlbeck and M. R. Abell, pp. 21-42. Baltimore: Williams & Wilkins.

Gross, N. J. 1977. Pulmonary effects of radiation therapy. *Am. Int. Med.* 86:81-92.

Hackett, R. L., and Sunderman, F. W. H., Jr. 1968. Pulmonary alveolar reactions to nickel carbonyl. *Arch. Environ. Health* 16:349-357.

Hackney, J. D., Evans, M. J., and Christie, B. R. 1975. Effects of 60% and 80% oxygen on cell division in alveoli of squirrel monkeys. *Aviat. Space Environ. Med.* 46:791-794.

Harris, C. C. 1978. *Pathogenesis and Therapy of Lung Cancer,* vol. 10, *Lung Biology in Health and Disease.* New York: Dekker.

Heppleston, A. G. 1975. The fibrogenic action of silica. *Br. Med. Bull.* 25:282-287.

Hirai, K. I., Witschi, H. P., and Côté, M. G. 1977. Electron microscope of butylated hydroxytoluene-induced lung damage in mice. *Exp. Mol. Pathol.* 27:295-308.

Kuhn, C. H., Senior, R. M., and Pierce, J. A. 1982. The pathogenesis of emphysema. In *Mechanisms in Respiratory Toxicology,* eds. H. P. Witschi and P. Nettesheim, vol. II, pp. 155-211. Boca Raton, Fla.: CRC.

Last, J. A., Jennings, M. D., Schwartz, L. W., and Cross, C. E. 1977. Glycoprotein secretion by tracheal explants cultured from rats exposed to ozone. *Am. Rev. Respir. Dis.* 116:695-703.

Last, J. A., Greenberg, D., and Castleman, W. L. 1979. Ozone-induced alterations in collagen metabolism of rat lungs. *Toxicol. Appl. Pharmacol.* 51:247-258.

MacFarland, H. N. 1976. Respiratory toxicology. *Essays Toxicol.* 7:121-154.

Menzel, D. B. 1976. The role of free radicals in the toxicity of air pollutants (nitrogen oxides and ozone). In *Free Radicals in Biology,* ed. W. A. Pryor, vol. II, pp. 181-202. New York: Academic.

Mudd, J. B., and Freeman, B. A. 1977. Reaction of ozone with biological membranes. In *Biochemical Effects of Air Pollutants,* ed. S. D. Lee, pp. 97-133. Ann Arbor, Mich.: Ann Arbor Science.

Murray, J. F. 1976. *The Normal Lung. The Basis for Diagnosis and Treatment of Pulmonary Disease.* Philadelphia: Saunders.

Mustafa, M. G., and Tierney, D. F. 1978. Biochemical and metabolic changes in the lung with oxygen, ozone and nitrogen dioxide toxicity. *Am. Rev. Respir. Dis.* 118:1061-1090.

National Research Council. 1974. Committee on Medical and Biological Effects of Environmental Pollutants. Chromium. Washington, D.C.: National Academy of Scineces.

National Research Council. 1975. Committee on Medical and Biological Effects of Environmental Pollutants. Nickel. Washington, D.C.: National Academy of Sciences.

National Research Council. 1977a. Committee on Medical and Biological Effects of Environmental Pollutants. Nitrogen oxides. Washington, D.C.: National Academy of Sciences.

National Research Council. 1977b. Committee on Medical and Biological Effects of Environmental Pollutants. Ozone and other photochemical oxidants. Washington, D.C.: National
Academy of Sciences.

National Research Council. 1978. Committee on Medical and Biological Effects of Environmental Pollutants. Sulfur oxides. Washington, D.C.: National Academy of Sciences.

Nettesheim, P., and Marchok, A. 1983. Neoplastic development in airway epithelium. *Adv.
Cancer Res.* 39:1–70.

Niewoehner, D. E., and Cosio, M. G. 1978. Chronic obstructive lung disease: The role of
airway disease with special emphasis on the pathology of the small airways. In *The Lung.
Structure, Function and Disease,* eds. W. M. Thurlbeck and M. R. Abell, pp. 160–179.
Baltimore: Williams & Wilkins.

Pasi, A. 1978. *The Toxicology of Paraquat, Diaquat and Morfamquat.* Bern: Hans Huber.

Philpot, R. M., Anderson, M. W., and Eling, T. E. 1977. Uptake, accumulation and metabolism of chemicals by the lung. In *Metabolic Function of the Lung,* eds. Y. S. Bakhle and
J. R. Vane, pp. 123–172. New York: Dekker.

Raabe, O. G. 1982. Deposition and clearance of inhaled aerosols. In *Mechanisms in Respiratory Toxicology,* eds. H. P. Witschi and P. Nettesheim, vol. I, pp. 2–76. Boca Raton, Fla.:
CRC.

Rall, D. P. 1974. Review of the health effects of sulfur oxides. *Environ. Health Perspect.*
8:97–121.

Reeves, A. L. 1977. Beryllium in the environment. *Toxicol. Annu.* 2:37–48.

Reid, L. 1978. The cell biology of mucus secretion in the lung. In *The Lung. Structure,
Function and Disease,* eds. W. M. Thurlbeck and M. R. Abell, pp. 138–150. Baltimore:
Williams & Wilkins.

Reiser, K. M., and Last, J. A. 1979. Silicosis and fibrogenesis: Fact and artifact. *Toxicology*
13:51–72.

Reiser, K. M., Hesterberg, T. W., Haschek, W. M., and Last, J. A. 1982. Experimental
silicosis. *Am. J. Pathol.* 107:176–185.

Rennard, S. I., Ferrans, V. J., Bradley, K. H., and Crystal, R. G. 1982. Lung connective
tissue. In *Mechanisms in Respiratory Toxicology,* eds. H. P. Witschi and P. Nettesheim,
vol. II, pp. 115–154. Boca Raton, Fla.: CRC.

Rose, M. S., and Smith, L. L. 1977. The relevance of paraquat accumulation by tissue. In
Biochemical Mechanisms of Paraquat Toxicity, ed. A. P. Autor, pp. 71–87. New York:
Academic.

Schwartz, L. W., Dungworth, D. L., Mustafa, M. G., Tarkington, B. K., and Tyler, W. S.
1976. Pulmonary responses of rats to ambient levels of ozone. *Lab. Invest.* 34:565–578.

Seaton, A. 1975a. Silicosis. In *Occupational Lung Disease,* eds. W. K. C. Morgan and A.
Seaton, pp. 80–111. Philadelphia: Saunders.

Seaton, A. 1975b. Asbestosis. In *Occupational Lung Disease,* eds. W. K. C. Morgan and A.
Seaton, pp. 124–148. Philadelphia: Saunders.

Selikoff, I. J., and Lee, D. H. K. 1978. *Asbestos and Disease.* New York: Academic.

Shimkin, M. B., and Stoner, G. D. 1975. Lung tumors in mice: Application to carcinogenesis
bioassay. *Adv. Cancer Res.* 21:1–58.

Smith, P. H., and Heath, D. 1974. Paraquat. *CRC Crit. Rev. Toxicol.* 4:411–455.

Snider, G. L., Hayes, J. A., and Korthy, A. L. 1978. Chronic interstitial pulmonary fibrosis produced in hamster by endotracheal bleomycin. *Am. Rev. Respir. Dis.* 117:1099–1108.

Sostman, H. D., Matthay, R. A., and Putnam, C. E. 1977. Cytotoxic drug-induced lung disease. *Am. J. Med.* 62:608–615.

Stokinger, H. E. 1966. *Beryllium: Its Industrial Hygiene Aspects.* New York: Academic.

Stuart, B. O. 1976. Deposition and clearance of inhaled particles. *Environ. Health Perspect.* 16:41–53.

Sunderman, F. W. H., Jr. 1978. Carcinogenic effects of metals. *Fed. Proc.* 37:40–46.

Swift, D. L., and Proctor, D. F. 1977. Access of air to the respiratory tract. In *Respiratory Defense Mechanisms,* part I, vol. 5, *Lung Biology in Health and Disease,* eds. J. D. Brain, D. F. Proctor, and L. M. Reid, pp. 63–94. New York: Dekker.

Tepper, L. B. 1972. Beryllium. *CRC Crit. Rev. Toxicol.* 1:235–259.

Weibel, E. 1973. Morphological basis of alveolar-capillary gas exchange. *Physiol. Rev.* 53:419–495.

Weibel, E. R., Gehr, P., Haies, D., Gil, J., and Bachofen, M. 1976. The cell population of the normal lung. In *Lung Cells in Disease,* eds. A. Bouhuys, pp. 3–16. Amsterdam: Elsevier/ North Holland.

Wilson, A. R., Fairshter, R. D., Gillespie, J. R., and Hackney, J. D. 1976. Evaluation of abnormal lung function. *Annu. Rev. Pharmacol. Toxicol.* 16:465–486.

Witschi, H. P., and Côté, M. G. 1977. Primary pulmonary responses to toxic agents. *CRC Crit. Rev. Toxicol.* 5:23–66.

Witschi, H. P., Kacew, S, Hirai, K. I., and Côté, M. G. 1977. *In vivo* oxidation of reduced nicotiamide-adenine dinucleotide diphosphate by paraquat and diquat in rat lung. *Chem. Biol. Interact.* 19:143–160.

Chapter 6

Renal Toxicology

William O. Berndt

INTRODUCTION

The kidney is more than an organ that removes waste products, although if it were only that, its importance as a target organ for toxic chemicals would be significant. However, in addition, it serves important homeostatic functions, such as regulation of body pH, and control of body-compartment volumes, osmolalities, and electrolyte composition. Also, the kidney manufactures substances with important regulatory functions, such as renin-angiotensin, prostaglandins, and erythropoietin. Finally, it is becoming increasingly clear that the kidney can metabolize xenobiotics, perhaps not as effectively as the liver, but to a significant extent. Hence, any substance that can interfere with normal renal function has the capability of disrupting important homeostatic, excretory, regulatory, and metabolic functions. Indeed, survival will be threatened if these disruptions are sustained for extended periods of time.

Many events that produce sustained deficits in renal function so do indirectly. For example, generalized trauma, extensive hemolysis, or cardiovascular shock may result in acute renal failure. Important extrarenal syndromes such as these will not be the focus of this review, however. Rather, the focus will be on those events that impinge directly on the kidney. In particular, the direct interaction of chemical substances on renal function and the consequences of such interactions will be examined.

This is not to suggest that generalized trauma, hemolysis, etc. are not important, but they will not be the subject of this analysis.

Several important reviews related to renal toxicology have been published recently. These should be consulted for more detailed presentation of some aspects of this topic, and for earlier reference material (Berndt, 1976a,b, 1979; Foulkes and Hammond, 1975; Foulkes, 1977; Hook et al., 1979; Magos and Clarkson, 1977). In addition, the reader should be aware that excellent reviews of renal physiology also are available and should be read as necessary (Brenner and Rector, 1981; Orloff and Berliner, 1973; Pitts, 1974; Sullivan and Grantham, 1982; Valtin, 1973, 1979). Also, a multitude of "Annual Reviews," "Proceedings of International Meetings," etc., are published frequently and should be sought out by the serious student of renal toxicology as well as those with a developing interest.

It is not the intent of this review to highlight the complexities of renal function, although to some extent this will be unavoidable. The diversity of renal function observed under physiological conditions is extreme, and this complicates an analysis of nephrotoxicity. Indeed, no one or two individual measurements of renal function will suffice to analyze thoroughly the actions of drugs or other chemical substances on renal function. The actions of chemicals are complex when reversible, and extremely so when potentially irreversible and life-threatening. Of course, with many nephrotoxins both irreversible and life-threatening events do occur. It is important to note, however, that many acute renal insults are reversible if sufficient time is allowed. Hence, under these circumstances artificial renal-function substitutes are essential.

In an attempt to clarify these issues, a brief review of renal anatomy and physiology will follow. Second, an examination of some of the techniques that are important in the analysis of nephrotoxicity also will be represented briefly. Finally, an attempt will be made to offer useful generalizations concerning mechanisms of nephrotoxicity as they pertain to a wide variety of substances with the potential for severe, if not permanent, disruption of renal function. A catalog of chemical nephrotoxins will not be given, but appropriate examples will be used, as they relate to mechanisms of action.

REVIEW OF RENAL FUNCTION

Anatomy

Two major tissue types exist in the kidney: vascular tissue and the tubular epithelia. The blood vessels and the tubular tissue are intertwined and present a complex arrangement that is essential to overall renal function. The intrarenal localization of the nephron with respect to the intrarenal vasculature is presented in Fig. 1.

The renal arteries supply the interlobar arteries, which in turn divide into the arcuate arteries. The interlobular arteries proceed from the cortico–medullary junction, and it is from these that the glomeruli arise. The renal circulation at this point develops into two capillary networks in series. The glomerulus is the first of these. In the mid-cortical and superficial cortical areas, the efferent arterioles that leave the

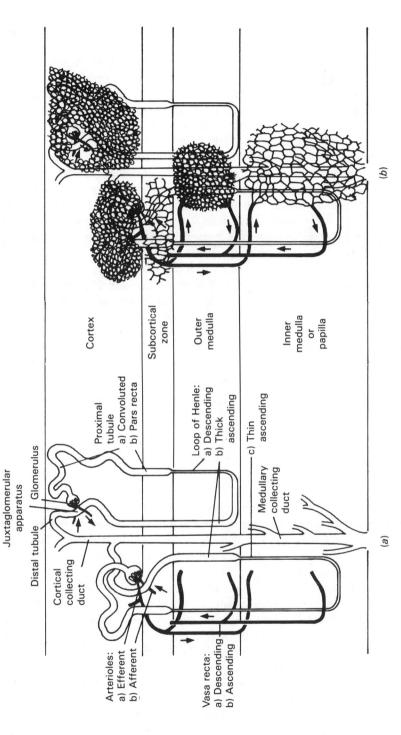

Juxtaglomerular
apparatus

Distal tubule   Glomerulus

Cortical
collecting
duct

Proximal
tubule
a) Convoluted
b) Pars recta

Loop of Henle:
a) Descending
b) Thick
   ascending

c) Thin
   ascending

Medullary
collecting
duct

Arterioles:
a) Efferent
b) Afferent

Vasa recta:
a) Descending
b) Ascending

Cortex

Subcortical
zone

Outer
medulla

Inner
medulla
or
papilla

(a)

(b)

Figure 1 Relationship of renal blood supply to cortical and juxtamedullary nephrons. *(From Valtin, 1973.)*

glomeruli form a capillary network, the peritubular capillaries, which surround the tubular tissue. It is this blood supply that supports the essential nephron functions of reabsorption and secretion. The vessels that emerge from the peritubular network are true veins and eventually leave the kidney by a route similar to that of the arteries.

The efferent arterioles from the juxtamedullary glomeruli branch into capillaries of approximately equal size, the vasa recta. Some of these vessels form capillary networks around the loops of Henle in the outer medullary regions. These networks are anatomically similar to those seen in the cortical areas. Other branches of vessels form bundles, and these pass deep into the medulla before developing into capillary networks or forming hairpin turns similar to those noted for the nephrons themselves (see below). These vessels travel in close association with the loops of Henle and form the countercurrent exchangers that support the countercurrent multiplication process.

As the vascular anatomy of the kidney varies from region to region, so does the distribution of blood flow. Normally the cortical regions receive the vast majority of the intrarenal blood, with lesser amounts being distributed to the inner cortex or outer medulla, the inner medulla, the renal papillae, the perirenal fat, and connective tissue. Studies on the intrarenal circulation have been performed with radioactive microspheres, with the washout of inert gases, and with other techniques. Usually xenon or krypton is used as the inert gas. The data from these procedures suggest that 80–85% of the total renal blood flow can be associated with perfusion of the cortical regions of the kidney. The medulla is thought to be perfused by 10–15% of the total renal blood flow. The remainder of the blood goes into other areas of the kidney. Certainly, the total renal blood flow and probably the intrarenal distribution of blood can be altered by chemical substances (e.g., vasoconstrictors or vasodilators), and hence, the renal vasculature may serve as an important site of action of nephrotoxic chemicals. However, direct evidence to show primary nephrotoxic effects related to actions on the renal or intrarenal vasculature is lacking.

The renal energy metabolism more or less parallels the intrarenal distribution of blood. For example, the large intrarenal blood distribution to the cortex suggests that this region of the kidney is highly oxygenated compared to the medulla or papilla, and the types of metabolism—that is, oxidative and glycolytic—are distributed appropriately (Lewy et al., 1973; Lee and Peter, 1969): a greater degree of glycolysis occurs in the medulla than cortex. However, this is not to suggest that glycolysis is a primary energy source for the medulla. For example, papillary tissue has high aerobic mitochondrial oxidative metabolism and high aerobic glycolytic metabolism (Cohen, 1979). Whatever the predominant energy source, either or both of these renal metabolic processes may be sites of action for nephrotoxic compounds. Although one can list many substances that alter energy metabolism, direct evidence that disruption of energy metabolism is primary in the production of nephrotoxicity has not been demonstrated. Indeed, one would anticipate that nephrotoxic effects on renal metabolism should be of long duration if not essentially irreversible, since nephrotoxic effects on renal function may be of long duration. For example, life-sustaining procedures often are needed for a human in acute renal failure to recover normal renal function.

If nephrotoxic compounds or other chemical substances are to be expected to act on renal metabolism, specific interactions with well-established metabolic pathways should be examined. Free fatty acids are metabolized in renal cortical areas, and whether or not this is the primary fuel for renal respiration (Pitts, 1974; Cohen and Kamm, 1981), it represents an important component of energy production in the kidney and probably serves as an important fuel for the reabsorption of sodium, chloride, and water by the nephrons. This is a complicated issue, however, since the extent of oxidative metabolism of fatty acids depends to a large extent on acid-base balance in the animal. Despite what is known about this and other renal metabolic pathways, it is very difficult to pinpoint a specific, single site of action within the energy-producing mechanisms in the kidney on which nephrotoxins might exert their effects, although it is well known that some compounds do interfere with energy production (see below). Probably better developed biochemical techniques and a better understanding of renal biochemistry will be necessary before this issue can be resolved.

The anatomy of the nephron is presented in Fig. 2. In general, mammals present two nephron populations. The first have relatively short loops of Henle, with the entire nephron confined to the cortical or cortical and outer medullary regions. The second are the juxtamedullary nephrons. In most mammalian species, all nephrons have their glomeruli and major segments of the proximal and distal tubules in the renal cortex. Only the loops of Henle of the juxtamedullary nephrons along with all collecting ducts course deeply into the medulla (Fig. 2). In addition to anatomical differences between the nephron populations, there are functional differences. For example, the glomerular filtration rate in the glomeruli close to the medulla is higher than that of the more superficial glomeruli.

In the superficial and mid-cortical regions, the nephrons have short loops of Henle with relatively longer proximal tubules, both the convoluted and straight parts (pars recta) of the proximal tubule. The juxtamedullary nephrons have longer loops of Henle and, hence, proximal and distal segments comprise proportionately less of the total nephron length. The frequency of occurrence of the juxtamedullary nephrons, the length of the thin loops, etc. vary considerably from species to species and will not be emphasized here. Suffice it to say that those animals whose environment requires extreme water conservation have longer loops of Henle (e.g., various desert rodents), and those that live in more moist climates have shorter or possibly no deep loops of Henle (hippopotamus, beaver). The greater the percentage of long loops in the kidney, the greater the renal concentrating ability. Humans, dogs, and most of the common laboratory rodents possess intermediate numbers of long loops and are intermediate in their urinary concentrating ability. Detailed gross anatomical considerations of nephron architecture were described by Sperber in the 1940s (Sperber, 1944) and served as the anatomical basis for the development of the countercurrent multiplication theory of urinary concentration first proposed by Wirz, Hargitay, and Kuhn in the 1950s (Wirz et al., 1951).

Physiology

After an examination of the anatomical diversity of the nephron, it will not be surprising to learn that this functional "unit" of the kidney is in reality a series of functional

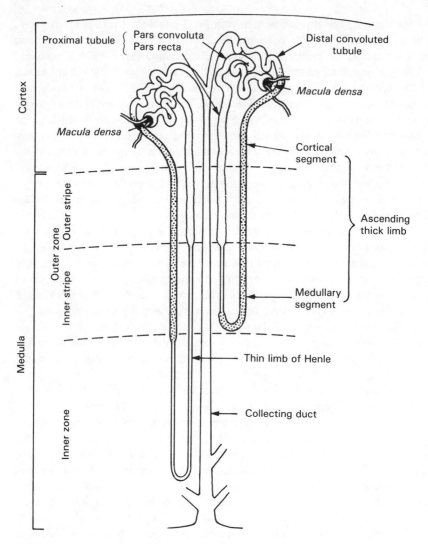

Figure 2 Structural organization of two nephron types, and the relationship of the segments of these nephrons in the various regions of the kidney. *(From Tisher, 1981.)*

units. In this brief examination of renal physiology, emphasis will be placed on those functions that are of particular interest in toxicological studies. These are highlighted in schematic representation of the nephron in Fig. 3.

The blood is delivered into the glomerulus under a significant hydrostatic pressure, which is the primary driving force for filtration (A, Fig. 3), although the overall filtration process is regulated by a variety of factors. The main driving force is opposed by colloid osmotic pressure of the capillary itself and the hydrostatic pressure of the capsular fluid, the so-called intracapsular pressure. Although the exact values of the net filtration pressure is still debated, many workers agree that at least 6–10 mm Hg is the resulting net pressure. This small pressure is sufficient to drive a virtually protein-free filtrate across the glomerular membranes into the initial segments of the proximal tubules. Except for large proteins and substances bound to those proteins, this tubular fluid has the same chemical composition as that of plasma.

The consequences of plasma protein binding on the concentration of small chemical substances in the tubular fluid are an important consideration for toxicologists. Only those substances in free solution will pass the glomerular filter; hence, for example, a substance bound 50% to plasma proteins has an effective filterable concentration of one-half its total plasma concentration. This may be an important consideration in terms of the duration of action of a chemical substance on the kidney or elsewhere, as well as in the consideration of the concentration to which the tubular cells are actually exposed. In addition, although the materials bound to the plasma proteins are neither filterable nor pharmacologically active at the time they are bound, almost all of these binding processes are reversible. Hence, as the binding process reverses, based on the laws of mass action, the bound drug becomes free to exert its toxicological effect as well as to be filtered at the glomerulus.

Finally, there are at least two additional important considerations. First, the glomerulus is not a perfect filter, in that small amounts of protein do appear in the proximal tubular fluid. This protein is reabsorbed later in the proximal tubule, so that in humans essentially no protein appears in the final urine. Most of the material that passes the filter is of relatively low molecular weight, for example, small proteins or peptides (Maack et al., 1979; Peterson et al., 1979). A healthy glomerulus will not permit passage of high-molecular-weight proteins. Second, it should be realized that the glomerular filtration system is not a static one. A variety of factors play a role in the regulation of the filtration process. For example, although molecular size is of great importance in the determination of the filterability of a substance, the effectiveness of size discrimination is modified by molecular charge (Orloff and Berliner, 1973; Tisher, 1977). For example, dextran sulfate molecules of the same molecular

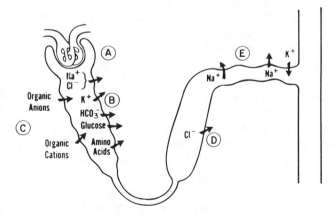

Figure 3 Schematic representation of nephron function. *(From Berndt, 1982.)*

weight as neutral dextran molecules are filtered less well. Probably this charge discrimination applies only to high-molecular-weight substances.

The proximal tubule of the nephron has proven to be a site of action for several chemical nephrotoxins (see below). In addition, large quantities of fluid and electrolytes are reabsorbed in this segment, and these activities are complemented by high levels of secretory activity (B, Fig. 3). The proximal tubule is in reality three segments. Proximal tubule segments SI, SII, and SIII are different anatomically as well as physiologically and biochemically (Tisher, 1981).

As much as 50–80% of the fluid and electrolytes filtered at the glomerulus are reabsorbed before the tubular fluid and its contents pass into the loop of Henle. The proximal tubular reabsorptive process is isosmotic. That is, the major constituents of the tubular fluid—sodium, chloride, and water—are reabsorbed from the tubular fluid in the same proportions as they exist in the plasma. Hence, the osmolality of the proximal tubular fluid is the same at the end of the tubule as it is at the beginning, despite a volume reduction of 50% or more. Apparently both active and passive reabsorptive processes are involved with sodium chloride transported by a coupled process. A very large proportion of the potassium in the glomerular filtrate is reabsorbed in the proximal tubules, as are large quantities of the filtered bicarbonate.

Several organic substances of importance are reabsorbed in the proximal tubules. For example, virtually all of the filtered glucose is reabsorbed in this segment of the nephron. In human subjects with diabetes mellitus, the appearance of large amounts of glucose in the urine is indicative of filtration of larger than normal amounts of glucose. The glucose concentration in the tubular fluid is so large that maximal reabsorptive capacity of the tubule is exceeded. Incidentally, in a nondiabetic subject who has ingested a nephrotoxin, glucose also may appear in the urine. Under these circumstances, the abnormal excretion of glucose is not a reflection of enhanced filtration because of elevated blood concentration of the sugar, but probably reflects damage to the proximal tubular reabsorptive mechanism.

Various amino acids are reabsorbed in this segment of the nephron as well. A variety of specific, active-transport systems exist that are, in part, selective for amino acid structure and charge. The details of these selective reabsorptive processes have been described elsewhere (Burg, 1981). Most investigations have been directed at dibasic amino acids and cystine in one group and imino acids and glycine in another. Although imino acids and glycine do appear to share some aspects of transport, there is not total overlap. Dibasic amino acids and cystine do not share the same transport system, as evidenced by lack of interaction and different developmental patterns (Burg, 1981). In general, all amino acids are reabsorbed well (virtually totally) during their transit through the proximal tubule.

Transport of organic substances into the tubular fluid also occurs in the proximal segment (C, Fig. 3). Classically, the secretory activities are represented by two general types of transport systems: the organic anion secretory process, and a similar one for organic cations. The organic anion process has been more thoroughly studied and is better understood. Although several subsets of organic anion transport processes may exist (Cohen and Kamm, 1981), the overall process is typified by the active tubular secretion of p-aminohippurate (PAH), which in many species is transported so efficiently that its clearance can be used for the measurement of total renal blood flow. The secretory process occurs in both the convoluted and straight segments of the proximal tubule. However, depending on the species, more or less transport occurs in one or another proximal tubule segment (i.e., SI, SII, or SIII). For example, in the rabbit the pars recta (SIII) segments seem to be more active for PAH secretion (Tune et al., 1969), while in the rat the SII and SIII segments appear equally active (Roch-Ramel and Weiner, 1980).

Because PAH excretion can be used to approximate renal plasma flow, it must be that the combined efforts of active tubular secretion and glomerular filtration remove virtually completely all the PAH entering the kidney in the arterial blood. For example, actual measurements show that in humans and the dog, PAH extraction is 80–90% complete. A word of caution: because the PAH clearance falls after the administration of a potential nephrotoxin, one should not conclude that this is a direct effect on renal blood flow. For PAH to be cleared from the blood, there must be an adequate blood supply to the kidney, but also the active tubular secretory process in the proximal tubule must be intact. A possible nephrotoxic effect could be either to alter total renal blood flow by an effect on the vasculature or to disrupt the active secretory process by an action on the proximal tubular epithelial cell. Either one or both of these effects might result in a decrease in the PAH clearance.

Organic cations such as tetraethylammonium (TEA) or N-methylnicotinamide (NMN) also are secreted actively. Unquestionably, this process occurs in the proximal tubule, although the details of the anatomical localization are not as well established as for the organic anions. Recent studies (McKinney, 1982) suggest, however, that SII and SIII segments are the predominant ones, at least in the rabbit. Furthermore, detailed species studies have not been done, and whether or not species differences exist with cations as with anions is not known.

Whatever the segmental localization of these transport systems, it is important to emphasize that these two active secretory processes are functionally separate and distinct despite being located in the same major segment of the nephron. Each transport system has its own competitors and inhibitors. PAH transport is inhibited by other organic anions such as probenecid or penicillin, while TEA or NMN transport is unaffected. These organic anion effects are thought to be competitive. TEA or NMN transport can be blocked by organic cations such as quinine, which have no effect on the transport of PAH. Also the dye cyanine #863 is an effective competitive inhibitor, while haloalkylamines such as phenoxybenzamine irreversibly inhibit cation transport. In the latter instance, irreversible alkylation of the transport carrier is thought to occur. It is likely that these compounds act by conversion to a reactive ethylenimonium intermediate that alkylates the active transport carrier. Irreversible inhibition of organic cation transport by haloalkylamines does not alter PAH transport (Ross et al., 1968; Holohan et al., 1976). Although, in general, metabolic inhibitors do not show selectivity for one transport system over another, some selective effects of nephrotoxic substances have been shown (see below).

As the tubular fluid moves into the loop of Henle, it enters that segment of the nephron primarily responsible for urinary concentration. The details of these mechanisms will not be discussed here, since they are presented elsewhere by many investigators (e.g., Orloff and Berliner, 1973; Valtin, 1973; Cohen and Kamm, 1981) and because the direct importance of these mechanisms to toxicology is not clear. It is important to be aware, however, that in the presence of high concentrations of antidiuretic hormone (ADH) in the blood, due to differential permeabilities of the limbs of the loop of Henle and the presence of certain important transport processes, the tubular fluid in Henle's loop, as well as the interstitial fluid surrounding the loop, becomes hyperosmotic with respect to plasma. These effects are magnified by the presence of antidiuretic hormone (ADH), and in the kidney of an animal producing a concentrated urine, a sizable gradient of osmolality develops from the cortex (low osmolality) to the medulla (high osmolality). When the tubular fluid in the collecting ducts passes through the kidney mass and encounters increasing osmolality from the cortex to papilla, passive removal of water occurs, which causes the production of relatively small volumes of hyperosmotic urine. This process of urinary concentration is assisted by (a) the hair-pin turn construction of the loops of Henle, which permits them to act as countercurrent multipliers; (b) the vasa recta, with a similar hair-pin configuration, acting as countercurrent exchangers; and (c) the overall anatomical relationships within the kidney, which permit the passage of the final tubular fluid through the region of high osmolar concentration. The countercurrent multiplication process is initiated by an active tubular transport mechanism located in the thick segment of the ascending limb of Henle's loop (D, Fig. 3). This transport process is apparently unique in the nephron in that chloride is moved actively rather than sodium, although the details of the process have not been resolved. This transport process has been shown to be unusually sensitive to certain diuretics (the so-called loop diuretics such as furosemide or ethacrynic acid) and may be an important site of action for nephrotoxic compounds, although direct data relating to the latter point are lacking.

Regardless of the details of the countercurrent multiplication process and regardless of whether or not nephrotoxins can act directly on active chloride transport in the ascending limb of Henle's loop to disrupt renal function, it is important to be aware that an early response to chemically induced nephrotoxicity is the excretion of a hypoosmotic urine. The lack of direct data that implicate an effect of nephrotoxins on the countercurrent multiplier process and the abundance of data that suggest the actions of nephrotoxins on the proximal tubule would lead one to conclude that the effects of chemical injury on urinary concentration is an indirect one. Perhaps the action on the proximal tubule permits sufficient disruption of renal function to allow washout of the cortico–medullary concentration gradient within the kidney, and by this means dissipation of the concentrating process. For example, diuretics that act on the proximal tubule can reduce the cortico–medullary gradient by washout of solutes in the medulla.

The distal tubule is as heterogenous a nephron segment as is the proximal tubule (E, Fig. 3). Both anatomical variability and functional variability are noted. For example, it appears to include as many as four distinct cell types between the macula densa and the first confluence of the "distal" segment with another tubule segment (Wright and Giebisch, 1978). This complex distal segment has been referred to as the cortical diluting segment, partly because active sodium transport occurs essentially independently of fluid movement, leading to formation of a dilute tubular fluid.

Late in the distal tubule (or perhaps in the collecting duct), potassium ion enters the tubular fluid. Although net secretion of potassium can occur by this process, the overwhelming body of evidence suggests that potassium entry into the nephron is primarily a passive event. Details of the mechanisms are not absolutely certain. Classically, potassium secretion was associated with a sodium reabsorptive process and referred to as a sodium–potassium exchange. Although the concept of a one-for-one exchange has been useful, there is little doubt that the active sodium reabsorptive component is not linked directly to the passive potassium secretory process. Apparently, the major role of the sodium reabsorption is to generate a favorable electrical gradient for potassium entry from the distal tubular cell. The electrical gradient coupled with the chemical gradient for potassium makes passive potassium entry into the tubular fluid very likely. Blockade of the sodium reabsorption with an appropriate diuretic or by the presence of nonreabsorbable anion will reduce or eliminate potassium secretion (Wright and Giebisch, 1978).

It is also in the distal segment of the nephron that urinary acidification occurs. This is an important consideration, in that alterations in tubular fluid pH may greatly affect passive reabsorption (nonionic diffusion) of organic compounds in the distal segment of the nephron (Valtin, 1973). Hence, a nephrotoxic substance with the proper pK_a might be recycled in the distal segment of the nephron through passive reabsorption of the unionized chemical moiety. This might then allow an enhanced exposure of the distal tubular cells to an undesirable chemical, as well as permit a prolonged stay of the substance in the blood.

MEASUREMENT OF NEPHROTOXICITY

A detailed consideration of renal methods applicable to toxicology has been published elsewhere (Berndt, 1982). Only a relatively brief discussion will be presented here.

As indicated above, the complexity of renal function precludes a single technique for the examination of renal function. Likewise, reliance on a single procedure to detect and analyze nephrotoxicity is inappropriate. Accordingly, several renal-function and transport measurements will be discussed briefly below. This battery of analyses will cover the entire spectrum of renal-function parameters and when employed in various combinations will allow for a relatively thorough understanding of kidney function as affected by nephrotoxins.

Specific techniques will be discussed below. A generalized approach to the problem of assessing renal function is presented in Fig. 4. This flowchart emphasizes the use of both whole animals and isolated renal tissue. For example, rats are pretreated with a suspected nephrotoxin and placed in metabolism cages. Urine can be collected daily for routine analyses. At the time the animals are sacrificed, blood can be collected for a variety of measurements. If desired, histological studies can be undertaken. The renal tissue obtained from the animals can be used in renal slice experiments, studies with the isolated perfused kidney, etc. Hence, data from intact animals and from isolated tissues can be obtained from the same experimental protocol utilizing the same test animals.

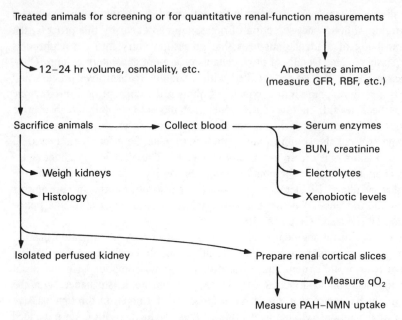

Treated animals for screening or for quantitative renal-function measurements

►12–24 hr volume, osmolality, etc.   Anesthetize animal
                                             (measure GFR, RBF, etc.)

Sacrifice animals ───────► Collect blood ───────► Serum enzymes

                                                ► BUN, creatinine

► Weigh kidneys   ► Electrolytes

► Histology   ► Xenobiotic levels

Isolated perfused kidney   ► Prepare renal cortical slices

                                                 ► Measure qO_2

                             Measure PAH–NMN uptake

Figure 4   Assessment of renal function in vivo and in vitro. *(From Berndt, 1982.)*

Clearance Measurements

The laboratory evaluation of overall renal function is facilitated greatly if small animals are used and these can be housed individually in metabolism cages. This permits the collection of timed urine samples, each of which can be evaluated for a variety of renal function parameters. Furthermore, this procedure offers the advantage of performing the studies in unanesthetized animals that have free access to food and water. Of course, the animals may have food and/or water restricted, depending on the experimental design. The rat produces a sufficient volume of urine so that accurate assessments of a variety of renal function parameters is possible. Mice also may be used, but usually several animals will have to be pooled in order to have enough urine per collection period if the test periods are of short duration.

    Always the easiest and sometimes the most informative analysis is that for urine volume. After appropriate control measurements, either the development of anuria or high-output renal failure is detected readily. Although urine output varies from animal to animal, daily urine volumes from one rat are quite reproducible.

    As indicated above, an inability to concentrate the urine is one of the earliest signs of renal dysfunction, and total solute concentration in the urine can be assessed easily with the volumes of urine produced in a normal, unanesthetized rat over 1–2 h. Usually this technique involves an estimation of freezing-point depression, although with modern technology most instruments are "direct-reading," so conversion from freezing-point depression to more recognizable concentration units (milliosmoles per liter) is automatic. An example of an effect of a nephrotoxin on urine osmolality and volume is depicted in Fig. 5 (Berndt, 1975). Potassium dichromate caused the rat to lose its ability to concentrate the urine, whether the animal was excreting a large or a small volume of urine. It is noteworthy that urine osmolality remained low even as other renal function parameters tended to recover. More precise clearance procedures can be accomplished in the anesthetized animal (see below). In these experiments, glomerular filtration and renal blood flow can be assessed quantitatively along with urine volume, sodium excretion, etc. Experiments of short duration can be conducted and acute effects of potential nephrotoxins can be determined.

Glomerular Integrity

Glomerular integrity may be assessed by several procedures. Direct measurement of the glomerular filtration rate can be determined even in the unanesthetized rat by monitoring creatinine clearance, but this is accomplished more accurately by measurement of inulin clearance in an anesthetized animal. Since the glomerulus is a primary means for restricting protein entry into the urine, assessment of urinary protein concentration will help determine the extent of glomerular integrity. The normal, healthy laboratory rat excretes small amounts of protein in the urine, and hence, it is important to have reliable control measurements on these animals before treatment with a suspected nephrotoxin. If quantitative assessment of urinary protein excretion is required, a number of precise analytical techniques are available. In most cases, at least for screening purposes, "dipstick" procedures will suffice. These procedures will give qualitative or semiquantitative measurements of urinary protein

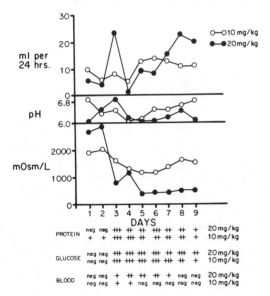

Figure 5   Effect of potassium dichromate on renal function in the rat. $K_2Cr_2O_7$ was administered as a single dose (10 or 20 mg/kg) after day 2. Both days 1 and 2 were control days. See text for further explanations. *(From Berndt, 1975.)*

and have been shown to distinguish easily between control animals and those treated with known nephrotoxins. An example of such data is given in Fig. 5.

Measurement of the blood urea nitrogen (BUN) is probably the most commonly used procedure for the assessment of glomerular function and is remarkably sensitive. As filtration slows or ceases, the BUN rises. Paralleling this rise is an increase in the plasma creatinine level. The relationship between the BUN or the plasma creatinine and glomerular filtration rate has been well established in chronic renal failure, and data from the human are depicted in Fig. 6 (Relman and Levinsky, 1971). The rectangular hyperbola depicted in the figure allow for accurate prediction of the extent of remaining renal function for a given value of the BUN. Although analyses such as these are most useful when the development of renal failure is relatively slow, the BUN has obvious utility in experimental, acutely induced renal failure as well. Control values for the BUN are well established for every commonly used laboratory animal, and even a single value considerably in excess of the known controls is predictive of renal dysfunction. Without a sequential analysis it may not be possible to determine the extent of remaining renal function based on BUN, but even so a single value is useful. Although there are some circumstances under which an elevated BUN may not be diagnostic of renal dysfunction, these are not encountered routinely in the acute situation in the experimental laboratory (Valtin, 1979).

From an analytical point of view, neither the BUN nor creatinine determination is particularly difficult. With creatinine there are concerns about nonspecific chromagens, but these can be avoided. For the BUN there are quite specific analytical methods. Indeed, a number of BUN kits are available commercially that greatly simplify the analysis. These usually employ accurate and sophisticated procedures that are simplified for routine use.

Tubular Function

Tubular function may be assessed by measurement of the urinary excretion of several substances. As indicated earlier, the reabsorptive capacity of the nephron for glucose may be diminished after a nephrotoxic insult. Once again, with the urine collected from an animal in a metabolism cage, rigid quantitative or "dipstick" semiquantitative assessments of urinary glucose excretion can be made. The excretion in the urine of any measurable amount of glucose, as detected by a "dipstick," is suggestive of some type of dysfunction. Whether this is a disruption of the reabsorptive process in the nephron or a diabetes mellitus-like syndrome would depend upon the experimental situation, and can be resolved readily by measurement of the plasma glucose concentration. Secretion of PAH or TEA, in general, is reduced by most nephrotoxins. Hence, after the administration of a nephrotoxic substance a reduction in glucose reabsorption is the difficulty, while a decrease in net secretory capacity for PAH or TEA is observed. Both sets of data indicate an effect of the potential toxin under study on the proximal segment of the nephron.

It is important to realize that with whole-animal clearance procedures, alterations in PAH secretion or glucose reabsorption after a nephrotoxin do not necessarily mean that the compound has acted specifically on the transport processes. The effects lead-

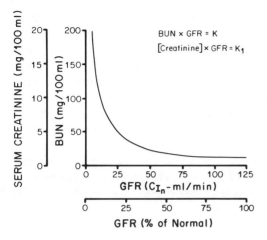

Figure 6 Relationship between serum creatinine or BUN and glomeruler filtration rate. *(From Relman and Levinsky, 1971.)*

ing to reduced PAH secretion or glucose reabsorption may be indirect. Hence, even if direct effects on selected transport processes can be exerted by a nephrotoxin, the specificity of these effects cannot be assessed by in vivo experiments. Clearly, whole-animal excretion experiments such as those suggested above will allow a description of the characteristics of a nephrotoxicity, determination of the temporal relationships of the renal failure, etc., but these procedures are less than ideal for a determination of mechanistic events. In general, assessment of mechanisms requires more sophisticated and precise techniques, often at the cellular or subcellular level.

Clearance experiments in anesthetized animals offer several advantages over those described above. For example, the anesthetized animal can be controlled carefully with respect to problems of fluid balance, achievement of desired blood levels of a given chemical substance, elimination of problems of accurate urine collection, assessment of early toxic events, etc. In general, precision is greatly enhanced by this approach, although to some extent flexibility is lost. Precise assessment of renal-function parameters, such as inulin clearance or PAH clearance, is possible over relatively short time periods. Test compounds can be administered acutely. In addition, animals that have been pretreated chronically with a suspected nephrotoxin can be studied with the same approach, although, obviously, they cannot be used as their own controls. Hence, with anesthetized animals more precise measurements are possible for the determination of population values or control and treated animals than with unanesthetized animals. With the latter approach, however, each animal can serve as its own control.

Micropuncture Techniques

These highly sophisticated techniques permit assessment of nephron function rather then whole-kidney function. By perfusion of discrete segments of a nephron or measurement or renal function in a single nephron in an animal treated with a nephro-toxin, precise measurements of individual nephron function are possible, such as measurement of PAH secretion, glomerular function, tubular flow rate, sodium reab-sorption, potassium reabsorption, and so forth. The difficulty with these procedures, however, is that the techniques are highly specialized, extremely expensive to estab-lish, and very demanding technically.

Detailed reviews of micropuncture methodology and its pitfalls and usefulness are available (Roch-Ramel and Peters, 1979), and no elaborate discussion will be attempted here. Suffice it to say that although the techniques offer a tremendous opportunity for a better understanding of the effects of nephrotoxins, extreme care must be taken. The greatest likelihood of success will come from micropuncture experts developing an interest in renal toxicology, rather than toxicologists attempting an immediate mastery of micropuncture.

Renal Cortical-Slice Procedure

This technique and its utility in the assessment of renal transport processes as they relate to overall renal function is reviewed in detail elsewhere (Berndt, 1976b, 1982). The following summarizes important aspects of the technique.

Renal cortex slices may be prepared freehand or with the aid of a Stadie–Riggs microtome. Small slices or tissue fragments can be obtained from a McIlwain tissue slicer. The slices or fragments prepared by these procedures (0.2–0.5 mm in thick-ness) are incubated in a balanced salt solution at a known temperature and with appropriate oxygenation. In general, a temperature of 25 °C is used, even though this is not physiological. Nonetheless, for many transport studies the lower temperature seems to permit better survival of the slices for longer periods of time. These tissues will accumulate a variety of foreign organic compounds, both anions and cations. The uptake processes appear to be the in vitro counterparts of in vivo renal tubular secre-tion. At least three general lines of evidence support the in vitro–in vivo comparison.

1   From the literature, it is clear that substances added in vitro that enhance the accumulation of an organic anion, such as PAH, by renal cortex slices, will, in general, increase the maximal transport rate for that anion in vivo. Additionally, substances that decrease uptake in vitro also decrease in vivo transport, whether these are specific transport or metabolic inhibitors.

2   Transport studies in different species serve to amplify the in vitro–in vivo comparison. For example, diatrizoate, a urographic agent, which is accumulated actively by rabbit renal cortex slices, also is secreted actively by the intact rabbit kidney. In contrast, dog renal cortex slices do not show net accumulation of diatri-zoate, and whole-animal excretion studies (both clearance and stop-flow experiments) fail to demonstrate net tubular secretion.

3   Finally, the association between in vivo and in vitro function for organic anion transport is well substantiated by studies on the development of renal function in the newborn. Organic anion transport, whether assessed in vivo or in vitro, is absent or minimal in the newborn. Furthermore, organic anion transport, once again,

whether assessed in vivo or in vitro, was inducible in the newborn by pretreatment of the pregnant dam with compounds such as penicillin. Both in vivo and in vitro transport develop over the same time scale as renal function develops in the newborn.

Hence, renal cortex slices may be used to assess the accumulation of various organic anions and the effect of various nephrotoxins on this accumulation process. The data obtained from such studies appear to be directly transferable to the in vivo situation. In addition, animals that have been pretreated chronically with a potential nephrotoxin can have their kidneys used for organic anion accumulation studies at various times after pretreatment.

Although the details of organic cation transport are less well understood, it is probable that the same in vivo–in vitro relationship exists. Most of the slice studies that have been done were similar in design to those for the original organic anion studies. Few nephrologists doubt that in vitro organic cation accumulation is the equivalent of the in vivo secretory process. For example, in vivo secretion occurs in the proximal tubule and in vitro uptake occurs in renal cortex, not renal medulla. Furthermore, similar effects of inhibitors, both metabolic and competitive, are noted.

The in vivo–in vitro association, at least with organic anions, is completely consistent with what is known about the cellular handling of these substances. In mammals, the active tubular secretory step is located on the peritubular surface of the cell, which allows for the intracellular accumulation of large quantities of the anion under study. Under in vivo conditions, the anion diffuses passively or moves passively by a mediated process into the fluid in the tubular lumen, and hence into the final urine. With the in vitro studies, since there is no tubular fluid flow, the renal slice retains high concentrations of the organic anion under study. Hence, in each case, the critical measurement is of peritubular cell-membrane transport of the organic anion (and probably the organic cation). It is only a question of whether one assesses the transport by examining urine concentration of the anion (or cation) or its tissue concentration.

The renal-slice technique offers several advantages over studies on intact animals. Specific transport studies can be undertaken without unwanted influences of alterations in glomerular filtration rate or renal blood flow, either of which may affect the availability of metabolites, substrates, etc., to the renal tubular cells and hence indirectly affect transport. Noxious agents also may be tested in vitro without unwanted actions on other physiological systems. In addition, precise control over parameters such as temperature and gas atmosphere can be maintained. Finally, and not insignificantly, large numbers of experimental variables can be tested with the renal tissue from a single animal under in vitro conditions. In vivo, such studies would require many animals.

MECHANISMS OF NEPHROTOXICITY: PHYSIOLOGICAL EVENTS

The complexities involved in a description or definition of nephrotoxicity are no less noteworthy than the complexities of renal function itself. In the simplest terms, acute renal failure (ARF) results when there is an abrupt, frequently reversible impairment or cessation of renal function that results in an inability of the kidney to perform its usual homeostatic activities. This definition is suitable whether urinary output falls or whether it increases. Usually, anuria or oliguria results, although there are well-documented reports of so-called "high-output" renal failure. Which ever type of renal failure occurs, renal regulatory function is lost and the condition may be serious enough to be inconsistent with survival. Accordingly, the physician usually has to intervene with extraordinary measures to sustain life until renal function returns to normal.

A variety of causes exist for the production of ARF. For example, ureteral obstruction or sustained, systemic hypotension could result in an acute interruption of renal function. However, for the purposes of this discussion, the focus will be on those events that operate within the kidney to produce ARF. In general, acute disruption of renal blood flow, the administration of chemical nephrotoxins, etc. will produce acute tubular necrosis (ATN) as the hallmark of this type of acute renal failure. Some exceptions to this will be noted below. Some chemical compounds—for example, certain tetracycline degradation products—will produce a reversible Fanconi-like syndrome (Hook et al., 1979). Even with this syndrome, acute tubular necrosis is seen, although the disruption of renal function is more gradual than with acute renal failure.

The lack of predictability of the onset of ARF is important. Although acute traumatic insults, severe surgically induced hypotension, etc. are likely to result in an impairment, if not cessation, of renal function, the ability of chemicals to produce such events is far less predictable. Certainly, large doses of heavy metals, such as mercury, can be expected to disrupt renal function as well as produce other toxic effects. However, the administration of drugs in usual therapeutic doses or the chronic exposure to modest doses or concentrations of environmental pollutants may or may not be troublesome. Certain drugs used for visualization of the gallbladder (cholecystographic agents), for example, are administered in relatively large doses and with considerable frequency in the United States every year. Although suspicious and unpredictable disruption of renal function has occurred as a sequel to administration of these radiopaque substances, direct evidence of the nephrotoxic potential of such compounds is lacking. If these compounds are potentially nephrotoxic, it is unclear why such a low incidence occurs, although it may relate to the circumstances of their administration as well as to the compounds themselves. Although some antibiotics can be shown to be nephrotoxic after every administration when given in high enough doses, the underlying mechanisms whereby some individuals are susceptible to these effects, even in normal therapeutic doses, remain unknown. Hence, repeated use of various therapeutic agents and exposure in the environment to "new" contaminants may lead to a greater incidence of renal failure, but the predictability of these events probably will not be improved over the present.

Susceptibility of the Kidney to Chemical Nephrotoxins

Whatever the expression of the acute renal failure syndrome, the kidney is unusually sensitive to the effects of a wide variety of chemical substances to which it is exposed. From the medical viewpoint, advantage has been taken of this fact with the development of several classes of diuretics. The actions here, however, are reversible and highly desirable.

Several explanations have been offered for the unusual sensitivity of the kidney to exogenous chemicals. First, the kidneys constitute only approximately 1% of the body weight yet receive approximately one quarter of the cardiac output. Because of this high perfusion rate, the kidneys are exposed to large quantities of whatever chemical substances are dissolved in the blood. This may be the most important factor. Second, the renal architecture is such that the filtration and secretory processes expose the renal tubular cells to ample amounts of substances. For instance, proximal tubular cells of the nephron might be exposed both on the luminal surface and from the peritubular vascular network. The tubular surfaces may be exposed to chemical substances from the glomerular filtrate and, in addition, transport of some compounds by the cells themselves also may occur. Third, and perhaps of considerable importance, is the phenomenon of urinary concentration. Many chemical substances may become highly concentrated in the tubular fluid by means of the normal countercurrent multiplier process responsible for urinary concentration. Hence, as water is reabsorbed and the tubular fluid volume reduced, concentrations of certain chemicals may become a hundred- or a thousandfold higher than in the plasma, depending on whether or not the substances can pass readily across the tubular epithelia. Some studies have suggested that a therapeutic advantage might be obtained from this concentrative process. For example, antiobiotics might develop high tubular fluid concentrations, and this might facilitate their desirable pharmacological effect. Enhanced tubular fluid or tissue concentrations of harmful xenobiotics may have important implications for toxicology as well. Of course, as indicated, the importance of this mechanism will depend on the extent to which a xenobiotic will be concentrated in the tubular fluid, and to some extent that will depend on how readily the compound crosses the tubular epithelium. Although extensive studies along these lines have not been undertaken, the few investigations available highlight the importance of this event—for example, see Duggin and Mudge (1976).

Mechanisms of Anuria or Oliguria

Although it would appear that a clear-cut answer should be available for the mechanism underlying the failure to produce urine after a nephrotoxic insult, many years of study have failed to reveal an unequivocal explanation. Indeed, it may be possible that more than one mechanism is involved and that all of the theories presently of interest are correct, with one predominating over another because of certain experimental or clinical circumstances. For example, differences in experimental design, such as different doses, might favor one set of physiological events over another, hence highlighting one renal failure mechanism over another.

One theory (tubular obstruction theory, Fig. 7) states that the renal tubules become occluded by debris that has sloughed into the tubular lumen from the damaged tubular epithelia. This obstruction would in turn raise the intratubular pressure, so that eventually the elevated pressure will equal the net filtration pressure and termi-

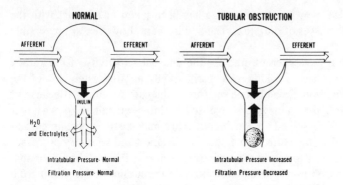

Figure 7 Renal tubular obstruction as a cause for anuria. See text for explanation.

nate glomerular filtration. This hypothesis is supported by a variety of experimental data:

1 Proteinaceous cases have been found frequently in the tubular lumina.

2 In *some* micropuncture studies it has been possible to demonstrate an elevated intraluminal pressure.

3 Some lumina have been found to be dilated as opposed to collapsed. This is thought to indicate an increased volume within the lumina and, hence, an increased pressure.

Not all the experimental data support this hypothesis, however. For example, data that support tubular obstruction come from a very few models of acute renal failure. In addition, although in some studies it has been possible to measure an increased intratubular pressure, in most studies this has not been possible. Finally, it should be noted that several investigators have demonstrated that the casts that have been observed in tubular lumina can be washed out with fluid pressures considerably below those generated by normal glomerular filtration. Hence, a few centimeters of water pressure could relieve the presumed obstruction.

As indicated above, more than one action may be involved, and it is possible that the role of tubular obstruction is to initiate in the glomerular vessels vasomotor changes that lead to a secondary reduction in glomerular filtration. That is, initially tubular obstruction occurs, which causes a disruption in glomerular function. Direct evidence for this proposal is lacking, however.

The passive back-flow or back-leak hypothesis has been investigated over many years and is supported by a variety of data. This proposal suggests that oliguria and/or anuria develop because of leakiness along the length of the nephron due to direct effects of the nephrotoxin on tubular permeability (Fig. 8). Because morphological evidence suggests that proximal tubular tissue is affected as much or more than any other segment of the nephron, it is usually thought that it is in the proximal tubule that the leakiness develops. Hence, no urine is formed because after filtration the tubular fluid leaks out of the nephron into the interstitium before it can traverse the length of the nephron to form the final urine. This hypothesis implies that glomerular filtration remains essentially normal in the face of the nephrotoxic insult, and whether or not an obstruction occurs is more or less irrelevant.

Several lines of evidence support this hypothesis.

1 The earliest observations were made by Dr. A. N. Richards in 1929. In these pioneering micropuncture experiments, studies were performed on frogs that had been treated with mercuric chloride. During a time when Richards could see a normal or greater than normal blood flow through the glomerulus and could collect a normal quantity of filtrate from Bowman's space by micropuncture, there was no urine being formed (Richards, 1929). Admittedly, these were very early micropuncture experiments, and some will argue that technical problems may have led to artifacts.

2 Bank et al. (1967) have demonstrated that lissamine green and inulin can leak from the nephron after the administration of a nephrotoxin. For instance, microinjection of inulin into the proximal tubule of a single nephron can be recovered completely from the final urine on the injected side when the kidney is healthy. No inulin appears on the contra-lateral side. After administration of a nephrotoxin, as little as 50% or less of the microinjected inulin can be recovered. The portion that was not recovered in the urine on the injected side was thought to have leaked out of the tubule and to have made its way into the systemic circulation, since the inulin eventually appeared in the urine from the kidney that was not injected.

3 Measurements of single-nephron glomerular filtration rate (SNGFR) have proven useful in dealing with this complicated issue. SNGFR is computed exactly as is whole-kidney glomerular filtration rate, except that the sampling is done from a single tubule that is fed by a single glomerulus. Theoretically, the same SNGFR should be calculated from samples collected from the distal segment of the nephron as from the proximal segment if technical adjustments are made to accommodate differences in flow rate. Indeed, in control animals with healthy renal function, identical SNGFRs were calculated by Bank and co-workers. Inulin was used as the nonreabsorbed solute in these studies. In rats pretreated with mercuric chloride, the SNGFR calculated from the early proximal tubule was the same as that for control rats.

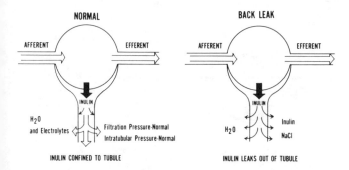

Figure 8 Back-leak as a cause of anuria. See text for explanation.

However, SNGFRs calculated from data obtained from late proximal or distal micro-punctures were significantly lower in mercury-treated rats than in controls, and significantly lower than the SNGFR values calculated from the early proximal punctures in the mercury treated rats. These observations are consistent with the leakage of inulin out of the nephron as it courses from the glomerulus to the collecting ducts. Micropuncture samples taken close to the glomerulus contained as much inulin as plasma, but samples taken far from the glomerulus had considerably reduced inulin content.

4   Abundant data exist to demonstrate that various nephrotoxins (e.g., metals, certain halogenated hydrocarbons) have direct effects on the renal tubular epithelium. For example, chromium can be shown to disrupt the normal inorganic electrolyte relationships within a renal cortex slice, as well as interfere with the active accumulation of a number of organic compounds. The magnitude of the effect is dependent on concentration of metal and presumably represents a direct attack on the transport processes in the renal tubular cells or on energy-producing mechanisms that support the transport. Of course, it is not clear how alterations in certain transport processes produced in vitro might relate to gross permeability changes in the intact nephron, but these data do demonstrate a direct effect of nephrotoxins on the tubular epithelium.

5   Zalme and colleagues (1976) have demonstrated an effect of mercury on renal brush border enzymes at a time thought to be far too early to be the result of vascular disruption. Although it may be difficult to argue about precise temporal relationships, few would argue that these data demonstrated a direct effect of a nephrotoxin on the proximal tubular epithelium.

Data that do not support this hypothesis are those that directly contradict the results of the experiments described above. Many of these data will be highlighted as

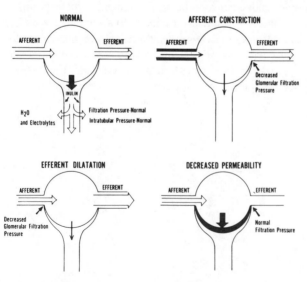

Figure 9   Alterations in glomerular events as a cause of anuria. See text for explanation.

explanations in support of an effect of nephrotoxins on the renal vasculature. Explanations for the discrepancies obtained from one laboratory versus another frequently are lacking or are incomplete.

The third proposal to explain the development of nephrotoxin-induced oliguria or anuria relates to the effects of these substances of the renal vasculature and has been summarized by Oken (1972). Stated simple, this proposal suggests that the primary event responsible for the lack of urine formation is a cessation or reduction of glomerular filtration, with the resultant decrease in tubular fluid flow (Fig. 9). The precise nature of the vascular action of substances that produce nephrotoxicity is unclear. Some workers have suggested marked afferent arteriolar vasoconstriction coupled with efferent arteriolar vasodilatation. This combination of effects would be consistent with the reduced filtration fraction observed in acute renal failure in humans. Another suggestion is that perfusion through the capillary remains unchanged, with the toxic effect being the result of an alteration in the filtration process. That is to say, the damage may be to the filtration mechanism itself, rather than to perfusion of the glomerular capillaries. This last hypothesis must be questioned, however, since it is clear that nephrotoxic substances can promote an intrarenal redistribution of blood (see below) and, hence, effects on flow do occur. Furthermore, proposals that deal with tubular events affecting glomerular activity more easily relate to alterations in renal vessel resistance, blood flow, etc., rather than to changes in glomerular capillary permeability. This is not to suggest that changes in glomerular capillary permeability may not be important, but it is to note that most data suggest other mechanisms.

A major complicating factor in the understanding of the mechanisms involved in nephrotoxin-induced anuria is the chemical diversity of the toxins that produce acute renal failure. For example, heavy metals such as mercury, chromium, or uranium, organic solvents such as carbon tetrachloride, and a variety of drugs, such as antibiotics, all produce approximately the same anatomical and physiological alterations. It would be appealing, therefore, to propose a common mechanism of action for this diverse group of chemicals that would ultimately lead to anuria or oliguria and the associated acute tubular necrosis. An action on the intrarenal vasculature might be such a mechanism.

Another attractive aspect of this proposal is that it is possible to suggest intrarenal mechanisms whereby glomerular filtration might be terminated under certain adverse conditions. For example, when there is damage to the renal tubular epithelium (whether by ischemia, a direct action on tubular cells, or some other means), the proximal tubule, and probably the loop of Henle, exhibit a reduced capacity to reabsorb sodium chloride. Hence, more sodium chloride than normal is delivered to the beginning of the distal tubule where the juxtaglomerular apparatus (JGA) is located. Whatever the nature of the sensing mechanism possessed by the JGA, it is clear that this apparatus can detect the increased delivery of sodium chloride and in response to this secrete renin. Ultimately, this leads to the production of angiotensin II. The locally produced angiotensin II would then cause constriction of the afferent arteriole belonging to that particular JGA-glomerulus complex, and this would reduce or abolish glomerular filtration in that particular nephron. To the extent that nephrons are damaged within a given kidney, more or less complete shutdown of whole kidney filtration could occur by this proposed mechanism.

Evidence in direct support of this hypothesis is as follows:

1 Data exist that demonstrate an intrarenal redistribution of blood after administration or injection of a nephrotoxin. For example, in humans, poisoning with carbon tetrachloride leads to a virtual blanching of outer cortical regions, with an increased blood flow through the outer medullary zone.

2 Direct measurement by micropuncture techniques have demonstrated a failure of glomerular filtration after the administration of large doses of mercuric chloride. In these studies, SNGFR decreased, as did intratubular pressure [see Oken (1972) for a summary of these data and those cited in Hook et al. (1979) above]. It is data such as these that directly contradict data in support of the back-leak hypothesis.

3 Certain drugs, such as indomethacin, seem to enhance the nephrotoxicity produced in some acute renal failure models, presumably by removal of the vasodilatory protection of the normally produced prostaglandins. This is an effect associated with antiinflammatory drugs, and is not a nonspecific effect.

4 The prior administration of salt loads, a maneuver known to deplete the kidney of renin, tends to reduce the severity of the acute renal failure caused by certain nephrotoxins, or at least to hasten recovery after the renal shutdown. These data are important for this hypothesis and have been debated considerably.

Not all data support this hypothesis. Of greatest concern to most investigators is the inability to prevent experimentally induced acute renal failure through inhibition

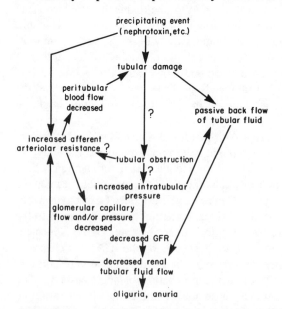

Figure 10 Summary of vascular and nonvascular factors potentially involved in anuric acute renal failure.

of renin release, formation of angiotensin, or formation of the angiotensin-converting enzyme. It is because of complications of this sort that many workers now suggest that the ultimate cause of the oliguria or anuria in acute renal failure is a combination of the above events.

Depicted in Fig. 10 is a schematic representation of the factors discussed above. It is conceivable that initially the nephrotoxin agent, either through the production of direct renal ischemia or direct renal tubular damage, initiates the events that lead to the acute renal failure syndrome. This effect is amplified and sustained through prolonged vasoconstriction, which can lead to a decreased GFR and a reduced peritubular blood flow. This latter effect enhances the direct tubular damage, leading to a greater degree of back-leak. Probably most workers would agree that a primary event in the production of acute renal failure is the vascular one. However, depending on the particular experimental model under study, homeostatic mechanisms in effect at the time the nephrotoxin is administered, etc., one or another anuric mechanism might predominate in a given situation. That is to say, glycerol-induced acute renal failure is not the same as mercury-induced renal failure. Hence, in one instance a predominance of the vascular events may be obvious, while with another enhanced tubular leakiness may become more important. Differences in doses, times of administration, or other alterations in the experimental protocols may be just as important.

Mechanisms Involved in "High-Output" Renal Failure

Although superficial explanations can be offered for the loss of the homeostatic function of the kidney coupled with high urine output, as one delves further into the problem it becomes exceedingly complex. For example, based on what is known about the effects of certain diuretics it is conceivable that nephrotoxins could more or less mimic these actions by a selective interference with active chloride transport in the thick ascending limb of Henle's loop, which in turn, of course, would lead to an increased urine output. However, this is a relatively naive supposition if one explores the actions of the loop diuretics. These agents act at a selective site, but in so doing do not cause a total disruption of homeostatic mechanisms within the kidney and certainly do not alter glomerular function, cause an elevation of BUN, etc. The key is that with high-output renal failure, as with oliguria or anuria, a complete disruption of the balance function of the kidney is observed. Even though potentially reversible, this is the most striking feature of acute renal failure.

Possibly, a combination of events occurs in the high output syndrome. An action on the thick ascending limb of Henle's loop might account for the large volume of urine being excreted. This might be coupled with an effect of the nephrotoxin on the distal tubule and collecting-duct permeabilities to water, which would explain the resistance of this syndrome to antidiuretic hormone. The lack of clear morphological evidence, however, to suggest an action of most nephrotoxins on the distal segment of the nephron makes this explanation unlikely. Alteration of proximal tubular and/or glomerular events seems essential as the major component in the high-output syndrome, as with anuric failure. Therefore, the best explanation of high-output failure may be that although glomerular filtration rate may be greatly reduced, there also is a significant deficit in nephron reabsorption so that sizable quantities of the filtered fluid are excreted. Such a pattern would be facilitated if back-leak were minimal, but also could occur if significant back-leak existed and normal reabsorptive processes were minimal or nonexistent.

This possibility has been investigated in the work of Phillips, Hayes, and Berndt (Phillips et al., 1980; Berndt et al., 1980; Berndt, 1983). Citrinin, a nephrotoxin of fungal origin, causes a high output syndrome in the Sprague-Dawley rat. These animals produced 24-h urine volumes of 4–8 times greater than normal after a single dose of citrinin, and these were sustained for several days. However, if a rat pretreated with citrinin was anesthetized and glomerular filtration rate (GFR) was measured with insulin, the GFR was found to be greatly reduced, as was the minute-to-minute urine output. Both the GRF and urine flow were reduced by as much as 10-fold. The total 24-h urine output based on the urinary excretion per minute in the anesthetized rat predicted quite precisely the 24-h urine volumes measured in the conscious animal. Hence, although the glomerular filtration rate was reduced in high-output failure, there was also a great reabsorptive deficit, so that as much as 15–20% of the filtered fluid load was excreted. In normal rats, 99 + % of the filtered fluid was reabsorbed. Precise quantitative studies to substantiate these arguments are difficult to accomplish. Nonetheless, the semiquantitative approach presented above is totally consistent with existing data.

MECHANISMS OF NEPHROTOXICITY: BIOCHEMICAL EVENTS

Modern renal toxicology is relatively new, and certain deficiencies are obvious in both conceptual and mechanistic areas. Frequently, precise descriptions of the fundamental changes elicited by toxic chemicals are lacking. Partly, this has been because the application of well-understood membrane effects of chemicals has been applied only recently to the kidney. In addition, the role of renal xenobiotic metabolism is only now being developed. A few generalities are possible with respect to cellular or subcellular events, however, and some of these will be discussed below.

Cell Membrane Effects

The cell membrane may serve as a protective barrier in many organ systems. As such it may be expected to have the first encounter with foreign substances that appear in the cellular environment, whether supplied in blood or tubular fluid. Heavy metals, for example, are known to alter brush-border enzymes in kidney very early after administration (Stroo and Hook, 1977). Although some selectivity exists with respect to the actions of the heavy metals, both mercury and chromium can produce these effects. Another example of such effects comes from the work of Ganote et al. (1974). These investigators attempted an ultrastructural and metabolic study of the time course of mercuric chloride-induced nephrotoxicity. Although by no means unequivocal, it appears that some of the earliest effects observed (loss of brush-border enzymes, disruption of cellular electrolytes, etc.) could be interpreted to be membrane effects rather than effects related directly to tissue metabolism.

These observations were best delineated by the work of McDowell et al. (1976) and Zalme et al. (1976). In these studies the investigators examined the time course of tubular dysfunction after the administration of a moderate nephrotoxic dose of mercuric chloride. The earliest time studied was 15 min after administration of mercury. Urinary excretion of brush-border enzymes was increased at 15 min but returned to normal in a few hours. Only modest morphological changes were observed at 3 h associated with tubular membranes, with severe necrosis of pars recta cells noted at 24 h. Primarily, morphological changes were observed in the pars recta segment of the nephron, with only modest damage seen in the pars convoluta.

All of these observations support the concept that metals (and perhaps other xenobiotics) act first on cell membranes. Rothstein (1973) suggested this attribute of "geographical specificity" of metal–ligand interactions: that is, the first interactions are with membrane ligands, with intracellular interactions occurring secondarily. Hence, release of brush-border enzymes would be expected before changes in mitochondrial structure or function. Of course, to demonstrate these precise relationships it is often necessary to select both dose and times of study very carefully. Too large a dose could overwhelm both membrane and intracellular activities, resulting in no discernment of cellular sites of action. Studies too late in the course of the toxic reaction would not reveal the selective events seen only at the earliest times. Clearly, to delineate "geographical specificity," careful time-course studies are required.

Not only metals act on cell membranes. Unquestionably, membrane effects are known to occur with certain antibiotic compounds; indeed, both the bacteriocidal and the nephrotoxic actions of the polymixins have been attributed to their surface-active properties. These compounds are known to disrupt the functional organization of the membrane, which may lead to the inability of the membrane to serve as an osmotic barrier. Probably amphotericin B also is active, at least in part, by a similar means, and this also may account for some of its nephrotoxic effects. Although some workers have demonstrated that gentamicin can produce inhibition of mitochondrial respiration, which presumably would lead to a depressed energy production, the time sequence of these events suggests that this is not a primary action. Indeed, the temporal sequence is not unlike that observed with mercuric chloride or other nephrotoxins, and suggests that the initial event may be an attack on the integrity of the cell membrane rather than an action on metabolism. Membrane permeability changes caused by gentamicin may, in fact, lead to a depressed mitochondrial function. The chemistry of specific membrane interactions aside, Kaloyanides and colleagues have proposed that gentamicin and related substances enter cells by specific interactions leading to disruption of lysosomal activity (a second membrane interaction), with the ultimate mitochondrial disruption occurring as a result of lysosomal enzyme attack (Kaloyanides and Pastoriza-Munoz, 1980).

The above are offered as examples of what may be important mechanisms of action of nephrotoxic substances. Conceivably such compounds could disrupt either the peritubular or the luminal membranes in the proximal tubule (because these are the first cells exposed to the nephrotoxin), and this could ultimately alter energy production through changes in mitochondrial function, leading to a final development of the necrotic syndrome. Changes in mitochondrial function might occur because of direct effects of the toxin or because the enhanced membrane permeability permits a pertubation of the intracellular environment. Gross alterations of membrane structure could lead ultimately to an inability of the membrane to serve as an osmotic barrier, and this could in turn contribute to cell lysis. In addition, disruption of the membrane structure may be responsible for the "leakiness" of the proximal nephron segment hypothesized for some models of acute renal failure. This could lead to the enhanced transfer out of the nephron of glomerular filtrate, as proposed in the "back-leak" theory.

Intracellular Interactions

It is well established that heavy metals and some organic compounds can react with sulfhydryl-containing substances in the kidney and other organs. Usually the sulfhydryl interaction is expressed in alterations of tissue glutathione concentrations or more precisely nonprotein sulfhydryl groups (NPSG), but, of course, reaction with glutathione itself is not the critical event in the production of cellular damage. On the contrary, the critical nature of glutathione comes from its ability to protect other sulfhydryl-containing substances in kidney and liver tissue by reacting with various xenobiotics. It is thought that the nonglututhione sulfhydryl-containing substances have important roles in preserving cellular homeostasis.

Interactions of glutathione (NPSG) with ligands are complex, however. Richardson and Murphy (1975) demonstrated a close correlation between renal glutathione concentrations and the accumulation of methylmercury. The role of this interaction in the cellular economy was unclear in that it might have served as a protective mechanism or a process for methylmercury accumulations by renal tubular cells. Metals are known to interact with other intracellular ligands as well, for example, cadmium with metallothionein.

With various organic compounds, once glutathione is sufficiently depleted, then a potentially toxic substance may be able to interact with the more critical sulfhydryl groups in the intracellular environment (Mudge et al., 1978). The exact nature of the substances with which the toxins might interact to produce nephrotoxicity is poorly defined. Covalent binding of some substances to macromolecular structures (proteins, nucleic acids) within the kidney has been demonstrated, but the underlying relationships that lead to nephrotoxicity are not completely understood (see below). Even when quantitative descriptions are possible concerning the numbers of groups of reactive substances available for binding, their precise relationship to the nephrotoxic phenomenon remains unclear (Magos and Clarkson, 1977). Indeed, at the extreme it might be suggested that the covalent interactions are irrelevant to the nephrotoxic response. Although few would share such a radical position, it does tend to emphasize how little is known about these fundamental toxicological mechanisms.

Although exact intracellular tissue sites with which important chemical reactions might occur are poorly defined, some generalities are possible. Examples are given next that highlight known or potential intracellular sites of reactivity with nephrotoxic substances.

Energetic Mechanisms Once a toxin enters a cell by passage through the cell membrane, a likely target for disruption of cell function might be the energy-producing mechanisms. Either glycolytic or oxidative pathways could be involved, which would in turn lead to a failure of energy supply and an eventual failure of the processes that utilize that energy, for example, transport processes.

Although gentamicin probably has important effects on the cell membrane, as noted above there also is evidence to suggest that with sufficient cellular deterioration mitochondrial function is compromised as well. Reduced mitochondrial respiration has been reported, a deficiency that subsequently may cause a complete disruption of energy-dependent systems in intermediary metabolism (Vera-Roman et al., 1975; Kluwe and Hook, 1978). It should be pointed out, however, that the effects of gentamicin on the mitochondrial function may or may not be primary events. Conceivably, failure of the energy supply may be secondary to other effects, but unquestionably these are demonstrable effects of nephrotoxic compounds and at the very least would contribute to the production of the nephrotoxic syndrome.

Another aminoglycoside antibiotic, kanamycin, appears to have a more direct effect on energy metabolism. High doses of this antibiotic have been found in the kidney and the perilymph of the inner ear. It was possible to correlate the presence of the antibiotic with an inhibition of the Embden–Meyerhof glycolytic pathway (Tachibana et al., 1976). Glycolytic pathways in other tissues were unaffected, as were the hexose monophosphate enzymes in the kidney. Hence, the effect of kanamycin appears to be directed at energy metabolism and to be relatively specific. A precise understanding of the mechanisms that dictate this unusual degree of specificity is lacking, as is a clear explanation of the distribution of these substances.

Tetracycline and especially its degradation products, epitetracycline and anhydrotetracycline, have been shown to alter mitochondrial structure and function. After administration of these substances, mitochondrial swelling occurs and respiration is compromised. These effects are not unique to the tetracycline compounds but are seen for a number of nephrotoxic substances, for example, heavy metals. Once again, it is not clear that these effects are primary causes of the nephrotoxicity produced by the tetracycline breakdown products, but they may well be contributory. Indeed, it is noteworthy that certain heavy metals and the tetracycline products produce similar effects on energy production by mitochondria, but cause different effects on renal function. For example, mercury produces acute renal failure with acute tubular necrosis, while the tetracycline compounds produce a Fanconi-like syndrome. This may be further evidence that the effects on energy metabolism are secondary events—that is, the result rather than the cause of the renal dysfunction. Indeed, a clear definition of cause-and-effect relationships is difficult with many nephrotoxins as well as other toxic xenobiotics.

Lipid Interactions A paucity of data exists concerning the role of lipid peroxidation in the development of nephrotoxicity. It is generally accepted that in carbon tetrachloride-induced hepatotoxicity lipid peroxidation plays a central role. Homolytic cleavage of CCl_4 to the trichloromethyl free radical has been suggested to be a very early event, if not the initiating one, in this process, with this free radical then generating other reactive compounds through the lipid peroxidative process. In general, substances that enhance CCl_4 metabolism seem to enhance hepatotoxicity, while those compounds that retard metabolism appear to reduce hepatotoxicity. The next step in the toxicological process is for the free radicals to react with vulnerable tissue sites, an event readily demonstrable with CCl_4 as well as other toxins. For example, it is known that $^{14}CCl_4$ will bind in a so-called covalent manner to lipids and proteins in the liver.

Carbon tetrachloride nephrotoxicity is at least as complicated as hepatoxicity. Direct evidence does not exist to date to implicate lipid peroxidation as a mechanism for CCl_4-induced nephrotoxicity. However, preliminary evidence suggests that CCl_4 metabolism is important for the production of nephrotoxicity (Hook et al., 1979), and by analogy to the liver, this might be suggestive of a similar mechanism of action. The problem is complicated further by sizable species variations in the renal response to CCl_4.

Protein Interactions A number of nephrotoxic compounds can be demonstrated to interact with tissue proteins. It is presumed that these interactions are of a covalent nature and are responsible for the development of necrosis, although the details of this relationship are not understood. Incidentally, covalent binding in studies of this sort is defined functionally. As an example, Mudge et al. (1978), as well as many others, used an exhaustive extraction technique. With this procedure an attempt is made to remove all "loosely bound" nephrotoxins, leaving only that material that coprecipitates with protein in trichloroacetic acid. Since the nephrotoxin is not removable by exhaustive extraction in various solvents, it is concluded to be covalently bound to the proteins with which it coprecipitated. Direct evidence of covalent bonding has not been forthcoming in renal studies, although isolation of specific ligands to which compounds have bound is being pursued in several liver studies.

Regardless of the specific substances that might interact with proteins, the importance of intrarenal metabolism of these substances cannot be overemphasized. As indicated earlier, three important subsegments of the proximal tubule have been delineated. The SIII segment comprises the straight portion of the proximal tubule, located in the medullary ray and outer stripe of the outer medulla. Many studies have been done in the rat, and the SIII cells are morphologically distinct from those in the other proximal subsegments: the cells have less height, less well developed and organized mitochondria, and more endoplasmic reticulum than SI or SII cells.

Consideration of renal xenobiotic metabolism requires a focus on SIII cells, however. The kidney apparently contains fewer cytochrome P-450s than the liver, but what is available would appear to exist predominantly in the SIII segment (Dees et al., 1980, 1982). Although the entire proximal tubule contains components of the mixed-function oxidase system, immunofluorescence techniques suggest the major localization to be in SIII. Because this segment comprises only a small part of the nephron (perhaps no more than 15%) it is not surprising that over all renal cytochrome P-450 activity is low. However, should xenobiotic metabolism that leads to a toxic metabolite occur in this nephron segment, significant pars recta damage should be expected.

A number of halogenated hydrocarbons have been shown to produce experimental nephrotoxicity. Reid (1973) found that bromobenzene in rats and mice produced severe renal necrosis at varying times after its administration. By a combination of histopathological, autoradiographic, and exhaustive extraction studies, Reid demonstrated that the [^{14}C]bromobenzene was covalently bound to renal proteins. Further, the localization of the ^{14}C label was primarily in the proximal tubules, and the areas showing binding also showed necrosis. Glomeruli were not damaged and showed little or no binding of the ^{14}C. Interestingly, this study also presented some of the first information to suggest that conversion to an active metabolite in the kidney may be important for the production of nephrotoxicity. Little or no binding of the [^{14}C]bromobenzene or evidence of microsomal damage could be obtained with in vitro experiments, suggesting that in vivo metabolism was essential. If the bromobenzene must be converted to a highly spontaneously reactive intermediate in order to exert its effects, it seems unlikely that the site of the reaction would be the liver. If chemical activation occurred in the liver and renal damage resulted, the reactive metabolite would have to retain its reactivity while in transit from the liver to the kidney. The chemical nature of such a highly spontaneously reactive, yet organ-specific, toxin has not been identified. Indeed, a highly spontaneously reactive intermediate would be expected to react with structures in the vicinity of its production. However, these first studies by Reid ended with the conclusion that the liver was the site of conversion to a reactive compound that acts in the kidney. Perhaps this conclusion was offered to emphasize that the nature of the so-called reactive intermediate is often unknown—indeed, speculative. For example, in this situation one might speculate that bromobenzene could be converted in the liver to a metabolite that would have sufficient stability to arrive at the kidney, because the final activation of the metabolite occurred in the kidney. Hence, the specificity of action would then relate either to the relative selectivity of the tissue organelle or molecule with which the bromobenzene metabolite interacts, or to the ability of the kidney to activate the bromobenzene metabolite to a spontaneously reactive intermediate.

Studies with chloroform demonstrated a metabolism-dependent renal necrosis in the mouse. Once again, covalent binding of the ^{14}CHCl$_3$ could be associated with the areas of necrosis in the tissue, but maximum binding occurred far in advance of the development of histological damage. This latter result is entirely consistent with the production of some reactive metabolite that interacts with vulnerable renal macromolecules. This interaction then sets in motion an as-yet-undefined sequence of events that terminates in the development of necrosis.

Several 2-substituted furans—for example, the diuretic furosemide—apparently can be activated to substances that will produce renal and/or hepatic necrosis. These effects are seen only after extremely large doses of furosemide are administered. Requirements for the activating reaction differ in the kidney from that in the liver, and this, along with other evidence, suggests that metabolism in the kidney itself is an important consideration.

The antibiotic cephaloridine has been shown to be nephrotoxic. This compound, according to Tune et al. (1977), is transported into the proximal tubular cells by the organic anion transport system. Once it has accumulated to sufficiently high concentrations in the intracellular environment, it produces a toxic effect. High intracellular concentrations of this compound are possible, even though it is transported actively into the cell, because it crosses the luminal membrane very poorly, unlike PAH, for example, which traverses the luminal membrane readily. The usual passive entry (whether mediated or by simple diffusion) into the luminal fluid of substances transported by the organic anion transport process appears to fail with cephaloridine. The exact mechanisms involved intracellularly are unclear. However, evidence for covalent bonding of various thiophenes, including cephaloridine, to renal proteins has been offered by McMurtry and Mitchell (1977), but the exact meaning of these observations is unclear. In any event, whatever the sequence of events beyond the initial binding phenomenon, cephaloridine, as with so many other nephrotoxins, seems to be able to undergo what is thought to be the initiating step in the production of nephrotoxicity. Although this may represent an example of a substance that must be activated in renal tissue before it exerts its nephrotoxic effect, the details of the requirements for the activation process are poorly defined at this time.

Other actions of cephaloridine also have been suggested. Studies by Silverblatt et al. (1970) indicated abnormal mitochondrial structure soon after cephaloridine administration. This led Tune and colleagues to examine possible effects of cephaloridine and other cephalosporin antibiotics on renal mitochondrial function (Tune et al., 1979; Tune and Fravert, 1980). Both in vitro and after in vivo administration, cephaloridine decreased the respiratory control ratio significantly, suggesting a loss of mitochondrial integrity. The in vitro effects occurred promptly after addition of the antibiotic and at concentrations of cephaloridine actually achieved after administration to intact animals. Further, these in vitro effects suggest a direct action of cephaloridine rather than an action mediated by a metabolite.

Finally, a few comments about the nephrotoxic analgesics are appropriate. Studies on analgesic nephropathy are complex because there is great difficulty in mimicking in the experimental laboratory the human medullary or papillary necrosis thought to be associated with phenacetin consumption (and perhaps other compounds) by humans. Acute cortical necrosis is possible with acetaminophen when administered in a high dose in the appropriate species. However, whether or not this acute cortical syndrome bears any relationship to the chronic medullary or papillary events noted in humans is doubtful. It is clear, however, that acetaminophen and its known conjugates behave rather differently within the kidney. Duggin and Mudge (1976) were able to demonstrate that acetaminophen itself could penetrate into the cells of the medullary tissue of dogs, whereas the conjugates could not. It was suggested, therefore, that acetaminophen itself might be responsible for the cytotoxicity, or possibly a metabolite produced intracellularly in the kidney. Data do not exist to differentiate between these two possibilities, or to indicate whether either possibility is correct as far as medullary disease is concerned.

Acute tubular necrosis of the cortical proximal tubule may result from exposure to a number of reactive substances. For example, aminophenols, quinones, quinoneimines, and even catechols might result from intrarenal metabolism of the large variety of substances that traverse the kidney, and perhaps these compounds or further metabolites might undergo covalent binding or produce the other effects necessary to initiate the toxic process (Mudge, 1982). The degree of severity of the toxicity would depend on the chemical compound involved and whether or not conversion to a reactive substance is possible. In any event, biochemical lesions as demonstrated by covalent binding can be associated with the development of necrosis (usually not on identical time scales) and are thought to be related as cause and effect.

Newton et al. (1982) have examined the possible nephrotoxic effects of *p*-aminophenol (PAP), a metabolite of acetaminophen. Carpenter and Mudge (1981) and Gemborys and Mudge (1981) noted the presence of PAP in studies on mouse kidney and earlier Calder et al. (1971, 1975, 1979) investigated possible nephrotoxic effects of PAP. Calder et al. (1979) noted that nephrotoxic effects of PAP probably were related to the formation of a reactive intermediate. Newton et al. (1982) investigated the relevance of these matters to acetaminophen nephrotoxicity. They identified PAP as an acetaminophen metabolite in the Fischer-344 rat, a strain of rat in which acetaminophen is nephrotoxic. Furthermore, PAP formation in the kidney was demonstrated by the use of the isolated perfused kidney. Hence, these studies afford direct evidence for one toxic metabolite of acetaminophen that may account for the nephrotoxic response.

Specific suggestions concerning the underlying mechanisms that might be involved in the production of nephrotoxicity once covalent bonding has occurred are lacking. Whether or not this irreversible interaction causes a failure of energy production, a disruption of the cell membranes from the inside out, permanent disruption of protein synthetic mechanisms, interference with lysosomal function, or any combination of these or other processes is quite unclear. All of these might be envisioned to take time after the initial insult, and all of them might be sufficient to result in irreversible damage. Quite clearly, many if not all of the above events have been observed, but it is not always clear whether these cause the nephrotoxic response or are the result of it. Hence, although the events occur, their role(s) in the nephrotoxicity response remains obscure.

RECAPITULATION

Several features of renal function must be kept in mind in an analysis of the effects of potential nephrotoxins. The functional unit of the kidney, the nephron, is in reality a series of functional units. Each segment of the nephron subserves a different physiological role, and it should be anticipated, therefore, that the effects produced by exogenous chemicals will vary depending in part on the section in the nephron on which they act. The preponderance of effects seems to be in the proximal tubule, where acute tubular necrosis occurs. However, analgesic nephropathy is clearly a medullary event and apparently bears little direct relationship to the acute necrotic syndromes seen in the cortex.

A clear single definition of nephrotoxicity is lacking because the event(s) is (are) as complex as the renal function itself. Although attempts are made routinely to develop and describe "simple" screening procedures for substances with effects on the kidney, these are generally unsatisfactory or at least have significant limitations. A multitude of physiological parameters need to be monitored in order, first, to establish that renal dysfunction has occurred, and second, to describe it. Unfortunately, many of the more powerful tools for analysis of renal function have not been and are not now being applied to a study of renal toxicity. Use of the isolated perfused nephron technique to establish a quantitative description of the actions of nephrotoxins on individual nephron segments is lacking in the literature. This technique has proven extremely valuable in understanding basic physiological, cellular, and subcellular events within the kidney, and should be utilized more frequently by toxicologists.

Only slightly more commonly used are techniques that allow direct assessment of renal transport parameters (e.g., micropuncture procedures) and the relationship of these to overall renal function. Techniques exist whereby one can examine the effects of a variety of chemical substances on the transport of both organic and inorganic compounds by the kidney and the actions of nephrotoxins on these transport processes. To establish fundamental membrane effects of nephrotoxins, however, specific studies directed at the use of isolated membrane vesicles and the effects of nephrotoxins on transport processes in these are essential.

Despite many years of intense study of the response of physiological parameters to nephrotoxins, a clear understanding of the mechanisms of oliguric or high-output renal failure is unavailable. Probably two major factors contribute to oliguria or anuria: back-leak out of the nephron, and intrarenal vascular disruption. Which one of these events predominates in a given experimental model is not clear. Further, more study is needed to determine the factors that cause predominance of one or the other mechanism. High-output renal failure, although described in the experimental as well as clinical literature, is even more poorly understood in terms of mechanism.

At the cellular or subcellular level, studies are only now developing that may yield insights into mechanisms of action. Effects of nephrotoxins on membrane function (plasma membrane, intracellular membranes) are developing and seem to be a promising direction for the future. Possible actions of nephrotoxins on energetic mechanisms also are being explored. It does appear that a preoccupation with purely descriptive studies (morphological and otherwise) is giving way to more sophisticated attempts at establishing underlying mechanisms. Until a clear-cut understanding of the fundamental events that underlie the disruption of renal function in several experimental models is possible, it will not be possible to develop appropriate remedies.

Finally, it should be noted that although most investigations concerning nephrotoxic compounds revolve around those substances that are humanmade, there exists an abundance of "naturally occurring" nephrotoxins of which we should be aware. For example, many fungal toxins are known to affect renal function (Elling et al., 1975; Krogh, 1976; Berndt et al., 1980). These substances are widespread in the environment and are probably a greater source of human contamination than is generally realized. Most of these compounds that have been studied demonstrate effects at most levels of assessment not unlike those produced by other nephrotoxic substances, although details of these effects vary somewhat. The role of naturally occurring substances in the production of disease states and their potential interaction with other, known nephrotoxic pollutants (e.g., organic solvents, many metals, etc.) may prove a fruitful area of study for the future. The large background of information on the heavy metal, solvent, etc. models for acute renal failure should be useful in the development of a better understanding of the nephrotoxicity produced by newly discovered substances. Once again, however, it must be emphasized that fundamental mechanisms must be understood before the relationship of these effects to basic physiology is known or before appropriate remedies can be sought.

REFERENCES

Bank, N., Mutz, B. F., and Aynedjian, H. S. 1967. The role of "leakage" of tubular fluid in anuria due to mercury poisoning. *J. Clin Invest.* 46:695–704.

Berndt, W. O. 1975. The effect of potassium dichromate on renal tubular transport processes. *Toxicol. Appl. Pharmacol.* 32:40–52.

Berndt, W. O. 1976a. Renal function tests: What do they mean? A review of renal anatomy, biochemistry, and physiology. *Environ. Health Perspect.* 15:55–71.

Berndt, W. O. 1976b. Use of the tissue slice technique for evaluation of renal transport processes. *Environ. Health Perspect.* 15:73–88.

Berndt, W. O. 1979. Effects of toxic chemicals on renal transport processes. *Fed. Proc.* 38:2226–2233.

Berndt, W. O. 1982. Renal methods in toxicology. In *Principles and Methods in Toxicology,* eds. A. W. Hayes and R. Dixon, pp. 447–474. New York: Raven.

Berndt, W. O. 1983. The nephrotoxicity of mycotoxins and botanicals. In *Nephrotoxicity, Assessment and Pathogenesis,* eds. P. Bach, F. W. Bonner, J. W. Bridges, and E. A. Lock, pp. 378–395. New York: Wiley.

Berndt, W. O., Hayes, A. W., and Phillips, R. D. 1980. Effects of mycotoxins on renal function: Mycotoxic nephropathy. *Kid. Int.* 18:656–664.

Brenner, B. M., and Rector, F. C., eds. 1981. *The Kidney,* vol. I and II. Philadelphia: Saunders.

Burg, M. B. 1981. Renal handling of sodium, chloride, water, amino acids and glucose. In *The Kidney,* 2d ed., eds. B. M. Brenner and F. C. Rector, vol. I, pp. 330–370. Philadelphia: W. B. Saunders.

Calder, I. C., Funder, C. C., Green, C. R., Ham, K.N., and Tange, J. D. 1971. Comparative nephrotoxicity of aspirin and phenacetin derivatives. *Br. Med. J.* 4:518–521.

Calder, I. C., Williams, P. J., Woods, R. A., Funder, C. C., Green, C. R., Ham, K. N., and Tange, J. D. 1975. Nephrotoxicity and molecular structure. *Xenobiotica* 5:303–307.

Calder, I. C., Yong, A. C., Woods, R. A., Crowe, C. A., Ham, K.N., and Tange, J.D. 1979. The nephrotoxicity of *p*-aminophenol. II. The effect of metabolic inhibitors and inducers. *Chem. Biol. Interact.* 27:245–254.

Carpenter, H. C., and Mudge, G. H. 1981. Acetaminophen nephrotoxicity: Studies on renal acetylation and deacetylation. *J. Pharmacol. Exp. Ther.* 218:161–167.

Cohen, J. J. 1979. Is the function of the renal papilla coupled exclusively to an anaerobic pattern of metabolism? *Am. J. Physiol.* 236:F423–F433.

Cohen, J. J., and Kamm, D. E. 1981. Renal metabolism: Relation to renal function. In *The Kidney,* eds. B. M. Brenner and F. C. Rector, vol. I, pp. 144–249. Philadelphia: Saunders.

Dees, J. H., Coe, L. D., Yasukochi, Y., and Masters, B. S. 1980. Immunofluorescence, NADPH-cytochrome C (P-450) reductase in rat and minipig tissues injected with phenobarbital. *Science* 208:1473–1475.

Dees, J. H., Parkhill, L. K. Okita, R. T., Yashuchochi, Y., and Masters, B. S. 1982. Localization of NADPH-cytochrome P-450 reductase and cytochrome P-450 in animal kidneys. In *Nephrotoxicity, Assessment and Pathogenesis,* eds. P. H. Bach, F. W. Bonner, F. W. Bridges, and E. A. Lock, pp. 246–249. New York: Wiley Heyden.

Duggin, G. G., and Mudge, G. H. 1976. Analgesic nephropathy: Renal distribution of acetaminophen and its conjugates. *J. Pharmacol. Exp. Ther.* 199:1–9.

Elling, F., Hald, B., Jacobsen, C., and Krogh, P. 1975. Spontaneous cases of nephropathy in poultry associated with ochratoxin A. *Acta Pathol. Microbiol. Scand. [A]* 83:739–744.

Foulkes, E. C. 1977. Mechanism of renal excretion of environmental agents. In *Handbook of Physiology, section 9: Reactions to Environmental Agents,* ed. D. H. K. Lee, pp. 495–503. Baltimore: Williams & Wilkins.

Foulkes, E. C., and Hammond, P. B. 1975. Toxicology of the kidney. In *Toxicology, The Basic Science of Poisons,* eds. L. J. Cassarett and J. Doull, pp. 190–201. New York: Macmillan.

Ganote, C. E., Reimer, K. A., and Jennings, R. B. 1974. Acute mercuric chloride nephrotoxicity. An electron microscopic and metabolic study. *Lab. Invest.* 31:633–647.

Gemborys, M. W., and Mudge, G. H. 1981. Formation and deposition of the minor metabolites of acetaminophen in the hamster. *Drug. Metab. Dispos.* 9:340–351.

Holohan, P. D., Pessah, N. I., Warkentin, and D. Ross, C. R. 1976. The purification of an organic cation-specific binding protein found by kidney. *Mol. Phamacol.* 12:494–503.

Hook, J. B., McCormack, K. M., and Kluwe, W. M. 1979. Biochemical mechanisms of nephrotoxicity. In *Review in Biochemical Toxicology,* eds. E. Hodgson, J. R. Bend, and R. M. Philpot, vol. 1, pp. 53–78. New York: Elsevier North Holland.

Kaloyanides, G., and Pastoriza-Munoz, E. 1980. Aminoglycoside nephrotoxicity. *Kid. Int.* 18:571–582.

Kluwe, W. M., and Hook, J. B. 1978. Functional nephrotoxicity of gentamicin in the rat. *Toxicol. Appl. Pharmacol.* 45:163–175.

Krogh, P. 1976. Epidemiology of mycotoxic procine nephropathy. *Nord. Vet. Med.* 28:452–458.

Lee, J. B., and Peter H. M. 1969. Effect of oxygen tension on glucose metabolism in rabbit kidney cortex and medulla. *Am. J. Physiol.* 217:1464–1471.

Lewy, P. R., Quintanilla, A., Levin, A. W., and Kessler, R. H. 1973. Renal energy metabolism and sodium reabsorption. *Annu. Rev. Med.* 24:365–384.

Maack, T., Johnson, V. Kau, S. T., Figueiredo, J., and Sigulem, D. 1979. Renal filtration, transport, and metabolism of low-molecular-weight proteins: A review. *Kid. Int.* 16:251–270.

Magos, L., and Clarkson, T. W. 1977. Renal injury and urinary excretion. In *Handbook of Physiology, section 9: Reactions to Environmental Agents,* ed. D. H. K. Lee, pp. 503–513. Baltimore: Williams & Wilkins.

McDowell, E. M., Nagle, R. B., Zalme, R. C., McNeil, J. S., Flamenbaum, W., and Trump, B. F. 1976. Studies on the pathophysiology of acute renal failure. I. Correlation of ultrastructure and function in the proximal tubules of the rat following administration of mercuric chloride. *Virchows Arch. [Cell Pathol.]* 22:173–196.

McKinney, T. D. 1982. Heterogeneity of organic base secretion by proximal tubules. *Am. J. Physiol.* 243:F404–F407.

McMurtry, R. J., and Mitchell, J. R. 1977. Renal and hepatic necrosis after metabolic activation of 2-substituted furans and thiophenes, including furosemide and cephaloridine. *Toxicol. Appl. Pharmacol.* 42:285–300.

Mudge, G. H. 1982. Analgesic nephropathy: Renal drug distribution and metabolism. In

Nephrotoxic Mechanisms of Drugs and Environmental Toxins, ed. G. A. Porter, pp. 209–227. New York: Plenum Medical.

Mudge, G. H., Gemborys, M. W., and Duggin, G. G. 1978. Covalent binding of metabolites of acetaminophen to kidney protein and depletion of renal glutathione. *J. Pharmacol. Exp. Ther.* 206:218–226.

Newton, J. F., Kuo, C.-H., Gemborys, M.W., Mudge, G. H., and Hook, J. B. 1982. Nephrotoxicity of *p*-aminophenol, a metabolite of acetamiophen, in the Fischer 344 rat. *Toxicol. Appl. Pharmacol.* 65:336–344.

Oken, D. E. 1972. Modern concepts of the role of nephrotoxic agents in the pathogenesis of acute renal failure. *Prog. Biochem. Pharmacol.* 7:219–247.

Orloff, J., and Berliner, R. W. 1973. *Handbook of Physiology, section 8: Renal Physiology.* Baltimore: Williams & Wilkins.

Peterson, D. R., Oparil, S., and Pullman, T. N. 1979. Renal tubular transport and catabolism of proteins and peptides. *Kid. Int.* 16:271–278.

Phillips, R. D., Hayes, A. W., Berndt, W. O., and Williams, W. L. 1980. Effects of citrinin on renal function and structure. *Toxicology* 16:123–137.

Pitts, R. F. 1974. Physiology of the Kidney and Body Fluids, Chapter 13. Chicago: Year Book Medical.

Reid, W. D. 1973. Mechanism of renal necrosis produced by bromobenzene or chlorobenzene. *Exp. Mol. Pathol.* 19:197–214.

Relman, A. S., and Levinsky, N. G. 1971. Clinical examination of renal function. In *Diseases of the Kidney,* eds. M. B. Strauss and L. G. Welt, 2d ed., pp. 87–137. Boston: Little, Brown.

Richards, A. N. 1929. Direct observations of change in function of the renal tubule caused by certain poisons. *Trans. Assoc. Am. Physicians* 44:64–73.

Richardson, R. J., and Murphy, S. D. 1975. Effects of glutathione depletion on tissue disposition of methylmercury in rats. *Toxicol. Appl. Pharmacol.* 31:505–519.

Roch-Ramel, F., and Peters, G. 1979. Micropuncture techniques as a tool in renal pharmacology. *Annu. Rev. Pharmacol. Toxicol.* 19:323–345.

Roch-Ramel, F., and Weiner, I. M. 1980. Renal excretion of urate: Factors determining the action of drugs. *Kid. Int.* 18:665–676.

Ross, C. R., Pessah, N. I., and Farah, A. 1968. Inhibitory effects of β-haloalkylamines on the renal transport of *N*-methylnicotinamide. *J. Pharmacol. Exp. Ther.* 160:375–385.

Rothstein, A. 1973. Mercaptans—Biological targets for mercurials. In *Mercury, Mercurials and Mercaptans,* eds. W. W. Miller and T. W. Clarkson, pp. 68–98. Springfield, Ill.: Thomas.

Silverblatt, F., Turck, M., and Bulger, R. 1970. Nephrotoxicity due to cephaloridine: A light and electron-microscopic study in rabbits. *J. Infect. Dis.* 122:33–34.

Sperber, I. 1944. Studies on the mammalian kidney. *Zool. Bidrag Uppsala* 22:249–341.

Stroo, W. E., and Hook, J. B. 1977. Enzymes of renal origin as indictors of nephrotoxicity. *Toxicol. Appl. Pharmacol.* 39:423–434.

Sullivan, L. P., and Grantham, J. J. 1982. *Physiology of the Kidney,* 2d ed. Philadelphia: Lea and Febiger.

Tachibana, M., Mizukoshi, O., and Kuriyama, K. 1976. Inhibitory effects of kanamycin on glycolysis in cochlea and kidney—Possible involvement in the formation of oto- and nephrotoxicities. *Biochem. Pharmacol.* 25:2297–2301.

Tisher, C. C. 1977. Glomerular morphology and its relation to glomerular filtration. In *Renal Function,* eds. G. H. Giebisch and E. F. Purcell, pp. 3–55. New York: Josiah Macy Foundation.

Tisher, C. C. 1981. Anatomy of the kidney. In *The Kidney,* 2d ed., vol. 1, eds. B. M. Brenner and F. C. Rector, pp. 3–76. Philadelphia: Saunders.

Tune, B. M., and Fravert, D. 1980. Mechanisms of cephaloridine nephrotoxicity: A comparison of cephaloridine and cephaloglycin. *Kid. Int.* 18:591–600.

Tune, B. M., Burg, M. B., and Patlak, C. S. 1969. Characteristics of *p*-aminohippurate transport in proximal renal tubules. *Am. J. Physiol.* 207:1057–1063.

Tune, B. M., Wu, K. Y., and Kempson, R. L. 1977. Inhibition of transport and prevention of toxicity of cephaloridine in the kidney. Dose-responsiveness of the rabbit and guinea pig to probenecid. *J. Pharmacol. Exp. Ther.* 202:466–471.

Tune, B. M., Wu, K. Y., Fravert, D., and Holtzman, D. 1979. Effect of cephaloridine on respiration by renal cortical mitochondria. *J. Pharmacol. Exp. Ther.* 210:98–110.

Valtin, H. 1973. *Renal Function: Mechanism Preserving Fluid and Solute Balance in Health.* Boston: Little, Brown.

Valtin, H. 1979. *Renal Dysfunction: Mechanisms Involved in Fluid and Solute Imbalance.* Boston: Little, Brown.

Vera-Roman, J., Krishnakantha, T. P., and Cuppage, F. E. 1975. Gentamicin nephrotoxicity in rats. I. Acute biochemical and ultrastructural effects. *Lab. Invest.* 33:412–417.

Wirz, H., Hargitay, B., and Kuhn, W. 1951. Lokalisation des konzentrierungs progresses in der niere durch direkte kryoskopie. *Helv. Physiol. Pharmacol. Acta* 9:196–207.

Wright, F. S., and Giebisch, G. 1978. Renal potassium transport: Contributions of individual nephron segments and populations. *Am. J. Physiol.* 235:F515–F527.

Zalme, R. C., McDowell, E. M., Nagle, R. B., McNeil, J. S., Flamenbaum, W., and Trump, B. F. Studies of the pathophysiology of acute renal failure. II. *Virchows Arch. (Cell Pathol.)* 22:197–216.

Chapter 7

Reproductive and Perinatal Toxicology

Richard K. Miller
Carol K. Kellogg
Risa A. Saltzman

INTRODUCTION

The appearance of birth defects is often the harbinger of alarm and concern for human exposures to chemicals, drugs, or other environmental agents. Such passionate exclaimers indicate our willingness to endure physical injury to ourselves but not our children, either born or unborn.

In selected cases, adult forms of toxicity are present earlier and at lower exposure levels than is the reproductive and/or developmental toxicity for a particular compound. In other cases, reproductive toxicity may be expressed at lower doses than other adult forms of toxicity. Koeter (1983) reported in a review of the literature that

The authors most gratefully acknowledge the many suggestions and helpful comments offered by Dr. Raymond Baggs, Dr. M. James Cosentino, Dr. Willem Faber, Dr. Arthur Levin, Dr. Eberhard Muechler, Dr. Henry Thiede, and Dr. Tacey White. The manuscript preparation was most capably performed by Jacqulyn White, and the graphic arts were created by Susan Morgan and Donald Stedman. We are particularly indebted to the editors for their patience and encouragement. The original research described was supported in part by the following grants: NIH ES02774, ES01247, CA22335, MH31850. R. K. Miller was also supported by a National Institutes of Health Fogarty Senior International Fellowship during part of the development for this work, and C. K. Kellogg was recipient of a research award from Hoffmann-LaRoche, Inc.

35% (13 out of 37) of the compounds evaluated were more sensitive in the reproduction studies than in the subchronic toxicity testing studies. It is noteworthy that the U.S. Toxic Substance Control Act (TSCA) requires four levels of testing, depending on the nature of the chemical, its proposed use, and frequency of use (Ellison, 1977). Reproductive testing is only required when the product is already in use (level IV). The mission of this chapter is to identify agents that may modify reproduction and development through both basic and clinical approaches to these problems.

Approximately 40% of all human pregnancies are lost before the third trimester. This large pregnancy loss has been considered a natural selection or "filter" to reduce the number of birth defects. Between 2 and 4% of all neonates have a documented physical defect at birth. This incidence increases to approximately 8–10% by the first year of life. Such statistics represent the background incidence of reproductive and developmental problems in the human population.

Unfortunately, all of our scientific and medical knowledge and intense desire to prevent these losses cannot eliminate the human factor in the equation. In the 1940s, vitamin A, in excess or deficiency, was the first agent to be identified as producing birth defects and therefore established an environmental contribution to reproductive problems. The early 1960s brought the world's attention to thalidomide. In the late 1960s and early 1970s, attention was focused on anticonvulsants, alcohol, diethylstilbestrol, coumarin, aminopterin, dibromochloropropane, and methylmercury. However, in the 1980s, a new human experiment was undertaken. A vitamin analog was marketed that was considered to have a very high potential for being teratogenic but was the only effective therapy for cystic acne. The bottles were labeled potential teratogen, the physicians informed; however, human nature presented what has been called the thalidomide of the 1980s. This drug, 13-*cis*-retinoic acid, has been associated with a syndrome of responses that appear to be related to abnormalities in neural crest-cell development and have many similarities to the malformations noted in animal model systems. Therefore, where does all of our testing, our epidemiology, our good medical practice bring us? Can prevention of these effects be achieved? Education is perhaps the only answer, with an acknowledgement that confounding variables (e.g., intercurrent disease, genetics, and polypharmacy) can contribute to these toxic effects.

For the human, numerous agents have been proposed to be reproductive and/or perinatal toxins based on case reports and animal studies. Yet only a few such selective agents have been so confirmed. For example, in the male, dibromochloropropane (a pesticide) and cholinergic drugs can inhibit spermatogenesis or libido. Estrogens can alter the menstrual cycle, induce miscarriages, or produce malformations and transplacental carcinogenesis. Some agents, like thalidomide, the antinausient, selectively alter gross structural development but not mental development, in comparison with methylmercury, the fungicide, which does the reverse.

If we know the mechanism of toxic action for these agents, then perhaps we can investigate the structure–activity relationships and metabolism for these compounds. What must be firmly entrenched in one's mind is that the ED50 or LD50 in males or nonpregnant females may not have any relationship to the pharmacokinetics, ED50, or LD50 in the pregnant female. Thus, constant vigilance in establishing criteria for such reproductive and developmental toxicity testing is critical for each compound and extrapolations to or from nonpregnant animals may not be assumed.

This chapter is divided into two major sections: reproductive toxicology; male and female, and perinatal toxicology from conception to the neonatal period. In each of these sections, the physiology, examples of toxic response, and methods for evaluation of toxicity are presented.

REPRODUCTIVE TOXICOLOGY

The reproductive process is a continuum of events from embryonic development through mature function of these organ systems (Fig. 1). The development of the female and male reproductive tracts and the effects of toxins on that developmental process is discussed in the perinatal section of this chapter. Therefore, the reproductive toxicology section is devoted only to the adult organ system and the impact of chemicals and physical agents on these processes.

Female Reproduction

For adequate reproductive function, the hypothalamic–pituitary–gonadal–reproductive axis must be intact, with the appropriate signals and responses occurring to produce ovulation. The environment of the uterine and fallopian tube must be conducive for fertilization and continued growth of the embryo. The central nervous system (CNS)–gonadal–reproductive tract axis can be disrupted by xenobiotic agents as well as excess or insufficient amounts of endogenous signals such as estrogens (Herbst and Bern, 1981). There are normally three levels of control for the female reproductive system: (1) the hypothalamic–pituitary axis, (2) the ovary with its endocrine and ovulatory functions, and (3) the reproductive tract.

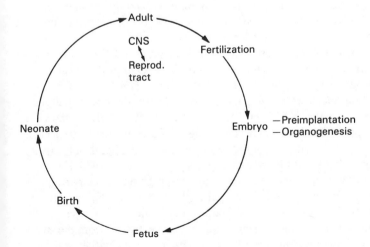

Figure 1 The continuum of perinatal pharmacology and toxicology.

Hypothalamus–Pituitary The female reproductive process requires the cyclical production of gonadotropins by the pituitary. Inhibition of these hypothalamic-pituitary functions can be expressed as amenorrhea, suppression of estrus, and reduced fertility. The three most commonly studied pituitary gonadotropins are follicle-stimulating hormone (FSH), luteinizing hormone (LH) and prolactin. The release of these gonadotropins is controlled by feedback loops in the hypothalamus. Chemicals that reversibly disrupt these pathways also alter fertility in a reversible manner, while chemicals that alter gonadal function directly may produce permanent infertility and/or genetic defects (Smith, 1983). Stress and exercise also can affect these systems, resulting in amenorrhea (Cumming and Rebar, 1983).

The hypothalamic control of gonadotropin release includes both adrenergic and dopaminergic neuronal influences. Anesthetics, analgesics, sedatives, and tranquilizers have been associated with reversible alterations in fertility (Smith, 1983). In particular, marijuana is disruptive to normal reproductive functions by inhibiting the secretion of both LH and FSH. This effect of delta-9-tetrahydrocannabinol was persistent (12–24 h) following a single administration, even when the blood levels of marijuana had decreased. This depression in gonadotropin release by the pituitary can be reversed following the administration of LHRH (luteinizing-hormone releasing hormone), a hypothalamic gonadotropin releasing factor. As evidence of these interactions, female monkeys treated chronically with marijuana did not exhibit any estrogen rises or LH surges (Smith et al., 1979).

The pituitary gonadotropins do supply substantial regulation of the ovary; however, the ovary through the release of estrogens does feedback directly to the hypothalamus and also to the reproductive tract (Fig. 2). These actions of both estrogens and progesterone by the ovary during the preovulatory and luteal phases of the ovarian cycle can be directly altered by environmental chemicals.

Ovary The ovary represents the focal point for female reproductive capacity. The ovary can control the proliferation of the endometrium and the function of the fallopian tube, yet its own function can be finely tuned and manipulated. To understand the function of the ovary, one must appreciate its origins.

The ovary begins with the migration of the primordial germ cells from the germinal ridge. If these germ cells do not reach the gonad by 8 weeks of gestation, they die (Forsberg and Kalland, 1981). In the human at 4 months of gestation, there are approximately 7 million oocytes. At this stage of development, the primordial germ cells differentiate into oogonia, which proliferate. After mitotic division, the cells remain attached to each other by cytoplasmic bridges. These intercellular bridges have been postulated as an explanation for the nest of follicles that appear in the ovary and as the reason for follicles with more than one oocyte (Mattison, 1983a).

As the oocytes develop and enter meiosis, they recruit granulosa cells from the stroma. This process of folliculogenesis is critical to the survival of the oocytes, yet the mechanisms involved in this process are poorly understood. If oocytes cannot recruit granulosa cells and a basement membrane, they are extruded from the ovary or become atretic. Since the total number of oocytes that the ovary will ever have is determined at this stage, any alteration in folliculogenesis may have a substantial

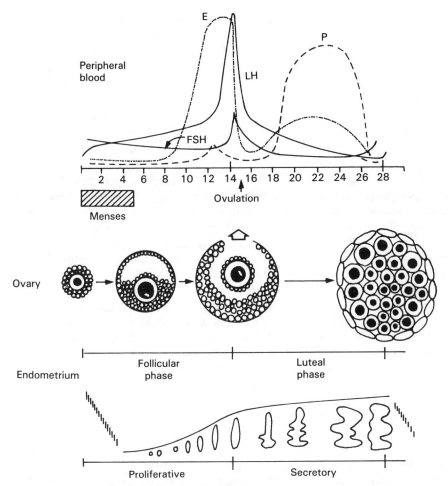

Figure 2   The endocrine and cellular events involved in the menstrual cycle along the pituitary–ovarian–uterine axis. Under the influence of follicle-stimulating hormone (FSH), the dominant follicle grows and secretes increasing quantities of estrogen (E) into the circulation. Estrogen secreted by the dominant follicle feeds back on the hypothalamus and pituitary, decreasing
FSH secretion. The increasing levels of E also stimulate proliferation of the endometrium. A
continued increase in the level of circulating E ultimately leads to the surge of luteinizing hormone, which is followed by ovulation. After ovulation, the morphology of the follicle changes,
with formation of the corpus luteum. The major secretory product of the corpus luteum is
progesterone (P). Increasing quantities of P stimulate the release of secretory granules into
endometrial glands, proliferation of endometrial stromal cells, and spiral arterioles in preparation
for implantation. *(From Mattison, 1982.)*

impact on the number of oocytes available for fertilization during the reproductive
life of the mammal. At birth there are approximately 1 million oocytes, and 200,000
at puberty. Of these oocytes, only 400 will yield mature ova during the reproductive
years (Weir and Rowlands, 1977; Mattison et al., 1983).

Follicles are developed from oocytes, which undergo meiosis but become arrested during the first meiotic division. Meiosis does not resume until just prior to ovulation. This suspension of meiosis can persist for 35 years or more (Schwartz and Mayaux, 1982). It is during this prolonged period of suspended meiosis that the primary oocyte may be susceptible to the toxic actions of environmental agents and drugs (Mattison, 1983a). Complete destruction of the oocytes in the prepubertal female can result in primary amenorrhea, while complete destruction of oocytes after puberty will produce premature menopause/ovarian failure and infertility (Chapman et al., 1979; Mattison, 1983c). The actual duration of reproductive capacity is only weakly dependent on oocyte number, but the rate of atresia appears to have the greatest impact (Mattison, 1982).

The susceptibility of the ovary to permanent injury appears to be limited to a specific period. The ovaries of prepubertal females are more resistant to damage and long-term toxicity from cancer chemotherapy (Arneil, 1972; Chapman, 1983; Himellstein-Brau et al., 1978; Shalet, 1980; Siris et al., 1976), when compared to those of pubertal or adult women. Women in their late 20s and older have increasing risks of complete ovarian failure following exposure to such multiple cytotoxic drug therapies as nitrogen mustard, vinblastine, procarbazine, and prednisolone (Chapman, 1983; Chapman et al., 1979; Horning et al., 1981; Schilsky et al., 1981). Ovarian failure is associated with chronically high levels of FSH and LH, as well as depressed levels of estradiol and progesterone with intermittent surges of LH and beta-endorphins. These biochemical events are accompanied by amenorrhea, hot flashes, insomnia, irritability, and depressed libido (Berman and Craig, 1985). For such cytotoxic agents, this age-dependent response of the ovary to toxic insult offers the possibility of modifying the gonadal toxicity of chemotherapeutic agent without affecting the anticancer action. Chapman (1983) proposes that hormonal suppression of the adult gonad may simulate the prepubertal ovary and therefore offer the ovary protection against the direct toxicity of these agents as well as from radiation (Dobson and Felten, 1983). Such protection of the ovary does not appear possible for exposure to other chemicals, such as polycyclic aromatic hydrocarbons.

Besides being teratogens, mutagens, and carcinogens, polycyclic aromatic hydro-carbons (PAH) can be toxic to the ovary and oocyte. This oocyte toxicity is strain-, species-, age-, dose-, and metabolism-dependent (Dobson and Felten, 1983; Mattison et al., 1983). A broad range of dose–response relationships for PAHs and other compounds is induced in the primordial oocyte of the mouse (Fig. 3). The relative oocyte killing effectiveness–oocyte toxicity index (the ratio of the whole animal dose that kills two but not more than three out of five animals to the oocyte LD50) is similar to the mutagenicity and carcinogenicity of these PAHs [dimethylbenzanthra-cene > 3-methylcholanthrene > benzo(a)pyrene] (Dobson and Felten, 1983).

As with toxins in other organs systems, the toxic response of the reproductive system for xenobiotic exposure may be the result of (1) direct interactions of the agent on the organ or cells or (2) an indirect action of the agent, either on other cellular or physiological processes or via reactive intermediates of the parent compound. Many of the direct-acting agents are structural analogs of endogenous substances, such as diethylstilbestrol, 6-mercaptopurine, or DDT, and so may interfere directly with these cellular functions. Agents may also directly affect these cell types without mimicking

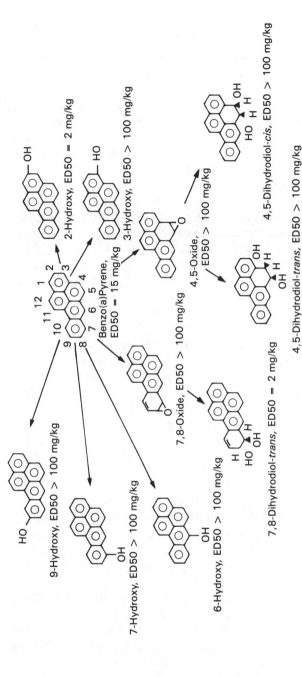

Figure 3 Oocyte destruction of benzo(a)pyrene and 10 derivatives. C57BL/6N mice were treated intraperitoneally with the indicated PAH at doses ranging from 1 to 100 mg/kg, and the ED50 for oocyte destruction was determined. *(From Mattison et al., 1983.)*

the actions of endogenous substances (e.g., gamma radiation, mercury, lead, and cadmium) (Herbst and Bern, 1981; Kupfer, 1982; Dobson and Felten, 1983; Wide, 1983; Clarkson et al., 1983).

Indirectly acting reproductive toxins represent the class of substances that provide multiple means for toxic interaction and often account for the great species, strain, and age differences in toxic response. Metabolic activations of chemicals to reactive intermediates have been mechanisms proposed for chemically induced toxicity, such as cyclophosphamide metabolism to nitrogen mustards. In many instances, it appears to be local cellular production of such reactive intermediates. Such local cellular production of metabolites has been noted for the developing reproductive tract for compounds like diethylstilbestrol (Metzler, 1981, 1984; Miller et al., 1982). The ovary has microsomal monooxygenases, epoxide hydrases, and transferases capable of metabolizing xenobiotics (Heinriesh and Juchau, 1980; Mattison and Thorgeirsson, 1978, 1979; Sims and Grover, 1974). The relative levels of the enzymes in the female reproductive tract can modify the production of such reactive intermediates, their detoxification, and the repair processes within any given cell type.

Benzo(a)pyrene is an example of such a reproductive toxin, teratogen, and fetal toxin. Specific toxic actions of this PAH involve the ovary, preimplantation embryo, postimplantation embryo, and fetus. Benzo(a)pyrene can be oxidatively metabolized to many different metabolites (both toxic and nontoxic). To solve the puzzle of toxicity, one must determine whether the ovarian toxicity produced by benzo(a)pyrene is from within the ovary and if so by what enzymes leading to the production of which selected metabolites. The pathway of benzo(a)pyrene metabolism for at least 10 metabolites is summarized in Fig. 3. When xenobiotic metabolism is considered, both the metabolites and enzymes have been traced as indices of local toxic effect (Gelboin, 1980). In particular for benzo(a)pyrene, the enzymatic activity of arylhydrocarbon hydroxylase (AHH) has been followed through development (Nebert and Gelboin, 1969; Nebert, 1981). Yet in the case of ovarian toxicity, AHH is not a good predictor of strain or species differences for PAHs (Mattison, 1979; Mattison and Nightingale, 1980; Mattison et al., 1980, 1983b). One reason for these differences in ovarian response to PAH may be that extraovarian sites may produce the toxic metabolites. This possibility was eliminated by direct injection of benzo(a)pyrene into one ovary, which produced oocyte toxicity while the control ovary was not affected (Shiromizu and Mattison, 1982).

Thus, a local ovarian response was identified. To determine whether benzo(a)pyrene or some of its metabolites are ovotoxic, the ED50 dose that produced oocyte destruction was found to be selective for the 2-hydroxy and 7,8-dihydrodiol transderivatives of benzo(a)pyrene. Since these metabolites are not formed via AHH in the ovary, as has been noted for other tissues (Gelboin, 1980), other ovarian enzymes must produce the 7,8-dihydrodiol-9,10-epoxide. If this metabolite of benzo(a)pyrene is an ultimate toxin in the ovary, then three different enzymes processes are involved: (1) formation of the 7,8-epoxide, (2) hydration of the 7,8-dihydrodiol, and (3) oxidation to the 7,8-dihydrodiol-9,10-epoxide (Mattison et al., 1983b). Thus, such a complex series of metabolic steps can provide for the dramatic differences in species and strain suspectibility to PAH destruction of oocytes.

Polycyclic aromatic hydrocarbons are ubiquitous in the environment, for example, in cigarette smoke. The relationship between smoking and reproductive history has been identified. An association has been reported between the number of cigarettes smoked per day and the early onset of menopausee (Jick et al., 1977; Mattison and Thorgeirsson, 1978). Since menopause is an indication of oocyte depletion, the ovary has been identified as a target site for toxicity in both animal and human.

The reproductive tract in the female provides the conduit for the transfer of the egg, its fertilization and nurture. Hormonal imbalances, physical defects (blocked fallopian tubes, bicornuate uterus), immunologic alterations and infections can be causes for infertility. In addition, the cause of some infertility has not been identified and may be related to xenobiotic exposure. Many problems with the fallopian tubes (oviducts) and uterus are congenital. Singularly, the one compound most associated with such reproductive toxicity is prenatal exposure to diethylstilbestrol. The similarities between the human and the rodent are striking for such reproductive failure (Table 1).

Immunological factors have also been implicated in the patient with repeated pregnancy loss. The role of xenobiotic drugs in this process has not been well established. However, as noted in the in vitro teratology section, plasma from patients who have repeated miscarriages does kill mouse blastocysts in culture and produce malformations in rat embryos (Chavez and McIntyre, 1984; Muechler et al., 1984). Similar observations have been noted for baboons who have a high-risk reproductive history (Carey et al., 1983).

One critical area of reproductive physiology not well evaluated in relationship to xenobiotic toxicity is the role the endometrium plays in the implantation process. The preimplantation embryo and the endometrium appear to exchange "signals" before and during the implantation process (Moulton et al., 1983). Besides the hormonal control, via the pituitary and ovary, the local control by the endometrium of implantation may be a site for xenobiotic interference. Such problem areas are now being highlighted because of the control over fertilization and the preimplantation embryo as related to the in vitro fertilization programs for infertility patients. The use of hormonal induction with gonadotropins is further evidence of such specific hormonal control over the ovulation process. The stimulation of multiple follicles and the release of multiple ova could be considered an adverse effect of fertility drugs such as clomophine citrate or pergonal. However, for the in vitro fertilization program, the release of multiple eggs is essential.

Assessment of Female Reproductive Function
Human Among the most important assessments for infertility and reproductive toxicity evaluations is the reproductive history, which includes a detailed account of menstruation, number of pregnancies, number of early miscarriages, number of pregnancy losses, stillbirths, perinatal mortality, number of live births, and sex of the offspring. To be included are any maternal disease, nutritional status, social and therapeutic drug use, and detailed evaluation of any environment exposures (Table 2), including caffeine use and smoking, as well as stress factors involved in every day life including the amount of strenuous exercise.

Table 1   Summary of Abnormalities following Prenatal Exposure to Diethylstilbestrol in Human and Rat/Mouse

Human[a]	Rat/Mouse[b]
Female anatomical abnormalities	
Vagina	
Adenosis	Adenosis
Adenocarcinoma	Adenocarcinoma
Squamous-cell dysplasia	Squamous-cell carcinoma
	Hyperkeratosis
	Hypospadias
	Calculi
	Vaginitis
Cervix	
Hoods	
Stenosis	
Incompetence	
Uterus/fallopian tube	
T-shaped uterus	Endometrial hyperplasia
"Withered" fallopian tube	Uncoiled tubes
	Salpingitis
External genitalia	
	Patent vagina at birth
	Persistent cleft phallus
	Perineal excoriation
Female functional abnormalities	
Menstrual irregularities	Noncycling
Spontaneous abortions	Infertility
Ectopic pregnancy	
Premature delivery	
Male anatomical abnormalities	
Meatal stenosis	
Hypospadias	
Epididymal cysts	
Hypotrophic testes	Hypotrophic testes
Leydig-cell hyperplasia	
Cryptorchidism	Cryptorchidism
Microphallus	Microphallus
Testicular agenesis	Undescended testes
	Tumors of the rete
Male functional abnormalities	
Altered semen analysis	
Azoospermia	Azoospermia
Decreased sperm penetration in hamster-egg sperm penetration assay	

[a]Data for the human was derived from Stillman (1982); Herbst and Bern (1981); Kaufman (1984); and Bibbo et al. (1975).
[b]Data for the rat was derived from Greene et al. (1940), Miller et al. (1982), R. B. Baggs and R. K. Miller (unpublished data), and for mouse from McLachlan (1981), and McLachlan et al. (1980, 1981, 1982 and unpublished).

Table 2 Selected List of Female Reproductive Toxins Noted in Various Species

Androgens	Halogenated polycyclic hydrocarbons
Azathiotine	Lead
Amphetamine	Narcotics
Busulfan	Marijuana
Benzo(a)pyrene	Mercury
Bleomycin	Morphine
Cadmium	3-Methylcholanthrene
Chlorambucil	Nitrosamines
Cyclohexylamine	Phenothiazine
Cyclophosphamide	Progestins
Diethylstilbestrol	Radiation
7,12-Dimethylbenzanthracene	Reserpine
17β-estradiol	6-Mercaptopurine
Ethanol	Vinblastine
Ethylnitrosourea	

Another evaluative step is hormonal status during the menstrual cycle. Multiple samples of blood are drawn preovulation and postovulation as well as at the time of ovulation. These samples are assessed for steroid levels (17β-estradiol and progesterone) and gonadotropins (follicular stimulating hormones and luteinizing hormones). Such hormone analysis can indicate potential sites of toxicity, whether in the brain or in the ovary. Laporoscopic examination of the tubes and ovary can also be most helpful in assessing infertility problems. These procedures are often coupled with a hysterosalpinogram (radiographic examination of the uterus and tubes) and endometrial biopsies (Table 3).

Animal In animal studies, many of the above procedures are performed but in a more rigorous and terminal manner. As in the human, functional tests are often the primary screening tools for determining reproductive deficiencies. Among these screens are multigenerational studies looking at the reproductive capacity for at least two to three generations following exposure throughout the life spans. These tests are often implemented differently depending on the intended use of a particular agent. A dose–response relationship is determined based usually on a control group and three experimental dosage groups. Since compounds may be drugs, pesticides, or food additives, the method of administration can be oral, either intragastric, in the food and drinking water, or by injection.

The copulatory behavior is evaluated to determine whether the female is appropriately responsive to the male (lordosis). A mating index is determined based upon the number of estrous cycles required to produce pregnancy and the number of copulations and is helpful in determining the reproductive behavior of the female. The fertility index (the number of females conceiving divided by the number of females exposed to fertile males) gives one of the best indications of overall reproductive capacity. The final assessment though is an evaluation of the full-term pregnancies and the number of live births divided by the number of conceptions. These techniques

Table 3   Potential Sites of Action and Mechanisms of Damage for Toxins in the Female Reproductive System and Methods for Evaluating Such Effects[a]

Site of action	Potentially altered mechanism	Evaluative tests
Hypothalamus	Synthesis and secretion gonadotropin-releasing hormone (GnRH)	Hormone assay
	Receptors for LH, FSH, and steroids	Receptor analyses
	Neurotransmission	None at present
Anterior pituitary gland	Synthesis and secretion of LH and FSH	Hormone assay; GnRH challenge
	Receptor for GnRH, LH, FSH, and steroids	Receptor analyses
Ovary	Oocyte toxicity and increased atresia	Oocytes counts/ morphology
Number of LH or FSH receptors	Receptors in follicular or granulosa cells	Receptor analyses
	E_2 and P synthesis and secretion	Hormone assay or in vitro tests
	Abnormal meiosis; sensitivity to lutealysis	In vitro tests
Ovum	Altered zona pellucida	Sperm penetration
	Surface protein interacting with sperm	Biochemical analyses
	Implantation/corpora lutea ratio	
	Metabolic processes DNA, protein synthesis	In vitro
Fallopian tubes (oviducts)	Ciliagenesis and function of cilia; fimbria movement	In vitro tests/ morphology
	Number of E_2, P, and T receptors	Receptor analyses
	Sperm and ovum transport	Recovery count
	Fluid environment	Biochemical analyses
Uterus	Protein and glycoprotein secretion	Biochemical analyses
	Number of E_2 and P receptors	Receptor analyses
	Prostaglandins secretions	Prostaglandin assays
	Luminal fluid	Biochemical analyses
	Sperm survival and transport	Recovery and count
	Exposure of sperm and embryo to agents in uterine secretions	Assay for agent in vitro tests
	Endometrial staging	Morphology
	Parturition	Incidence of dystocia
Cervix	Mucus effects on sperm	In vitro tests
Vagina	Exposure of sperm to agent and secretion	Assay for agent
Mammary gland	Secretion of agent in milk	Assay for agent
	Altered milk composition	Biochemical analyses
	Decreased milk yield	Volume collection and examination of offspring

[a]Adapted from Amann (1982).

coupled with forced breeding can provide for the direct assessment of reproductive capacity. Such procedures have been implemented for evaluating the reproductive toxicity of diethylstilbestrol (McLachlan and Dixon, 1976). To follow up on these functional tests, hormonal evaluations as performed in the human can be performed. However, instead of obtaining vaginal or cervical biopsies, usually a necropsy is performed with evaluation of gross pathology, including organ weights especially for the reproductive tract and other endocrine organs, such as adrenals and pituitary, and histology of the pituitary, adrenals, ovaries, oviducts, uterus, cervix, and vagina are performed with multiple stains to assess the status of these tissues. One important comparison for reproductive status is to match the stage of estrus in the reproductive tract with the stage in the ovary.

Increasing use of the monitoring of uterine and vaginal fluids/mucus and the determination of steroid receptors in the oviductal, uterine, and vaginal tissue has also been useful. Histologically, oocyte counts and staging of the follicular development have become a routine evaluation.

Male Reproduction

In 1951, MacLeod and Gold published a study reporting sperm counts in a thousand men of known fertility. Forty-four percent of the subjects had sperm counts of over 100 million/ml of ejaculate and 5% had counts of less than 20 million/ml. Data published in 1974 by Nelson and Bunge on sperm counts in fertile men seeking elective vasectomy sharply contrasted with this report. Only 7% of the 386 men evaluated had sperm counts greater than 100 million/ml; 20% had counts below 20 million/ml. In 1975, Rehan et al. reported the results of sperm-count evaluation in 1300 men of known fertility seeking elective vasectomy. Twenty-four percent of the men had sperm counts of over 100 million/ml, whereas 7% had counts falling below 20 million/ml. Although some variation in methods could contribute to the differences among these reports, a decrease in the percentage of men with sperm counts of over 100 million/ml is apparent over this 24-year period. Sperm count, although not the only parameter by which to assess fertility, is an important determinant of reproductive success.

As technology advances, the number of chemical and physical agents to which humans may be exposed occupationally, environmentally, or therapeutically increases. Could this downward shift in sperm count be partially in response to man's increased exposure to potential reproductive toxins? Male reproductive toxicity can be manifested in many ways; effects such as abnormalities in sperm production and function, decreased libido, and impotence have been reported following exposure to reproductive toxins (Tables 4 and 5). These effects share a common endpoint, that is, impaired reproductive capacity.

Male reproductive capacity involves the formation of fertile spermatozoa (spermatogenesis and sperm maturation), delivery of the germ cell to the female tract (including formation of seminal plasma, libido, erection, and ejaculation), and functional changes in the spermatozoa before ovum penetration (capacitation). It can be

**Table 4 Selected Agents Reported to Have
Adverse Effects on the Male Reproductive System
in the Human[a]**

Alcohol	Elevated temperatures
Cadmium	Gossypol
Carbon disulfide	High altitudes
Chlorambucil	Ionizing radiation
Clomiphene	Lead
Cyclophosphamide	Marijuana
Cyproterone acetate	Medroxyprogesterone acetate
Dibromochloropropane	Testosterone ethanate
Diethylstilbestrol	Vinyl chloride

[a]Compiled from Mendelson et al. (1977), Manson and
Simons (1979), Council on Environmental Quality (1981),
and Wyrobeck et al. (1983).

evaluated in vivo and in vitro, as well as noninvasively, to determine the effects of
chemical exposure (Table 6).

During the 1970s, an agricultural nematocide, dibromochloropropane (DBCP),
was reported to be a reproductive hazard in workmen (Whorton et al., 1977; Potashnik et al., 1978). The major effects observed in these exposed males were azoospermia, oligospermia, and elevations in serum concentrations of luteinizing hor-

**Table 5 Selected Agents Reported to Have Adverse Effects on the Male
Reproductive System in Animal Models[a]**

Alcohol	Ethylene oxide
Aminopterin	Ethylnitrosourea
Benzene	Fluoroacetamide
Benzo(a)pyrene	Gossypol
Busulfan	Hexamethylphosphoramide (HMPA)
Cadmium chloride	Ionizing radiation
α-Chlorohydrin	Lead
Clomiphene	Marijuana
Colchicine	Methadone
Cyclophosphamide	Methyl mercury
Diamines	Methylmethane sulfonate
Dibromochloropropane (DBCP)	Morphine
Dichlorodiphenyltrichloroethane (DDT)	Nitrous oxide
Dichlorvos	Procarbazine
Diethylstilbestrol (DES)	Triethylenemelamine (TEM)
Estradiol	Vinblastine sulfate
Ethylene dibromide	

[a]Compiled from Hunt (1979), Council on Environmental Quality (1981), and Wyrobek et al.
(1983).

Table 6 Potential Sites of Action and Mechanisms of Damage for Toxins in the Male Reproductive System and Methods for Evaluating Such Effects[a]

Site of action	Potentially altered mechanisms	Evaluative tests
Hypothalamus	Synthesis and secretion of GnRH	Hormone assay
	Receptors for LH, FSH, and steroids	Receptor analyses
	Neurotransmission	None at present
Anterior pituitary gland	Synthesis and secretion of LH and FSH	Hormone assay; GnRH challenge
	Receptor for GnRH, LH, FSH, and steroids	Receptor analyses
Testis	Receptors for LH on Leydig cells	Receptor analyses
	Testosterone synthesis and secretion	In vitro production; gross/histopathological exam; mating trials/libido; hormone assay
	Vascular bed and blood flow	Morphology; marker dyes
	Blood–testis barrier	Morphology; marker dyes
	Receptors for FSH on Sertoli cells	Receptor analyses
	Receptors for steroids	Receptor analyses
	Secretion of inhibin or androgen-binding protein (ABP)	In vitro production; serum assay; testicular fluid assay via micropuncture
	Sertoli-cell function	In vitro function: production of ABP and other proteins, support of spermatogenic development
	Death of reserve spermatogonia	Germ-cell counts; serial mating
	Spermatogenesis	Germ cell counts; histopathology; mating trials; spermatozoan morphology, count, motility, function; semen evaluation; cytogenetics
Efferent ducts	Vascular bed	Morphology; marker dyes
	Resorption of tubular fluid	Micropuncture

(See footnote on p. 210.)

Table 6   Potential Sites of Action and Mechanisms of Damage for Toxins in the Male Reproductive System and Methods for Evaluating Such Effects[a] (Continued)

Site of action	Potentially altered mechanisms	Evaluative tests
Epididymis	Resorption of tubular fluid	Micropuncture; sperm maturation
	Concentration of blood constituents	Micropuncture; sperm maturation; biochemical analyses
	Enzyme activity; secretions	Micropuncture; biochemical analyses
	Transfer of agent to luminal fluid	Assay for agent
	Smooth muscle contractility	Response to drugs in vivo or in vitro
	Sperm transport	Sperm in ejaculate
Ductus deferens	Smooth-muscle contractility	Response to drugs in vivo or in vitro
	Sperm transport	Sperm in ejaculate
Accessory sex glands; semen	Secretion of seminal components	Assay for seminal components directly or indirectly by assaying semen characteristics; semen volume; gland gross/histopathological exam; sperm function
	Secretion of agent into seminal fluid	Assay for agent
Seminal spermatozoa	Spermatozoan function	Motility; count/density; morphology; metabolism; capacitation and penetration (in vivo or in vitro)

[a]Adapted from Amann (1982).

mone (LH) and follicle-stimulating hormone (FSH). These changes occurred without alterations in serum testosterone or loss of libido, difficulty in erection or ejaculation, testicular atrophy, epididymal alterations, or changes in secondary sex characteristics. Testicular biopsies demonstrated a loss of spermatogonia and an almost complete atrophy of the seminiferous tubular epithelium without inflammation or severe fibrosis; Leydig cells, however, were intact. In some reports, oligospermia was observed in the presence of normal gonadotropin levels (Sandifer et al., 1979). An increased incidence of Y-chromosome nondysjunction without structural aberrations in the genome of peripheral lymphocytes was also reported (Kapp et al., 1979). Recovery from this reproductive toxicity of DBCP, as determined by an increase in ejaculate sperm density, was observed within 18–21 months following cessation of the occupational exposure (Lantz et al., 1981).

Similar reproductive toxicity was also noted in laboratory animals. Torkelson et al. (1961) reported that chronic exposure of rats to DBCP by inhalation caused testicular atrophy, decreased testicular weight, degeneration of seminiferous tubule epithelium, increased Sertoli-cell numbers, oligospermia, and abnormal sperm forms. Additional reports following acute and chronic exposure to DBCP confirmed the testicular and epididymal effects, including desquamation of germ cells from seminiferous tubules, disruption of seminiferous tubular architecture, a decrease in epididymal spermatozoa, and sloughing and degeneration of the caput epididymal epithelium; 30 days after acute exposure, although the epididymal epithelium had a normal appearance, some of the seminiferous tubules were still devoid of germ cells and the reduction in the number of epididymal spermatozoa had persisted accompanied by interstitial edema (Kluwe, 1981a,b). Effects on germ-cell DNA in rats and mice, in terms of the induction of dominant lethal mutation (Teramoto et al., 1980) and unscheduled DNA synthesis (Lee and Suzuki, 1979), respectively, have been reported. Although oral exposure to DBCP induced testicular aryl hydrocarbon hydroxylase and epoxide hydrolase activities in rats (Suzuki and Lee, 1981), the role of metabolism in DBCP toxicity is uncertain (Kluwe et al., 1983).

In 1977, a federal standard was established for occupational exposure to DBCP. Two points are of particular interest concerning DBCP: (1) why were the initial animal studies not well appreciated in setting risk standards to prevent human exposure, and (2) how can we evaluate other agents for comparable reproductive risk? As with all of reproductive and perinatal toxicity testing, if the mechanism of toxic action is not appreciated, then the species extrapolation may not be accurate. Since hepatotoxicity and testicular toxicity were observed at comparable dosages in laboratory animals, it was believed that if no hepatotoxicity was observed in the human then perhaps testicular toxicity would also be minimal. Unfortunately, in humans, it appears that the testes is more sensitive to the toxic effects of DBCP. Such examples reinforce the necessity of detailed reproductive and perinatal toxicity evaluations with the pharmacokinetics, pharmacodynamics, and mechanism of toxic action on the particular organ system evaluated. Comparisons among species may lead to a differential organ sensitivity for a particular agent. For DBCP, the testes in humans appear to be more sensitive than the liver. Such examples illustrate the importance of monitoring xenobiotics for potential reproductive hazards based on both experimental and human exposure data to detect effects that may occur at any level of reproductive function. function.

Following a brief review of the reproductive system, the evaluation of male reproductive capacity will be discussed in terms of spermatogenesis, seminal plasma, reproductive behavior, capacitation, and penetration.

Biology of Male Reproduction   The testes are composed of a series of highly convoluted seminiferous tubules, which are arranged in lobules. The tubules are supported by loose connective tissue containing testicular lymphatics, vasculature, and interstitial (Leydig) cells. Lining the tubules are two different cell populations: germ cells and Sertoli cells.

Germ cells of the testis are proliferative and migrate from the basement membrane of the tubule to the lumen during the course of their maturation. Spermatogenesis (the development of spermatogonia into spermatozoa) has three stages (Fig. 4): spermatocytogenesis, meiosis, and spermiogenesis. During spermatocytogenesis, type A spermatogonia mature and undergo mitotic division to primary spermatocytes. Type A spermatogonia are a self-renewing population of stem cells that can divide and differentiate into type B spermatogonia, each in turn committed to dividing into two primary spermatocytes. The first meiotic division results in the formation of two haploid secondary spermatocytes from each primary spermatocyte. Following the second meiotic division, two spermatids are formed from each secondary spermatocyte (Fig. 4a).

Spermiogenesis (differentiation of spermatids into spermatozoa) involves several functional and morphological changes (Fig. 4b). During this process, the spermatid remains buried in a cleft on the luminal edge of the Sertoli cell, held in place by a specialization in the surface membrane of the latter cell type (Fig. 5) (Russell, 1977). Golgi vesicles form the enzyme-rich acrosomal cap of the spermatozoon. The flagellum develops as a centriolar outgrowth and its distal portion extends into the tubule lumen. The spermatid nucleus condenses and elongates and undergoes a change in protein composition, becoming rich in arginine residues. Cytoplasm is extruded and phagocytized by the Sertoli cell. Upon the completion of this differentiation process, the spermatid is released from the Sertoli cell into the tubule lumen (spermiation) as a spermatozoon. The exact mechanism of this release is unknown.

Spermatogenic cells may exhibit differential sensitivities to xenobiotic toxins, reflecting not only differences in mechanisms of compound toxicity but also differences in the inherent characteristics of the germ cells due to their stage of development. Consider the effects of the alkylating agents methylmethane sulfonate (MMS) and busulfan, as determined by dominant lethal studies. Methylmethane sulfonate caused lethal mutations in spermatids and spermatozoa, while busulfan had such effects only in prespermiogenic cell types (Fig. 6). Selective localization of these agents in specific cells types was not evident following autoradiographic studies. Differences in DNA repair capabilities between the cell types have been proposed to account for the cell specificity of MMS-induced dominant lethality, as previous studies had indicated that spermatids and spermatozoa were unable to repair the single-strand DNA breaks induced by this monofunctional alkylating agent (Lee and Dixon, 1978; Lee, 1983). In the case of busulfan treatment, the lethally mutated prespermiogenic cells did not exhibit single-strand breaks. DNA cross-linking resulting from exposure to this bifunctional alkylator may interfere with DNA replicative processes beyond the scope of cell repair capabilities (Lee, 1983). The lack of such mutation in the older cell types was hypothesized to be due to the inability of bifunctional alkylators to penetrate in their DNA nucleophilic sites.

Further maturation in the epididymis confers fertility upon the spermatozoa. Progressive motility increases. Glucose metabolism becomes more anaerobic, and lipid metabolism is altered. Alterations in plasma membrane surface characteristics

Spermatogenesis

(a)

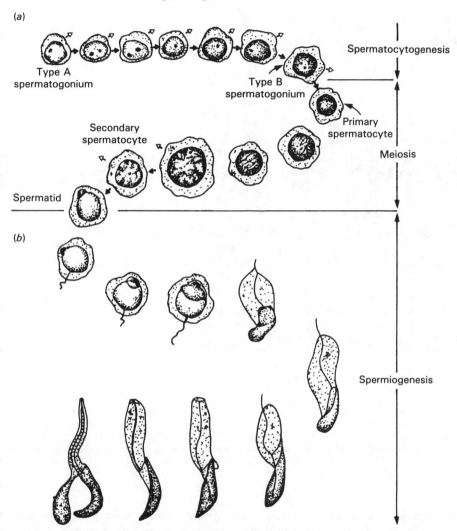

Type A
spermatogonium

Type B
spermatogonium

Primary
spermatocyte

Secondary
spermatocyte

Spermatid

(b)

Spermatocytogenesis

Meiosis

Spermiogenesis

Figure 4 Spermatogenesis (the differentiation of a spermatogonium into a spermatozoon) in the rat. The arrows point to the progeny of mitotic or meiotic processes; the open arrows indicate the daughter cells whose passage through this cycle is not illustrated. (a) Type A spermatogonia divide into type B spermatogonia, which, in turn, divide to form primary spermatocytes. Meiotic division results in the formation of the secondary spermatocyte and then the spermatid. (b) Spermiogenesis is the final step in the spermatogenic process. The spermatid undergoes a series of functional and morphological changes, including formation of an acrosome, a flagellum, and an elongate condensed nucleus, and loss of cytoplasm. When this process is completed, the spermatid is released from the Sertoli cell into the tubule lumen as a spermatozoon. *(Adapted from L. D. Russell, 1983.)*

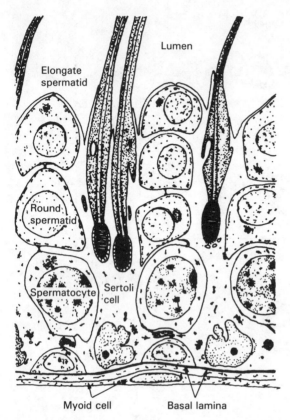

Figure 5 Relationship of spermatogenic cells and Sertoli cells within the seminiferous tubule. Tight intercellular junctions of the Sertoli cells form the blood–testis barrier (paired arrows). As spermatogenic cells mature and migrate towards the lumen of the tubule, they must travel through these regions. During spermiogenesis, the spermatids are embedded in the luminal end of the Sertoli cell with the distal portion of their flagella extending into the tubule. They are held in place by specializations in the surface characteristics of the membrane of the Sertoli cell (open arrows). *(From L. D. Russell, 1983.)*

include changes in pH and differential charge density over the surface of the spermatozoon. There is an increase in disulfide linkages in the nuclear chromatin and tail elements (Bedford, 1975). α-Chlorohydrin, an antifertility agent, acts reversibly at the level of the epididymis to inhibit the fertilizing capacity of spermatozoa (Ericsson and Baker, 1970; Tsunoda and Chang, 1976). This agent interferes with spermatozoan metabolism (Edwards et al., 1976; Mohri et al., 1975), but whether this is the mechanism of infertility is uncertain. At higher doses, an increased percentage of morphologically abnormal spermatozoa is seen in the epididymis, in addition to exfoliation and vacuolar degeneration of epididymal tubular epithelium, formation of epididymal sperm granulomas, and vacuolar degeneration of seminiferous tubule epithelium to the point of tubular atrophy (Ericsson and Baker, 1970; Kluwe et al., 1983).

The epididymis has been investigated as a potential target site for male contraceptives. Altering epididymal function for this purpose has two advantages: (1) the period of latency prior to infertility and subsequent reversal of such infertility would be relatively short due to the time course of epididymal spermatozoan maturation, and (2) by not interfering with testicular function, the infertility associated with such an agent would be more likely to be reversible and would minimize potential genetic and systemic effects. Sulfasalazine, a sulfonamide currently used for the treatment of inflammatory bowel disease and ulcerative colitis, is an agent that appears to reversibly affect male fertility at the level of the epididymis (Cosentino et al., 1984). Gossypol, another agent currently being evaluated as a potential male contraceptive, may also be functioning at the level of the epididymis to reduce male fertility (Segal, 1985).

The rate of passage of a spermatogonium through spermatogenesis and the time required for epididymal maturation vary among species. In the human, 62 and 21 days are required, respectively; in the rat, these processes occur in 48 and 12 days,

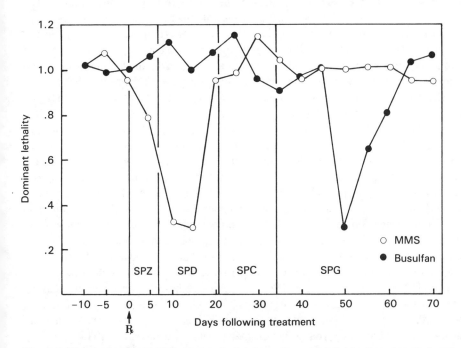

Figure 6 Dominant lethality following a single intraperitoneal administration of methylmethane sulfonate (MMS), 45 mg/kg body weight, or busulfan, 21.7 mg/kg body weight, in mice serially mated. Lethality is expressed as the ratio of the total number of live embryos from the matings of treated males to the total number of live embryos of control paternal geneology. The agents were administered on day 0 (arrow). The time course of spermatogenic cell development in the mouse is plotted on the same axis as the day following treatment on which the animal was mated. For example, the spermatozoa ejaculated from an animal mated 30 days following treatment would have been spermatocytes at the time of exposure. SPZ, spermatozoa; SPD, spermatids; SPC, spermatocytes; SPG, spermatogonia including stem cells. Each point represents 10 mice. *(Data from Lee and Dixon , 1978; Lee, 1983.)*

respectively. Once the spermatozoa have been ejaculated, they undergo capacitation, which involves alterations in sperm surface characteristics and metabolism. This process is essential for the subsequent release of acrosomal enzymes and ovum penetration (Chang and Hunter, 1975).

Sertoli cells, irregularly columnar somatic cells extending from the basement membrane to the lumen of the seminiferous tubule, play many roles in the maintenance of testicular function. Sertoli cells produce and secret androgen-binding protein (ABP), inhibin (a peptide involved in the negative feedback control of FSH release from the pituitary), and testicular fluid (containing proteins, ions, steroids, and ABP). The supportive role of the Sertoli cell is both nutritional and physical. The tight intercellular junctions at the bases of the Sertoli cells form the blood–testis barrier (Fig. 5), through which macromolecules in the blood must cross in order to enter the tubule; permeability is determined by compound size, lipophilicity, and ionic characteristics (Okumura et al., 1975). As the germ cells migrate, they must transit through this junctional region (Fig. 5). Late spermatocytes and spermatids, which reside on the luminal side of the barrier, can thus be protected from circulating toxins. The blood–testis barrier also serves an immunological function to prevent the development of an autoimmune response to the antigenic germ cells (Neaves, 1977). Sertoli cells also have phagocytic capabilities and, in this way, can remove both extruded spermatid cytoplasmic droplets and abnormal germ cells from the tubule (Setchell and Waites, 1975; Steinberger and Steinberger, 1975; Rich and de Kretser, 1983).

The ejaculate (semen) is composed of accessory gland secretions, testicular and epididymal fluids, and spermatozoa. In the human, 60% of this volume is from the seminal vesicles. This gland's secretions are high in fructose, prostaglandins, fibrinogen, and protein. Thirty percent of the ejaculate volume is from the prostate gland. Prostatic fluid contains zinc, citric acid, acid phosphatase, clotting enzymes, and fibrinolysin. The remaining 10% of this volume is made up of the mucoid secretions of the bulbourethral gland and testicular and epididymal fluids. Glycerolphosphorylcholine, carnitine, and mucoproteins are characteristic substituents of epididymal fluid (Manson and Simons, 1979). Semen composition is not consistent throughout the ejaculation, as the accessory glands secrete in succession: bulbourethral gland, prostate gland, and then seminal vesicles (and testicular and epididymal fluids). Both the total number and the concentration of spermatozoa are greatest in the first portion of the ejaculate (Tauber et al., 1975). Exogenous chemicals can enter the seminal plasma at the level of the testis (by crossing the blood–testis barrier), epididymis, efferent ducts, or accessory sex glands to potentially alter the components of seminal plasma and affect spermatozoan function (Mann and Lutwak-Mann, 1983).

Testicular activity is regulated by several hormones. Hypothalamic gonadotropin-releasing hormone (GnRH) stimulates the release of two pituitary gonadotropins: follicle-stimulating hormone (FSH) and luteinizing hormone (LH), also known as interstitial cell-stimulating hormone (ICSH). FSH is required in the initiation of spermatogenesis, although its role in the maintenance of this process is not clear. FSH stimulates Sertoli cell production of androgen-binding protein (diZerega and Sherins, 1981). Inhibin, a Sertoli-cell product, has a negative feedback function on the anterior pituitary to modulate FSH levels. LH acts on Leydig cells to stimulate testosterone synthesis and release. Testosterone is necessary for the transformation of primary spermatocytes to secondary spermatocytes and for epididymal spermatozoa maturation; it is also important in the maintenance of the accessory sex glands and secondary sex characteristics. Testosterone also plays role in the negative feedback regulation of gonadotropin release via the hypothalamus and the pituitary.

Hormonal regulation of the male reproductive system can be altered at several different levels of function of the hypothalamic–pituitary–gonadal axis. Centrally acting neuropharmacologic agents, including anesthestics, analgesics, tranquilizers, antidepressants, antipsychotics, and stimulants, can impair reproductive function by affecting the control of gonadotropin release and subsequently, as a potential secondary effect, steroid synthesis and release (Smith, 1982). Drugs of abuse such as marijuana, narcotics, and alcohol (Smith, 1983) may also act in this capacity, as previously noted for the female. Agents that can interfere directly with steroid metabolism or activity include exogenous steroids (e.g., anabolic steroids, antiandrogens, and estrogenic compounds) and alcohol (Smith, 1982; Waller et al., 1985).

The vascular bed of the testis is not immune to the effects of exogenous agents. Parenteral administration of cadmium is known to result in testicular necrosis and evidence indicates that the initial (and possibly primary) effect is on the testicular vasculature. Autoradiography has shown that testicular cadmium is concentrated in the interstitial tissue (Berlin and Ullberg, 1963). Parizek (1960) reported complete necrosis of the testes of the rat following a single parental injection of cadmium salts, with initial effects including interstitial edema and hyperemia followed by hemorrhage. These effects were accompanied by a decrease in testis size, desquamation of seminiferous tubule epithelium, and a decrease in accessory sex-gland weight. Gunn et al. (1963) observed interstitial edema in both the testis and the caput epididymis within 6 h of cadmium exposure; at that time, the veins of the pampiniform plexus were dilated and congested. Within 24h tubular elements in both the testes and the epididymis had undergone degeneration. Setchell and Waites (1970) reported an initial increase and then a sustained decrease in testicular blood flow following cadmium exposure, accompanied by an increase in testicular capillary permeability. Dilation of testicular endothelial clefts has been observed as early as 15–30 min following intravenous cadmium exposure (Gabbiani et al., 1974). Located primarily in arterioles, the resulting cavities were as large as 5000 Å in diameter, in some cases damaging the endothelial cell membranes; the microvasculature of the epididymis showed similar effects within that same timeframe. In trying to determine the mechanism of cadmium-induced testicular toxicity, it must be noted that the role of zinc in normal testicular function and the protective action of zinc against this toxicity (Parizek, 1960; Gunn et al., 1963; Webb, 1972) do not allow for the interference of cadmium in zinc metabolism to be eliminated as a potential mechanism for this agent's testicular effects.

Interaction of xenobiotic agents, such as polycyclic aromatic hydrocarbons, with testicular tissue may be mediated by enzymatic activation or detoxication due to the presence of significant levels of aryl hydrocarbon hydroxylase, epoxide hydrase, glutathione S-transferase, and cytochrome P-450 in that organ. Studies in the rat indicate that enzyme activities and P-450 content are differentially concentrated between two testicular cell types. Epoxide hydrase and glutathione S-transferase activities are twofold greater in spermatogenic cells than in interstitial cells; in contrast, aryl hydrocarbon hydroxylase activity and cytochrome P-450 content are greater in the interstitial cells than in the germ cells. Although the levels of these enzymes are not as great as those found in hepatic tissue, the proximity of the generated metabolites to the potential target cells of the testis identifies a role for such metabolic capabilities in modifying organ toxicity (Mukhtar et al., 1978).

A gross evaluation of the male reproductive tract can reveal effects on that organ system following exposure to xenobiotic toxins. Testicular size has been correlated with parameters of that organ's function, including serum hormone levels, sperm numbers, and sperm quality (M. J. Cosentino, personal communication) and so may be used in assessing the functional status of that organ. Prenatal exposure to diethylstilbestrol (DES), a synthetic estrogen, produces in the human male reproductive-tract anomalies such as hypoplastic testes, microphallus, cryptorchidism, and epididymal cysts, as well as oligo- and azoospermia (Table 1) (Gill et al., 1979, 1981). Male mice exposed to DES in utero also exhibit cryptorchidism and epididymal cysts, in addition to nodular enlargements of the accessory sex glands (Table 1) (M. C. McLachlan et al., 1975). Although changes in gross parameters may reflect direct organ damage or indirect effects due to interference with related physiological mechanisms, manifestations of damage can also become apparent by the analysis of reproductive capacity.

Assessment of Male Reproductive Function

Analysis of Spermatogenesis During spermatogenesis, every spermatogonium has the potential to divide and mature into eight spermatozoa, each capable of determining half of the genotype of the conceptus. Functional or genetic damage to these cells during their differentiation threatens reproductive success.

Spermatogenic cells can be obtained from the testes and epididymis by tissue biopsy, micropuncture, or homogenation; spermatozoa can also be collected in the urine by anastomosing the ductus deferens to the bladder (Vreeburg et al., 1974), or in the ejaculate. Separation of the major spermatogenic cell types in a cell suspension prepared from testicular tissue can be achieved by velocity sedimentation (Lee and Dixon, 1972). The results of comparing the number of each type of cell and the ratio of these numbers in control and treated situations can suggest direct cytotoxicity of target cells and mechanisms of damage. A similar analysis can be done on a cross-sectional slice of seminiferous tubule to evaluate intact cells as well as those that are degenerating and/or phagocytized.

Quantitative and qualitative analysis of spermatozoa in the ejaculate is particularly important in the evaluation of human reproductive function, as this is the most accessible sample indicative of spermatogenic function. The number of sperm in the sample can reflect toxic effects on developmental or maturational processes; considerations in the evaluation of this parameter include testicular size and the period of abstinence prior to sample collection. Although there is no concentration of sperm in the semen that will guarantee fertilization of the ovum, a decrease in human male fertility is often seen at a concentration of less than 20 million spermatozoa per milliliter of ejaculate (MacLeod and Wang, 1979). Morphological changes, such as head and tail defects, can affect motility, which can be studied in either seminal plasma or cervical mucus. However, whether such changes can result in heritable defects in the offspring is uncertain (Wyrobek et al., 1984). Alterations in functional parameters such as respiration, metabolism, acrosomal enzyme levels and activities, and resistance to stress reflect changes in germ-cell survivability and, ultimately, fertility (Eliasson, 1978).

Direct germ-cell evaluation is also a means of assessing genetic damage resulting from exposure to a mutagenic agent. Cytogenetic analysis of germ cells harvested at any stage of their development can identify cell types susceptible to an agent's mutagenicity. For example, the double Y-body test (also known as the YFF test) identifies meiotic nondysjunction of the Y chromosome in human spermatozoa. A fluorescent stain indicates the presence of the Y chromosome; such fluorescence does not occur in rodent sperm (Wyrobek et al., 1983). It is important, however, not to limit an analysis to spermatozoa, as this may underestimate the number and types of mutated cells. Spermatogenic cells at various stages of development have different capacities for DNA repair (Lee and Dixon, 1978). Also, Sertoli cells are capable of phagocytizing genetically abnormal germ cells.

In Vivo Assays of Fertility   In vivo assays of fertility can be performed in conjunction with in vitro spermatogenic cell evaluation to identify deleterious effects on the male reproductive system in the rodent model.

A serial pattern of mating treated males to untreated females can be useful in identifying the stage(s) of spermatogenic cell development affected by an agent. The animals are housed together for a duration of time to include one or more estrous cycles; housing the male with multiple females will increase the number of female reproductive cycles to which he is exposed. Females are checked daily during this time for vaginal sperm plugs to ensure that the agent has had no adverse effects on libido or ejaculation. This mating protocol is repeated for the duration of spermatogenesis to be evaluated. The time course of male fertility following treatment, as determined by the percent of females impregnated, is compared to the time course of spermatogenic cell development. The later in its development a spermatogenic cell is at the time of exposure, the earlier that cell will appear in the ejaculate as a mature spermatozoon (Fig. 6). A decrease in fertility immediately after treatment would indicate damage to epididymal spermatozoa; delayed recovery of fertility (longer than the time for an affected spermatogonium to complete spermatogenesis) suggests effects on the reserve stem-cell population (Lee and Dixon, 1972). Data generated in vivo on affected cell types can be confirmed by corroboration with that derived from in vitro examination of the spermatogenic cells.

Mating trials can also be used to indicate the presence of certain genetic lesions. Three tests commonly used towards that end are the dominant lethal, heritable translocation, and specific locus assays. These breeding protocols can be done by serial mating to aid in identifying target cell types.

Dominant Lethal Assay   In the dominant lethal assay (Bateman, 1977), treated males are mated to untreated females. These dams are euthanatized at midgestation, and the numbers of corpora lutea and live, dead, and resorbed conceptuses are recorded. Fetal lethality is considered to represent lethal germ-cell mutation in the male genome induced by exposure to the agent in question. Such mutations generally result from gross chromosomal changes such as nondysjunction or alteration in structure or ploidy (Brusick, 1978). This protocol, however, does not allow for verification of the genetic origin of the lethality.

Induction of dominant lethal mutations following exposure to the alkylating agents methylmethane sulfonate (MMS) and busulfan has been examined under a serial mating protocol (Lee and Dixon, 1978; Lee, 1983). The occurrence of this type of mutation was expressed as the ratio of the total number of live embryos from the matings of treated males to the total number of live embryos of control paternal geneology. The MMS (45 mg/kg body weight, ip) affected only spermatozoa and spermatids, as seen by a decrease in the lethality ratio for embryos conceived immediately following treatment and for 25 days thereafter (Fig. 6). Busulfan (21.7 mg/kg body weight, ip), however, resulted in lethal mutations in embryos conceived between 45 and 65 days following treatment, indicating spermatogonial effects (Fig. 6). Lee (1983) suggests differential cell sensitivity, including DNA repair capabilities, to account for cell specificity, in addition to the alkylating characteristics of each compound. Induction of dominant level mutations has also been determined in vitro by harvesting two-cell embryos and monitoring their growth and differentiation in culture (Goldstein, 1984).

Heritable Translocation Assay Following mating to treated males, the unexposed dams are allowed to litter in the heritable translocation assay (Leonard, 1977). The male F_1 progeny, having been exposed in utero, are then mated to untreated females. These dams are euthanatized at midgestation. Fertility of the F_1 males is evaluated to determine whether heritable alterations in the F_0 male genotype, specifically clastogenic effects involving the balanced translocation of genetic material, have affected reproductive capacity. A reduction in fertility, as determined by the number of living embryos per litter, identifies males who may be translocation heterozygotes. The presence of such an alteration of genome can be verified by cytogenetic analysis of F_1 germ cells (Brusick, 1978).

Under such a protocol, Generoso et al. (1982) mated male mice treated with triethylenemelamine (TEM) to unexposed females at 2 time intervals following treatment, 1.0–2.5 h and 11.5–14.5 days, corresponding to the evaluation of mature spermatozoa and of spermatids, respectively. Although the frequency of heritable translocation was significant in both groups of F_1 progeny, such mutations were induced to nearly a fivefold greater extent in spermatids than in mature sperm in the germ cells of the F_0 males. Generoso et al. (1982) suggested the longevity of the premutational lesion, as determined by the stage of development at which the cell was exposed, to play a role in the rate of mutation induction.

Specific Locus Assay The specific locus assay detects heritable point mutations occurring within a set of marker loci (Searle, 1977). The male parental strain is homozygous wild-type at all the marker loci, and the female parental strain is homozygous recessive for these traits. Following the mating of a treated male to an untreated female, the offspring are examined for the phenotypic expression of the recessive traits, indicating the transmission of a mutation from the male genome at that locus. The alleles monitored are usually those that are visibly expressed in the pheno-type, such as coat color and color distribution, eye color, hair structure, and ear morphology, although biochemical traits can also be examined. The genotype of the mutated allele can be confirmed by mating the F_1 progeny to animals homozygous at the locus in question (L. B. Russell et al., 1981).

Ethylnitrosourea (ENU) is a potent inducer of mutation in mouse spermatogonia. Administration of this compound (250 mg/kg body weight, ip) results in a point mutation frequency 87 times greater than the frequency that would occur spontane-ously in the strains tested. Mutations occurred in at least five of the seven loci tested in offspring that had been conceived from spermatozoa exposed to ENU at the sper-matogonial stage of development (W. L. Russell et al., 1979).

Analysis of Seminal Plasma In determining the effects of potential reproduc-tive toxins, seminal plasma should be evaluated not only as a vehicle, but also as a source of nutrients and other substances imperative for the survivability and fertility of the spermatozoa. Ejaculate can be collected whole or in fractions, as a split ejacu-late, to isolate the product of each gland. In the case of the human, since 90% of the ejaculate volume is derived from the seminal vesicles and prostate, volume changes may reflect damage to either of these two glands. Alterations in semen chemistry, determined either by measurement of the amounts of specific seminal plasma compo-nents or by effects on semen characteristics such as liquefaction, viscosity, and pH, can identify target glands. Glandular dysfunction can also be reflected in changes in accessory gland weight or volume (Eliasson, 1978).

Analysis of Reproductive Behavior Whether mating can even occur is a key question in evaluating reproductive toxicity. In both humans and animals, changes in mating patterns, such as a decrease in libido or inability to achieve and maintain erection or complete ejaculation, should be monitored following exposure to a sus-pected reproductive toxin. In the human, this can be accomplished by obtaining a complete reproductive history. In the rodent, confirmation of intromission and ejacu-lation can involve the observation of coitus and/or the presence of a vaginal plug or sperm in the vagina. Effects may be manifested due to direct tissue damage or due to indirect effects via alterations in the hypothalamic–pituitary-gonadal axis, through hormonal influences on libido and impotence, or in the neuromuscular system, as both sympathetic and parasympathetic nerves are involved in erection and ejaculation. Examples of agents that interfere with the hormonal control of male reproductive processes have already been discussed; agents that act at the neural level to adversely affect male reproductive function include antihypertensives, antipsychotics, and anti-depressants (Horowitz and Goble, 1979; Smith, 1982; Waller et al., 1985).

Analysis of Capacitation and Penetration Impairment of spermatozoan capaci-tation and penetration of the ovum can result from germ-cell insult during spermato-genesis, changes in seminal plasma composition, or direct damage to the spermato-zoa. Capacitation and penetration can be examined in vitro following either in vivo or in vitro exposure of spermatozoa. Sperm capacitated in vivo can be harvested for use in in vitro fertilization studies. In vitro penetration of ova can be evaluated by moni-toring the percent of ova penetrated and their subsequent development. Human sperm have been tested in this capacity using zona-free golden hamster (*Mesocricetus aura-*

tus) eggs; such heterologous fertilization can aid in testing human male fertility (Karp et al., 1981). Artificial insemination allows for the potential effects of an agent on libido to be bypassed while examining sperm fertility. Immunological interference with fertilization in the human has been examined in vitro by identifying the presence and characteristics of sperm-directed antibodies in the plasma or serum of infertile couples and on the plasma membrane of the sperm of infertile men to determine how such factors might impair reproduction (Bronson et al., 1981; Haas et al., 1982).

Concluding Comments on Female and Male Reproductive Toxicity

Due to the complexity of interactions at the various levels of control and function of the reproductive system, indirect tissue insult may be as detrimental to reproductive function as direct organ damage. As with the evaluation of any other organ system, a means of extrapolation from animal data to the human condition must be devised in order to identify reproductive toxins and elucidate their sites and mechanisms of action. Can some of these toxic effects on both male and female reproductive capacity actually be utilized to an advantage as contraceptives? Although they are expensive to perform, in vivo assays of reproductive capacity are invaluable sources of data that can be used to answer a key question in reproductive toxicity evaluation: that is, is the ability to produce normal offspring impaired?

The diversity and complexity of reproductive biology in the male and female provides many sites for interference. The goal of this section has been to identify sites of control for the reproductive process in both sexes such that future human and animal studies may help to further elucidate mechanisms of reproductive toxicity.

PERINATAL TOXICOLOGY

Perinatal toxicology is the study of aberrant or toxic responses to environmental agents or drug therapy following exposure any time from conception through the neonatal period. Recognition that environmental agents and drugs can alter the development of the conceptus has only been achieved since the 1940s, and most of the emphasis for study and concern has been concentrated on the postimplantation embryo—the period of organogenesis, and not on the other periods of development. The sites for such toxicological effects include the mother, placenta, and embryo/fetus. As gestation progresses from conception through delivery, there are multiple changes occurring in each of these complex systems. This section reviews preimplantation embryogenesis, postimplantation embryogenesis, fetal development, in vivo animal experimentation, in vitro experimentation, and current knowledge related to human investigations.

It is essential to appreciate that the toxicity of an agent, whether it is directed toward the mother, placenta, or embryo/fetus, may be entirely different depending on the day when the compound is administered during gestation, the dose, the species, and the route of administration. Even though a compound may have a single mechanism of action, the complexity of the changes that occur in the mother during gestation (Table 7), in the placenta (Table 8), and in the conceptus (Table 9) may lead to entirely different responses. An example of such a compound is ethylnitrosourea (ENU).

As noted in Fig. 7, the period of primary organogenesis is from implantation until 8–12 weeks of gestation in the human, from implantation until day 13–14 in the rat, and both pre- and postnatal in the opossum. This demarcation is entirely based upon structural (especially skeletal) features. It has become increasingly apparent that many organ systems, especially endocrine, immune, reproductive, and the central nervous system (CNS), continue to develop well into the fetal and postnatal period. Additionally, substantial functional impairment of the organism may occur if exposure occurs during the fetal period.

Ethylnitrosourea is classified as a direct-acting alkylating agent and is also a

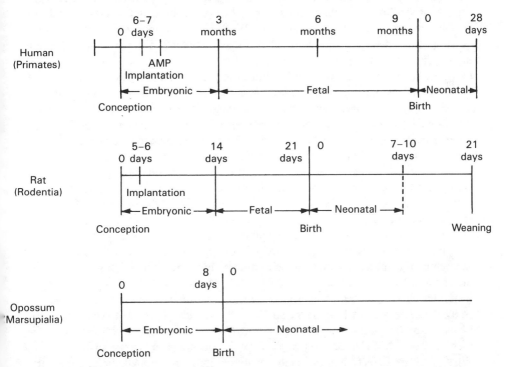

Figure 7 Comparative perinatal development in the human, rat, and opossum. The periods of development are defined for each species. LMP, last menstrual period; AMP, anticipated menstrual period. The menstrual cycle in the average human female is 28 days, with ovulation occurring about 14 days. As noted for the rat, since in utero development is abbreviated compared to the human (21–22 days versus 9 months), the maturation of the rat newborn is substantially different than in the human. Thus, it has been proposed that the 7- to 10-day-old rat neonate may be more comparable to the human at birth. The opossum presents an entirely different development pattern: there is no chorioallantoic placenta, and the neonate is still in an embryonic form. Even with these differences, the effects of chemicals in all three species can be established; however, the timing of exposures, route of administration, and developmental stage must be considered when comparing effects among species. For additional information concerning the opossum, see Jurgelski et al. (1974). *(From Miller, 1983.)*

direct-acting carcinogen in the adult. Spontaneously, ethylnitrosourea forms a highly reactive, electropositive intermediate (ethyldiazonium hydroxide) that forms covalent bonds with electron-rich molecules (e.g., DNA, RNA, and protein) (Rice, 1984). Ethylnitrosourea produces all of these effects within its biological half life of 7–8 min. Depending on the day of gestation when ethylnitrosourea is administered, ENU can produce multiple responses. In the rat, if ENU is administered during preimplantation, embryo lethality is noted. When ethylnitrosourea is administered during organogenesis (especially days 9–11 of gestation), hydrocephaly, exencephaly, and anophthalmia are observed. During late gestation (in the fetal period), a single injection of ethylnitrosourea results in an increasing incidence (up to 100%) of adult-onset neurogenic tumors in the offspring (Napalkov, 1973). The incidence of such neurogenic tumors is 50-fold greater following prenatal exposure when compared to administration of ENU to the adult. Thus, within a given species a different clustering of effects (or syndrome) is demonstrated depending on the dose and specific time during gestation when the agent is administered. When prenatal exposure to ENU occurs in other species, the types of tumors induced may be notably different (hamster, brain; mouse, liver, lungs, brain, and lymph; monkey, connective tissue; opossum, kidney, eye, peripheral nerve; rabbit, kidney, brain) (c.f. Miller, 1983; Rice, 1984).

Not only can the tissues of the fetus be affected directly but also those of placenta and the mother. Besides transplacental carcinogenicity in the offspring, ethylnitrosourea induces gestational choriocarcinoma (trophoblast invading and proliferating in nonuterine tissue, e.g., in maternal lung of female patus monkeys) (Rice et al., 1981; Rice, 1984). This highly invasive carcinoma can be lethal.

If we consider this single genotoxic, direct-acting, alkylating agent (ENU) as a compound with a presumed known mechanism of action, then an understanding of its developmental toxicology should be easily achieved. Yet the diversity of toxic responses in the embryo/fetus, placenta, and mother in different species epitomizes the difficulties we face in assuring the manufacturer, the regulator, the concerned public, and, most importantly the parents-to-be that the therapy required or the environment around them will not compromise their children and future generations. In fact, from the above information concerning ENU, what effects would you expect in the pregnant human? What doses do we study? During what time during gestation should we study the effects of such an agent and in what species? Is there a syndrome? How likely is that syndrome to occur in the human? What is the safety factor for not having a child with a birth defect even if two species do not demonstrate malformations? What is a birth defect? Is it the exencephaly of ENU, the anophthalmia, the embryo lethality, or the tumors in the offspring or in the mother? Should our concerns and our attention be directed toward producing normal progeny? Or should specific exposures to substances during pregnancy be offered if these agents are known to increase the intellectual capacity or athletic prowess of the child? Studies indicate that prenatal exposure to selected drugs can modify specific adult behaviors in animals (Simmons et al., 1984a,b) and in humans (Reinisch et al., 1981). With these opportunities for modifying the next generation by selective chemical exposure in utero, what then is toxicity and what is therapy? How does perinatal toxicity testing provide such a basis for decision-making?

In perinatal toxicology, three general areas of investigation have been emphasized: (1) the ability of chemicals to be metabolized to toxic products, which may then produce their effects in either mother and/or conceptus; (2) specific interactions with developing processes, such as cell–cell interactions necessary for appropriate organ development, or receptor-specific responses; and (3) organ-specific responses leading to lethality, or reduced functional or structural capacity, for instance in the central nervous system, reproductive system, and the placenta. No single set of experimental approaches can be applied to explore these problems. Most often a comprehensive evaluation of the distribution, metabolism, and interactions of a chemical must be completed for mother and conceptus before any understanding of mechanistic action can be established. These are common recommendations for the pharmacologist or toxicologist. Investigators not devoted to studies of perinatal toxicology, however, often do not appreciate that in many instances the conceptus can be a separately functioning organism from both a pharmacological and toxicological perspective. Therefore, such investigators cannot be content with extrapolating observations concerning drug distribution, metabolism, and interactions from the nonpregnant adult to the pregnant adult. For perinatal toxicology, the following tenets must be constantly emphasized:

1   There are dramatic and continuing changes in the physiology and biochemistry of pregnancy, which include both mother and conceptus and persist throughout the entire course of gestation.

2   There are two entirely separate and distinct genomes existing in the same organism (mother).

3   There are two separate and distinct blood supplies with a unique interface, the trophoblast.

4   There is rapid and selective growth of specific cell types in the conceptus at particular stages of gestation.

5   There are direct and indirect interactions among mother, embryo/fetus, and placenta (Miller and Kellogg, 1985).

With such sensitivity to the basic principles of toxicology, it is possible to assess the reasons by which certain responses in the pregnant female may differ fro that of the nonpregnant female, and equally important why the placenta–conceptus unit (whether embryo or fetus) may respond differently at one time from any other time in its life cycle. Yet to evaluate the effects of chemical exposure during pregnancy, the impact of such exposure not only on those cells, organs, or systems but also on the total development and life of the mother and conceptus must be established. How persistent are the effects? Are these effects due to the presence of the chemical at the time of exposure, or are these effects the result of permanent alterations in system function induced at the time of exposure without the persistence of the chemical? Does the conceptus have mechanisms to guard itself against such chemical invasions, or is it at the mercy of the mother to protect and sustain its growth and development?

The remaining sections of this chapter consider many of the questions raised above and attempt to answer them. This chapter cannot hope to provide the reader with a complete review of comparative embryology. The reader is referred to embryology texts by Moore (1985) and Tuchmann-Duplessis (1976). Even though many examples of chemical and physical interactions are presented, only a limited number of examples are discussed in detail to amplify how mother, placenta, and conceptus may be affected differentially during gestation. These examples are polycyclic aromatic hydrocarbons, ethylnitrosourea, cadmium, and diazepam.

These questions of pharmacodynamics are reviewed in the following three categories: (1) maternal factors, (2) placental factors, and (3) embryo/fetal factors.

Maternal Factors

As gestation progresses there are many complex alterations occurring in the pregnant mammal. As noted in Table 7, many of these physiologic changes during pregnancy have a substantial impact on the pharmacodynamics and kinetics for drugs and environmental agents. A number of therapeutic agents, such as phenytoin, digoxin, and lithium, must have the dosage levels adjusted during pregnancy to keep them within a therapeutic range because of an increased clearance. The two primary factors related to these pharmacokinetic considerations are altered renal function and plasma protein binding due to pregnancy-related influences.

For example, the teratogenicity of salicylate was dramatically increased when sodium benzoate was coadministered with a usually nonteratogenic dose of salicylate in the rat. In addition, the embryonic tissue levels of salicylate were also elevated. The resulting increased transfer to the embryo and increased teratogenicity are directly related to the competition for albumin binding between salicylate and the sodium benzoate in the maternal plasma (Kimmel et al., 1974). Placenta hormones, such as estrogens, will increase the concentration of circulating thyroid-binding globulins. Such increases reflect increased total thyroxine levels, while free thyroxine levels do not change.

Even though a chemical may be highly protein bound in the plasma ($>99.99\%$), the amount that is free may pass through the placental membranes and potentially bind to the fetal plasma proteins. In fact, the redistribution of selected water-soluble

Table 7 Physiological Changes in the Pregnant Human during Pregnancy that Affect the Disposition of Chemicals[a]

1. GI absorption—decreased gastric motility: increased transit times for chemicals.
2. Subcutaneous absorption—increased vasomotor instability: irratic absorption.
3. Maternal blood volume—increased by 20%: greater volume for distribution.
4. Plasma proteins—selectively increased, e.g., thyroid-binding globulin.
5. Blood-flow redistribution—increased blood flow to the uterus by 70–80%.
6. Nutrient metabolism—carbohydrate consumer (mother) converted to fatty-acid consumer.
7. Xenobiotic metabolism—selectively increased or decreased production of drug/chemical metabolites to either inactive or active products.
8. Renal function—increased GFR and excretion of water-soluble metabolites.

[a]For additional information see Stave (1978) and Kuemmerle and Brendel (1984).

agents to the fetus may be an important means of decreasing the adult body burden of a chemical. In both human and hamster studies, iophenoxic acid, a choleocysto-graphic dye, has a biological half-life of approximately 2.5 years. This dye is transferred across the placental membranes. Ten years after in utero exposure, children had comparable elevated levels of protein-bound iodine as did their mothers. These tremendously elevated levels of protein-bound iodine are excellent indices of the retained dye. Most of the pharmacokinetic patterns were attributed to the high plasma protein binding of iophenoxic acid, yet when calculated the decrease in the adult body burden of dye in the gall bladder following pregnancy was 20–30% (Shapiro, 1961; Miller et al., 1972). Thus, both drugs and environmental chemicals may have unique pharmacokinetic and pharmacodynamic patterns that are influenced by gestational status.

Binding and excretion are not the only explanations for selected increased toxicity during gestation. Chemicals are normally administered on an adult body-weight basis; however, both the maternal and fetal toxicity of an agent can be substantially altered based upon the ratio of uterine weight/maternal weight and the placental permeability of the chemical under study. These observations are especially true for rodents where the mass of the uterus late in gestation comprises a disproportionate percentage of the maternal weight. If a toxic agent rapidly penetrates into the fetus, then increased fetal toxicity and possibly decreased maternal toxicity may be observed, as for methylmercury. However, if the chemical does not easily reach the fetus then higher maternal tissue concentrations of the chemical may lead to increased maternal toxicity based on the distribution of the agent, as for cadmium (Magos and Webb, 1983). The site of toxic action may be the same as in the nonpregnant female, but the distribution of the chemical within the pregnant uterus may account for the exposure differences and therefore the variation in toxic response.

Metabolism of drugs and environmental chemicals by the mother can be an important detoxifying mechanism; however, through the induction of enzyme activity, increased metabolism of selected xenobiotics to bioreactive intermediates may lead to increased toxicity rather than inactivation. For example, cigarette smoking has been associated with increased embryonic and fetal lethality, placental pathology and intra-uterine growth retardation in human (Yerusholmy, 1971; Meyer and Tonascia, 1977; Buchet, 1978; Asmussan, 1979; Naeye, 1981; Papoz et al., 1982; McIntosh, 1984).

Such toxicity can be attributed to the many constituents of cigarette smoke: polycyclic aromatic hydrocarbons, carbon monoxide, cyanide, nicotine, and heavy metals (cadmium). Many of these compounds will inhibit normal cellular function, and the metabolism of these chemicals can produce additional alterations. Polycyclic aromatic hydrocarbons like benzo(a)pyrene are metabolized by selected maternal and fetal tissues (Welch et al., 1968; Pelkonen, 1980; Juchau, 1981; D. K. Manchester et al., 1984). Carbon monoxide induces biochemical and behavior defects resulting in altered growth and development (Longo, 1977). Not just cigarette smoke or auto emission but, also, for example, metabolism of selected solvents can generate carbon monoxide. Methylene chloride can be metabolized to carbon monoxide in the pregnant rat. Yet even though the methylene chloride concentration was greater in the maternal plasma compared with the fetal plasma, the levels of carbon monoxide in the fetal blood was in excess of the maternal blood concentrations of carbon monoxide (Anders and Sunram, 1982). Thus, metabolism of xenobiotics in utero can produce toxic intermediates. These results have also been noted for certain nitriles, especially acrylonitriles and laetrile. The metabolism of these nitriles will result in the production of cyanide and the production of malformations (Willhite et al., 1981, 1982). When thiosulfate, an antagonist of nitrile metabolism to cyanide, is administered, the teratogenicity is eliminated. Therefore, even if the parent compound is not toxic to the conceptus, the metabolites produced by the mother may directly affect the development of the conceptus and the survival of the mother.

Placental Factors

The placenta and associated extraembryonic membranes are both the conduit and the controller of pregnancy. The placenta regulates the transfer of nutrients, waste products, and xenobiotics, production, release and metabolism of both steroid and protein hormones, and the immunoresponsiveness of the concepto–placental unit (Miller et al., 1976, 1983; Klopper, 1980; Faulk, 1981; Waddell and Marlowe, 1981; Young et al., 1981; Kuemmerle and Brendel, 1984; Miller and Thiede, 1981, 1984; P. Webb et al., 1986).

Without the placenta, the gestational period would be no more than 8–10 days, as noted for the marsupial (e.g., opossum and kangaroo). During this in utero period the marsupial must depend upon the visceral yolk sac for survival as does the rodent in early gestation. The chorioallantoic placenta in the rodent does not play an important role until about day 12 of gestation. From that time on, there is an increasing dependence upon the chorioallantoic placenta for the presentation of oxygen and other nutrients. These extraembryonic membranes (chorioallantoic placenta, parietal yolk sac, and visceral yolk sac) are presented in Fig. 8. To study the direct effects of chemicals on the developing organism in most species, one must contend with the placenta and/or the visceral yolk sac; however, the newborn opossum has proven most useful for both teratogenic and carcinogenic testing without interaction of placenta during the period of organgenesis (Jurgelski et al., 1976, 1979). For most rodents, the only means of producing comparable results are with in vitro methods (see in vitro experimentation) or via administration of compounds directly into the fetus (Levin and Miller, 1980; Henry et al., 1984).

The visceral yolk sac is important for both marsupials and rodents throughout gestation. For the human, after 8–10 weeks of gestation, there is no defined role for this tissue. In the rodent and lagamorph, the visceral yolk sac is critical for immunological competence in the newborn with the passage of IgG proteins through this columnar epithelium and into the vitelline circulation (Fig. 8). The yolk sac has been implicated in perinatal toxicology for the rodent because, until day 11 of gestation, it is the primary supplier of nutrients. This condition, where the embryo relies on local nutrient supplies, has been described as histiotrophic nutrition (Beck, 1976, 1982). This histiotrophic activity can persist as the visceral yolk sac becomes everted and collects nutrients from the uterine environment. Such nutrient function can be inhibited by specific agents, such as trypan blue (Williams et al., 1975a,b, 1976; Beck,

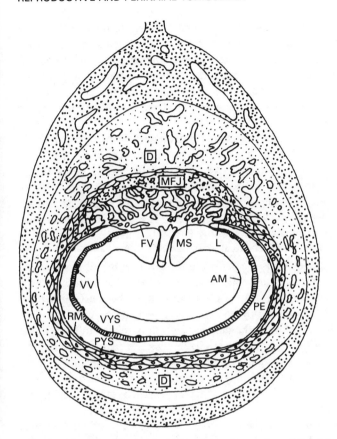

Figure 8 Schematic representation of a cross-section of the feto–placental unit of the rat at day 11 of pregnancy. The embryo is not depicted, but the umbilical vessels are shown and connected to the chorioallantoic placenta which consists of the labryinth (L) and the maternal–fetal junction (MFJ). The labyrinth or region for maximal maternal–fetal exchange has both the fetal vessels (FV) and the maternal blood space (MS). The other extraembryonic membranes that surround the conceptus are the amnion (AM), the visceral yolk sac (VYS), Reichart's membrane (RM), and the parietal yolk sac (PYS). Surrounding these extraembryonic membranes are the maternal decidua (D). This visceral yolk sac connects with the conceptus via the vitelline vessels (VV). This is the alternative circulation for maintaining the conceptus. On the embryonic side to the Reichart's membrane are the parietal endodermal cells (PE), which maintain the Reichart's membrane until days 17–18 of gestation, when both the Reichart's membranes and the parietal yolk sac rupture and retract to the periphery of the chorioallantoic placenta. *(From Miller et al., 1976 as redrawn from Anderson, 1959.)*

1982; Williams, 1982) antisera specific for yolk sac and kidney (Brent et al., 1961; New and Brent, 1972; Brent and Jensen, 1977; Freeman et al., 1981; Leung et al., 1985), and leupeptin (Freeman and Lloyd, 1983). These malformations and resorptions are apparently induced by inhibiting the histiotrophic activity, including endocytosis and catabolism of macromolecules (Freeman et al., 1981; Freeman and Lloyd, 1983; Freeman and Brown, 1985).

After day 11 of gestation in the rodent and lagamorph, the predominant mode of nutrition is hemotrophic, that is, the maternal and fetal circulations provide the major sustenance for the conceptus. At this time, the chorioallantoic placenta with its associated umbilical circulation play the predominate role even though the visceral yolk sac does persist throughout gestation. For the human, the chorioallantoic placenta is the critical organ from the time of implantation. The response of the chorioallantoic placenta to environmental insult can be quite varied, from alterations in selected enzyme activity to necrosis.

The placenta is selective in the xenobiotic metabolism performed. The polycyclic aromatic hydrocarbons [benzo(a)pyrene, dimethylbenzanthracene, N-fluorenylacetamide] are metabolized to reactive intermediates, while many drugs, such as phenytoin, do not appear to be so metabolized (Shah and Miller, 1985). Arylhydrocarbon hydroxylase in placentae from cigarette smokers is induced 8 to 10-fold when compared to nonsmokers (Welch et al., 1969). However, not all placentae from smokers have induced enzymes. Cytochrome P_1-450 has also been identified in the human placenta (Song et al., 1985; Jaiswal et al., 1985). Since benzo(a)pyrene is a constituent of cigarette smoke and is the substrate for this enzyme, it is suggested that benzo(a)pyrene and its metabolism by the conceptus may be related to its effects on fetal development. To date no dose–response relationship has been established for the effects of smoking and for benzo(a)pyrene as a teratogen and perinatal carcinogen. However, the induction of AHH in the human placenta is related to the number of cigarettes smoked per day and is saturated at 20–25 cigarettes/day (Gurtoo et al., 1983). It is difficult in all studies of human placental AHH to demonstrate a dose-response effect because of the variability in genetic composition and enzyme inducibility among individuals (Juchau, 1980, 1982; Gurtoo et al., 1983; D. M. Manchester et al., 1984). Metabolism of benzo(a)pyrene by the human placenta results in metabolites being covalently bound to DNA (Berry et al., 1977) and a positive mutagenic response in the Ames test (Jones et al., 1977). These data certainly indicate the potential for the human placenta to be a production site for toxic substances, especially when these enzymes are induced by environmental agents (Juchau, 1980; Juchau et al., 1986; Pelkonen, 1980). However, it is equally possible that the placenta acts as filter to prevent the passage of the reactive substances into the conceptus. Interestingly, fetal tissue (especially endothelium from the umbilical vein) was not induced in tissue from cigarette smokers as was the placenta, but the AHH activity of the endothelium could be induced in primary cultures. Perhaps the fetus is spared exposure to these low-level environmental pollutants via first-pass protection by the placenta (Manchester and Jacoby, 1984; Manchester et al., 1984).

Besides xenobiotic metabolism, direct effects of agents and manipulators on the placenta itself or via the circulations can compromise the development of the conceptus. Such vasoreactive interactions include prostaglandins, serotonin, cigarette smoke, and uterine vascular clamping (Rankin, 1978; Robson and Sullivan, 1966; Honey et al., 1967; Craig, 1966; Lehtovista and Forss, 1978; Brent and Franklin, 1960; Franklin and Brent, 1964; Bruce, 1972; Leist and Graviler, 1974). Other agents are also associated with alterations in placental function, ranging from decreased transport of nutrients to necrosis, [e.g., cadmium, nicotine, morphine, cocaine, lead, vitamin E deficiency, mycotoxins (T-2), endotoxins, feeding peroxidized lipids, mercury, polychlorinated biphenyls, and ethylnitrosourea] (Wir et al., 1986; Rowell, 1981; Sastry et al., 1977; Barnwell and Sastry, 1984; Gerber et al., 1978; Olson and Massaro, 1980; Kihlstrom, 1982; Rousseaux et al., 1985; Kaunitz et al., 1962; McKay and Huang, 1962). The only agent to date well documented as a placental toxin in multiple species (including human) and multiple studies is cadmium. Therefore, this heavy metal discussed here in greater depth as an example of a placental toxin.

Exposure to cadmium may occur via water, air, food or tobacco smoke. Even low-level exposures to cadmium result in a prolonged retention of cadmium in the body, especially the liver and kidney, but also the placenta. A nephrotoxic tissue concentration of cadmium is reported to be between 1500 and 2000 nmol/g (Frieberg et al., 1974). The placenta highly concentrates cadmium, and such concentrations of trace metals by the placenta have been suggested as exposure indices (cf. Miller, 1983). In particular, placentae from cigarette smokers concentrate cadmium to higher levels than placentae from nonsmokers, while the levels of lead, zinc, and copper were not significantly different (Lauwerys et al., 1978; Miller and Gardner, 1981; Kuhnert et al., 1982; Copius Peereboom-Stegeman et al., 1983; Miller, 1983). Perhaps some of the pathology noted for the placentae from smoking mothers may be related to the contributions of cadmium (Asmussen, 1979; Van der Veen and Fox, 1982; Copius Peereboom-Stegeman et al., 1983).

Cadmium when injected into hamsters on day 8 of gestation is highly teratogenic, resulting in facial malformations (cleft palate, anophthalmia, microphthalmia, exencephaly) and resorptions (Ferm and Carpenter, 1968; Ferm et al., 1969; Mulvihill et al., 1970). Malformations were also noted in the rat following administration on days 9, 10, and 11 of gestation and demonstrated different terata depending on the day of administration (Barr, 1972, 1973). Significant amounts of cadmium are detected in the day 8 embryo within 24 h following maternal administration (Ferm et al., 1969; Berlin and Ullberg, 1963; cf. Clarkson et al., 1983). These teratological and pharmacokinetic responses during organogenesis are substantially different from the responses noted late in gestation. Some of the differences in pharmacokinetics are partially attributed to the dominance of the visceral yolk sac early in gestation, which may provide better access of cadmium to the conceptus when compared to later in gestation, as has also been noted for trypan blue (Dencker et al., 1983).

Single injections of cadmium late in gestation to mice and rats will produce fetal lethality and placental necrosis within 18–24 h (Ahokas and Dilts, 1979; Samawickarama and Webb, 1979; Levin and Miller, 1980). These effects are not due to a direct effect on the fetus but rather an effect on the placenta (Levin and Miller, 1980). There are reductions in utero-placental blood flow by 12 h (Levin et al., 1981), but this is not the initial response to cadmium. The initial insult appears to be directly on the placenta, resulting in increased mitochondrial calcium levels and ultrastructural changes occurring within 4–6 h (Levin et al., 1981, 1983). These effects can be prevented by the prior administration of zinc (Ahokas and Dilts, 1980). In addition, cadmium inhibits the transfer of zinc from mother to conceptus in the rat (Samawickarama and Webb, 1981) and in the human (Wier et al., 1986). Even though amino acid transfer from mother to conceptus was not decreased, the transfer of cobalamin

Table 8   Biochemical and Physiological Processes Involving the Placenta
and Extraembryonic Membranes[a]

---

1. Control
   Production of hormones and proteins, which alter maternal and fetal physiology, e.g., hu-
       man chorionic gonadotropin, estrogens, interferon, progesterone, human placental
       lactogen, cACTH, cFSG, cTSH, interleukin I, and PAPP A.
   Receptor sites: beta-adrenergic, glucocorticoid, epidermal growth factor, immunoglobulin-
       IgG-F_c, insulin, low-density lipoproteins, opiate, somatomedin, testosterone, folate,
       transcobalamin II, transferrin atrial naturetic factor.
2. Metabolism
   Nutrients: glucose, lipids, low-density lipoproteins.
   Xenobiotics: phencyclidine, benzo(a)pyrene.
3. Transport
   Diffusional
       Simple: H_2O, antipyrine, creatinine, gases, L-glucose, urea.
       Facilitated: D-glucose.
   Active: sodium, potassium, calcium.
   Coupled: amino acids, creatine.
   Receptor-mediated endocytosis: immunoglobulins (IgG), vitamin B_{12}-transcobalamin-II, iron
       transferrin.

---

[a]Modified from tables in Miller et al. (1983).

was depressed following cadmium exposure (Danielsson and Dencker, 1984). Administration of metallothionein-cadmium did not produce the fetal lethality or placental
necrosis in the rat but did produce significant nephrotoxicity (Plautz et al., 1980,
1981). The pharmacokinetics of cadmium demonstrates a rapid rise and decline in the
maternal plasma levels from 20 nmol/ml to 1 nmol/ml, while the placenta concentrated cadmium to levels of 100 nmol/g (Levin et al., 1983). These placental levels of
cadmium were in excess of those noted for the kidney. Administration of cadmium
throughout pregnancy is also associated with morphological changes in the rat placenta (Copius Peereboom-Stegeman et al., 1983).

Utilizing a recirculating dual perfusion system for the isolated human placental
lobule, the placenta can be maintained functional and morphologically intact for periods in excess of 12 h (Miller et al., 1985). When cadmium was introduced into the
maternal circulation at concentrations comparable to the rodent studies, the human
placenta rapidly concentrated cadmium to levels similar to those noted in the rodent
studies. Within 8 h, placental necrosis, decreased hormone synthesis, and membrane
leakiness were demonstrated in a dose-related manner (Wier et al., 1986). It is apparent that cadmium can also be placentally toxic in the human at tissue levels comparable to those noted for the rodent. Cadmium can be highly concentrated by the placenta, producing direct cellular damage while limiting the passage of cadmium into
the fetal circulation.

Not only are the mother and embryo/fetus susceptible to the direct actions of
selected agents, but the placentae (whether chorioallantoic or visceral yolk sac) can
be more sensitive to specific chemicals, such as cadmium, trypan blue, and antisera,

than is the embryo directly or the adult. Placental toxicity can encompass enzyme induction, growth retardation, necrosis, fetal death, and the induction of trophoblastic neoplasia.

Embryo/Fetal Factors

The embryo and fetus represent two important stages in the life cycles of all mammals. Unfortunately, it is quite difficult to study these developmental processes in utero, since the conceptus is relatively inaccessible, especially in the human. Advances in the development of noninvasive procedures for the study of the human embryo/fetus have provided a new spectrum of evaluative procedures from ultrasonography, echo-cardiography, amniocentesis, chorionic biopsy, magnetic-resonance imaging (tomography), and in vitro fertilization, to fetal surgery and therapy. Yet the introduction of these diagnostic and surgical techniques are not without their own sets of risks. When these advances are coupled with the chemical and physical exposures in the workplace and the environment as well as medically, the conceptus, even though relatively inaccessible, is actually surrounded by potential problems throughout its in utero existence. As noted for ethylnitrosourea, administration of an agent at different stages of gestation may result in a spectrum of embryonic and fetal responses that may or may not be present at birth. This discussion of developmental toxicology is subdivided into the three primary periods of development: (1) preimplantation embryo, (2) postimplantation embryo, and (3) the fetus.

The Preimplantation Embryo The transit and development of the fertilized mammalian ovum in the tube and uterine fluid is a stage of development not widely investigated using toxicologic techniques. There is substantial difficulty in easily identifying effects of agents on this stage of development, except for lethality or reduced growth of these embryos. In fact, this preimplantation period has been classically defined as the "all or none period." This definition refers to either the survival and normal development of the embryo or lethality due to xenobiotic and nutrient modifications (cf. Brent and Harris, 1976; Wilson, 1977). The basis of this description has been primarily morphological: gross structural defects noted in the embryo and fetus. Beside substances like ethylnitrosourea and cancer chemotherapeutic agents, X-irradiation produces similar lethality (Brent and Gorson, 1972).

Generalizations about the preimplantation period are often oversimplifications. Cellular differentiation does occur early in this developmental period, giving rise to outer and inner cell masses, of which the former becomes the trophectoderm (placenta), and the latter becomes the embryo. During the past decade, increasing emphasis has been placed on whether xenobiotics can appear and accumulate in the preimplantation embryo (Fabro, 1973; Fabro et al., 1984).

Selective and sensitive disruption of single cells in the eight-cell frog embryo by antibodies to gap-junctional proteins can lead to specific unilateral malformations on the embryo (Warner et al., 1984). Certainly the amphibian eight-cell embryo and mammalian eight-cell embryo are not identical in form and determination; however, the potential of mammalian cells to respond to environmental manipulations has been reported. Agents such as nicotine, caffeine, and benzo(*a*)pyrene cause cell death or may induce persistent alterations in biochemical function. In addition to ovarian metabolism and toxicity, benzo(*a*)pyrene can be metabolized to reactive intermediates (diols and quinones) in the preimplantation embryo of the mouse. This metabolism of benzo(*a*)pyrene is inducible by 2,3,7,8-tetracholorodibenzo-*p*-dioxin (TCDD) and is definitely dose-dependent. Such examples of interactions of agents within the preimplantation embryo portend the persistence of other deficits that may be expressed in the fetus, newborn, or child. The strain dependence for the inducibility of arylhydrocarbon hydroxylase by TCDD further indicates and supports the concept that the embryo does have the potential for metabolizing compounds directly, as originally noted by Shum and associates (1979).

It is becoming more apparent that the preimplantation embryo in rodents may be affected by numerous agents, and even though survival may occur, substantial effects on the developing organism may be observed if selected biochemical processes are evaluated. Currently these graded and specific effects on development other than lethality require continued research for confirmation and extrapolation to the human.

Postimplantation Embryo The period of organogenesis has been typically called the teratogenic period because this is the time during development when most of the organ structure takes form but not necessarily function. Most testing for teratological effects concentrates on evaluating this period. As noted in Fig. 9, the development of many of the organs and structure in the rat does occur during this period. However, also note that substantial development occurs during the fetal period as well.

The postimplantation embryo represents a period during which selective cell proliferation, selective cell death, cell–cell interactions, cell migration, and nouvelle biosynthesis are all occurring. Such coordination of specific cell types, whether in the limb bud, palate, or pronephros, indicates the potential susceptibility of the postimplantation embryo to be permanently affected by physical or chemical exposures. There is no one mechanism of action associated with any one teratogen that routinely accounts for all of its actions, because there are so many potential mechanisms for disrupting development (Table 9). Thus, agents like ethylnitrosourea can have multiple effects depending on when the agent is administered.

In addition, a foundation in basic embryology provides the opportunity for best assessment of the interactions of agents on particular organ systems. Administering an agent like thalidomide to a rat after day 13 of gestation would not produce limb-reduction defects since the limb buds are developing much earlier (Fig. 9). If a study of vaginal malformations was of primary concern for a compound (e.g., estrogens), administration of the agent after day 18 of gestation in the rat would be the most sensitive time for inducing those lesions.

The dilemma presented to the scientist is to determine which organs are affected and which ones may express the greatest sensitivity for the expression of perinatal toxicity, and at which stage of gestation the agent must be administered. As noted in the human section of this chapter, clinicians have their primary concerns relating to the production of physical defects. Therefore, the period of organogenesis is the most

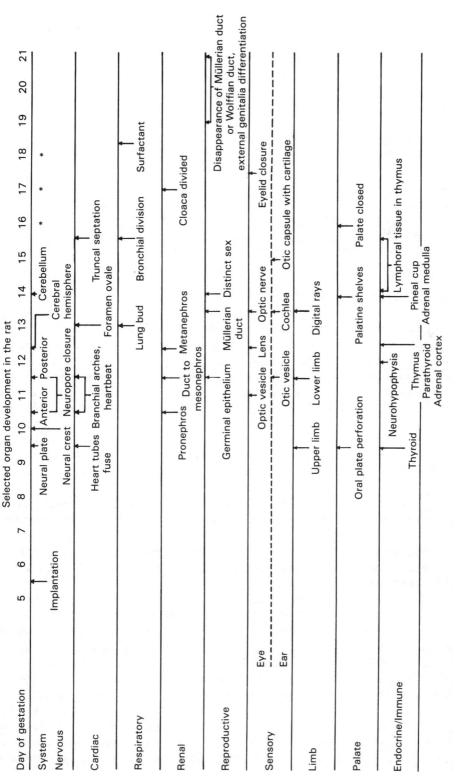

Figure 9 Selected organ system development in the rat when the day following mating is considered day 0 of gestation. Data collected from Witschi (1962) and Shepard (1980).

Table 9   Mechanisms for the Induction
of Abnormal Development in the Embryo/Fetus[a]

Mutations (gene expression)
Chromosomal breaks, nondysjunction
Mitotic interference
Altered nucleic acid integrity or function
Lack of normal precursors and substrates
Altered energy sources
Changed membrane characteristics
Osmolar imbalance
Enzyme activation/or inhibition
Receptor interaction

---

[a]Modified from Wilson (1977).

critical for such potential influences of environmental exposures. The appreciation of whether an agent is a teratogen or not often relates only to the incidence of the physical or functional defects and not to the underlying causes of such a defect. Thus, the quest is to combine risk-assessment tools and studies of mechanism of action for the particular agent or series of agents. The diversity of mechanisms of action precludes a uniform response for any chemical or affected organ concerning teratogenic outcome. One example of such diversity relates to the closure of the palate and its sensitivity to a spectrum of diverse agents as related to metabolism, receptor binding, genetic differences, species differences, and cell–cell interactions. Discussion of other organ systems [e.g., cardiovascular, pulmonary, skeletal (face and limb)] and teratogenic response can be reviewed in publications by Grabowski and Daston (1983), Wilson and Fraser (1977), Hoar (1976), Johnston et al. (1977a,b), Kochhar (1982), and Juchau (1981).

Besides cadmium, many other chemicals with diverse action produce clefting of the palate. Such chemicals include corticosteroids, diazepam, 6-aminonicotinamide, beta-2-thienylalanine, and TCDD (Pratt, 1984). The closure of the secondary palate provides the opportunity for studying epithelial–mesenchymal interactions, cellular adhesions, morphogenetic movement and programmed cell death, all in one system (cf. Transler and Fraser, 1977).

To amplify on the cellular complexity of each organ system, the development of the palate will be briefly described. From the oral aspects of the maxillary processes (Fig. 10a), bilateral outgrowths emerge to eventually form the palate. Epithelium covered by mesenchymal cells in a hyaluronate-rich matrix undergoes a complex series of morphogenetic movements: the processes move from a vertical position on each side of the tongue to a horizontal position over the tongue. As this migration is completed, the newly synthetized glycoconjugates are synthesized by the epithelium of the medial edge for these palatal processes, forming a seam. These cells eventually undergo autolysis, and form the secondary palate by merging the mesenchyme from the two formerly separate palatal processes. At this stage the nasal cavity above the palate is separate from the oral cavity. Among the modulators of these processes are

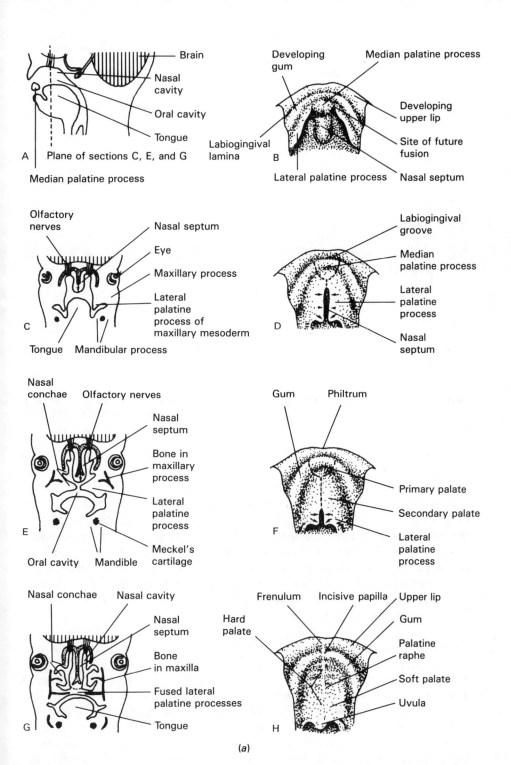

Figure 10 (a) The developmental aspects of palate development in the human. *(From Moore, 1985.)*

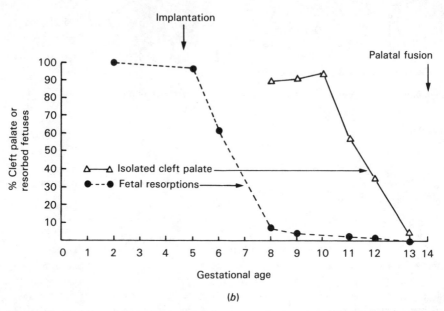

Figure 10 *(Continued)* (*b*) Incidence of cleft palate and resorptions following single administrations of 100 µg/kg (sc) of 2,3,7,8-tetrachlorodibenzo-*p*-dioxin in the pregnant B6 mouse. *(From Pratt et al., 1984.)*

cyclic AMP, prostaglandins, catecholamines, and an array of receptors (cf. Greene and Carbarino, 1984; Pratt, 1984).

One such receptor-mediated induction of cleft palate has been noted for 2,3,7,8-tetrachlorodibenzo-*p*-dioxin (TCDD) (Pratt et al., 1984) (Fig. 10*b*). Specific saturable binding of TCDD to maxillary cytosolic proteins has been established. The presence of TCDD in the palatal cells between days 8 and 12 in the B6 mouse appears to inhibit cell death in the medial epithelium, leading to cleft palate, while earlier administration (days 2–6) of TCDD produces a high incidence of resorptions. Such specificity of response indicates the sensitivity of selected tissues at specific times of development for identifiable receptors, whether in this case for TCDD or in other instances for glucocorticoids (cf. Pratt, 1984).

The Fetus   The fetal period of development may be as sensitive or even more sensitive to certain toxicological effects than any other time in the life of the organism. Evidence for such responses are certainly reflected in the 100% incidence of neurogenic tumors following the administration of ethylnitrosourea during the fetal period in the rat described above. Besides the increased susceptibility to carcinogenesis, certain organ systems, such as the central nervous system (CNS), and the reproductive, immune, and endocrine systems, are not completely developed during the embryonic period. Besides the morphological development of selected organ systems, as development progresses the fetal period reflects both the continued cell–cell interactions and a more integrated organ–organ interaction and dependence. This more sophisticated and interdependent relationship can be interrupted without the appearance of structural or life-threatening deficits, such as the neurochemical and physiological alterations in stress responses in adult rats exposed in utero to diazepam (see section on vulnerability of the central nervous system). Yet it is possible to produce structural alterations in the central nervous system (hydrocephalus) following administration of metals (tellurium) during days 15–20 in the rat (Perez et al., 1984). Also, the production of specific reproductive tract malformations in both the male and female can be produced when diethylstilbestrol is administered between days 18 and 20 of gestation in the rat (Table 1) (Baggs et al., 1983; Miller, 1983). Thus, concerning chemical exposure, the fetal period must be considered with serious reservations, as is the embryonic period.

Clinically, there are two major time periods during fetal development that can dramatically alter the postnatal outcome: (1) labor–delivery, and (2) prelabor-delivery. If agents are administered during labor, the effects on the fetus and mother can be substantially different from exposure only a few days earlier. Among the reasons for such responses is the influence of uterine contraction on the distribution of drugs to the conceptus and the response of the mother and placenta to such contractions. However, the major consideration relates to the fetus, who within a few hours is changing its physiological dependence upon the mother for sustenance, protection, and excretion (Stave, 1978). A drug administered during labor and delivery or near-term may not be entirely eliminated by the mother before birth, and therefore the neonate must now independently respond to the presence of this drug or environmental chemical. For example, when diazepam is administered just prior to delivery to control the convulsions of eclampsia, the neonate can be born with substantial body burdens of diazepam, which must be metabolized and excreted to be inactivated. If the diazepam is not excreted, it can have direct effects on the neonate, resulting in the "floppy baby" syndrome, which is characterized by hypotonia, apnea, and altered temperature regulation (Cree et al., 1973). In fact, the best means to reduce these effects of large body burdens in the neonate is via exchange transfusion. Such clinical recommendations are related to the actual development of the neonate. The more premature the birth of the child, the more important the developmental factors become whether for the human or animal model under investigation (Table 10) (Stave, 1978; Kuemmerle and Brendel, 1984; Fabro and Scialli, 1986).

Such factors play important roles related to the pharmacokinetics involved for any substance. Since there is quantitatively less albumin in the fetus and neonate, the amount of protein-bound chemical will be different if that compound is highly bound to albumin. If a substance like methylmercury or diazepam is highly lipophilic, then more of the agent will be distributed to the fetal brain than the adult brain for at least three reasons: (1) fat content is lower in the fetus, while the relative percentage of brain mass is much greater, giving the brain a disproportionate depot for these agents; (2) a much larger percentage of the cardiac output goes directly to the fetal brain than the adult brain; and (3) the metabolism of these agents is usually minimal by the fetus and neonate. In Table 11, these factors are expressed in relationship to the half-life of diazepam and its relative metabolism. The premature neonate would best represent the fetus. Obviously, with these pharmacokinetic parameters, an understanding of the exaggerated responses in the very premature neonate, as described above, can be appreciated.

Such neonatal problems related to chemical exposure near-delivery with an excess of chemical being left in the neonate following delivery have been noted for ethanol, hypotonia, apnea (Abel, 1980); for aspirin and warfarin, hemorrhage and for chlorpropamide and propranolol (Berkowitz, 1980). Furthermore, the metabolism of some chemicals may not reduce their toxicity but maintain or increase their effects depending on the types of metabolites formed [e.g., acrylonitrile (Willhite et al., 1981), benzo(a)pyrene (Shum et al., 1979), diazepam (Sher et al., 1972), diethylstilbestrol (Metzler, 1984), ethylnitrosourea (Ivankovic and Druckery, 1968; Kleihues, 1982), methylene chloride (Anders and Sunram, 1982), and laetrile (Willhite et al., 1981)]. The effects of these agents can be most specific, as with the estrogens on the reproductive tract, or rather general, as with ethylnitrosourea.

Table 10   Fetal/Neonatal Factors Modifying Therapy and Toxicity

Circulation (fetal to neonatal)
  Fetal channels (all closed in normal infant)
    Ductus arteriosus
    Ductus venous
    Foramen ovale
    Umbilical artery
    Umbilical vein
  Fetal hepatic channels (25% of umbilical venous filtered by liver)
    Hepatic artery
    Portal vein
    Umbilical vein
  Fetal pulmonary channels (blood flow; vascular resistance)
  Cardiac output (40% to fetal brain and heart)
Body composition
  Total body water (fetus > neonate > adult)
  Extracellular water (fetus > neonate > adult)
  Fat content (adult > child > neonate)
  Brain weight (fetus > neonate > adult)
Xenobiotic metabolism
  Monooxygenase activity (variable, generally adult > neonate > fetus)
  Conjugation activity (adult > neonate > fetus)
  Induction of enzymes possible (e.g., aryl hydrocarbon hydroxylase; glucuronyl
    transferase)
Plasma
  Albumin (adult > neonate, fetus)
  Immunoglobulins (adult > neonate, fetus)
  Selected proteins
    Alpha-fetoprotein (fetus > mother)
    Chorionic gonadotropin (mother > fetus)
    Placental lactogen (mother > fetus)

Table 11 Effect of Age and/or Inducting Agent on the Disposition of Diazepam[a]

Age group	Exposure to barbiturates[b]	Apparent half-life (h)	Percentage of total excreted of urinary metabolites	
			N-Desmethyl diazepam	Oxazepam
Premature neonate	No	75 ± 35	90–95	<1
	Yes	11	—[c]	—[c]
Full-term neonate	No	31 ± 2	66–90	0–13
	Yes	18 ± 1	18–21	37–58
Infants	No	10 ± 2	25–35	30–34
Children	No	17 ± 3	26–40	18–53

[a]Modified from Morselli (1977).
[b]Exposure of diazepam represents a single dose of diazepam either directly to the child or to the mother. When barbiturates were used, the exposure was either during intrauterine life or during the first days of extrauterine life.
[c]No data available.

The impact of these chemicals during the perinatal period can be diverse and yet quite specific. The remainder of this section concentrates on specific problem areas and organ systems: perinatal carcinogenesis, reproduction, immunology, and central nervous system.

Perinatal Carcinogenesis Perinatal carcinogenesis, one of the most ominous of all tumor-inducing processes, predisposes an unborn child to the latent development of life-threatening neoplasia. Recognition of such carcinogenic potential and the increased sensitivity of the fetus has been accepted only recently with the association of vaginal clear-cell adenocarcinoma in young women whose mothers had taken diethylstilbestrol between 8 and 18 weeks of pregnancy (Herbst and Bern, 1981). Yet the potential of such effects was first described in 1947 by Laren, when urethane was discovered to produce lung tumors in the progeny when given to the pregnant mothers. Today at least 50 compounds have been reported to have perinatal carcinogenic capabilities when administered to many different species (Table 12). Yet in comparison to the known number of carcinogens, this number of perinatal carcinogens is low. Part of the reason for fewer numbers of known perinatal carcinogens is the timing for the exposure and the length of time sometimes necessary to demonstrate many of these adult-onset types of tumors. In addition, many carcinogens may be embryo/fetal-lethal and therefore limit the ability for carcinogenicity testing. Also, the multivariate response of the fetus to chemical exposure presents many difficulties in determining whether the fetus is in fact more sensitive or responsive to tumor induction than is the adult, as is noted for ethylnitrosourea (Rice, 1981; Kleihues, 1982).

Whether maternal, placental, or fetal tissues are the site of xenobiotic metabolism

Table 12 Perinatal Carcinogens in Animal Models[a]

Aflatoxin B₁	Ethylurea plus sodium nitrite
o-Aminoazotoluene	N-Ethyl-N-nitrosobiuret
Azoethane	N-Ethyl-N-nitrosourea
Azoxyethane	Furylfuramide
Azoxymethane	4-Hydroxybutyl butylnitrosamine
Benzo(a)pyrene	2-Hydroxypropyl propylnitrosamine
bix(2-Hydroxypropyl)nitrosamine	Methoxyazomethanol
N-n-Butyl-N-nitrosourea	1-Methyl-2-benzylhydrazine
Carcinolipin	3-Methylcholanthrene
Cycad meal	Methyl methanesulfonate
Dibutylnitrosamine	N-Methyl-N-nitrosourea
3,3'-Dichlorobenzidine	N-Methyl-N-nitrosourethane
1,2-Diethylhydrazine	Methylpropylnitrosamine
Diethylnitrosamine	4-Nitroquinoline 1-oxide
3,3-Diethyl-1-phenyltriazene	Nitrosohexamethyleneimine
3,3-Diethyl-1-pyridyltriazene	Nitrosopiperidine
Diethylstilbestrol	2-Oxopropyl propylnitrosamine
Diethylsulphate	Procarbazine
4-Dimethylaminoazobenzene	Propane sulphate
7,12-Dimethylbenz(a)anthracene	N-n-Propyl-N-nitrosourea
Dimethylnitrosamine	Safrole
3,3-Dimethyl-1-phenyltriazene	o-Toluidine
Dimethylsulphate	Urethane
Dimethylnitrosamine	Vinyl chloride
Dipropylnitrosamine	
Ethyl methanesulfonate	

[a]The experimental animals are rat, mouse, hamster, gerbil, patas monkey, dog, pig, and opossum. Information compiled from reviews by Rice (1981), Kleihues (1982), and Miller (1983).

can be important in determining whether an agent can be a perinatal carcinogen. In some instances the fetus may be spared the carcinogenic effects of selected agents because of its reduced capacity to metabolize certain xenobiotics. In other instances, the fetus may be more susceptible because of specific enzymes being present that are not present in the adult. Cycasin can be a perinatal carcinogen via metabolism to methylazoxymethanol. This metabolism occurs in the fetal skin via β-glucosidase, which is not present in the adult skin (Spatz and Laquer, 1967; Laquer and Spatz, 1973). Thus, the presence of reactive compounds coupled with cell systems that are rapidly dividing are considered the essential factors by which the fetus may be more susceptible than the adult to tumor induction.

In many instances, a perinatal carcinogen is also an embryotoxin and teratogen, as noted for ethylnitrosourea and diethylstilbestrol. Such diversity of actions represents for many of these compounds both the general toxicity and the multiple sites for interaction in a developing organism.

Reproduction   As noted in Fig. 9, the development of the reproductive system in the rat is both pre- and postnatal. Structural defects can be produced well into the fetal period. The premier example for a developmental reproductive toxin is diethylstilbestrol. In 1940, Greene and associates reported impaired testicular descent in the rat. There is a wide range of both teratogenic and carcinogenic responses to the prenatal administration of diethylstilbestrol (Table 1). Infertility and poor reproductive history are related to structural abnormalities of the urogenital system, that is, oviduct, ovary, cervix, uterine, vagina, testes, phallus, and epididymis. Many of the reproductive-tract abnormalities noted in the human have been related in primates (Hendrickx et al., 1979; Johnson et al., 1981), hamsters (Rustia and Shubik, 1976), mice (Forsberg and Kallana, 1981; Bern and Talamantes, 1981; McLachlan, 1981), and rats (Greene et al., 1940; Napalkov and Anisimov, 1979; Boylan and Calhoon, 1979; Baggs et al., 1983; Miller, 1983). The origin of many of these urogenital abnormalities is in the Müllerian duct (Forsberg and Kalland, 1981).

When other natural estrogens are evaluated similar reproductive-tract abnormalities are not observed except at maternal toxic doses (Henry and Miller, 1985). A number of pharmacokinetic and pharmacodynamic considerations appear to limit the capability of an equally estrogenic compound 17β-estradiol from being as effective a teratogen and perinatal carcinogen as diethylstilbestrol in a number of species. Such factors include metabolism and protein binding. 17β-Estradiol is not metabolized to similar reactive intermediates as has been noted for diethylstilbestrol (Klopper, 1980; Slikker et al., 1982; Henry and Miller, 1985; Miller et al., 1982). In the pregnant rat, human, and primate, 17β-estradiol is converted to estrone by the placenta. Estrone is substantially less estrogenic than estradiol or DES. If estradiol is directly injected into rat fetuses, most of it is bound to plasma proteins and/or metabolized to estrone (Henry et al., 1984; Henry and Miller, 1985). The estradiol is bound to alpha-fetoprotein in the rat, while DES is not (Sheehan et al., 1980). Similar responses are not noted for human alpha-fetoprotein. Thus it appears that the metabolism and plasma binding of estradiol may be defense mechanisms for the fetus to reduce the potential toxicity of the natural estrogens. Thus the synthetic estrogens can produce their toxicity by avoiding inactivation and binding.

Exposure to diethylstilbestrol offers a unique opportunity for directly evaluating human and animals responses in sufficient numbers to determine effect and statistical significance even at a low incidence. These comparisons between human and animal data assist in developing new testing protocols for both functional and structural disorders and help to define sensitive windows of toxic response throughout in utero development and not just for organogenesis.

Perinatal Immunotoxicology   The immune system, as noted in Fig. 9, develops well into the fetal and neonatal periods. The sensitivity of this system to toxic insult has only recently been appreciated in the adult and even now is rarely well evaluated as an area for major effects due to perinatal exposures. As immunologists begin to understand more thoroughly this period of in utero development, the potential for alterations in immune development will be investigated.

The maturation of the thymus-derived lymphocytes (T cells), the bursa equivalent-derived lymphocytes (B cells), macrophages, and the complement system spans much of the prenatal and neonatal period. The origins of the lymphocyte precursors are located in the yolk sac during early embryogenesis. These precursors migrate to the liver, bone marrow, and eventually thymus and lymphoid tissue (Roberts and Chapman, 1981).

It is particularly interesting that many agents that affect the complex immune system during development have irreversible effects while administration of the agent to the adult results in reversible changes. Examples of such agents are busulfan (Pinto-Machado, 1970), cortisone (Kalland et al., 1978; Ways and Bern, 1979), cyclophosphamide (Glick, 1971; Linna et al., 1972), estrogens (Reilly et al., 1967; Luz et al., 1969; Luster et al., 1979; Kalland, 1980; Kalland et al., 1978, 1979; Ways and Bern, 1979), and TCDD (Vos and Moore, 1974; Faith and Moore, 1977; Thomas and Hindsall, 1979).

Such studies only reflect the possible interactions of xenobiotics with the immune system. Since the immune system has dominant roles in infections, carcinogenesis, and immune diseases, this fetal area of perinatal toxicity evaluation will be of great importance.

Central Nervous System Vulnerability

Considerable data have shown an enhanced susceptibility of the developing brain (compared to the mature brain and to other developing organs) to chemicals [e.g., alcohol (Streissguth et al., 1980), mercury (Clarkson et al., 1981), and phenytoin (Hanson, 1976)]. Considering the current state of our understanding of the molecular aspects of brain development, there is a logical rationale to support the hypothesis that exposure during development to agents that interact with the central nervous system (CNS) could exert long-lasting effects on the organism. For example, many of the drugs that may be administered during pregnancy, such as antihypertensive, sympathomimetic, antipsychotic, antidepressive, and anxiolytic agents, have as target sites critical components of chemically mediated neurotransmission (Table 13). Knowledge concerning the course of development of chemical transmission has increased considerably in recent years. Many sites on which these drugs act appear early in fetal development, and the fetal brain responds in a predictable manner to many psychoactive drugs (see below). Interference with specific mechanisms of chemical neurotransmission during development using selected neurotoxins has been demonstrated to alter the course of brain development with resulting functional consequences.

Chemical Neurotransmission Before considering the effect of chemical exposure on the development of mechanisms for chemical transmission, a brief discussion of chemical neurotransmission is in order. Chemical neurotransmission is the major means whereby neurons communicate with one another or with effector cells such as muscles and glands. This communication takes place in the synapse, a schematic diagram of which is presented in Fig. 11. The information flow across a synapse is

Table 13   Some Agents Utilized during Pregnancy and Their Actions in the Central or Peripheral Nervous System[a]

Drug	Effect
Antipsychotic agents	
Halperidol (Haldol)	DA receptor antagonists; some action at 5-HT
Phenothiazines (e.g., Thorazine)	and NE receptors.
Antidepressant agents	
Imipramine (Tofranil)	Block reuptake of released transmitter into
Amitriptyline (Elavil)	5-HT and NE neurons; induce down regulation of β receptors.
Ataractic drugs	
Chlordiazepoxide (Librium)	Agonists at specific benzodiazepine binding
Diazepam (Valium)	site; may influence GABA neurotransmission via GABA receptor.
Anticonvulsant agents	
Diazepam (Valium)	See above.
Phenobarbital	May bind to particular domain of GABA–receptor complex and influence GABA transmission.
Phenytoin (Dilantin)	May bind to GABA–receptor complex.
Valproic acid	
Antihypertensive agents	
Methyldopa (Aldomet)	Amine metabolite may act directly on adrenergic receptors in CNS.
Clonidine (Catapres)	Agonist at α_2 receptors.
Sympathomimetic agents	
Selective β_2 agonists	
Salbutamol (Albuterol)	Stimulate β_2 receptors
Terbutaline (Bricanyl)	
Amphetamine (Benzadrine)	Promote release of catecholamines; may block reuptake and MAO.
Methylxanthines	Precise action unclear; may act at adenosine
(caffeine)	sites, benzodiazepine binding sites.
Cold medications containing	Act like NE on adrenergic receptors;
ephedrine, phenylephrine	may release CA.
Analgesic agents	
Morphine	Agonists to opiate receptors.
Hydromorphine (Dilaudid)	
Methadone (Dolophine)	
Meperidine (Demerol)	
Codeine	

[a]Abbreviations: DA, dopamine; NE, norepinephrine; 5-HT, 5-hydroxytryptamine (serotonin); CA, catecholamine; MAO, monoamine oxidase.

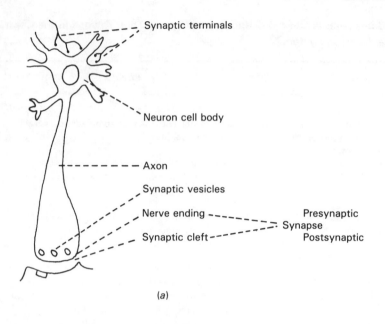

(a)

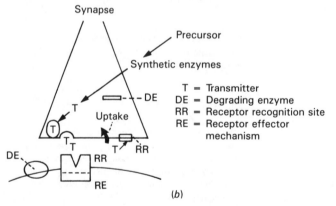

(b)

Figure 11 (a) Diagram of a neuron and synapse. (b) Synaptic mechanisms involved in the production and regulation of neurotransmission.

unidirectional, with information proceeding from the presynaptic to the postsynaptic side of the synapse. The information in the presynaptic cell reaches the synapse by way of conduction of an action potential along the axonal membrane. When the action potential reaches the synaptic ending, depolarization of the terminal initiates a series of processes; the classical culmination of these events is the movement of synaptic vesicles (which contain the transmitter) within the presynaptic ending toward the terminal membrane. Fusion of the vesicle membrane with the axonal membrane results in the release of the contents of the synaptic vesicle into the synaptic cleft (the space between the two cells). The transmitter can then interact with specialized receptor molecules in the postsynaptic membrane and initiate response within the postsynaptic cell.

Complex processes are present within both the pre- and postsynaptic cells to maintain chemical neurotransmission as outlined above. The amount of transmitter contained in a nerve terminal is usually maintained at a relatively constant level over a wide range of physiological activity, and this constancy is maintained by complex regulation of the mechanisms for production and utilization of transmitter (Fig. 11b). Transmitters are synthesized in the nerve ending by synthetic enzymes, either from precursor accumulated from the circulation or from precursor produced within the cell. Once a transmitter is synthesized, it is usually packaged in synaptic vesicles. This packaging prepares the transmitter for release and protects it from breakdown by degradative enzymes that may be present in the presynaptic nerve ending. Upon release, the transmitter may interact with receptors on either the pre- or postsynaptic side of the cleft. As indicated above, interaction with the postsynaptic receptor mediates the flow of information between cells. Interaction of a transmitter with presynaptic receptors can influence the synthesis and/or release of the transmitter itself, thereby sculpturing the time course of release relative to the amount of transmitter in the synaptic cleft. In general, transmitter released into the synaptic cleft is inactivated by active transport back into the presynaptic ending (reuptake). Enzymatic degradation of the transmitter in the cleft is also a means of inactivation, although this mechanism is limited as a primary inactivating mechanism to specific transmitters.

Compounds that are generally considered to be neurotransmitters fall into three categories: amines (dopamine, norepinephrine, epinephrine, serotonin, and acetylcholine); amino acids (γ-aminobutyric acid or GABA, glutamate, aspartate, glycine); and peptides. The latter category is growing daily in the number of feasible candidates, and any listing should be considered only representative at best. However, peptides known to reside in specific neurons in the CNS, include classic neuroendocrine peptides such as vasopressin, oxytocin, luteinizing-hormone releasing hormone (LHRH), thyrotropin-releasing hormone (TRH), somatostatin (SRIF), adrenocorticotrophic hormone (ACTH), and corticotropin-releasing factor (CRF); brain–gut peptides such as vasoactive intestinal peptide (VIP), cholecystokinin, and substance P; and the opioid peptides such as β-endorphin, met- and leu-enkephalin, and dynorphin.

The synthesis and inactivation as well as the regulation thereof for each transmitter is individualized to that particular system. However, each system is vulnerable to pharmacologic intervention, and such intervention can disrupt the process of transmission. Hence, interference with synthesis by agents that either interfere with the synthetic enzymes or alter substrate availability will decrease the amount of transmitter available for release. Following chronic exposure, this decrease in available transmitter may be followed by compensatory responses such as a change in the sensitivity of related receptors. Likewise, interference with degrading enzymes may increase the amount of available transmitter, but again compensatory responses, such as a decrease in receptor sensitivity or in the rate of synthesis, may result. Drugs that alter transmitter release may also activate compensatory changes, as do drugs that interfere with reuptake. A characteristic neural response, for example, to drugs that interfere with transmitter binding to its receptor is enhanced synthesis and release of that transmitter as a compensatory step to overcome the action of the drug. Therefore, in considering the consequences of drug exposure on organisms, one must consider the compensatory responses as well as the primary action. Compensatory responses may be particularly critical in the developing organism.

The above has been a very brief overview of the processes of chemical neurotransmission. The complexity of chemical transmission gives validity to the importance of this process in neural communication. A most critical function imparted to the brain by chemical transmission is that of inhibition; inhibition allows the precise patterning of neural activity in the brain. As the next section demonstrates, the development of the mechanisms of chemical transmission is a complex and very ordered process.

Development of Chemical Neurotransmission   The development of the brain is a precisely orchestrated event and follows the same basic sequence in all mammalian species. Development begins with induction of the neural plate and continues through cell proliferation, migration, aggregation, and differentiation of immature neurons to the establishment of synaptic connections. The final sculpturing of the brain involves selective cell death and the elimination of some connections [see Cowan (1979) for review]. While the course of brain development is similar across species, it must be remembered that the relationship of the various developmental events to birth differs across species. Hence, a rat is born with a more immature brain than a human, which has a more immature brain than a guinea pig.

As individual neurons undergo the process of differentiation, they develop those mechanisms necessary for chemical neurotransmission. Many cells develop their transmitters very early in the differentiation process, whereas other cells take on their transmitter characteristics sometime after the onset of morphologic differentiation. It may be that the timing or the appearance of chemical transmitters relative to the time of cell birth may predict developmental functions for specific transmitters.

Neurons that will utilize monoamines (such as the catecholamines and serotonin) as neurotransmitters are among the earliest cells to differentiate (Lauder and Bloom, 1974). The time course of development of the mechanisms underlying catecholamine neurotransmission in the rat is described in Fig. 12. Cell division of these neurons ceases shortly after neural tube closure. The presence of transmitter has been detected histochemically in these immature neurons soon after the onset of differentiation (the cessation of cell division), and the necessary enzymes for synthesis have also been detected. The formation of synaptic contacts by these cells begins late in gestation in the rat and continues at a more rapid rate postnatally with full development achieved somewhere around 4 weeks postnatal age (Lauder and Bloom, 1975). Just as catecholamines are some of the earliest transmitters to appear in early development, in some regions these neurons are also the earliest to begin synaptogenesis. Embryonic rat cortex is innervated by catecholamine-containing fibers (Schlumpf et al., 1980), and norepinephrine (NE) appears to occupy a much higher percentage of cortical synapses in the neonatal rat as compared to the adult (Coyle and Molliver, 1977). The catecholamine-containing neurons are also pharmacologically responsive early in gestation (Coyle and Henry, 1973). These early differentiating chemically defined neurons, therefore, may have important developmental functions such as regulation of cell proliferation (Patel et al., 1983) or as signals for differentiation (Lauder and Krebs, 1978). They are also target sites for any psychoactive agents (Table 13).

The catecholamine neurons have been shown to appear early in human development as well as in the rat (Fig. 12). Neural-tube closure is completed by 4 weeks of gestation in the human and catecholamine histofluorescence is detectable in some cells by 7 weeks of gestation, with marked fluorescence present by 10 weeks (Olson et al., 1973; Nobin and Bjorklund, 1973). These catecholaminergic neurons may play similar developmental roles in different mammalian species.

The development of catecholamine (CA) neurons has been described in some detail, as substantial information is known about their development. Other proposed transmitter candidates have also been identified in cells early in gestation in the rat (such as the peptides vasopressin, somatostatin, substance P, and leu-enkephalin). These substances may also have developmental functions. However, for certain pep-

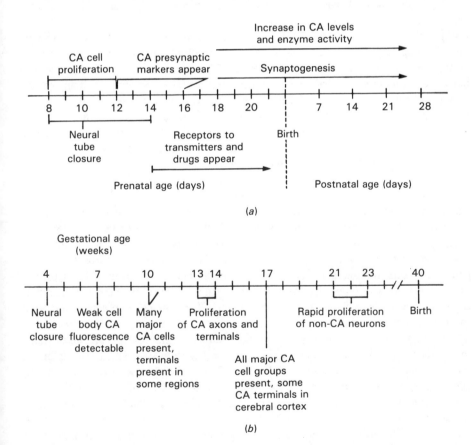

Figure 12 (a) Development of catecholamine neurons in the rat. (b) Development of catecholamine neurons in the human. CA, catecholamine.

tides, such as cholecystokinin, whereas the cells appear fairly early in gestation, fiber development appears to be mainly a postnatal event (Cho et al., 1983).

Interference with such neurons during certain stages of development would not be expected to have the same consequences as would interference with CA transmission. GABA is a transmitter subserving major inhibitory functions. While GABA-containing fibers have been identified in specific brain regions of the rat by embryonic day 12, its presence in cells known to utilize GABA as a transmitter in the adult brain occurs much later (Lauder et al., 1984). While some of the cells in which GABA will serve as a transmitter differentiate late (e.g., cerebellar basket and stellate cells), other cells, such as the Purkinje cells in the cerebellum, differentiate morphologically long before they appear to undertake transmitter differentiation. Additionally, presynpatic markers of GABA (its synthesizing enzyme) have not been detected until the end of the first postnatal week in rat cerebellum (Coyle and Enna, 1976). Again, the developmental function of GABA-containing neurons may be quite different from that of CA-containing neurons.

From the above discussion it should be apparent that pharmacologic substrates are shifting throughout neural development, as are neural interrelationships that determine the responses to drugs. Thus, while catecholamine (CA) neurons can be pharmacologically manipulated very early in development, the specific responses within the CA neurons themselves to chemical interference vary with development as the different components of chemical neurotransmission develop (Kellogg et al., 1979). Likewise, the functional responses of the organism to specific drugs varies with development as the individual component transmitter systems mature. Interference with NE neurons in the cortex may have a more profound effect in early development than later because of the predominance of NE input to the cortex at this stage prior to the appearance of other component transmitter systems.

Development of Transmitter Receptors   A major site of action of many centrally acting drugs listed in Table 13 is at a neurotransmitter receptor. With the increased understanding of molecular aspects of receptors, the perceived importance of receptors to neural function has increased immeasurably. It is apparent that intervention at the level of the receptor is a major mode of action for many neuroactive drugs, and also that neurologic and psychoactive disorders may result from receptor pathology. Because of the importance of receptors for neural function, the development of transmitter receptors will be considered separately from the development of the other mechanisms of chemical neurotransmission (presented above).

There appears to be little synchrony between the timing for appearance of transmitter receptors and their synaptic input. As indicated in Fig. 12, the receptors to many transmitters appear quite early in gestation in the rat. However, transmitters such as the catecholamines are present prior to the appearance of their receptors, and there is evidence that development of certain catecholamine receptors is dependent on transmitter input (Deskin et al., 1981). Other receptor molecules, such as the GABA receptor on cerebellar Purkinje cells, are present long before the appearance of GABA-containing terminals (Palacios and Kuhar, 1982; McLaughlin et al., 1975). Some of these early-appearing receptors (such as the GABA receptor) are linked to active effector mechanisms and if pharmacologically activated can elicit responses in the cells on which they reside (Woodward et al., 1972). On the other hand, other early-appearing receptors appear unable to mediate appropriate effector responses. While alpha-2 receptors are present on blood platelets in the full-term human fetus, epinephrine will not induce platelet aggregation in the term fetus (Jones et al., 1983). There is also some evidence that certain transmitter receptors during fetal life may have overlapping specificity with more than one transmitter (Freidhoff and Miller, 1983).

Information on the timing of appearance of transmitter receptors in the human brain is not available; however, since other mechanisms of chemical transmission appear in the human brain in a manner similar to their appearance in other species, it is likely that transmitter receptors are present during gestation in the human. A study in human brain tissue taken from birth to 2 years of age demonstrated that the receptors measured had adult-like characteristics, which suggests a prenatal course of development (Maggi et al., 1979).

The presence of a transmitter receptor linked to a functioning effector mechanism (even without the presence of a presynaptic input) could render cells on which the receptor resides vulnerable to exogenous agents that might bind to and activate that specific receptor. Additionally, the course of development of receptors that depend on transmitter input for proper development could be altered by drugs that interfere with transmitter synthesis or release. All the drugs listed in Table 13 could potentially alter receptor function at some level if administered during development.

Effects of Interference with Neurotransmitter Function during Development   Evidence that has been gathered from studies using specific neurotoxins to destroy selective neurotransmitter systems has provided important guidelines for conducting research on the effects of developmental exposure to centrally acting drugs and environmental chemicals that have relatively select modes of action. Injections of the neurotoxin, 6-hydroxydopamine (6-OHDA), to rats early in postnatal development or of its precursor 6-hydroxydopa (6-OHDOPA) during prenatal development have demonstrated restrictive responsiveness of the developing noradrenergic neurons. Hence, early postnatal exposure to 6-OHDA (days 1–3) induces a denervation of NE innervation to the cerebral cortex but a hyperinnervation of NE innervation to the brainstem and cerebellum (Jonsson and Sachs, 1976; Jaim-Etchenerry and Zieher, 1977). The NE innervation to the diencephalon is not altered. If 6-OHDA exposure is delayed until after day 3 (but before day 10), the NE innervation to the cerebellum will be denervated rather than hyperinnervated (Amaral et al., 1975). The selective changes in NE terminal growth following developmental exposure to the specific neurotoxin must be expressions of mechanisms related to normal development. These studies indicate, therefore, that the effects of any drug given during development can be expected to be very selective and dependent on the timing of exposure. A specific receptor antagonist or agonist, for example, should not be expected to exert the same effect on all neurons on which that receptor might be located, and therefore the functional consequences may vary depending on the time of exposure.

Studies utilizing specific neurotoxins have also indicated that functional changes that may occur after early developmental exposure to such agents will be discreet and best observed if the functional task to be evaluated is coordinated with the known anatomical distribution of the systems altered. Thus, while early postnatal exposure to 6-OHDA induces a profound depletion of NE terminals in the cerebral cortex, general behavioral tests failed to show any effect of the drugs (Isaacson et al., 1977). However, knowing the NE neurons innervate the visual cortex, Kasamatsu and Pettigrew (1976) demonstrated that perfusion of 6-OHDA into the visual cortex during development interfered with the usual cortical plasticity that kittens display in response to monocular occlusion.

In other studies, when the functional test was correlated with known neurochemical anatomy, the effects of early intervention with known transmitter systems have been shown to appear after a period of normal development. Hence, early 6-OHDA treatment has been shown to alter the development of cardiac function in a manner suggestive of an altered balance between the sympathetic and parasympathetic nervous system (Deskin et al., 1980). The CNS rather than the peripheral neurons themselves appeared to be responsible for the altered function. The deficits observed were not apparent until the second to third postnatal week, when tonic sympathetic control of the heart normally appears. This observation serves to illustrate the point that interference with CNS development can be expressed in physiologic dysfunction as well as behavioral alterations.

To evaluate the effects of developmental exposure to neuropsychoactive drugs and environmental chemicals, the above-mentioned observations must be kept in mind: (1) the effects of any one drug may be very selective, (2) functional tests should be carefully chosen, and (3) alterations may not appear until after a period of normal development.

Testing and Evaluation of CNS Effects following Developmental Exposure to Drugs and Environmental Chemicals   The above sections illustrated the prolonged and complicated course of neural development. Whereas some neurons have begun differentiation by the eighth week of gestation in the human, full maturation of the human brain is not complete until 6–8 years of age. As was also illustrated above, the responsiveness of the developing brain to chemical agents varies depending on the timing of exposure relative to developmental events. To determine the effects an agent may induce on neural development requires extensive evaluation using many approaches: anatomical, chemical, and physiological. To then determine whether altered neural activity is translated into alterations in the ability of the brain to perform (i.e., to regulate behavioral and physiological processes) is a task that requires considerable thought and planning. The consequences of altered neural function are not as obvious as alterations in reproductive function.

Several countries now specify that tests of psychological and behavioral processes be conducted in assessing the safety of new therapeutic compounds. The United Kingdom requires tests for "auditory, visual, and behavioral impairment." Japan has requirements for tests of "locomotion, learning, sensory functions, and emotionality." No standard test batteries are provided, primarily because there is no agreement on the best methods for the analyses required. While a screening battery of tests may be appropriate to evaluate effects of early developmental exposure to certain chemical agents, the generalized use of such tests does not seem to be appropriate when the specificity of neuronal interactions and functions is considered. As noted above, a general battery of tests did not detect functional impairment associated with early developmental exposure to the neurotoxin 6-OHDA (Isaacson et al., 1977), whereas specific testing designed with the knowledge of specific neural substrate–function relationships did detect impairments following early 6-OHDA exposure (Kasamatsu and Pettigrew, 1976). Likewise, the use of a test battery did not detect any functional impairments in animals exposed in utero to diazepam (Butcher and Vorhees, 1979), but tests designed specifically to evaluate the action of an anxiolytic compound demonstrated functional alterations following prenatal exposure to diazepam at doses as low as l/mg/kg·day (Simmons et al., 1984b; Kellogg et al., 1980).

As a guideline, the use of specific tests for individual compounds would appear to be most likely to detect functional alterations following developmental exposure to agents with a known mechanism of action and neural substrate interaction. Thus, tests of responsiveness to stress may detect neural effects of early exposure to anxiolytic compounds, while evaluation of seizure susceptibility may be more appropriate for evaluation of exposure to anticonvulsant drugs, and measures of cyclic behaviors such as sleep patterns most useful in evaluating the possible consequences of early developmental exposure to antidepressant agents. A screening battery would seem to have the greatest use in evaluating developmental exposures to agents in which there is little knowledge of how such compounds interact with the brain.

Adams and Buelke-Sam (1981) suggest that a test battery should provide information on the following endpoints: (1) physical growth, (2) reflex and motor development, (3) sensory function, (4) activity and reactivity levels, (5) learning and memory ability, and (6) neurotransmitter function. Additionally, behavioral dysfunctions should be evaluated across lifespans, since functional impairment may be revealed as developmental retardation, as an alteration in levels of responding in adulthood, or in an inability to meet stress challenges at any age such as those accompanying adolescence or the aging process.

Fechter and Mactutus (1984) have shown, for example, that animals exposed to low-level hypoxia during gestation are developmentally retarded in measures of learning and memory, as evidenced in the slower acquisition of avoidance behavior in developing rats, while young adults (3–4 months) show no impairment. Recent reports show that the deficits reappear in the animals prenatally exposed to hypoxia when the animals are tested after 1 year of age (Mactutus and Fechter, 1985). Considering the impact that the results of functional testing can have in determining compound safety, the extensive testing suggested by Adams and Buelke-Sam (1981) to be done in the context of longitudinal studies is essential.

The reader is referred to reports by Adams and Buelke-Sam (1981), Vorhees (1983), and Rodier (1978) for descriptions of tests generally recommended in screening for the effects of perinatal exposure to chemical agents. It is the goal of this presentation to discuss only some of the tests used, particularly in terms of providing guidelines for interpretation of results and selection of tests.

Measures of physical development generally include such measures as body weight, time of hair growth, ear and eye opening, and time of appearance of simple reflexes such as geotactic and body righting. The understanding has been generally accepted that if no difference is noted between exposed animals and controls on these measures, marked effects on more complex tests will not be evident (Sullivan, 1983), but this hypothesis must be viewed with caution.

Recent experimental studies evaluating the effects of prenatal exposure to compounds such as alcohol (Shoemaker et al., 1983), diazepam (Kellogg et al., 1983), cadmium (Newland et al., 1986), and lead (Jason and Kellogg, 1981) have shown marked functional and/or neural impairment when no reliable alterations in measures of physical development were observed or when the impairments could not be related to indices of physical development. Also, while animals exposed to chemical substances may show delays and retardation in measures of physical development, such alterations may reflect secondary responses to the exposure. Nutritional deficiencies will also induce developmental delays and growth retardation. Studies on the effects of prenatal exposure to ethanol are often plagued by interference with nutrition of the offspring for which proper controls are often not included. In many studies evaluating the effects of chemical exposure, interpretation of the results can be complicated by marked effects of the compounds on the nutritional status of the developing animal. For example, when lead exposure levels were kept low enough to eliminate the effects of lead on the body weight of developing animals, many of the effects previously attributed to the lead exposure were no longer evident, while other effects were found to emerge or persist at later ages (Jason and Kellogg, 1980).

Tests of motor function most generally involve measurement of simple locomotion in a horizontal plane. The use of locomotor tests in animals such as rats should be made at several ages during postnatal development, since rats tested in isolation show a rapid increase in locomotor activity around 12 days of age that peaks at 15–16 days and then decreases markedly, reaching adult levels by 18 days (Campbell et al., 1969). This phase of locomotor hyperactivity during development may reflect differential rates of maturation of specific excitatory and inhibitory systems, although the precise neural mechanisms involved are not understood. Prenatal exposure of rats to diazepam (Kellogg et al., 1980) and lead (Jason and Kellogg, 1981), for example, interfered with the developmental phase of locomotion but had no effect on locomotor activity after days 18–20. Interference with transient developmental behaviors may be predictive of later functional consequences. Failure to test for locomotion throughout development could result in missing effects of perinatal chemical exposure.

An important component of screening for CNS effects of perinatal chemical exposure should include tests of sensory function. In fact, analysis of CNS/functional teratology should begin with the analysis of sensory function, since behavior in any number of behavioral tests (e.g., tests of learning or emotional reactivity) requires that the organisms be able to extract information from its environment, and this function depends on the integrity of sensory systems. The failure of sensory systems to mature at a normal rate can be expected to interfere with the maturation of other behavioral functions. Very few direct neurophysiologic analyses of sensory function have been conducted in evaluation of the effects of early chemical exposure in experimental animals. One indirect approach used to evaluate sensory ability is the analysis of reflex modification (Hoffman and Ison, 1980). A reflex elicited by one stimulus is modified by the prior presentation or withdrawal of another, usually weaker stimulus. Using various sensory modalities to modify the acoustic startle reflex, Parisi and Ison (1979, 1981) have studied the maturation of visual, auditory, and cutaneous function in the rat. Others have used such a test to study the decay of sensorimotor function in the adult rat (Krauter et al., 1981). Such a simple test of sensory ability should be incorporated into drug evaluation studies. Analysis of acoustic inhibition of the acoustic startle reflex demonstrated no interference in the development of auditory function following prenatal exposure to diazepam (C. K. Kellogg, unpublished observations), whereas such exposure markedly delayed the noise facilitation of the acoustic startle reflex, a measure of arousal function (Kellogg et al., 1980). Therefore, measures of reflex modification can separate effects of drug exposure on primary sensory function from effects on other aspects of neural function.

The acoustic startle response can also be utilized to obtain information on more complex neural functions and behaviors. Evaluation of auditory temporal acuity in rats can be obtained by measuring the inhibition of the acoustic startle reflex incurred by the introduction of brief silent periods in an otherwise constant background noise presentation (Ison, 1982). In rats, the threshold for detection of these brief silent periods (gaps) correlates with the psychophysically defined threshold in humans (Ison and Pinckney, 1983). Studies of gap detection in humans show that individual differences in gap detection are related to speech perception in adults (Trinder, 1979) and to language and learning disabilities in children (McCroskey and Kidder, 1980). Thus, the test of gap detection addresses the need for developing tests of functional teratology in animals that have relevance to complex human functions. Such a test is easily quantifiable, requires no training or food or water deprivation of animals to encourage performance, and while the neural substrates underlying reflex modulation are not completely understood, the probability of identifying related substrates is greater than for understanding the substrates related to maze performance or avoidance behavior. Thus, there is a greater opportunity to understand the mechanisms affected by toxic exposure when reflex modulation is used as a functional test. Knowledge of underlying mechanisms is undoubtedly the key to successful extrapolation across species.

The lack of understanding of the neural mechanisms underlying most of the behavioral tests recommended in screening programs is a major problem of such tests. Prenatal exposure to many drugs may affect physical development or the development of locomotor activity, for example, but do they do so via the same mechanism(s)? The type of neural interference (if known) could predict overall functional impairment. Prenatal exposure to phenobarbital interferes with female reproductive function, but apparently at the level of the CNS rather than at the level of the reproductive organs themselves (Gupta et al., 1980). An assessment of neural alterations induced by certain chemical agents can greatly assist in the design of appropriate functional tests. The demonstration that prenatal exposure of rats to diazepam induced a rather selective effect on noradrenergic neurons innervating the hypothalamus (Simmons et al., 1984a) led to the analysis of central and peripheral responses of exposed offspring to restraint stress. It has long been known that catecholamine neurons in the hypothalamus are influenced by various stressors (Corrodi et al., 1968) and that these neurons exert a major influence over the stress-induced release of adrenocortico-trophic hormone and corticosterone (Fuxe et al., 1973; Hedge et al., 1976). Acute administration of diazepam to adult rats alters the response to stress within hypotha-lamic noradrenergic neurons and prevents stress-induced increases in plasma corti-costerone (Corrodi et al., 1971; Lahti and Borshun, 1975). Hence, it seemed highly probable that rats with altered function of noradrenergic neurons innervating the hypothalamus (induced by early exposure to diazepam) would have altered responses to stressors, as was found to be the case (Simmons et al., 1984b).

The observation that newborn rats prenatally exposed to ethanol have elevated plasma and brain corticosterone levels, compared to pair-fed controls (Taylor et al., 1982a), led the investigators to evaluate the offspring as adults for plasma corticoster-one responses to various stressors. They found that fetal exposure to alcohol pro-duced an increase in adult hypothalamic–pituitary–adrenal responsiveness to sensory or emotional stimuli (Taylor et al., 1982b, 1983). These effects appear related to the effects of fetal ethanol exposure on central neural mechanisms that regulate specific neuroendocrine functions rather than on the adrenal gland itself. Prenatal exposure to neuroleptic agents that are known to be antagonists at dopamine receptors induced a decrease in the density of dopamine receptors in specific brain regions of rat offspring that persisted into adulthood (Rosengarten and Friedhoff, 1979). Behaviors regulated by dopamine innervation to the involved brain region were also altered by the prena-tal exposure.

These examples serve to illustrate the concept that functional impairments conse-quent to prenatal drug exposure are likely to become more readily apparent when functional tests are coordinated with known neural alterations. Chemical exposure, especially if limited to specific periods of brain development, may induce very selec-tive alterations in neural function, such that most tests utilized in screening batters would not be sensitive enough to detect related functional alterations. The functional alterations, however, may be of major importance to the organism. A combination of both tests selected to correlate with a suspected mechanism of action and general screening tests may, however, be essential in order to reliably determine whether the developing CNS is affected by a chemical compound. The goal of these evaluations for possible effects of perinatal chemical exposure should be to detect alterations induced by even low levels of exposure.

Thus, all periods of development from the preimplantation embryo to the neonate are selectively responsive to environmental insult. The window for such response may be the loss of pregnancy before implantation, or the induction of gliaomas after exposure to ethylnitrosourea during the fetal period, or Wilms tumor of the kidney. To systematically explore the potential for induction of such perinatal toxicity, the fol-lowing section examines the in vivo and in vitro testing methods currently in use for determining such toxicity and examining the mechanisms by which this perinatal toxicity is produced.

Experimental Models

During the past 30 years almost as many different methods for studying the toxic and/ or teratogenic effects of agents during in utero development have been discussed or published as agents tested. As noted earlier, the reason for such a proliferation of study methods is primarily due to the multiple and multifactorial mechanisms by which such toxicity can be expressed in the developing organism. One of the difficulties in teratogenicity testing is the question of whether one is screening to reflect the human situation as a test system and therefore trying to extrapolate data from animal to human or whether the experimentation is being performed to determine the impact of this agent on various species, either in agriculture or for environmental impact statements.

The following two sections (in vivo and in vitro experimentation) are primarily written with the human in mind as a potential for comparison. However, there are numerous references made to other species, both aquatic and terrestrial. Therefore, even though a number of these tests will refer to the current requirements for teratologic testing and perinatal toxicity testing, for selected compounds, additional tests or perhaps the use of other species may be essential for determining the effect of the agents as well as their mechanisms of action.

Beside our need to use these protocols both as screening tools and documentation of developmental toxicity, it is also important to utilize other methods for determining the mechanisms by which these compounds are producing their insults. The preceding discussions, including species comparisons, must be evaluated with the developmental perspective in mind, such as different enzymatic responses required for the metabolism of xenobiotics and the differential growth and development of selected organ systems. In some instances, it even becomes difficult to separate in vivo and in vitro testing when one must consider species such as the chick, amphibian, and opossum. As we ask more sophisticated questions, the need for designing specific and elaborate experiments to answer these questions is inevitable. The following two sections are not presented as a comprehensive review of all methods used, but rather the general approaches utilized currently and references to selected variations.

In Vivo Experimentation   Substantial changes in the requirements for teratogenicity testing were introduced and established following the thalidomide incident of 1960. One of the most important documents concerning these issues was the Guidelines for Reproduction Studies for Safety Evaluation of Drugs for Human Use published in 1966 by the U.S. Food and Drug Administration. Similar protocols were adopted for food additives and pesticides in 1970. These testing protocols have been individually modified for certain compounds and have been utilized for environmental agents and adopted with modification for international use (Council on Environmental Quality, 1981). Reviews of these protocols and further modifications have been written by a number of investigators (Wilson and Fraser, 1977; Council on Environmental Quality, 1981; Manson et al., 1982).

There are two major components to these studies: multigenerational tests and

single generation tests. The multigenerational tests have been discussed in the reproductive toxicity section earlier and therefore will not be discussed in greater detail.
The single generation tests are among the most commonly used teratogenicity testing
protocols. Some confusion has developed in the designation of these tests based on
the similarity to clinical trials (i.e., phase I, II, and III studies). Therefore, the
preclinical teratogenicity studies are now designated as segment I, II, and III studies,
as noted in Fig. 13.

If an exposure to an agent is persistent and tends to accumulate in the body, then
a multigenerational study is most appropriate. For specific details concerning the
conduct of these studies, the reader is also referred to reviews by Ellison (1977),
Council on Environmental Quality (1981), and Manson et al. (1982). In reviewing
these multigenerational studies, it is essential that certain indices be kept in mind for
the statistical analysis and appropriate interpretation of such studies. These indices
are listed in Table 14. Many of these indices can also be applied to the single-
generation studies commonly known as the reproductive and teratology testing sequence.

One of the major features of this single-generation study is the use of two different species for evaluation. The rodent (typically mouse or rat) is used for more in-
depth evaluation. Rodents have been selected for the primary segment I and II screens
due to large litter size, a short gestational period, and an extensive literature relating
to these species. Of equal concern is the strain of these species that is selected to test
the compounds or agents. The second species must be a nonrodent and is usually a
lagomorph (e.g., rabbit). Other species, especially carnivores, are being proposed as
useful alternatives to the lagamorph for testing in segment III. A primary animal for
such consideration today is the ferret (*Teratology*, April 1982). Even before considering any of the details for the segment I, II, and III studies, the choice of species may
be among the most critical considerations in the evaluation for teratologic testing.
Species differences have been noted earlier but are reemphasized here. In attempting
to make extrapolations from animal to human, it is critical to choose an animal model
that has similarities to the human, especially in the area of xenobiotic metabolism,
distribution, and excretion. These factors are especially important for the action of
thalidomide and may partially account for some of the species differences. Consider-

**Table 14   Some Indices for Statistical Analyses in Multigenerational
Studies**

Fertility index = (number of pregnancies/number of matings) × 100
Gestation index
  (per litter) = number of live fetuses or newborns/litter
  (per fetus/newborn) = total number of liveborn/total born or fetuses
Viability index at a certain day (x)
  = (number of live pups at day x/number of pups following delivery
    at day y, where $y <$ initial x) × 100
  (x = 4, 7, 14, 21, 28 days)

Table 15   Assessment of Reproductive Toxicity

Preconception evaluations
  Animal weight
  Mating behavior
  Conception rate
Postconception evaluations
  Corpora luteal number
  Implantation number
  Size of litter
  Death, embryonic
  Death, fetal
  Live fetuses
  Incidence of malformations in live fetuses, external, internal
  Pup weight; crown rump weight
  Placental weight
  Maternal weight gain
    Date of conception
    Date of delivery
Postpartum evaluations
  Number of pups born
  Number of pups alive
  Number of pups dead
  Incidence of malformations, external, internal
  Weight of pups at delivery and growth rate
  Lactation
  Survival incidence from delivery through 21 days
  Time of developmental landmarks (eye opening, pinna opening, hair
    growth, vaginal opening)
  Functional testing (sensory, behavioral, physiological)
  Maternal weight gain

---

ations for testing chemicals should depend on the pharmacokinetics in the species for study as well as the gestational periods involved.

Reproductive and Teratology Testing Sequence

Segment I—Reproduction Studies   This test is the most comprehensive of the three segment tests for single generation evaluations. As noted in Fig. 13, exposure of the male and female occurs throughout gametogenesis. The exposure persists during mating, throughout pregnancy, and until weaning. Therefore, the evaluations conducted do assess the reproductive process from gonadal function through mating behavior, pregnancy loss, and incidence of teratogenesis, as well as difficulty in delivery, postnatal survival, growth, and development. Many functions and processes are involved during this exposure period, and numerous indices and evaluations can be routinely performed to assess the reproductive toxicity of any agent. The principle parameters are listed in Table 15.

With this particular protocol, when both the males and females are exposed premating, it is often difficult to examine all of these issues if, for example, the doses that are used for a particular compound produce a very high incidence of infertility. Segment I tests have been modified so that only the male or female may be exposed to examine where the reproductive toxicity may be occurring. Normally, 10 males and 20 females are used in this evaluation, and during the course of this experiment (Fig. 13) an additional 10 dams can be euthanatized during the fetal period, so that these assessments can be documented. In some instances, the assessments are performed on days 13 and 14 of gestation or near term at day 20 in the rat. The animals are euthanatized later in gestation, when one can determine whether gross, life-threatening malformations may be occurring that are not easily detected postnatally, because of cannabalism of deformed pups by the mother.

These evaluations provide the opportunity for determining a number of implantation sites in the uterine horn, which contains viable and dead embryos as well as metrial glands. The metrial glands reflect early resorptions following implantation. In addition, corpora luteal counts in the ovary can be compared with the number of implantation sites to determine whether there has been a high incidence of preimplantation loss. Corpora luteal counts are routinely performed in rats and are a bit more difficult to perform in mice. The preimplantation loss can be determined by subtracting the number of implantation sites in the uterus from the number of corpora lutea in the ovaries.

For postimplantation assessment, there are multiple endpoints to be evaluated. These include postimplantation loss, reflected as either embryonic or fetal death, and the incidence of malformations in the live fetuses. Since rodents do resorb their embryos and fetuses rather than abort them, this is an especially useful means for documenting embryonic and fetal lethality. Such postimplantation loss represents the number of implantation sites minus the number of live fetuses in the uterus. For fetal deaths, it is the number of dead fetuses that are not totally resorbed in the uterus divided by the number of implantation sites. The total postimplantation death rate is the total number of resorption sites and fetal deaths in the uterus divided by the number of implantation sites.

The evaluation of malformations utilizes the classical razor-blade slice technique following fixation and sectioning (Wilson and Warkany, 1965), skeletal staining techniques, and/or the immediate necrospy of the fetuses to assess both external and internal malformations. The data generated from these evaluations are then examined using two different experimental units. One unit is as an individual fetus and the other is as a litter effect. The reason for this dual evaluation is that under these experimental conditions, the individual fetuses are not exposed directly, but rather the mothers are the primary route of exposure. Therefore, there can be difficulties with a given dam producing a high incidence of embryonic losses and/or malformations while other dams do not demonstrate this generalized response. Therefore, examining the data both per fetus and per litter helps to distinguish whether there are maternal contributions that are unique for specific dams. This particular question has been thoroughly reviewed by Haseman and Hogan (1975).

Usually the 10 mothers not euthanatized are allowed to litter and the pups are evaluated immediately following delivery. The litters are culled to 8 pups by day 4 of life, as noted in Fig. 13. The culled pups are evaluated for malformations and the

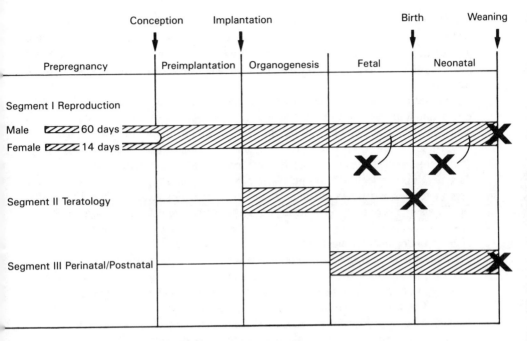

X = Euthanize dams and/or pups
▨ = Exposure to agent

Figure 13 Reproductive and teratology testing, single-generation studies. Segment I, reproduction, test species: rodent (e.g., rat). Exposure period: male, 60 days before mating; female, 14 days before mating, 21 days of gestation, 21 days of lactation. Number of animals: 10 males, 20 females. Exposure groups: at least two plus control. Segment II, teratology, at least two test species (one rodent, other nonrodent, e.g., rabbit, ferret). Exposure period: rat, 6–15 days of gestation; rabbit, 6–18 days of gestation. Number of animals: 20 pregnant rodents, 10 pregnant nonrodents. Exposure groups: at least three plus control. Segment III, perinatal/postnatal, test species: rodent (e.g., rat) or nonrodent. Exposure period: rat, 15 days of gestation through 21 days of lactation. Number of animals: 20 pregnant rodents. Exposure groups: at least two plus control.

remaining 8 pups remain with the mothers until day 21, when both the mothers and pups are euthanatized. During this postnatal period, the growth and development of the animals are assessed, as well as the dam's health status. Many of the functional aspects have already been discussed. Thus, at the end of 21 days, one will have an evaluation of fertility, gestational survival, and postnatal growth and development. Yet it is equally important to address the sensitivity of these assays as well as the results they are producing. Besides the question of species and/or strain, the question of dose is important.

Usually three exposure doses of the agent are selected in addition to the control group. The most difficult decision is selecting an appropriate high-dose exposure based on the subchronic testing of the compound in male and/or nonpregnant females. It is essential to separate maternal toxicity and its effects on development from a primary effect on the embryo. Therefore, one dose that produces some maternal toxicity should be included. One commonly used variable is the measurement of maternal weight and the documentation that the agent does reduce maternal weight greater than 10% of control values. The lowest dose should be selected because it produces the therapeutic effects without the toxic effects that would be expected in humans.

Following this testing, the investigator should be able to determine whether there is a major impact on fertility and assess the development of the conceptus and neonate. Obviously, any compound that directly affects fertility will reduce the ability of this segment I test to differentiate teratogenicity and neonatal toxicity. One difficulty with these segment I tests for reproductive toxicity is the selectivity and sensitivity to document toxic effects. Unfortunately, the power of the statistics based on the numbers of fetuses and litters available limit the investigator at best to the 5% level of significance. There must be a substantial response before one can be sure there is an effect. Therefore these tests need to be further investigated with a greater number of animals to document a much lower incidence of toxicity.

Segment II Testing—Teratology The segment II tests were devised specifically to screen agents for toxicity during the organogenesis period of development. Such tests are routinely performed in two species, a rodent and a nonrodent (usually the rabbit). The exposure periods in rats and mice are from day 6 through 15 and for rabbits day 6 through 18 of gestation. The day that pregnancy is documented either via the appearance of the vaginal plug or sperm in the female reproductive tract is designated day 0. It is essential to all investigations that this day of pregnancy is documented. Some investigators call it day 0.5 or day 1. This ambiguity in the literature can lead to confusion, especially when studies are conducted with single-day exposures. As noted earlier, since many organ systems proliferate rapidly during very specific periods, the single administration of an agent may result in an entirely different syndrome when administered 24 h apart.

Usually 20 pregnant female rats and 10 rabbits are used in these initial studies. These females are then euthanatized 1 day prior to delivery. All parameters (noted in Table 15) are evaluated. The interpretation of such data is dependent on a knowledge of the background incidence of defects and the species being studied. Besides the control group that is included during the course of the experiment, it is essential to know the background incidence of birth defects/structural defects for the strain. Once the data have been collected for all of these parameters (gross structural, internal and external viscera, and skeletal exams), a composite data pool can then be developed for each exposure group.

One of the points for major concern is the classification of major and minor malformations. Major defects such as phocomelia or cardiac defects (atrial–septal communication) are examples of serious alterations in development. A minor defect or variant may be a wavy rib. If a wavy rib is the only defect noted after an intensive evaluation, then certainly the risk assessment would not be as alarming as if the response was a cardiac malformation. There should be a dose–response relationship for the induction of these defects. The appearance of birth defects only at the lower dose in these studies with no increase in fetal lethality at high doses would raise a question about the relationship between the exposure of the agent and its ability to

produce birth defects. Additional information concerning the specific types of evaluations for documenting malformations and the analytical tests performed can be found
in reviews by Wilson and Warkany (1965), Palmer (1977), and Manson et al. (1982).

Segment III Testing—Perinatal/Postnatal Depending on the organ systems
evaluated and the species examined, organogenesis does not stop at 14, 15, or 18
days. It is a continuum of events from conception through postnatal life. Even though
the organ may be physically present, it may not have completed its differentiation, as
noted for the central nervous system (see previous section) or the reproductive tract,
as seen with the production of female hypospadias following exposure to agents
between 18 and 20 days in the rat. As noted in Fig. 13, segment III testing involves
exposure during both the fetal and neonatal periods, emphasizing an evaluation on
fetal development/delivery, lactation, and neonatal survival. Usually the animals are
studied until weaning. However, variations have been included in this phase of testing
to evaluate adult behavior as well as survival. The behavioral assessments often
include testing in early development as well as in the adult and have been discussed in
the previous section. Reproductive performance is another key evaluation in the
adult.

Interestingly though, decreased neonatal survival may be a good index that major
defects may be occurring due to prenatal exposure to an agent. Such defects, as
cardiac, can be readily documented in both segment I and II studies. Since most
cardiac defects are induced during organogenesis, the exposure and toxic response for
a segment III study may not reflect cardiac defects, but rather other developmental
deficits in maturation. Lung maturation and the potential induction of hyaline membrane disease or respiratory distress syndrome due to a delayed maturation of the type
II pneumocytes in the lung by an environmental exposure would certainly compromise postnatal survival. Cadmium has been shown in the rat to produce such an effect
(Daston et al., 1982). As noted earlier for ethylnitrosourea, among the major toxicities related to prenatal exposure is the production of tumors, whether adult or juvenile
onset.

Prenatal exposure to diethylstilbestrol is highly associated with the production of
carcinomas in the female genital tract of young women (Table 1), and such assessments of carcinogenicity during development have become important, especially
since a developing organism may be much more sensitive than is the adult. The use of
such perinatal testing for carcinogenesis evaluation was perhaps best exemplified in
the carcinogenicity testing for saccharin (Arnold et al., 1980). As previously discussed under fetal factors, multiple mechanisms for the induction of carcinogenesis
can occur. There currently is no way to determine whether the compound will result
in the rapid appearance of tumors such as Wilm's tumor or the delayed appearance of
tumors such as schwanomas. Therefore as recommended, all bioassays for carcinogens should be pursued for 2 years.

At the onset of segment I or segment II studies, the selection of progeny to be
studied for 2 years must be determined. Conventional carcinogenesis testing requires
50 test animals of each sex. As discussed in the segment I protocols, often the most
sensitive and valid experimental unit may be the litter. If that unit is to be used, then
single pups must be identified from 50 litters and followed for 2 years. If there are no

litter effects, then this evaluation may add increased statistical power. Further evaluations have used smaller number of litters and multiple pups from each litter. Actually, the least expensive component of the study is the reproductive and teratology section. However, the carcinogenesis component of this study provides for the intensive evaluation of these animals for other parameters besides carcinogenesis. Guidelines for such evaluations of carcinogenesis have been proposed and implemented (Food and Drug Administration, 1971; Health and Welfare Canada, 1975; Rice, 1979).

In vivo experimentation is the hallmark of reproductive and teratogenicity testing. The multigenerational and single-generation tests just described represent the current standards for screening compounds. By definition, screening means trying to identify compounds with the greatest likelihood of producing a problem. This in no way establishes the mechanisms by which such compounds may be producing the effects, as described in the mechanism section. In addition, the sensitivity of the selected organ systems and the overlapping toxicity may mask some especially important toxic responses if the compounds are administered at different times during pregnancy. Therefore, once agents have been identified as having potential toxicity, individualized in vivo studies as well as in vitro studies can then be designed to determine the exact nature of the toxicity and the potential mechanisms involved. In vivo studies resulting from single maternal injections at specific critical periods in the developmental process based on the organ development for that species, as well as the pharmacokinetics involved, may require the animals to be pretreated with other chemicals, such as inducers of xenobiotic metabolism or other known teratogens, to determine if there is potentiation. This particular area has not been widely addressed in screening but may be an important component of teratogenic response in the human. Other methods for exposing the conceptus include direct embryonic or fetal injections. These types of studies can help document direct toxicity in the conceptus or indicate maternal mediation (Levin and Miller, 1980). Pharmacokinetic parameters may also be species-specific, which limits the toxicity of selected compounds such as natural estrogens versus synthetic estrogens in the rat (Henry et al., 1984).

Once a chemical has been suspected to be a reproductive toxin, then in vitro studies are often undertaken to determine the mechanisms of action for toxic response. Due to the expensive nature of in vivo studies, it has been proposed that in vitro methods be developed as prescreens to determine the potential toxicity of compounds, especially for therapeutic agents to determine the relative potential of toxicity for these agents or for performing the in vivo screens. Such in vitro prescreens are currently under development and may, in the next 10 years, become critical tools in the area of reproductive teratogenicity testing. However, a combination of in vivo and in vitro testing will be essential for years to come.

In Vitro Experimentation   In vitro teratogenicity testing can involve many different culture techniques, utilizing either mammalian or nonmammalian tissues. Wilson (1978) described the essential characteristics of an ideal in vitro teratogenicity screen to include (1) use of biological subjects available in large numbers; (2) involvement of some aspects of progressive development; (3) relevance to known mechanisms of teratogenicity; and (4) easily performed yielding interpretable results. He indicated that it would also be desirable for the system to use an intact organism capable of absorbing, circulating, and excreting chemicals, giving a minimal number of false negatives, and reacting to varied types of agents. Applicability of a technique could then be determined by the period of development to be studied, the endpoints desired, and the inherent limitations of that system (Fig. 14, Table 16). Perhaps the greatest difficulty with all of these efforts, however, has been in firmly establishing these limitations.

The advantages of in vitro testing are manyfold. Control of dose and time of exposure and elimination of maternal factors can facilitate the collection, evaluation, and interpretation of teratogenicity data. Although the very nature of an in vitro protocol is its main disadvantage, by choosing the best test system for the parameter to be examined, in vitro test systems can be useful in the determination of teratogenesis and the elucidation of the mechanisms by which terata occur. Both mammalian and nonmammalian in vitro systems of evaluating teratogenicity will be reviewed in this section.

Mammalian Culture Systems   Preimplantation Embryo Culture: Preimplantation embryos can be explanted as early as the one- to two-cell stage and maintained in culture until the time of implantation. This period of embryonic development has been considered the "all or none" period, in that insult to the conceptus is either lethal or is repaired by the rapid proliferation of undifferentiated cells so that no malformations are manifested (Brent and Harris, 1976; Wilson and Fraser, 1977).

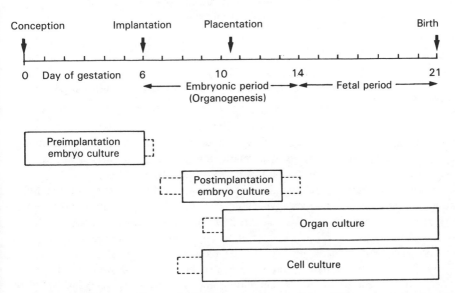

Figure 14 Applicability of mammalian culture techniques during different gestational periods for the study of teratogenicity (and normal development) in vitro. Such applicability is determined by the period of development to be studied, the endpoints desired, and the inherent limitations of each technique. Dashed lines outline periods when use of the indicated technique may be limited. The gestational period indicated is in the rat.

Table 16   Selected in Vitro Testing Systems for Assessing Teratogenic Risk Using Mammalian and Nonmammalian Tissues

Testing system	Endpoints evaluated[a]
Mammalian	
Embryo culture	
Preimplantation	Blastocyst development; trophoblast development and attachment to culture dish
Postimplantation	Heartbeat; circulation; energy metabolism; organ differentiation; protein and DNA content; crown–rump length
Organ culture	Growth; biochemical, cellular, and morphogenetic differentiation; cellular interactions
Cell culture	Cell differentiation; cell migration; cell–matrix interactions; intercellular relationships
Nonmammalian	
Drosophila melanogaster	Differentiation of embryonic cells; malformations in adults exposed as larvae
Hydra attenuata ("artificial embryo")	Regeneration of the adult form; adult toxic dose/developmentally toxic dose (A/D ratio)
Xenopus laevis	Growth, motility, pigmentation, and malformations in tadpoles exposed as embryos
Chick embryotoxicity screening test (CHEST)	Growth; malformations; organ differentiation

[a]The endpoints indicated for these techniques are those that have been cited in the literature. The potential applicability of other endpoints of evaluation to each technique should be considered.

Although no gross morphological deviations in development may occur, more subtle responses such as intrauterine growth retardation can result from the exposure of offspring to exogenous toxins during this period (Fabro et al., 1984).

Passage of exogenous compounds from maternal circulation into the uterine fluid and into the preimplantation blastocyst can occur and depends on compound lipophilicity, size, and ionic characteristics (Fabro, 1973). The preimplantation mouse blastocyst is capable of metabolically bioactivating xenobiotic compounds such as polycyclic aromatic hydrocarbons due to the development of mixed-function oxidase activity. This enzyme system's activity can also be induced above basal level by exposure of the blastocyst to certain environmental chemicals, such as 2,3,7,8-tetrachlorochlorodibenzo-p-dioxin. At this stage, however, the embryos have not yet developed detoxifying enzyme systems (Filler and Lew, 1981).

Analysis of human sera in the culture medium of mouse preimplantation blastocyst (obtained 5 days postcoitum) indicated that serum from women with poor obstetrical histories prevented trophoblast-cell outgrowth and attachment to the culture dish; inner-cell-mass growth was not affected. Serum from women with normal obstetrical histories and from men caused no adverse effects in this system (Chavez and McIntyre, 1984). The potential role of this embryo system in the determination of abortifacient and teratogenic risk due to endogenous or exogenous serum factors gives it an important place in in vitro fertilization studies.

Postimplantation Embryo Culture: Postimplantation embryos are explanted for culture during the organogenic period. Parameters of the viability and growth of the conceptus include heartbeat, circulation, energy metabolism, organ differentiation, and protein/DNA content (New, 1978a). Embryos explanted before the formation of the chorioallantoic placenta resemble their in vivo counterparts in both the rate of differentiation and protein synthesis for at least 48 h in culture; those explanted after placentation differentiate to a similar extent as their in vivo littermates, but their overall growth occurs more slowly (New, 1978b).

The major limitation in culturing the postimplantation embryo is believed to be due to the inability to maintain adequate delivery of oxygen and other nutrients to the conceptus due to its increasing size and metabolic demands; in vivo, the chorioallantoic placenta begins to assume this function during midorganogenesis (New, 1978b). Continuous oxygenation of the culture environs, rather than gassing at set intervals, may extend the viability of the conceptus (as determined by the criteria of heartbeat and circulation). Under these conditions, organ differentiation is comparable to that in vivo, although a corresponding level of overall growth, as determined by protein and DNA content, cannot be achieved (Tarlatzis et al., 1984).

Although the postimplantation embryo may possess its own bioactivating enzyme systems, effects of a chemical exposure may be due to maternal bioactivation. This maternal factor can be evaluated in vitro by addition of the metabolites, if they are known, or of a metabolizing enzyme system to the culture medium. In the case of the mixed-function oxidase system, addition of the S9 fraction of liver homogenate (which contains microsomal enzymes capable of metabolizing exogenous and endogenous compounds), along with the necessary cofactors, to the medium can mimic in vivo metabolism.

Cyclophosphamide (CP) is a compound that requires cytochrome P-450-dependent metabolism to elicit its teratogenic effects. In experiments leading toward that end, Fantel et al. (1979) found that the addition of CP to the medium had no effect on the growth and differentiation of day 10 rat embryos (sperm positive is day 0) following a 24-h incubation period (Fig. 15). When the S9 fraction of liver homogenate and cofactors were also added, a CP concentration-dependent decrease in somite number, crown–rump length, and protein concentration and an increase in malformation incidence were seen. Kitchin et al. (1981) examined the role of cytochrome P-450 metabolism in the teratogenicity of CP. No adverse effects were seen on the growth and development of day 10 rat embryos (sperm positive is day 0) coincubated with CP and cumene hydroperoxide-pretreated (and so cytochrome P-450 depleted) microsomes; coincubation of embryos with CP and control microsomes, however, resulted in a decrease in embryonic and yolk sac growth as well as a significant incidence of malformation.

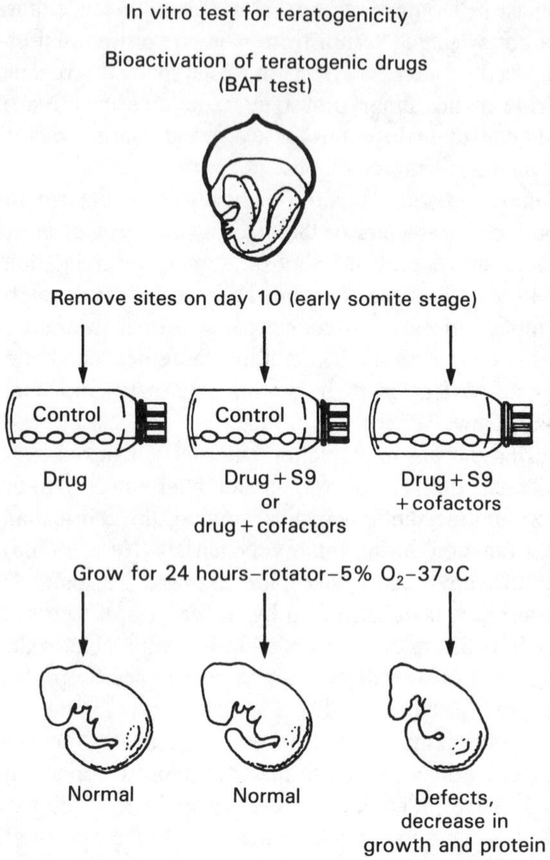

In vitro test for teratogenicity

Bioactivation of teratogenic drugs
(BAT test)

Remove sites on day 10 (early somite stage)

| Drug | Drug + S9 or drug + cofactors | Drug + S9 + cofactors |

Grow for 24 hours–rotator–5% O_2–37°C

| Normal | Normal | Defects, decrease in growth and protein |

Figure 15 An experimental protocol for testing the role of bioactivation in chemical terato-genicity in the rat embryo in vitro. Embryos are explanted at the early somite stage (day 10 of gestation; sperm positive is day 0). Three control experiments are performed by incubating the embryos for 24 h with the following additions to the medium: drug alone, drug plus S9 hepatic microsomal supernatant, or drug plus S9 cofactors (NADPH and glucose 6-phosphate). To test for metabolism-mediated teratogenicity, embryos are cultured in medium containing drug plus S9 plus cofactors. *(From Shepard et al., 1983.)*

Teratogenicity of serum can also be evaluated in this system by including blood products in the culture medium. Klein et al. (1980) analyzed the effects of serum from cyclophosphamide-treated rats on rat embryos to establish a time course for the presence of a teratogenic entity. Serum harvested soon after treatment was more teratogenic than that harvested at a later time point. The addition of high levels of cyclophosphamide directly to the culture medium, however, did not cause malforma-tions. These data not only support the role of metabolism in this compound's terato-genicity but indicate the potential of this culture system in monitoring the teratogenic activity of serum. Serum from monkeys with histories of fetal wastage failed to allow normal growth and development of rat embryos in culture, while that from monkeys with normal reproductive histories did not show this effect (Klein et al., 1982; Carey et al., 1983); similar results were obtained from culturing rat embryos in serum from women with poor reproductive histories (Carey et al., 1983; Muechler et al., 1984). These findings suggest the presence of endogenous abortifacient/teratogenic factors. Studies on human sera showed that serum from females undergoing cancer chemotherapy or anticonulsant treatment did not support the growth of rat embryos as did serum obtained from control subjects (Chatot et al., 1980). This culture method may provide a screen for human exposure to potentially teratogenic agents and for the presence of endogenous abortifacient factors.

Organ Culture: The response of a specific developing organ to insult can be evaluated by isolating that organ in culture. Organ culture allows for the tissue to be studied more directly while maintaining its structural and intercellular relationships. A multitude of tissue types have been evaluated in this system, including limb buds (Kochhar, 1982), palatal shelves (Tyler and Pratt, 1980), kidney (Preminger et al., 1980), genital tract (Newbold et al., 1981), heart (Ingwall et al., 1980), inner ear (Davis and Hawrisiak, 1981), and lung (Gross et al., 1978; Miner, 1979). The organ is usually explanted during mid to late organogenesis and maintained in culture into the fetal period; in mouse limb bud culture, a greater extent of differentiation can be achieved by culturing an older explant (Neubert, 1982).

Overall growth, biochemical, cellular, and morphogenetic differentiation, and specific cell interactions can be monitored in this culture system. These parameters may be evaluated in terms of developmental landmarks specific for that organ or in terms of specific processes that occur in embryonic development with which a teratogen may interfere. The role of metabolism in chemical teratogenicity can be examined by including a metabolizing enzyme system in the culture medium. For example, in the evaluation of cyclophosphamide teratogenicity, neither cyclophosphamide nor the metabolizing enzyme system had deleterious effects on mouse limb bud development; coincubation of both cyclophosphamide and the enzyme system with that tissue, however, resulted in abnormal development of limb cartilage, implicating maternal bioactivation in the teratogenicity of that drug (Manson and Smith, 1977, 1979).

Cell Culture: Cell cultures can be utilized to monitor growth and differentiation at a cellular level. In the micromass culture technique, dispersed cells from an embryonic organ, grown at high density, maintain the capacity to differentiate. Effects on cell differentiation, cell migration, cell–matrix interactions, and intercellular relationships can be examined following either in vivo or in vitro exposure to an agent to identify potential teratogens that may act through these mechanisms. Metabolizing enzyme systems can be included in the medium to evaluate the role of biotransformation in xenobiotic teratogenicity. Rat embryonic neuroepithelium and limb bud cells (Flint, 1983; Flint and Orton, 1984) and chick cranial neural crest cells and limb bud mesenchyme cells (Wilk et al., 1980) are among the cell types that have been studied in this system.

Rotation-mediated aggregate cell culture is another means of evaluating teratogenicity at the cellular level. In contrast to the monolayer culture, the aggregates formed are spherical (spheroids) with histotypic organization and thus allow for a three-dimensional analysis of the cellular response. Differentiation of rodent fetal brain cells cultured under such conditions is biochemically and morphologically similar to that in vivo, resulting in the formation of a spheroid of neuronal and glial cells capable of synthesizing neurotransmitters characteristic of the area from which the tissue was derived. In addition, cell migration and proliferation and intercellular relationships, including recognition, can be monitored (Trapp and Richelson, 1980).

Cultured cell lines, such as the ascitic mouse ovarian tumor cell (Braun et al., 1982; Braun and Weinreb, 1984) and the mouse neuroblastoma cell (Mummery et al., 1984), have also been used as teratogenicity screening tests. In the former, potential teratogens are identified by their ability to inhibit the attachment of the tumor cells to concanavalin-A-coated culture dishes. Attachment of the cell to the lectin is similar to the receptor–ligand interaction of embryonic cells to one another and to their matrices. Interference with this process in vitro suggests potential teratogenic activity by the same mechanism in vivo. Bioactivation can be simulated by the addition of hepatic microsomes (and cofactors) to the medium. Teratogenic screening by the neuroblastoma assay evaluates the ability of a compound to interfere in cell growth and differentiation. Because this transformed cell line retains its ability to differentiate, compounds added to the culture system, with or without a microsomal fraction, can be evaluated for inhibition or inappropriate induction of cell differentiation.

Nonmammlian Culture Systems In vitro teratogenicity testing is not limited to mammalian tissues. Nonmammalian tissues, from species at several different levels of the evolutionary scale, can be utilized in this capacity. Their applicability in screening for teratogenic risk lies in the similarities between the developmental processes of mammalian and nonmammalian organisms. Teratogenesis may result from the manifestations of such processes as inhibition of cellular proliferation, destruction of specific cell populations (or inhibition of such preprogrammed activity), and interference in cell–cell interaction (Wilson, 1977). An agent that interferes with any of these processes in developing nonmammalian tissue may have teratogenic potential in the mammalian conceptus by affecting that same process; cellular mechanisms of teratogenicity can be similar among the various species despite differences in their maternal–fetal environments. Like other in vitro testing systems, such nonmammalian tests are generally less expensive and more rapid to perform than in vivo mammalian tests.

Drosophila melanogaster has been evaluated for use in teratogenicity testing. Embryonic cell cultures prepared from homogenized eggs of that species can be exposed to the agent in question via incubation medium. This technique detects teratogens by their ability to interfere with muscle or neuron differentiation in culture. The effects of the addition of a metabolizing enzyme system or of human or animal serum have also been evaluated in this culture (Bournais-Vardiabasis et al., 1983). Intact eggs can also be utilized by exposing them to the testing agent throughout the metamorphosis period (egg to pupa). When the larva become adults, they are examined for external morphological alterations, including bristle, eye, leg, wing, thorax, and abdomen abnormalities (Shuler et al., 1982).

Hydra attenuata, a freshwater coelenterate, has been used as an "artificial embyro" in teratogenicity testing. It is the lowest species with complex cells and organs but the highest that can totally regenerate an adult form from a randomly reassociated pellet of dissociated adult cells. To regenerate the adult, the cells undergo processes similar to those that occur in embryonic development (e.g., changes in size and shape, programmed cell death, and formation of specialized junctions and organ fields). The teratogenic hazard is determined by the ratio of the adult toxic dose A to the developmentally toxic dose D. A high A/D ratio indicates high teratogenic risk; a low A/D indicates low teratogenic risk, as developmental toxicity would be manifested only at a dose greater than the adult toxic dose (Johnson and Gabel, 1983; E. M. Johnson, 1984). Table 17 indicates the developmental toxicity index for several chemicals, as tested in mammalian and hydra systems.

Embryos of the amphibian *Xenopus laevis* can be used to screen agents for teratogenicity following exposure in their incubation medium. Growth, motility, pigmentation, and malformation incidence can be monitored at the embryo stage or later in development when the embryo has become a free-swimming tadpole (Schultz et al., 1982; Nakatsuji, 1983). The use of this animal as a model for fetal alcohol syndrome has been suggested by Nakatsuji (1983), as tadpoles exposed to ethanol as embryos showed craniofacial malformations similar to those described for this syndrome in mammals. The *X. laevis* embryos have also been used in the evaluation of the role of cell–cell communication in embryonic development. Warner et al. (1984)

Table 17 Developmental Toxicity Index A/D Ratio) of Compounds in Mammalian Bioassays and Hydra Assays[a]

	Developmental toxicity index	
Chemical	Mammals	Hydra
Aspirin	1.7	1.3
Benzene	0.6	0.4
Caffeine	< 2.0	1.5
Colchicine	8	10
Diethyl phthalate	2.5	2.5
Ethyl alcohol	2	1.5
Formaldehyde	1.0	1.0
Isoniazid	46	20
Methotrexate-D: biologically inactive	?[b]	?[b]
Methotrexate-L: folate antagonist	4	7
Retinal acetate	2	2
Vitamin A acid	2	2

[a]The A/D ratio determines teratogenic risk relative to the adult toxic dose. Dividing the dose that causes overt toxicity in the adult of a species by the dose that is toxic to its developing embryo yields the A/D ratio. A large A/D ratio indicates that the compound interrupts development at a dose below that causing adult toxicity and so may present significant teratogenic risk (in the mammal, however, adult toxicity may present a hazard). (Adapted from Johnson and Gabel, 1983.)

[b]No mammalian data are available for this optical isomer which had no effect on either the hydra adult or "embryo" even at its limit of solubility.

blocked gap-junction communication by injecting antibody to that structure into a specific cell in the eight-cell stage embryo. This exposure resulted in tadpoles with a characteristic set of malformations, which were often associated with the side of the embryo that had been injected.

In the chick embryotoxicity screening test (CHEST), chick embryos are exposed in ovo to the proposed teratogen. The embryotoxic dose range is determined by measuring trunk length as an indicator of the intactness of the caudal morphogenetic system (Jelinek, 1977). This system has also been proposed for use in determining dose–effect relationships, including identification of sensitive developmental periods and malformations and their potential mechanisms (Jelinek and Kistler, 1981).

Perinatal Toxicology in the Human

The question of reproductive loss and birth defects in the human has been a difficult issue to resolve when evaluated in relationship to environmental exposures and drug therapy. Since the 1950s a number of registries for health surveillance have specifically evaluated birth defects and stillbirths. Since that time, most states and nations have implemented some form of surveillance related to birth defects. Many of these registries have taken data from the birth certificates as minimum information, while some have actually performed rather in-depth monitoring. Examples of such programs are the British Columbia Registry (Miller and Lowry, 1977), the Perinatal Collaborative Study (Heinonen et al., 1977), Finnish Registry (Saxen, 1984), Swedish Registry (Kallen and Winberg, 1968), the Centers for Disease Control in Atlanta, Georgia (Ordero and Oakley, 1983), and state government programs (New York, Georgia, Washington, California, and Florida) using vital statistics (Polednak and Janerich, 1983). An international perspective began in 1974 through the International Clearing House for Birth Defects monitoring systems (ICBDNCS). This program currently includes 24 countries collaborating to evaluate 11 types of malformations that are selected for regular exchange; data from other types of malformations are also collected.

New services for the dissemination of teratology information directly to patients and care providers are rapidly developing on an independent basis nationally. These services range from a single consultant to a complex organization of physicians, counselors, and volunteers. It is hoped that besides supplying counsel, these teratology information services will collect valuable patient outcome information. The Reproductive Toxicology Center in Washington, D.C. (Fabro, 1983), has been supplying such council and collecting data for the past few years. The more recently developed programs are primarily telephone-based services, as in San Diego, Philadelphia, and Boston, interacting with both the public and the care providers (Chernoff et al., 1986).

Many other individuals registries have been developed on a private basis, such as the Kaieser Permente Clinic Studies (Milkovich and Van den Berg, 1974), as well as individual registries for specific compounds, such as lithium, diethylstilbestrol, and isotretinoin. It is critical to note that quite often the question of birth defects is raised because of unique syndromes or their associations and clustering of defects that are related by case reports to particular environmental exposures or drug therapies. Unfortunately, these are often the least reliable data for basing patient care because they represent usually single case reports; however, perhaps it is the best means to raise questions in the medical literature concerning the safety of any agent. Case reports and registry follow-up are invaluable because the pregnant women is truly a pharmacologic orphan when a drug is initially marketed.

Unfortunately for postmarketing drug surveillance, the least reliable documentation related to drug administration is during pregnancy. This is true whether examining the resultant benefits of such therapy or risks to both mother and progeny. These difficulties are directly related to four areas:

1 Usually a low rate of drug utilization by pregnant women because they are in general a young, healthy population.
2 The definition of teratogenesis/birth defect, its incidence in human population, and means to assess these variables in utero, at birth and as the child matures.
3 The effects of intercurrent disease, environmental factors, other therapy, and social factors (recreational drug use).
4 The resources and reporting systems available for evaluating prenatal effects of chemicals (Miller, 1985).

Table 18 provides a selection of environmental and drug exposures that indicates the limitations of our knowledge as well as the difficulty in establishing the question of risk during different stages of pregnancy. As noted in Fig. 7, the developmental sequences for human and other species are not identical. Throughout gestation and into the neonatal period, many organ systems are maturing and substantial cell–cell interactions are occurring, especially in organ systems like the central nervous system, immune system, endocrine system, reproductive system, and urogenital system. Therefore, in the human our concern for chemical and environmental exposure is no longer just for the first trimester but rather for all trimesters. In addition, some studies are finding a better association between chemical exposure and physical abnormalities when prepregnancy usage of an agent is used as the index (Hanson et al., 1978).

Again, our considerations are for reproductive outcome in terms of both pregnancy loss and induction of abnormalities in the offspring, whether they be functional or physical deformities. Therefore, our definition, as noted earlier, for teratogenesis is constantly changing based on more sophisticated methods, and documented alterations at birth or within the first few years of life are not sufficient (Table 19). This has become especially important when one considers questions like the latency of vaginal adenocarcinoma associated with exposure to diethylstilbestrol in utero in both animal model and human.

As noted above, there is great difficulty, both from the epidemiological point of view and from the bench-top laboratory point of view, in gathering sufficient data regarding human exposures and effects to ensure a documented mechanistic evaluation.

Table 18 Exposure to Drugs and Environmental Agents[a,b]

Category/agent	First trimester	Second and third trimesters	Labor–delivery
Allergy			
Antihistamines			
Chlorpheniramine (Chlor-Trimeton)	U	U	U
Pheniramine (Triaminic)	U	U	U
Diphenhydramine (Benadryl)	U	U	U
Tripelennamine (PB7)	U	U	U
Methapyrilene (Histadyl)	U	U	U
Brompheniramine (Dimetane)	Q malformations	U	U
Medizine (Antivert)	U/A	U	U
Cydizine (Marezine)	U/A	U	U
Doxylamine (Benedectin)	U	U	U
Sympathomimetic drugs			
Phenylephrine (Dimetane)	U	U	U
Phenylpropanolamine (Ornade)	U	U	U
Ephedrine (Tedral)	U	U	U
Pseudoephedrine (Actifed)	U	U	U
Epinephrine (Adrenalin)	S malformations	U	U
Corticosteroids			
Hydrocortisone	U/A	U	U/lung maturity
Prednisone (Meticorten)	U/A	Q IUGR	U/lung maturity
Dexamethasone (Decadron)	U	U	U
Bedomethansone (Vanceril)	U	U	U
Betamethasone (Celestone)	U	U	U/lung maturity
Cromolyn (Intal)	U	U	U

Drug			
Analgesics			
Narcotics			
Codeine	U		
Meperidine (Demerol)	U/A		K neonatal respiratory depression; K decreases fetal heart rate
Morphine	U/A	K chronic neonatal withdrawal; K IUGR	K neonatal respiratory depression
Heroin	U/A	K increased neonatal mortality; K premature labor	K fetal heart rate
Nonnarcotic analgesics			
Aspirin	U/A	U	K closure of ductus; K fetal bleeding; K increases gestation
Indomethacin (Indocin)	U	U	K closure of ductus; K fetal bleeding; K increases gestation
Acetaminophen (Tylenol)	U	U	U
Propoxyphene (Darvon)	U/A	U	U
Anesthetics			
General anesthetics (chronic)	Q malformation; Q abortion	Q abortion	U
Local anesthetics			
Mepivacaine (Carbocaine)	U	U	S fetal bradycardia
Bupivacaine	U	U	U
Chloroprocaine	U	U	S fetal bradycardia
Lidocaine	U	U	K fetal acidosis, depression, fetal bradycardia

(See footnotes on p. 282.)

Table 18 Exposure to Drugs and Environmental Agents[a,b] (Continued)

Category/agent	First trimester	Second and third trimesters	Labor–delivery
Antibiotics			
Penicillin (Penicillin G)	U maternal allergic responses	U	U
Ampicillin (Polycillin)	U maternal allergic responses	U	U
Chloramphenicol (Chloro-mycetin)	U	K neonatal gray baby	K neonatal gray baby
Streptomycin	K 8th nerve damage, micromedia, multiple	K 8th nerve damage	U
Gentamicin (Garamycin)	S 8th nerve	S 8th nerve	U
Kanamycin (Kantrex)	S 8th nerve	S 8th nerve	U
Nitrofurantoin (Furadantin)	U	K hyperbilirubinemia	K hyperbilirubinemia
		K hemolytic anemia	K hemolytic anemia
Sulfonamides (Gantrisin)	U	K hyperbilirubinemia	K hyperbilirubinemia
Tetracycline (Achromycin)	K inhibition of bone growth	K stain deciduous teeth	K stain deciduous teeth
	S micromedia	K inhibition of bone growth	
	S syndactyl	S ethanol hypoplasia	
Sulfamethoxazole (Bactrim, Septra)	Q/A malformation	U	U
Trimethoprim (Bactrim, Septra)	Q/A malformation	U	U
Metranidazole (Flagyl)	U/A—tumors	U	U
Anticoagulants			
Heparin (Panheprin)	U	U	U
Warfarin (Panwarfarin)	D/K syndrome, stippled cartilage, midline facial depression, blindness	K IUGR, mental retardation	K neonatal hemorrhage
Bishydroxycoumarin	K syndrome (see Warfarin)	K IUGR, mental retardation hemorrhage	K neonatal hemorrhage

276

Anticonvulsants

Drug			
Phenytoin (Dilantin)	D cardiac K syndrome, midline hypoplasia, ptosis, wide mouth, inner epicanthal folds, short neck, mild webbing, hypoplasia nails, short phalanges	S IUGR S mental retardation	S neonatal hemorrhage
Trimethadione (Tridione)	D cardiac K syndrome, abnormal facies, V-shaped eyebrows, cardiac, cleft palate	S mental retardation	U
Paramethadione (Paradione)	D cardiac K syndrome, abnormal facies, V-shaped eyebrows, cardiac, cleft palate	S mental retardation	
Phenobarbital (Valpin 50-PB)	D cardiac	U/A increases metabolism of drug	K withdrawal
Diazepam (Valium)	S malformations D cardiac S cleft lip palate K neural tube defects	Q withdrawal	K neonatal hypotonia, apnea
Valproate			
Antidiabetic drugs			
Insulin	D skeletal malformations	U	U
Chlorpropamide (Diabinase)	U/A—CNS	K neonatal hypoglycemia	K neonatal hypoglycemia
Tolbutamide (Orinase)	U/A—CNS	K neonatal hypoglycemia	K neonatal hypoglycemia
Antihypertensive drugs			
Methyldopa (Aldomet)	U	D stillbirths	D stillbirths, neonatal death
Hydralazine (Apresoline)	U/A—skeletal	U	U
Clofibrate (Attomid-S)	U	U	U
Diazoxide (Hyperstat)	U/A	Q hyperbilirubinemia, thrombocytopenia, hypoglycemia (IUGR)	Q hyperbilirubinemia, thrombocytopenia, hypoglycemia (IUGR)

(See footnotes on p. 282.)

Table 18 Exposure to Drugs and Environmental Agents[a,b] (Continued)

Category/agent	First trimester	Second and third trimesters	Labor–delivery
Antimalarial drugs			
Quinine (Quinamin)	S malformations, abortion, 8th nerve damage	S deafness, thrombocytopenia	U thrombocytopenia
Primaquine (Aralen)	U	U	U
Pentaquine	U	U	U
Chloroquine (Aralen)	S 8th nerve damage	S 8th nerve damage	U
Antithyroid drugs			
[125]Iodide	K goiter, thyroid ablation >10 weeks	K goiter, thyroid ablation	U
Propylthiouracil (PTU)	Q mental status, K goiter	Q mental status, K goiter	U
Methimazole (Tapazole)	K goiter	K goiter	U
Antitubercular drugs (usually combinations)			
Ethambutol (Myambutol)	U	U	U
Rifampin	U/A–CNS	U	U
Streptomycin	See antibiotics		
Dihydrostreptomycin	See antibiotics		
Isoniazid (INH)	Q CNS	U	U
Ethionamide (Trecator-SC)	U/A	U	U
Aminosalicylic acid	U	U	U
Drugs acting on the central nervous system			
Lysergic acid (LSD)	Q CNS, limb	U	U
Marijuana (THC)	U	U	U
Phenthiazines (Thorazine)	Q general malformations	U	U
Lithium (Lithnate)	S cardiac malformations	U	U
Thalidomide	K malformations, phocomelia	U	U
Haloperidol (Haldol)	Q malformations	U	U
Reserpine	U/A	U/A	K neonatal nasal congestion
			K neonatal depression

	U/A malformations		
Propranolol (Inderal)		K IUGR K decreases fetal cardiac output K neonatal hypoglycemia	K neonatal galactocemia K decreases cardiac output, K fetal hypoglycemia
Beta agonists			
Ritodrine	U	K inhibits uterine contractions	K inhibition labor
Terbutaline	U	K fetal tachycardia	K fetal tachycardia
Solbutamol	U		
Isoproterenol	U	U	U
Anticholinergics	Q	K fetal bradycardia	K fetal bradycardia
Ataractic drugs			
Meprobanate (Miltown)	Q general malformations	U	U
Chlordiazepoxide (Librium)	Q general malformations	U	U
Diazepam (Valium)	S cleft palate	Q neonatal withdrawal	K neonatal respiratory depression K apnea, hypotonia
Antidepressant drugs			
Imipramine (Tofranil)	Q general malformations	U	U
Amitriptyline (Elavil)	U	U	U
Cytotoxic drugs			
Busulfan (Myleran)	S multiple anomalies		
Cyclophosphamide (Cytoxan)	}	}	
Mercaptopurine (Purinethol)	S IUGR	S IUGR	
Idoxuridine (Stoxil)	S abortion	S abortion	
Fluorouracil (Adrucil)			
Folic acid antagonists			
Aminopterin	K multiple anomalies K craniofacial K/A abortion K IUGR	K IUGR K mental retardation K abortion	K IUGR K mental retardation

(See footnotes on p. 282.)

279

Table 18 Exposure to Drugs and Environmental Agents[a,b] *(Continued)*

Category/agent	First trimester	Second and third trimesters	Labor–delivery
Pyrimethamine	U/A/D—high risk	U	U
Methotrexate	K multiple anomalies	K IUGR	U
	K craniofacial		
	K IUGR		
Diuretics			
Acetazolamide (Diamox)	U/A malformations	U	U
Thiazides (Diuril,	S maternal K+ and water	S fetal neonatal jaundice	S fetal neonatal jaundice
Hydrodiuril)	imbalance	S fetal thrombocytopenia	S thrombocytopenia
	U	S ion imbalances	S ion imbalances
Immunosuppressants			
Corticosteroids	See corticosteroids		
Azathioprine (Imitran)	Q adrenal hypoplasia	Q hypoplasia	U
Steroids			
Clomiphene (Clomid)	Q/D neural tube, assorted	U	U
	anomalies, Down's syndrome		
Diethylstilbestrol (DES)	K vaginal tumors	K/A vaginal tumors	U
	K/A uterine and cervical	K/A uterine malformations	
	malformations		
	K/A adenosis	K/A adenosis	
	K/A male genital malformations	K/A male genital malformations	
		Q behavior	
Orally administered	Q VACTERL syndrome	U	U
contraceptives			
Synthetic progestins	S limb reduction	Q behavior	U
	K masculinization of female fetus		
Androgens	K masculinization of female fetus	U	U

Agent			
Miscellaneous			
X Irradiation			
Diagnostic	Q leukemia	Q leukemia	Q leukemia
High dose	K malformations	K IUGR, K CNS, K gonadal, Q leukemia	
Microwaves (thermal)	U/A skeletal malformations	U/A abortion	U
Ultrasound (diagnostic)	U	U	U
Radioisotopes			
^{125}I	See antithyroid drugs		
^{99m}Te			
Isotretinoin	K spontaneous abortions, malformed ears, cardiac defects, CNS malformations	U	U
Ethanol (chronic, binge)	K/A syndrome, midline hypoplasia, microcephaly, low-set ears, cardiac, female genital	K IUGR, mental retardation neonatal withdrawal, decreases fetal breathing	U
	U	U	K neonatal depression
Gasoline	Q malformations	U	U
Hyperthermia	Q/A malformations, abortions	U/A IUGR, abortion	U
2,4,5-T (agent orange)	Q malformations	U	U
	A unknown		
Vinyl chloride	U	U	U
Tobacco smoking	K IUGR	K IUGR	K increases perinatal mortality
		K increases perinatal mortality	K decreases fetal breathing
		K decreases fetal breathing	
Disulfram (Antabuse) with ethanol	U alone	U alone	U alone
		S severe reaction with ETOH	Severe cardiovascular reaction with ETOH

(See footnotes on p. 282.)

Table 18 Exposure to Drugs and Environmental Agents[a,b] *(Continued)*

Category/agent	First trimester	Second and third trimesters	Labor–delivery
Methylmercury	K mental retardation	K mental retardation	U
Polychlorinated biphenyl	K skin discoloration	K skin discoloration	U
TCDD (Dioxin)	Q/A malformations	U	U
Mebendazole (Vermox)	U/A high risk	U	U
Caffeine	Q increases reproductive loss	Q increases reproductive loss	K fetal tachycardia
	A malformations		

[a]Modified from Miller (1981); with Council on Environmental Quality (1981), Brendel et al. (1985), and Council on Scientific Affairs (1985).
[b]This partial list of drugs used during pregnancy is divided into therapeutic classes. If there are no currently known effects on the conceptus or a lack of reported studies, these drugs are listed as unknown (U). Since long-term follow-ups of progeny have not been completed, caution should be considered with all therapy. In some instances the drug has been associated with an increase in abnormalities in the conceptus and is therefore also listed as disease-related (D). If no human data are available and animal data indicate abnormalities, A is used. A representative trade name is associated with each generic drug. Symbols: K, known effects; S, suspected effects; Q, questionable effects/sporadic case report(s); U, unknown effects or no reported adverse effects; D, maternal disease-related effects; A, animal-documented effects.

Table 19 Criteria for Recognizing a New Teratogen/Perinatal Toxin in Humans[a]

1. An abrupt increase in the incidence of a particular defect or association of defects (syndrome), which may be structural, biochemical, or functional in nature.
2. Coincidence of this increase with a known environmental change, such as widespread use of a new drug.
3. Proven exposure to this environmental change during a particular stage of gestation yielding the characteristically defective syndrome.
4. Absence of other factors common to all pregnancies yielding infants with the characteristic defects, such as other drug use, intercurrent disease, or genetics.

[a]Modified from Wilson (1972).

With human observations, the low numbers of patients exposed to an agent have presented the greatest difficulty for establishing a true incidence of effect. This is especially true when a potential incidence for a defect can be much less than 1% of the exposed population. One of the major problems is evaluating the utilization of drugs in the pregnant women. In general, young women are in good health and do not require routine medications, as disease processes do not normally appear until later in life. At least in the United States there are currently no drugs other than vitamins recommended for use during early pregnancy. However, this lack of organic disease does not mean that the social environment does not extract its own use of chemical modifiers, from aspirin to benzodiazepines, from caffeine to cocaine, from nicotine to marijuana. Actually, drug use during pregnancy has substantially changed during the past 15 years. A study of 245 pregnant patients followed from conception onward revealed that recreational drugs have become the predominant chemicals used during the first trimester, even though 98% of the patients eventually did use vitamins (Rayburn, 1982). Such vitamin usage often represents the influence of prenatal care. All of the drugs used in these patients and the percentage of mothers taking these compounds are listed in Tables 20 and 21. It is interesting to note that a number of these agents can affect the central nervous system (e.g., benzodiazepines, marijuana, anticonvulsants, anesthestics, and narcotics).

For the epidemiologist, a group of 245 patients is certainly too small to even estimate a potential risk of exposure to these agents. In many instances, one needs tens of thousands of patients to begin to approach any teratologic evaluation. Therefore in our risk assessment using rodent model systems (described in the animal teratology section), the number of fetuses involved ranged from 200 to 400; the sensitivity of this system is certainly 1% or better in attempting to detect any incidence of malformations. This evaluation is based on an individual fetal analysis, and certainly the incidence for the detection limit is much higher for litter analysis. Let us take into account the question of sufficient numbers to document human exposure and the risk of birth defects.

Usually no single hospital, region, or even state can supply sufficient numbers of patients to identify and establish the relationship between a chemical exposure and a birth defect if the incidence of the defect is much less than 1%. Therefore in most instances one is attempting to establish a much higher incidence than 1 per 100. During the past 14 years at least seven fetal drug syndromes have been proposed, based on exposures to aminopterin (Warkany, 1978), alcohol (Lemoine et al., 1967; K. L. Jones et al., 1973; Sclarren and Smith, 1978), phenytoin (Hanson, 1976), trimethadione (Goldman and Yaffee, 1978), warfarin (Wakany, 1976), diethylstilbestrol (Herbst and Bern, 1981), and isotretinoin (Stern et al., 1984). What is critical to note is whether all of these compounds can meet the original definitions established by Wilson and Warkany in 1965 for defining the criteria for teratogenic agents developed (Table 19). In fact, only two drugs to date fulfill even one of the major criteria— that is, the introduction of a new drug or chemical into the marketplace and the occurrence of a syndrome of birth defects. Those two drugs are thalidomide, identified in the 1950s, and isotretinoin, identified in the 1980s. The other drugs and chemicals have been in use for many years and require substantial continued evaluation.

Table 20   Frequency of Drug Use in 245 Pregnant Patients at Conception during the Antepartum Period from Two Hospitals in Michigan[a]

Drug	Mothers taking drugs (%)
Iron or vitamins	98
Analgesics, mild	75
Cold and cough preparations[b]	41
Antacids	33
Antibiotics	15
Antiemetics	12
Marijuana	13
Oral contraceptives	10
Anesthetics, local	7
Antifungal vaginal preparations	4
Aminophylline	5
Diuretics	5
Benzodiazepines	4
Thyroid supplements	2
Anticonvulsants	2
Anesthetics, general	2
Cocaine, heroin, methadone, quaaludes (methaqualone)	2
Fertility drugs	1
Anticoagulants	1
Cardiovascular, antihypertensive	1
Tocolytic drugs	1
Glucocorticoids	1

[a]From Rayburn et al. (1982).
[b]Includes decongestants and antihistamines.

Table 21 Number of Drugs Taken per Patient and Drugs Used Most Commonly before and during Pregnancy in a Maternity Population from Two Hospitals in Michigan, January and February 1982[a]

Time of gestation	Drugs taken per patient: mean (range)[b]	Drugs taken most commonly
Prepregnancy	0.4 (0–2)	Oral contraceptives Marijuana Diet pills
Conception	0.5 (0–4)	Oral contraceptives Marijuana Diet pills
First trimester	1.9 (0–5)	Vitamins or iron Antibiotics
Second and third trimester	2.2 (0–5)	Vitamins or iron Antibiotics Antacids Decongestants Analgesics, mild

[a]From Rayburn et al. (1982).
[b]Excludes alcohol, caffeinated beverages, and cigarette smoking.

Perhaps the best example of an agent requiring more testing is ethanol. Although both French and American investigators reported the dysmorphology, growth retardation, and mental retardation associated with chronic ingestion of large amounts of ethanol during pregnancy, the full extent of ethanol toxicity is not understood (Table 19). Yet it is interesting to note that it was not until the 1960s or 1970s that such a syndrome was well defined. Most people had attributed it to other environmental and social issues and not specifically to alcohol. If the animal studies present difficulties for interpretation, then the polygenetic heterogeneous human population presents even more difficulties for the epidemiologists.

Why only 10% of the exposed human population demonstrates the complete phenytoin syndrome while an additional 30% demonstrates some components of that syndrome raises the possibility of a multicomponent relationship to the induction of malformations. As noted in the animal studies (Martz et al., 1977), the metabolism of the compound (e.g., phenytoin) to more reactive intermediates, which are the teratogenic agents, may be a possibility. If that is the case, is it the mother producing these metabolites that is affecting the embryo, or is it that the embryonic tissues are producing such toxicants, which affect their own development directly? If it is the embryonic tissues, perhaps this could be one explanation why mothers who are taking the same agent during two consecutive pregnancies have one child with the teratogenic syndrome while the other child apparently does not. Substantial evaluations need to be conducted in determining the biotransformation by mother and conceptus. A means for examining metabolism-mediated teratogenicity can be obtained using some of the in vitro studies where serum from these patients can be evaluated in rodent tissue culture studies using the 8- to 9-day-old rat embryo or the preimplantation mouse embryo to determine toxicity both in the area of preimplantation biology and in the development of a conceptus.

For extensive discussions of human investigations and postmarketing surveillance, the reader is referred to volumes by Wilson and Fraser (1977), Mattison (1983b), and Miller (1985).

SUMMARY

To become immersed in the issues of reproductive and/or perinatal toxicology, one must have an understanding of general toxicology, embryology, and reproductive physiology and neurobiology. The breadth of interactions and specific organ–system responses provide for almost an infinite variety of mechanisms of toxic action that may or may not have any similarity to the effects of an agent on the adult organism. Therefore, just as with the thalidomide or 13–*cis*-retinoic acid, the species differences, the dose responses, the diversity of responses, and applicability to the human by definition make the pregnant female and her conceptus pharmacologic and toxicologic orphans.

First must come recognition of the problems. In the 1960s, both the lay and the medical communities were sensitized to the environmental impact of chemicals like thalidomide, ethanol, and phenytoin, and to the development of structural defects. The 1970s attuned us to the risks of perinatal carcinogenesis from drugs like diethylstilbestrol. The 1980s have increased our awareness of the permanent and transient alterations in central nervous system function due to prenatal exposure to a wide range of agents and how behavior can be permanently manipulated due to in utero exposure to specific agents. The immune system and our assessments of species comparisons and in vitro monitoring, besides the above issues will most likely be the concerns of the 1990s. Selected exposures like that of diethylstilbestrol provide at this time a larger pool for evaluation of the human than is currently available from all animal studies. Examples like DES will require critical epidemiological as well as definitive clinical evaluations to understand the mechanisms involved in these teratogenic processes. These clinical and basic approaches in concert provide the foundation for rational regulatory and clinical judgments. This field of medical research encompasses all of us, and therefore a systematic and reasoned approach without a strict dependence on the principles of adult toxicity may provide for the resolutions necessary for an understanding of reproductive and perinatal toxicology.

If the rapid and continued development of this field combining obstetrics, pediatrics, pharmacology, toxicology, reproductive endocrinology, and all of the basic sciences during the past 25 years of investigation indicates how our sensitivity toward reproductive loss, birth defects, and altered development has multiplied, then the future carries our hopes for the eradication of such problems.

REFERENCES

Abel, E. L. 1980. Fetal alcohol syndrome: Behavioral teratology, *Psychol. Bull.* 87:29–50.

Adams, J., and Buelke-Sam, J. 1981. Behavioral assessment of the postnatal animal: Testing and methods development. In *Developmental Toxicology,* eds. C. A. Kimmel and J. Buelke-Sam, pp. 233–258. New York: Raven.

Ahokas, R. A., and Dilts, P. V. 1979. Cadmium uptake by the rat embryo as a function of gestational age. *Am. J. Obstet. Gynecol.* 135:219–222.

Ahokas, R. A., Dilts, P. V., and Lahaye, E. 1980. Cadmium-induced fetal growth retardation. *Amer. J. Obstet. Gynecol.* 136:216–221.

AMA Division of Drugs. 1983. *AMA Drug Evaluations,* 5th ed. Chicago: American Medical Association.

Amann, R. P. 1982. Use of animal models for detecting specific alterations in reproduction. *Fundam. Appl. Toxicol.* 2:13–26.

Amaral, D. G., Foss, J. A., Kellogg, C., and Woodward, D. J. 1975. Effects of subcutaneous administration of 6-hydroxydopamine in neonatal rats on dendritic morphology in the hippocampus. *Soc. Neurosci. Abstr.* 1:789.

Anders, M., and Sunram, J. 1982. Transplacental passage of dichloromethane and carbon monoxide. *Toxicol. Lett.*

Anderson, J. 1959. The placental barrier to gamma-globulins in the rat. *Amer. J. Anat.* 104:403–430.

Aranda, J. V., and Stern, L. 1983. Clinical aspects of development pharmacology and toxicology. *Pharmacol. Ther.* 20:1.

Arneil, C. C. 1972. Cyclophosphamide and a pubertal testes. *Lancet* II:1259–1260.

Arnold, D. L., Moodie, C. A., Griff, H. C., Charbonneau, F. M., Stavric, B., Collins, B. T., McGuire, T. F., Munro, I. C., and Blake, B. A. 1980. In vivo teratogenicity testing. In *Proc. Workshop on Methodology for Assessing Reproductive Hazards in the Work Place,* eds. P. F. Infante and M. F. Legator, pp. 219–226. U.S. Department of Health and Human Services, publication 81-100, Washington, D.C.

Asmussen, I. 1979. Effects of maternal smoking on the fetal cardiovascular system. *Cardiovasc. Med.* 4:777–790.

Baggs, R. B., Harnish, P. T., and Miller, R. K. 1983. Radiologic diagnosis of diethylstilbestrol induced teratogenesis in rats. *Lab. Anim. Sci.* 33:451–453.

Barlow, S. M., and Sullivan, F. M. 1982. *Reproductive Hazards of Industrial Chemicals.* London: Academic.

Barnwell, S. L., and Sastry, B. V. R. 1984. Depression of amino acid uptake in human placental villus by cocaine, morphine and nicotine. *Trophoblast Res.* 1:101–120.

Barrach, H. J., and Neubert, D. 1980. Significance of organ culture techniques for evaluation of prenatal toxicity. *Arch. Toxicol.* 45:161–187.

Bateman, A. J. 1977. The dominant lethal assay in the male mouse. In *Handbook of Mutagenicity Test Procedures,* eds. B. J. Kilbey, M. Legator, W. Nichols, and C. Ramel, pp. 325–334. New York: Elsevier Scientific.

Beck, F. 1976. Comparative placental pathology and function. *Environ. Hlth. Persp.* 18:5–12.

Beck, F. 1982. Model of teratology research. In *Developmental Toxicology,* ed. K. Snell, pp. 11–32. New York: Praeger.

Bedford, J. M. 1975. Maturation, transport, and fate of spermatozoa in the epididymis. In *Handbook of Physiology,* section 7, eds. D. W. Hamilton and R. O. Greep, vol. 5, pp. 303–317. Baltimore: Williams & Wilkins.

Berglund, F., Flodh, H., Lundborg, P., Prame, B., and Sannerstendt, R. 1985. Drug use during pregnancy and breast feeding: A classification system for drug information. *Acta Obstet. Gynecol. Scand. Suppl.* 126:5–55.

Bergsma, D., ed. 1979. *Birth Defects Compendium.* New York: Liss.

Berkowitz, R. L. 1980. Anti-hypertensive drugs in the pregnant parent. *Obstet. Gynecol. Survey* 35:191–204.

Berlin, M., and Ullberg, S. 1963. The fate of CD[109] in the mouse. *Arch. Environ. Health* 7:72–79.

Berman, R. L., and Craig, J. A. 1985. Current perspectives on gynecology. *CIBA Clin. Symp.* 37:1–32.

Bern, H. A., and Talamantes, F. J. 1981. Neonatal mouse models and their relation to disease in human female. In *Developmental Effects of DES in Pregnancy,* eds. A. L. Herbert and H. A. Bern, pp. 129–145. New York: Thieme-Stratton.

Berry, D. L., Zachariah, P. K., Slaga, R., and Juchau, M. R. 1977. Analysis of biotransformation of benzo(a)pyrene in human fetal and placental tissues with high-pressure liquid chromatography. *Eur. J. Cancer* 13:667–675.

Bibbo, M., Naqebb, M. A., Baccarini, I., Gill, W., Newton, M., Sleepr, K. M., Sonek, M., and Wied, G. L. 1975. Follow-up study of male and female offspring of DES-exposed mothers. *J. Reprod. Med.* 15:29–32.

Bormschein, R. N. 1980. The role of behavioral assessment in standard in vivo teratogenicity testing. In *Proc. Workshop on Methodology for Assessing Reproductive Hazards in the Work Place,* eds. P. F. Infante and M. F. Legator, pp. 227–246. U.S. Department of Health and Human Services, publication 81-100, Washington, D.C.

Bournais-Vardiabasis, N., Teplitz, R., Chernoff, G. F., and Seecof, R. L. 1983. Detection of teratogens in the *Drosophila* embryonic culture test: Assay of 100 chemicals. *Teratology* 28:109–122.

Boylan, E. S., and Calhoon, R. E. 1979. Mammary tumorogenesis in the rat following prenatal exposure to diethylstilbesterol and postnatal treatment with 7,12-dimethylbenz(a)anthracene. *J. Toxicol. Environ. Hlth.* 5:1059–1071.

Braun, A. G., Buckner, C. A., Emerson, D. J., and Nichinson, B. B. 1982. Quantitative correspondence between the in vivo and in vitro activity of teratogenic agents. *Proc. Natl. Acad. Sci. USA* 79:2056–2060.

Braun, A. G., and Weinreb, S. L. 1984. Teratogen metabolism: Activation of thalidomide and thalidomide analogues to products that inhibit the attachment of cells to concanavalin A coated plastic surfaces. *Biochem. Pharmacol.* 33:1471–1477.

Brendel, L., Duhamel, R. C., and Shepard, T. 1985. Embryo toxic drugs. *Biol. Res. Pregy. Perinatol.* 6:1–54.

Brent, R. L., Averich, E., and Brapiewski, V. A. 1961. Production of congenital malformations using tissue antibodies. *Proc. Soc. Exp. Biol. Med.* 106:523–526.

Brent, R. L., and Harris, M. L., eds. 1976. Prevention of embryonic, fetal and perinatal disease. DHEW publication NIH 76-853, Washington, D.C.

Brent, R. L., and Jensen, M. 1977. Immunological aspects of development. In *Handbook of Teratology,* eds. J. Wilson and C. Fraser, pp. 339–396. New York: Plenum.

Briggs, G. G., Bodendorfer, T. W., Freeman, R. K., and Yaffe, S. J. 1983. *Drugs in Pregnancy and Lactation. A Reference Guide to Fetal and Neonatal Risk.* Baltimore: Williams & Wilkins.

Bronson, R., Cooper, G., and Rosenfield, D. 1981. Ability of antibody-bound human sperm to penetrate zona-free hamster ova in vitro. *Fertil. Steril.* 36:778–783.

Brown, M. A., and F. E. Fabro. 1982. The in vitro approach to teratogenicity testing. In *Developmental Toxicology,* pp. 31–58. New York: Praeger.

Brusick, D. J. 1978. Alterations of germ cells leading to mutagenesis and their detection. *Environ. Health Perspect.* 24:105–112.

Buchet, J. P., Hubermont, G., and Lauwerys, R. 1978. Placental transfer of lead, mercury, cadmium and carbon monoxide. *Environ. Res.* 15:494–503.

Butcher, R. E., and Vorhees, C. V. 1979. A preliminary test battery for the investigation of the behavioral teratology of selected psychotrophic drugs. *Neurobehav. Toxicol. Suppl.* 1:207–212.

Campbell, B. A., Lytle, L. D., and Fibiger, H. C. 1969. Ontogeny of adrenergic arousal and cholinergic inhibitory mechanisms in the rat. *Science* 166:637–638.

Carey, S. W., Klein, N. W., Frederickson, W. T., Scakett, G. P., Greenstein, R. M., Sehgal, P., and Elliott, M. 1983. Analysis of sera from monkeys with histories of fetal wastage and the identification of teratogenicity in sera from human chronic spontaneous aborters using rat embryo cultures. *Trophoblast Res.* 1:347–360.

Chang, M. C., and Hunter, R. H. F. 1975. Capacitation of mammalian sperm: Biological and experimental aspects. In *Handbook of Physiology,* section 7, eds. D. W. Hamilton and R. O. Greep, vol. 5, pp. 339–351. Baltimore: Williams & Wilkins.

Chapman, R. N. 1983. Gonadal injury resulting from chemotherapy. *Am. J. Ind. Med.* 4:149–161.

Chapman, R. N., Sutcliffe, S. B., and Malpas, J. S. 1979. Cytotoxic-induced ovarian failure in women with Hodgkin's disease: I. Hormone function. *J. Am. Med. Assoc.* 245:1877–1881.

Chatot, C. L., Klein, N. W., Piatek, J., and Pierro, L. J. 1980. Successful culture of rat embryos on human serum: Use in the detection of teratogens. *Science* 207:1471–1473.

Chavez, D. J., and McIntyre, J. A. 1984. Sera from women with histories of repeated pregnancy losses cause abnormalities in mouse peri-implantation blastocysts. *J. Reprod. Immunol.* 6:273–281.

Chernoff, G., Jones, J., and Kelley, C. 1986. The California teratogen: Five and one-half years of operational experience. *J. Perinatal,* in press.

Cho, H. E., Shiotani, Y., Shiosaka, S., Inagaki, S., Kubota, Y., Kujama, H., Umegaki, K., Tatashi, K., Hashimura, E., Hamaoka, T., and Tohyama, M. 1983. Ontogeny of cholecystokinin-8-containing neuron system of the rat: An immunohistochemical analysis. I. Forebrain and upper brainstem. *J. Comp. Neurol.* 218:25–41.

Clarkson, T. W., Cox, C., Marsh, D. O., Myers, G. J., Al-Tikriti, S. K., Amin-Zaky, L., and Dabbagh, R. 1981. Dose-response relationship for adult and prenatal exposures to methylmercury. In *Measurement of Risks,* eds. G. G. Berg and H. D. Maillie, pp. 111–130. New York: Plenum.

Copius Peereboom-Stegeman, J., Van der Velde, W., and Dessing, J. 1985. Influence of cadmium on placental structure. *Ecotoxicol. and Environ. Safety* 7:79–86.

Clarkson, T. W., Nordberg, G., and Sager, P. 1983. *Reproductive and Developmental Toxicity of Metals.* New York: Plenum.

Cordero, J. F., and Oakley, G. P. 1983. Drug exposure during pregnancy: Some epidemiologic considerations. *Clin. Obstet. Gynecol.* 26:418.

Corrodi, H., Fuxe, K., and Hokfelt, T. 1968. The effect of immobilization stress on the activity of central monoamine neurons. *Life. Sci.* 7:107–112.

Corrodi, H., Fuxe, K., Lidbrisk, P., and Olsen, L. 1971. Minor tranquillizers, stress, and central catecholamine neurons. *Brain Res.* 29:1–16.

Cosentino, M. J., Chey, W. Y., Takihara, H., Cockett, A. T. K. 1984. The effects of sulfasalazine on human male fertility potential and seminal prostaglandins. *J. Urol.* 132:682–686.

Council on Environmental Quality. 1981. *Chemical Hazards to Human Reproduction.* U.S. Government Printing Office, Washington, D.C.

Council on Scientific Affairs. 1985. Effects of toxic chemicals on the reproductive system. *J. Am. Med. Assoc.* 253:3431–3437.

Cowan, W. M. 1979. The development of the brain. *Sci. Am.* 241:112–133.

Coyle, J. T., and Enna, S.J. 1976. Neurochemical aspects of the ontogenesis of CABAergic neurons in rat brain. *Brain Res.* 111:119–133.

Coyle, J. T., and Henry, D. 1973. Catecholamines in fetal and newborn rat brain. *J. Neurochem.* 21:61–67.

Coyle, J. T., and Molliver, M. E. 1977. Major innervation of newborn rat cortex by monoaminergic neurons. *Science* 96:444–446.

Cree, J., Meyer, J., and Hailey, D. 1973. Diazepam in labor. *Brit. Med. J.* 4:251–255.

Cumming, D. C., and Rebar, R. W. 1983. Exercise and reproductive function in women. *Am. J. Ind. Med.* 4:113–125.

Danielsson, B. R. G., and Dencker, L. 1984. Effects of cadmium on the placental uptake and transport to the fetus of nutrients. *Biol. Res. Pregnancy* 5:93–101.

Daston, G. 1982. Toxic effects of cadmium on the developing lung. *J. Toc. Environ. Hlth.* 9:51–61.

Davis, G. L., and Hawrisiak, M. M. 1981. In vitro cultivation of the fetal guinea pig inner ear. *Ann. Otol. Rhinol. Laryngol.* 90:246–250.

Dencker, L., Danielsson, B., Khoyat, A., and Lingren, A. 1983. Disposition of metals in the embryo and fetus. In *Reproductive and Developmental Toxicity of Metals,* eds. T. Clarkson, G. Nordberg, and P. Sager, pp. 261–286. New York: Plenum.

Deskin, R., Mills, E., Whitmore, W. L., Seidler, F. J., and Slotkin, T. A. 1980. Maturation of sympathetic neurotransmission in the rat heart. IV. The effect of neonatal central catecholaminergic lesions. *J. Pharmacol. Exp. Ther.* 215:342–347.

Deskin, R., Seidler, F. J., Whitmore, W. L., and Slotkin, T. A. 1981. Development of α-noradrenergic and dopaminergic receptor systems depends on maturation of their presynaptic nerve terminals in rat brains. *J. Neurochem.* 36:1683–1690.

di Sant'Agnese, P. A., Jensen, K., Levin, A. A., and Miller, R. K. 1983. Placental toxicity of cadmium: An ultrastructural study. *Placenta* 4:149–163.

diZerega, G. S., and Sherins, R.J. 1981. Endocrine control of adult testicular function. In *The Testis,* eds. H. Burger and D. deKrester, pp. 127–140. New York: Raven.

Dobson, R. L., and Felton, J. S. 1983. Female germ cell loss from radiation and chemical exposures. *Am. J. Ind. Med.* 4:175–190.

Edwards, E. M., Dacheux, J.-L., and Waites, G. M. H. 1976. Effects of alpha-chlorhydrin on the metabolism of testicular and epididymal spermatozoa of rams. *J. Reprod. Fertil.* 48:265–270.

Eliasson, R. 1978. Semen analysis. *Environ. Health Perspect.* 24:81–85.

Ellison, T. 1977. Toxicologic effects testing. In *Guide Book: Toxic Substances Control Act,* ed. G. S. Dominguez, pp. 8.1–8.22. Ohio: CRC.

Ericsson, R. J., and Baker, V.F. 1970. Male antifertility compounds: Biological properties of U-5897 and U-15,646. *J. Reprod. Fertil.* 21:267–273.

Fabro, S. 1973. Passage of drugs and other chemicals into the uterine fluids and preimplantation blastocyst. In *Fetal Pharmacology,* ed. L. Boreus, pp. 443–461. New York: Raven.

Fabro, S. 1983. Reproductive toxicology: State of the art. *Am. J. Ind. Med.* 4:391.

Fabro, S., McLachlan, J. A., and Dames, N.M. 1984. Chemical exposure of embryos during the preimplantation stages of pregnancy: Mortality rate and intrauterine development. *Am. J. Obstet. Gynecol.* 148:929–938.

Fabro, S., and Scialli, A., eds. 1986. *Principles of Drug Action during Pregnancy.* New York: Marcel Dekker, Inc.

Fantel, A. G., Greenaway, J. C., Juchau, M. R., and Shepard, T. H. 1979. Teratogenic bioactivation of cyclophosphamide in vitro. *Life Sci.* 25:67–72.

Faulk, W. P. 1981. Trophoblast and extraembryonic membranes in the immunobiology of human pregnancy. In *Placenta: Receptors, Pathology and Toxicology,* eds. R. K. Miller and H. A. Thiede, pp. 3–22. London: Saunders.

Fechter, L. D., and Mactutus, C. F. 1984. Prenatal carbon monoxide exposure: Learning and memory deficits in avoidance performances. *Science* 223:409–410.

Ferm, V., and Carpenter, S. 1968. The relationship of cadmium and zinc in experimental mammalian teratogenesis. *Lab. Invest.* 18:429–432.

Ferm, V., Hanlon, D., and Urban, J. 1969. The permeability of the hamster placenta to radioactive cadmium. *J. Embryol. Exp. Morph.* 22:107–133.

Filler, R., and Lew, K. J. 1981. Developmental onset of mixed-function oxidase activity in preimplantation mouse embryos. *Proc. Natl. Acad. Sci. USA* 78:6991–6995.

Fletcher, J. 1974. Attitudes toward defective newborns. *Hastings Cent. Stud.* 2:21.

Flint, O. P. 1983. A micromass culture method for rat embryonic neural cells. *J. Cell Sci.* 61:247–262.

Flint, O. P., and Orton, T. C. 1984. An in vitro assay for teratogens with cultures of rat embryo midbrain and limb bud cells. *Toxicol. Appl. Pharmacol.* 76:383–395.

Food and Drug Administration. 1971. Advisory Committee on Protocols for Safety Evaluation. Panel on Carcinogenesis Report on Cancer Testing in the Safety Evaluation of Food Additives and Pesticides. *Toxicol. Appl. Pharmacol.* 20:418–438.

Forsberg, J. G., and Kalland, T. 1981. Embryology of the genital tract in humans and rodents. In *Developmental Effects of Diethylstilbestrol (DES) in Pregnancy,* eds. A. L. Herbst and H. A. Bern, pp. 4–25. New York: Thieme-Stratton.

Freeman, S. J., Beck, F., and Lloyd, J. B. 1981. The role of the visceral yolk sac in mediating protein utilization by rat embryos cultured in vitro. *J. Embryol. Exp. Morphol.* 66:223–234.

Freeman, S. J., Brent, R. L., and Lloyd, J. B. 1982. The effect of teratogenic antiserum in yolk sac function in rat embryos cultured in vitro. *J. Embryol. Exp. Morphol.* 71:63–74.

Freeman, S. J., and Brown, N. A. 1985. Inhibition of proteolysis in rat yolk sac as a cause of teratogenesis effects of leupeptin in vitro and in vivo. *J. Embryol. Exp. Morphol.* 78:183–193.

Frieberg, L., Piscator, M., Nordberg, G., and Kjellstrom, T. 1974. *Cadmium in the Environment.* Cleveland, Ohio: Chemical Rubber.

Fried, P. A. 1982. Marihuana use by pregnant women and effects on offspring. *Neurobehav. Toxicol. Teratol.* 4:451.

Friedhoff, A. J., and Miller, J. C. 1983. Prenatal psychotrophic drug exposure and development of central dopaminergic and cholinergic neurotransmitter systems. *Monogr. Neural Sci.* 9:91–98.

Fuxe, K., Hokfelt, T., Jonsson, G., and Lofstrom, A. 1973. Brain and the pituitary–adrenal interaction studies on central monoamine neurons. In *Brain–Pituitary–Adrenal Interrelationships,* eds. A. Brodish and E. S. Redgetel, pp. 239–269. Basel: Karger.

Gabbiani, G., Badonnel, M.-C., Mathewson, S. M., and Ryan, G. B. 1974. Acute cadmium intoxication: Early selective lesions of endothelial clefts. *Lab. Invest.* 30:686–695.

Garbowski, C. T., and Daston, G. T. 1983. Functional teratology of the cardiovascular and other organ systems. *Issues Rev. Teratol.* 1:285–308.

Gelboin, H. B. 1980. Benzo(a)pyrene metabolism activation and carcinogenesis: Role in regulation of mixed function oxidases and related enzymes. *Physiol. Rev.* 60:1107–1166.

Generoso, W. M., Cain, K. T., Cornett, C. V., Russell, E. W., Hellwig, C.S., and Horton, C. Y. 1982. Difference in the ratio of dominant-lethal mutations to heritable translocations produced in mouse spermatids and fully mature sperm after treatment with triethylenemelamine (TEM). *Genetics* 100:633–640.

Gerber, G., Maes, J., and Deroo, J. 1978. Effect of dietary lead on placental blood flow and fetal uptake of alpha-aminoisobutyricate. *Arch. Toxicol.* 41:125–131.

Gill, W. B., Schumacher, G. F. B., Bibbo, M., Straus, F. H., II, and Schoenberg, H. W. 1979. Association of diethylstilbestrol exposure in utero with cryptorchidism, testicular hypoplasia and semen abnormalities. *J. Urol.* 122:36–39.

Gill, W. B., Schumacher, G. F. B., Hubby, M. M., and Blough, R. R. 1981. Male genital tract changes in humans following intrauterine exposure to diethylstilbestrol. In *Developmental Effects of Diethylstilbestrol (DES) in Pregnancy,* eds. A. L. Herbst and H. A. Bern, pp. 103–119. New York: Thieme-Stratton.

Glick, B. 1971. Morphologic changes and humoral immunity in cyclophosphamide-treated chicks. *Transplantation* 11:433–439.

Goldman, A. S., and Yaffe, S. J. 1978. Fetal trimethadione syndrome. *Teratology* 17:103.

Goldstein, L. S. 1984. Dominant lethal mutations induced in mouse spermatogonia by antineoplastic drugs. *Mutat. Res.* 140:193–197.

Grabowski, C. T. 1977. Altered electrolight and fluid balance. In *Handbook of Teratology,* J. C. Wilson and F. C. Fraser, vol. 2, pp. 753–770. New York: Plenum.

Crabowski, C., and Daston, G. 1983. Functional teratology of the cardiovascular and other organ systems. *Issues Rev. Teratology* 1:285–308.

Greene, R. R., Burrill, M. W., and Ivy, A. C. 1940. Experimental intersexuality. *Am. J. Anat.* 67:305–313.

Greene, R. M., and Carbarino, M. P. 1984. Role of cyclic AMP, prostaglandins, and catecholamines during normal palatal development. *Curr. Top. Dev. Biol.* 19:65–79.

Gross, I., Walker Smith, G. J., Maniscalco, W. M., Czajka, M. R., Wilson, C. M., and Rooney, S. A. 1978. An organ culture model for the study of biochemical development of fetal rat lung. *J. Appl. Physiol.* 45:355–362.

Gruenwald, P. 1963. Chronic fetal distress and placental insufficiency. *Biol. Neonat.* 5:215–226.

Gunn, S. A., Gould, T. C., and Anderson, W. A. D. 1963. The selective injurious response of testicular and epididymal blood vessels to cadmium and its prevention by zinc. *Am. J. Pathol.* 42:685–702.

Gupta, C., Sonawane, B. R., Yaffe, S. J., and Shapiro, B. H. 1980. Phenobarbital exposure in utero: Alterations in female reproductive function in rats. *Science* 208:508–510.

Gurtoo, H., Williams, C., Gottlied, J. 1983. Population distribution of benzo(a)pyrene metabolism in smokers. *Int. J. Cancer* 31:29–37.

Haas, G. G., Jr., Weiss-Wik, R., and Wolf, D. P. 1982. Identification of antisperm antibodies on sperm of infertile men. *Fertil. Steril.* 38:54–61.

Hansen, T. W., Myrianthopoulos, N. C., Harvey, M. A., and Smith, D. W. 1976. Risks to the offspring of women treated with hydantoin anticonvulsants. *J. Pediatr.* 89:662–665.

Hanson, J. W. 1976. Fetal hydantoin syndrome. *Teratology* 13:185.

Hanson, J. W., Streissguth, A. P., and Smith, D. W. 1978. The effects of moderate alcohol consumption during pregnancy on fetal growth and morphogenesis. *J. Pediatr.* 92:457.

Harada, M. 1978. Congenital minamata disease. *Teratology* 18:285.

Haseman, J. K., and Hogen, M. D. 1975. Selection of the experimental unit in teratology studies. *Teratology* 12:165–172.

Health and Welfare Canada. 1975. The testing of chemicals for carcinogenicity, mutagenicity, and teratogenicity, p. 183. Administrative Health and Welfare, Ottawa.

Hedge, G. A., Van Ree, J. M., and Versteed, D. H. G. 1976. Correlation between hypothalamic catecholamine synthesis and either stress-induced ACTH secretion. *Neuroendocrinology* 21:236–246.

Heinonen, O. P., Slone, D., and Shapiro, S. 1977. Birth defects and drugs in pregnancy. Littleton, Mass.: PSG.

Heinriesh, W. L., and Juchau, M. R. 1980. Extra hepatic drug metabolism: The gonads. In *Extra Hepatic Metabolism of Drugs and Other Foreign Chemicals,* eds. T. E. Graham, pp. 313–332. New York: Medical and Scientific.

Hendrickx, A. J. 1984. Disorders of fertilization transport and implantation. Reproduction. In *The New Frontier in Occupational and Environmental Health Research,* eds. J. E. Lockey, J. K. Lemasters, and W. R. Keye, Jr., pp. 211–227. New York: Liss.

Hendrickx, A., Benirschke, K., Thompson, R. S., Ahern, J. K., Lucas, W. O., Oi, R. H. 1979. The effects of prenatal diethylstilbestrol exposure on the genitalia of pubertal mucaca mulatta. *J. Reprod. Med.* 22:233–240.

Henry, E. C., and Miller, R. K. 1985. Comparison of the disposition of DES and estradiol in the fetal rat: Correlation with teratogenic potency. *Biochem. Pharmacol.*

Henry, E. C., Miller, R. K., and Baggs, R. B. 1984. Direct fetal injections of diethylstilbestrol in 17β-estradiol: A method for investigating their teratogenicity. *Teratology* 29:297–304.

Herbst, A. L., and Bern, H. A., eds. 1981. *Developmental Effects of DES in Pregnancy.* New York: Thieme and Stratton.

Herbst, A. L., Ulfelder, H., and Poskanzer, D. C. 1971. Adenocarcinoma of the vagina: Association of maternal stilbestrol therapy with tumor appearance in young women. *N. Engl. J. Med.* 284:878.

Himelstein-Braw, R., Peters, H., and Faber, M. 1978. Morphological study of the ovaries of leukemic children. *Br. J. Can.* 38:82–87.

Hoar, R. M. 1976. Comparative developmental aspects of selected organ systems. II. Gastrointestinal and urogenital systems. *Environ. Health Perspect.* 18:61–66.

Hoffman, H. S., and Ison, J. R. 1980. Principles of reflex modification in the domain of startle. I. Some empirical findings and their implications for how the nervous system processes sensory information. *Psychol. Rev.* 87:175–189.

Horning, S. J., Ophopte, R. T., Kaplan, H. S., and Rosenberg, S. A. 1981. Female reproductive potential after treatment for Hodgkin's disease. *N. Engl. J. Med.* 304:1377–1382.

Horowitz, J. D., and Goble, A. J. 1979. Drugs and impaired male sexual function. *Drugs* 18:206–217.

Ingwall, J. S., Roeske, W. R., and Wildenthal, K. 1980. The fetal mouse heart in organ culture: Maintenance of the differentiated state. *Methods Cell Biol.* 21A:167–186.

Isaacson, R. L., Street, W. J., Petit, T. D., and Dunn, A. J. 1977. Neonatal treatment with 6-OH-DA affects the brain NE content but not behavior. *Physiol. Psychol.* 5:49–52.

Ison, J.R. 1982. Temporal activity in auditory function in the rat: Reflex inhibition by brief gaps in noise. *J. Comp. Physiol. Psychol.* 96:945–954.

Ison, J. R., and Pinckney, L. A. 1983. Reflex inhibition in humans: Sensitivity to brief silent periods in white noise. *Percept. Psychophys.* 34:84–88.

Ivankovic, S., and Druckery, H. 1968. Transplacentore erzengung maligner tumoren des nervensystems. I Athylnitrosoharnstoff (ANH) and BDIX-Ratten. *Z Krebsforsch* 71:320–360.

Jaim-Etchenerry, G., and Zieher, L. M. 1977. Differential effects of various 6-hydroxydopa treatments on the development of central and peripheral nonadrenergic neurons. *Eur. J. Pharmacol.* 45:105–116.

Jaiswal, A. K., Gonzalez, F. J., and Nebert, D. W. 1985. Human dioxin-inducible cytochrome P₁-450: Complimentary DNA and amino acid sequence. *Science* 228:80–82.

Jason, K. M., and Kellogg, C. K. 1980. Behavioral neurotoxicity of lead. In *Lead Toxicity,* eds. R. L. Singhal and J. A. Thomas, pp. 241–271. Baltimore: Urban and Schwarzengerg.

Jason, K. M., and Kellogg, C. K. 1981. Neonatal lead exposure: Effects on development of behavior and striatal dopamine neurons. *Pharmacol. Biochem. Behav.* 15:641–649.

Jelinek, R. 1977. The chick embryotoxicity screening test (CHEST). In *Methods in Prenatal Toxicology,* eds. D. Neubert, H.-J. Merker, and T. E. Kwasigroch, pp. 381–386. Stuttgart: Thieme.

Jelinek, R., and Kistler, A. 1981. Effect of retinoic acid upon the chick embryonic morphogenetic systems. I. The embryotoxicity dose range. *Teratology* 23:191–195.

Jick, H., Porter, J., and Morrison, A. S. 1977. Relation between smoking and age of natural menopause. *Lancet* I:1354–1355.

Johnson, E. M. 1984. Mechanisms of teratogenesis: The extrapolation of the results of animal studies to man. In *Pregnant Women at Work,* ed. G. Chamberlain, pp. 135–151. London: Royal Society of Medicine/Macmillan.

Johnson, E. M., and Gabel, B. E. G. 1983. The role of an artificial embryo in detecting potential teratogenic hazards. In *Handbook of Experimental Pharmacology,* eds. E. M. Johnson and D. M. Kochhar, vol. 65, pp. 335–348. Berlin: Springer-Verlag.

Johnson, E. M., and Gabel, B. 1983. An artificial "embryo" for detection of abnormal developmental biology. *Fund. Appl. Tox.* 3:243–249.

Johnson, L. D., Palmer, A. E., King, N. W., Jr., and Hertig, A. T. 1981. Vaginal adenosis in cebus apella monkeys exposed to DES in utero. *Obstet. Gynecol.* 57:629–635.

Johnson, P. 1986. Biochemical and immunological aspects of the human trophoblast cell surface. *Trophoblast Res.* 2, in press.

Johnston, M. C., Morris, G. M., Kushner, D. C., and Bingoe, G. J. 1977a. Abnormal organogenesis of facial structures. In *Handbook of Teratology,* eds. J. G. Wilson and F. C. Fraser, vol. 2, pp. 421–450. New York: Plenum.

Johnston, M. C., Morris, G. M., Kushner, D. C., and Bingle, G. J. 1977b. Normal organogenesis of facial structures. In *Handbook of Teratology,* eds. J. G. Wilson and F. C. Fraser, vol. 2, pp. 421–451. New York: Plenum.

Jones, A. H., Fantel, A., Kocan, R. A., and Juchau, M. R. 1977. Bioactivation of procarcinogens in mutagens in human fetal and placental tissues. *Life Sci.* 21:1831–1837.

Jones, C. R., Hamilton, C. A., and Reid, J. L. 1983. Development of platelet a₂ adrenoreceptors and catecholamine production in man. *Prog. Neuropsychopharmacol. Biol. Psychiatry* (Suppl.).

Jones, K. L., Smith, D. W., Ulleland, C. N., and Streissguth, A. P. 1973. Patterns of malformations in offspring of chronic alcoholic mothers. *Lancet* I:1267.

Jonsson, G., and Sachs, C. 1976. Regional changes in (³H)-noradrenaline uptake, catecholamines and catecholamine synthetic and catabolic enzymes in the rat brain following neonatal 6-hydroxydopamine treatment. *Med. Biol.* 54:286–297.

Juchau, M. R. 1980. Drug transformation in the placenta. *Pharmacol. Ther.* 8:501–524.

Juchau, M., ed. 1981. *The biochemical Basis of Chemical Teratogenesis.* New York: Elsevier.

Juchau, M. R. 1982. The role of the placenta in developmental toxicology. In *Development Toxicology,* ed. K. Snell, pp. 187–210. New York: Praeger.

Juchau, M. R., Namkung, M. J., and Rettie, A. 1986. P-450 Cytochromes in the human placenta: Oxidations of xenobiotics and endogenous steriods. *Trophoblast Res.* in press.

Juchau, M. R. 1986. Function of P-450 hemoproteins in placental tissues. *Trophoblast Res.* 2, in press.

Jurgelski, W., Forsythe, W., and Dahl, D. 1974. The opossum as a biochemical model. *Lab. Anim. Sci.* 24:407–411.

Jurgelski, W., Hudson, P., and Falk, H. 1976. Embryonal neoplasm in the oppossum. *Science* 193:375–403.

Jurgelski, W., Hudson, P., and Falk, H. 1979. Tissue differentiation and susceptibility to embryonal tumor induction by ethylnitrosourea in the opossum. In *Perinatal Carcinogenesis,* ed. J. Rice, pp. 123–158. Washington: NCI Monograph.

Kalland, T. 1980. Alterations of antibody response in female mice after neonatal exposure to diethylstilbestrol. *J. Immunol.* 124:194–198.

Kalland, T., Forsberg, T., and Forsberg, J. 1978. Effect of estrogen and corticosterone on the lymphoid system in neonatal mice. *Exp. Mol. Pathol.* 28:76–95.

Kallen, B., and Winberg, J. 1968. Dealing with suspicions of malformation frequency. *Acta Paediatr. Scand. Suppl.* 275:66–74.

Kalter, H., and Warkany, J. 1983. Congenital malformations. *N. Engl. J. Med.* 308:424.

Kapp, R. W., Jr., Picciano, D. J., and Jacobson, C. B. 1979. Y-chromosomal nondisjunction in dibromochloropropane-exposed workmen. *Mutat. Res.* 64:47–51.

Karp, L. E., Williamson, R. A., Moore, D. E., Shy, K. K., Plymate, S. R., and Smith, W. D. 1981. Sperm penetration assay: Useful test in evaluation of male fertility. *Obstet. Gynecol.* 57:620–623.

Kasamatsu, T., and Pettigrew, J. D. 1976. Depletion of brain catecholamines: Failure of ocular dominance shift after monocular occulsion in kittens. *Science* 194:206–209.

Kaufman, R. H., Noller, K., Adam, E., Irwin, J., Gray, M., Jefferies, J. A., and Hilton, J. 1984. Upper genital tract abnormalities and pregnancy outcome in diethylstilbestrol-exposed progeny. *Am. J. Obstet. Gynecol.* 148:973.

Kaunitz, J., Mallins, D., and McKay, D. 1962. Studies of the generalized Shwartzman reaction by diet. *J. Expt. Med.* 115:127–136.

Kavlok, R. J., Chernoff, M., and Rogers, C. H. 1985. The effect of acute maternal toxicity on fetal development in the mouse. *Teratog. Carcinog. Mutagen.* 5:3–13.

Kavlock, R. J. The ontogeny of the hydropenia response in neonatal rats and its application in developmental toxicology studies. In *Environmental Factors and Human Growth and Developmental,* eds. V. R. Hunt, M. K. Smith, and D. Wert, pp. 173–186. Springs Harbor, Me.: Plain Springs Harbor Laboratory.

Kavlok, R. J., Chernoff, M., and Rogers, C. H. 1985. The effect of acute maternal toxicity on fetal development in the mouse. *Teratog. Carcinog. Mutagen.* 5:3–13.

Kellogg, C., DiRaddo, J., and Roch, J. 1979. Age-related characteristics of the in vitro accumulation of ^{3}H-NE. In *Catecholamines: Basic and Clinical Frontiers,* eds. E. Usdin and I. Kopin, pp. 833–835. New York: Pegamon.

Kellogg, C., Tervo, D., Ison, J., Parisi, T., and Miller, R. K. 1980. Prenatal exposure to diazepam alters behavioral development in rats. *Science* 207:205–207.

Kellogg, C., Ison, J. R., and Miller, R. K. 1983. Prenatal diazepam exposure: Effects on auditory temporal resolution in rats. *Psychopharmacology* 79:332–337.

Kelse, F. O. 1982. Regulatory aspects of teratology: Role of the food and drug administration. *Teratology* 25:193–199.

Kihlstrom, I. 1982. Placental transport of the non-metabolizable a-aminoisobutyric acid in guinea pigs given a commercial chlorobiphenyl preparation or a defined pure chlorobiphenyl. *Acta. Pharm. Toxicol.* 51:428–433.

Kimmel, C., Wilson, J., and Schumacher, H. 1971. Studies on the metabolism and identification of the causative agent in aspirin teratogenesis in the rat. *Teratology* 4:15–24.

Kitchin, K. T., Schmid, B. P., and Sanyal, M. K. 1981. Teratogenicity of cyclophosphamide in a coupled microsomal activity/embryo culture system. *Biochem. Pharmacol.* 30:59–64.

Kleihues, P. 1982. Developmental carcinogenicity. In *Developmental Toxicity,* ed. K. Snell, pp. 211–246. New York: Praeger.

Klein, N. W., Vogler, M. A., Chatot, C. L., and Pierro, L. J. 1980. The use of cultured rat embryos to evaluate the teratogenic activity of serum: Cadmium and cyclophosphamide. *Teratology* 21:199–208.

Klein, N. W., Plenefish, J. D., Carey, S. W., Frederickson, W. T., Sackett, G. P., Burbacher, T. M., and Parker, R. M. 1982. Serum from monkeys with histories of fetal wastage causes abnormalities in cultured rat embryos. *Science* 215:66–69.

Klingberg, M. A., Papier, C. M., and Hart, J. 1983. Birth defects monitoring. *Am. J. Ind. Med.* 4:309.

Klopper, A. 1980. New placental proteins. *Placenta* 2:77–89.

Kluwe, W. M. 1981b. Acute toxicity of 1,2-dibromo-3-chloropropane in the F344 male rat: II. Development and repair of the renal, epididymal, testicular, and hepatic lesions. *Toxicol. Appl. Pharmacol.* 59:84–95.

Kluwe, W. M., Gupta, B. N., and Lamb, J. C. 1983. The comparative effects of 1,2-dibromo-3-chloropropane (DBCP) and its metabolites, 3-chloro-1,2-propaneoxide (epichlorohydrin), 3-chloro-1,2-propane-diol (alphachlorohydrin), and oxalic acid, on the urogenital system of male rats. *Toxicol. Appl. Pharmacol.* 70:67–86.

Kochhar, D. M. 1982. Embryonic limb bud organ culture in assessment of teratogenicity of environmental agents. *Teratog. Carcinog. Mutagen.* 2:303–312.

Koeter, H. B. W. M. 1983. Relevance of parameters related to fertility and reproduction in toxicity testing. In *Reproductive Toxicology,* ed. D. R. Mattison, pp. 81–86. New York: Liss.

Kohler, E., Merker, H. P. J., Ahmke, W., and Oojnorwicz, F. 1972. Gross kinetics in the mare and embryos during the stage of differentiation. *Naunyn-Schmiedebergs Arch. Pharmackol.* 272:69–81.

Krauter, E. E., Wallace, J. E., and Campbell, B. A. 1981. Sensory-motor function in the aging rat. *Behav. Neural. Biol.* 31:367–392.

Kuemmerle, H. P., and Brendel, K. 1984. *Clinical Pharmacology in Pregnancy.* New York: Thieme-Stratton.

Kuhnert, P., Kuhnert, B., Bottoms, S., and Erhard, T. 1982. Cadmium levels in maternal blood, fetal cord blood, and placental tissues of pregnant women who smoke. *Amer. J. Obstet. Gyn.* 142:1021–1025.

Kupfer, D. 1982. Studies on short and long-range estrogenic action of chlorinated hydrocarbon pesticides. In *Environmental Factors and Human Growth and Developmental,* eds. V. R. Hunt, M. K. Smith, and D. Wert, pp. 379–389. Plain Springs Harbor Laboratory, Me.: Plain Springs Harbor.

Lahti, R. A., and Borshun, G. 1975. Effects of various doses of minor tranquilizers on plasma corticosterone in stressed rats. *Res. Commun. Chem. Pathol. Pharmacol.* 11:595–603.

Lantz, G. D., Cunningham, G. R., Huckins, C., and Lipshultz, L. I. 1981. Recovery from sever oligospermia after exposure to dibromochloropropane. *Fertil. Steril.* 35:46–53.

Laquer, G. L., and Spatz, M. 1973. Transplacental induction of tumors and malformations in rats with cycasin and methoxyazomethanol. In *Transplacental Carcinogenesis,* eds. L. Tomatis and U. Mohr, pp. 59–64. Lyon: International Agency for Research on Cancer.

Lasagna, L. 1979. Toxicological barriers to providing better drugs. *Arch. Toxicol.* 43:27.

Lauder, J. M., and Bloom, F. E. 1974. Ontogeny of monoamine neurons in the locus coeruleus, raphe nuclei, and substantia signs of the rat. I. Cell differentiation. *J. Comp. Neurol.* 155:469–492.

Lauder, J. M., and Bloom, F. E. 1975. Ontogeny of monoamine neurons in the locus coerulus, raphe nuclei, and substantia nigra in the rat. II. Synaptogenesis. *J. Comp. Neurol.* 163:251–264.

Lauder, J. M., and Krebs, H. 1978. Serotonin as a differentiation signal in early neurogenesis. *Dev. Neurosci.* 1:13–30.

Lauder, J. M., Towle, A. C., Han, V. K. M., and Henderson, P. 1984. Ontogeny of GABAergic neurons in the rat brain: An immunocytochemical study. *Soc. Neurosci. Abstr.* 10:645.

Lauwerys, R., Buchet, J., Roels, H., and Hubermont, G. 1978. Placental transfer of lead, mercury, cadmium and carbon monoxide, I. *Environ. Res.* 15:278–289.

Lee, I. P. 1983. Adaptive biochemical repair response toward germ cell DNA damage. *Am. J. Ind. Med.* 4:135–147.

Lee, I. P., and Dixon, R. L. 1972. Effects of procarbazine on spermatogenesis determined by velocity sedimentation cell separation technique and serial mating. *J. Pharmacol. Exp. Ther.* 181:219–226.

Lee, I. P., and Dixon, R. L. 1978. Factors influencing reproduction and genetic toxic effects on male gonads. *Environ. Health Perspect.* 24:117–127.

Lee, I. P., and Suzuki, K. 1979. Induction of unscheduled DNA synthesis in mouse germ cells following 1,2-dibromo-3-chloropropane (DBCP) exposure. *Mutat. Res.* 68:169–173.

Legator, L. S., and Ward, J. B., Jr. 1984. Genetic toxicology—relevant studies with animals and humans. In *Reproduction: The New Frontier in Occupational and Environmental Health Research,* eds. J. E. Lockey, G. K. Lemasters, and W. R. Keye, Jr, pp. 491–525. New York: Liss.

Lemoine, P., Harouseau, H., Borteyru, J. P., and Mennet, J. C. 1967. Les enfants de parents alcooliques: Anomalies observees a propos de 127 cas. *Arch. Fr. Pediatr.* 25:820.

Lenz, W. 1961. Klinische missbildungen nach medikament-einnahme während der gradvidität. *Dtsch. Med. Wochenschr.* 86:2555.

Leonard, A. 1977. Tests for heritable translocations in male mammals. In *Handbook of Mutagenicity Test Procedures,* eds. B. J. Kilbey, M. Legator, W. Nichols, and C. Ramel, pp. 293–299. New York: Elsevier Scientific.

Leung, C. C. K., Lee, C., Cheewatrakoolpong, B., and Hilton, D. 1985. Abnormal embryonic development induced by antibodies to rat visceral yolk sac endoderm: Isolation of the antigen and localization to microvilli membrane. *Dev. Biol.* 107:432–441.

Levin, S. M. 1983. Problems and pitfalls in conducting epidemiological research in the areas of reproductive toxicology. *Am. J. Ind. Med.* 4:349.

Levin, A. A., and Miller, R. K. 1980. Fetal toxicity of cadmium: Maternal vs. fetal injections. *Teratology* 22:105–110.

Levin, A. A., and Miller, R. K. 1981. Fetal toxicity of cadmium in the rat: Decreased uteroplacental blood flow. *Toxicol. Appl. Pharmacol.* 58:297–306.

Levin, A. A., Plautz, J. R., di Sant'Agnese, P. A., and Miller, R. K. 1981. Cadmium: Placental mechanisms of fetal toxicity. *Placenta* 3:303–318.

Levin, A. A., Miller, R. K., and di Sant'Agnese, P. A. 1983. Heavy metal alterations of placental function: A mechanism for the induction of fetal toxicity by cadmium. In Developmental and Reproductive Toxicity of Metals, eds. T. Clarkson, G. Nordberg, and P. Sager, pp. 633–654. New York: Plenum.

Linna, T. J., Frommel, D., and Good, R. A. 1972. Effects of early cyclophosphamide treatment on the development of lymphoid organs and immunological functions in the chicken. *Int. Arch. Allergy Appl. Immunol.* 42:20–39.

Longo, L. 1977. The biological effects of carbon dioxide on the pregnant woman, fetus and newborn infant. *Am. J. Obstet. Gynecol.* 129:69–78.

Luster, M., Faith, R., McLachlan, J., and Clark, G. 1979. Effect in utero exposure to diethylstilbestrol on the immune response in mice. *Toxicol. Appl. Pharmacol.* 47:279–285.

Luz, N., Margues, M., Ayub, A., and Correa, P. 1969. Effects of estradiol upon the thymus and lymphoid organs of immature female rats. *Am. J. Obstet. Gynecol.* 105:525–528.

MacLeod, J., and Gold, R. Z. 1951. The male factor in fertility and infertility. II. Spermatozoon counts in 1000 men of known fertility and in 1000 cases of infertile marriage. *J. Urol.* 66:436–449.

MacLeod, J., and Wang, Y. 1979. Male fertility potential in terms of semen quality: A review of the past, a study of the present. *Fertil. Steril.* 31:103–116.

Mactutus, C. F., and Fechter, L. D. 1985. Moderate prenatal carbon monoxide exposure produces persistent and apparently permanent memory deficits in rats. *Teratology* 31:1–12.

Maggi, A., Schmidt, M. J., Ghetti, B., and Enna, S. J. 1979. Effects of aging on neurotransmitter receptor binding in rat and human brain. *Life Sci.* 24:367–374.

Manchester, D., and Jacoby, E. 1984. Decreased placental monooxygenase activities associated with birth defects. *Teratology* 30:31–37.

Manchester, D. K., Parker, D. B., and Bowmen, C. M. 1984. Maternal smoking increases xenobiotic metabolism in placenta but not umbilical vein endothelium. *Pediatr. Res.* 18:1071–1075.

Mann, T., and Lutwak-mann, C. 1983. Passage of chemicals into human and animal semen: Mechanisms and significance. *CRC Crit. Rev. Toxicol.* 11:1–14.

Manson, J. M. 1984. Current mechanisms of environmental agents by cause associated with adverse female reproductive outcome. In *Reproduction: The New Frontier in Occupational and Environmental Health Research,* eds. J. E. Lockey, G. K. Lemasters, and W. R. Keye, Jr., pp. 237–248. New York: Liss.

Manson, J. M., and Simons, R. 1979. Influence of environmental agents on male reproductive failure. In *Work and the Health of Women,* ed. V. R. Hunt, pp. 155–179. Boca Raton, Fla.: CRC.

Manson, J. M., and Smith, C. C. 1977. Influence of cyclophosphamide on mouse limb development. *Teratology* 15:291–300.

Manson, J. M., and Smith, C. C. 1979. In vitro metabolism of cyclophosphamide in limb bud culture. *Teratology* 19:149–158.

Manson, J. M., Zenick, H., and Costlow, R. D. 1982. Teratology test methods in laboratory animals. In *Principles and Methods of Toxicology,* ed. A. W. Hayes, pp. 141–184. New York: Raven.

Marsh, D., Myers, G., Clarkson, T., Amin-Zaki, L., Tikiriti, S., and Majeed, M. 1980. Fetal methyl mercury poisoning. *Ann. Neurol.* 7:348.

Martz, C., Failinger, C., and Blake, D. A. 1977. Phenytoin teratogenesis: Correlation between embryopathic effect and covalent binding of putative arene oxide metabolite. *J. Pharmacol. Exp. Ther.* 203:231.

Mattison, D. R. 1979. Differences in sensitivity of rat and mouse primordial oocytes to destruction by polycyclic armonatic hydrocarbons. *Chem. Biol. Interact.* 28:133–137.

Mattison, D. R. 1982. The effects of smoking on fertility from gonadogenesis to implantation. *Environ. Res.* 28:410–433.

Matison, D. R. 1983a. The mechanisms of action of reproductive toxins. *Am. J. Ind. Med.* 4:65–79.

Mattison, D. R., ed. 1983b. *Reproductive Toxicology.* New York: Liss.

Mattison, D.R. 1983c. Ovarian toxicity: Effects on sexual maturation, reproduction, and menopause. In *Reproductive and Developmental Toxicity of Metals,* eds. T. W. Clarkson, G. F. Nordberg, and P. R. Sager, pp. 317–342. New York: Plenum.

Mattison, D. R., and Thorgeirsson, S. S. 1978. Gonadal aryl hydrocarbon hydroxylase in rats and mice. *Can. Res.* 38:1368–1373.

Mattison, D. R., and Thorgeirsson, S. S. 1979. Ovarian aryl hydrocarbon hydroxylase activity in primortio oocyte toxicity of polycyclic aromatic hydrocarbons in mice. *Can. Res.* 39:3471–3475.

Mattison, D. R., Gates, A. H., Leonard, A. P., Wide, M., Hemminki, K., and Copius-Peereboom-Stegeman, J. 1983a. Reproductive and developmental toxicity of metals: Female reproductive system. In *Reproductive and Developmental Toxicity of Metals,* eds. T. Clarkson, G. Nordberg, and P. Sager, pp. 43–91. New York: Plenum.

Mattison, D. R., and Nightingale, M. S. 1980. The biochemical and genetic characteristics of murine ovarian aryl hydrocarbon (benzo(a)pyrene) hydroxylase activity and its relationship to primordial oocyte destruction by polycyclic aromatic hydrocarbons. *Tox. Appl. Pharm.* 56:399–408.

Mattison, D. R., Shiromizu, K., and Nightingale, M. S. 1983b. Oocyte destruction by polycyclic aromatic hydrocarbons. *Am. J. Ind. Med.* 4:191–202.

McBride, W. 1961. Thalidomide and congenital abnormalities. *Lancet* II:1358.

McCroskey, R. L., and Kidder, H. C. 1980. Auditory fusion among learning disabled, reading disabled, and normal children. *J. Learn. Disabil.* 13:18–25.

McIntosh, I. D. 1984. Smoking and pregnancy: Attributable risks and public health implications. *Can. J. Public Health* 75:141–148.

McKay, D., and Huang, T. 1962. Studies of the generalized Shwartzman reaction produced by diet. *J. Expt. Med.* 115:1117–1126.

McLachlan, J. A. 1981. Rodent models for perinatal exposure to diethylstilbestrol and their relation to human disease in the male. In *Developmental Effects of Diethylstilbestrol in Pregnancy,* eds. A. L. Herbst and H. A. Bern, pp. 148–157. New York: Thieme-Stratton.

McLachlan, J. A., Newbold, R. R., and Bullock, B. 1975. Reproductive tract lesions in male mice exposed prenatally to diethylstilbestrol. *Science* 190:991–992.

McLachlan, J. A., Newhold, R. R., and Bullock, B. C. 1980. Long term effects on the female mouse genital tract associated with prenatal exposure to diethylstilbestrol. *Cancer Res.* 40:3988–3999.

McLachlan, J. A., Newbold, R. R., Korach, K. S., Lam, J. C., IV, and Suzuki, Y. 1981. Transplacental toxicology: Prenatal factors influencing postnatal fertility. In *Developmental Toxicology,* eds. C. A. Kimmell and J. Buelke-Sam, pp. 213–232. New York: Raven.

McLachlan, J. A., Wong, A., Barrett, J. C. 1982. Morphologic and neoplastic transformation of syrian hamster embryo fibroblasts by diethylstilbestrol and its analogs. *Cancer Res.*

McLachlan, M. C., and Dixon, R. L. 1976. Transplacental toxicity of diethylstilbestrol: A special problem in safety evaluation. In *New Concepts and Safety Evaluation,* eds. M. A. Mehlamen, R. E. Shapiro, and H. Blumenthal, pp. 423–448. Washington, D.C.: Hemisphere.

McLaughlin, B. J., Wood, J. G., Saito, K., Roberts, E., and Wu, J. X. 1975. The fine structural localization of glutamate decarboxylase in developing axonal processes and presynaptic terminals of rodent cerebellum. *Brain Res.* 85:355–371.

Mendelson, J. H., Mello, N. K., and Ellingboe, J. 1977. Effects of acute alcohol intake on pituitary-gonadal hormones in normal human males. *J. Pharmacol. Exp. Ther.* 202:676–682.

Metzler, M. 1981. The metabolism of diethylstilbestrol. *CRC Crit. Rev. Biochem.* 10:171–213.

Metzler, M. 1984. Biochemical toxicology of diethylstilbestrol. In *Review of Biochemical Toxicology,* eds. E. Hodgson, J. R. Bend, and R. M. Philpot, pp. 191–220. New York: Elsevier.

Meyer, M. B., and Tonascia, J. 1977. Maternal smoking, pregnancy complications and perinatal mortality. *Amer. J. Obstet. Gyn.* 128:494–498.

Milkovich, L., and van den Berg, D. J. 1974. Effects of prenatal metrobamate and chlordiazepoxide on embryonic and fetal development. *N. Engl. J. Med.* 291:268.

Miller, R. K. 1981. Drugs during pregnancy: A therapeutic dilemma. *Rational Drug Therap.* 15:1–10.

Miller, R. K. 1983. Perinatal toxicology: Its recognition and fundamentals. *Am. J. Ind. Med.* 4:205–244.

Miller, R. K. 1985. Drugs and pregnancy—Documentation, evaluation and recommendations. In *Clinical and Social Pharmacology Postmarketing Period,* eds. J. L. Alloza, Cantor Editio, and W. Aulendorf, pp. 102–113. Germany.

Miller, R. K., Ferm, V., and Mudge, G. 1972. Placental transfer and tissue distribution of iophenoxic acid in the hamster. *Amer. J. Obstet. Gynecol.* 114:259–266.

Miller, R. K., and Gardner, K. 1981. Cadmium in the human placenta: Relationship to smoking. *Teratology* 23:51A.

Miller, R. K., Heckmann, M. E., and McKenzie, R. C. 1982. Diethylstilbestrol: Placental transfer metabolism, covalent binding and fetal distribution in the Wistar rat. *J. Pharmacol. Exp. Ther.* 220:358–365.

Miller, R. K., and Kellogg, C. K. 1985. The pharmacodynamics of prenatal chemical exposure. In *Prenatal Drug Exposure: Kinetics and Dynamics,* eds. N. Chiang and C. C. Lee, pp. 39–57. NIDA Research Monograph 60.

Miller, R. K., Koszalka, T. R., and Brent, R. L. 1976. Transport mechanisms for molecules across placenta membranes. In *Cell Surface Reviews,* eds. G. Poste and G. Nicolson, pp. 145–223.

Miller, R. K., Mattison, D. R., Filler, R. S., and Rice, J. M. 1985. Reproductive and developmental toxicology. In *Pharmacotherapy during Pregnancy,* eds. T. Eskes and M. Finster, pp. 215–224. London: Butterworths.

Miller, R. K., Ng, W. W., and Levin, A. A. 1983. The placenta: Relevance to toxicology. In *Reproductive and Developmental Toxicity of Metals,* eds. T. Clarkson, G. Nordberg, and P. Sager, pp. 569–605. New York: Plenum.

Miller, R. K., and Thiede, H. A. 1981. *Placenta: Receptors, Pathology and Toxicology.* London: Saunders.

Miller, R. K., and Thiede, H. A. 1984. *Fetal Nutrition, Metabolism and Immunology.* New York: Plenum.

Miller, R. K., and Thiede, H. A. 1986. *The Cell Biology and Pharmacology of the Placenta: Technics and Applications.* New York: Plenum.

Minor, R. R. 1979. Organ cultures of embryonic lung tissues. *J. Pediatr.* 95:910–916.

Mohri, H., Suter, D. A. I., Brown-Woodman, P. D. C., White, I. G., and Ridley, D. D. 1975. Identification of the biochemical lesion produced by alpha-chlorohydrin in spermatozoa. *Nature (Lond.)* 225:75–77.

Monie, R. W. 1965. Comparative development of rat, chick, and human embryos. In *2nd Teratology Workshop Manual (Suppl.),* pp. 146–162. Calif.: Pharmaceutical Manufacturers Assoc.

Monie, R. W. 1976. Comparative development of the nervous, respiratory, and cardiovascular systems. *Environ. Health Perspect.* 18:55–60.

Moore, K. E., ed. 1985. *The Developing Human.* Toronto: Saunders.

Morselli, P. L. 1977. *Drug Disposition during Pregnancy.* New York: Spectrum.

Moulton, B. 1984. Epithelial cell function during blastocyst implantation. *J. Biosci.* 6:11–21.

Muechler, E., Mariona, F. G., Miller, R. K., Gilles, P. A., Rhinehardt, E. A., Klein, N. W., and Greenstein, R. M. 1984. The culture of rat embryos and sera from women with histories of spontaneous abortion. *Fertil. Steril.* 41:22S.

Mukhtar, H., Lee, I. P., Foureman, G. L., and Bend, J. R. 1978. Epoxide metabolizing enzyme activities in rat testes: Postnatal development and relative activity in interstitial and spermatogenic cell compartments. *Chem. Biol. Interact.* 22:153–165.

Mulvihill, J., Gamm, S., and Ferm, V. 1970. Facial malformation in normal and cadmium-treated golden hamsters. *J. Embryol. Exp. Morph.* 24:393–403.

Mummery, C. L., Van Den Brink, C. E., Van Der Saag, P. T., and De Laat, S. W. 1984. A short-term screening test for teratogens using differentiating neuroblastoma cells in vitro. *Teratology* 29:271–279.

Nakatsuji, N. 1983. Craniofacial malformations in *Xenopus laevis* tadpoles caused by the exposure of early embryos to ethanol. *Teratology* 28:299–305.

Naeye, R. L. 1981. Common environmental influences on the fetus. In *Perinatal Diseases,* eds. R. Naeye, J. Kissane, and N. Kaufman, pp. 52–66. Baltimore: Williams & Wilkins.

Napalkov, N. P. 1973. Some general considerations of the problem of transplacental carcinogenesis. In *Transplacental Carcinogenesis,* eds. L. Tomatis and U. Mohr, pp. 1–10. Lyon: WHO-IARC.

Napalkov, N. P., and V. N. Anisimov. 1979. Transplacental effect of diethylstilbestrol in female rats. *Cancer Let.* 6:107–114.

Neaves, W. B. 1977. The blood-testis barrier. In *The Testis,* eds. A. D. Johnson and W. R. Gomes, vol. 4, pp. 125–162. New York: Academic.

Nebert, D. W. 1981. Birth defects and the potential of genetic differences in drug metabolism. *Birth Defects Orig. Artic. Ser.* 17:51–70.

Nebert, D. W., and Gelboin, H. B. 1969. The in vivo and in vitro induction of aryl hydrocarbon hydroxylase in the mammalian cells of different species. *Arch. Biochem. Biophys.* 1234:76–83.

Nelson, C. M. K., and Bunge, R. G. 1974. Semen analysis: Evidence for changing parameters of male fertility potential. *Fertil. Steril.* 25:503–507.

Neubert, D. 1982. The use of culture techniques in studies on prenatal toxicity. *Pharmacol. Thera.* 18:397–434.

New, D. A. T. 1978a. Whole embryo explants and transplants. In *Handbook of Teratology,* eds. J. G. Wilson and F. C. Fraser, vol. 4, pp. 95–133. New York: Plenum.

New, D. A. T. 1978b. Whole-embryo culture and the study of mammalian embryos during organogenesis. *Biol. Rev.* 53:81–122.

New, D. A. T., and Brent, R. L. 1972. Effect of yolk sac antibody on rat embryos grown in culture. *J. Embryol. Exp. Morphol.* 27:543–553.

Newbold, R. R., Carter, D. B., Harris, S. E., and McLachlan, J. A. 1981. Molecular differentiation of the mouse genital tract: Serum-free organ culture system for morphological and biochemical correlations. *In Vitro* 17:51–54.

Newland, M. C., Ng, W. W., Baggs, R., Weiss, B., and Miller, R. K. 1986. Delayed behavioral toxicity of acute perinatal exposure to cadmium. *Teratology,* in press.

Nishimura, H. 1983. Problems in human teratology. *Issues Rev. Teratol.* 1:1–18.

Nishimura, H., and Shiota, K. 1977. Summary of comparative embryology and teratology. In

Handbook of Teratology, eds. J. G. Wilson and F. C. Fraser, vol. 3, pp. 119–154. New York: Plenum.

Nobin, A., and Bjorklund, A. 1973. Topography of the monoamine neuron systems in the human brain as revealed in fetuses. *Acta Physiol. Scand. Suppl.* 388:1–38.

Oakley, G. P. 1979. Drug influences on malformations. *Clin. Perinatol.* 6:403.

Olsen, F., and Massaro, E. 1980. Developmental pattern of cAMP, adenyl cyclase, and cAMP phosphodiesterase in the palate, lung and liver of the fetal mouse. *Teratology* 22:155–166.

Okumura, K., Lee, I. P., and Dixon, R. L. 1975. Permeability of selected drugs and chemicals across the blood-testis barrier of the rat. *J. Pharmacol. Exp. Ther.* 194:89–95.

Olson, L., Bareus, L. O., and Seiger, A. 1973. Histochemical demonstration and mapping of 5-hydroxytryptamine and catecholamine-containing neuron systems in human fetal brain. *Z. Anat. Entwicklungs. Gesch.* 139:259–282.

Ounsted, M. K., Moar, V. A., Good, F. J., Redman, C. W. G. 1980. Hypertension during pregnancy with and without specific treatment. The children at the age of 4 years. *Br. J. Obstet. Gynecol.* 87:19.

Palacios, J. M., and Kuhar, M. J. 1982. Ontogeny of high affinity GABA and benzodiazepine receptors in the rat cerebellum: An autoradiographic study. *Dev. Brain Res.* 2:531–539.

Palmer, A. 1977. The design of subprimate animal studies. *Handbook of Teratology* 4:215–253.

Papoz, L., Lschivege, E., Pequingnot, G., Barrat, J., and Schwartz, D. 1982. Matrnal smoking and birth weight in relation to dietary habits. *Am. J. Obstet. Gynecol.* 142:870–876.

Parisi, T., and Ison, J.R. 1979. Development of the acoustic startle response in the rat: Ontogenetic changes in the magnitude of inhibition by prepulse stimulation. *Dev. PsychoBiol.* 12:219–230.

Parisi, T., and Ison, J. R. 1981. Ontogeny of control over the startle reflex by visual stimulation in the rat. *Dev. PsychoBiol.* 14:311–316.

Parizek, J. 1960. Sterilization of the male by cadmium salts. *J. Reprod. Fertil.* 1:294–309.

Patel, A. J., Barochovsky, O., Borges, S., and Lewis, P. D. 1983. Effects of neurotropic drugs on brain cell replication in vivo and in vitro. *Monogr. Neural. Sci.* 9:99–110.

Pelkonen, O. 1980. Environmental influences on human fetal and placental xenobiotic metabolism. *Eur. J. Clin. Pharmacol.* 18:17–24.

Perez-D'Gregorio, R., Miller, R. K., and Ng, W. W. 1984. Fetal toxicity of tellurium dioxide in the Wister rat. *Teratology* 29:50A.

Pinto-Machado, J. 1970. Influence of prenatal administration of busulfan on the postnatal development of mice. Production of a syndrome including hypoplasia of the thymus. *Teratology* 3:363–370.

Plautz, J. R., Levin, A. A., and Miller, R. K. 1980. Fetal and maternal toxicity of cadmium, metallothionein and its distribution in the pregnant Wistar rat. *Teratol.* 26:61.

Plautz, J. R., Levin, A. A., and Miller, R. K. 1981. Fetal placental distributions of cadmium, metallionein and cadmium chloride in the Wistar rat. *Teratol.* 23:56.

Polednak, A. P., and Janerich, D. T. 1983. Uses of available record systems in epidemiology studies of reproductive toxicity. *Am. J. Ind. Med.* 4:329.

Potashnik, G., Ben-Aderet, N., Israeli, R., Yanai-Inbar, I., and Sober, I. 1978. Suppressive effect of 1,2-dibromo-3-chloropropane on human spermatogenesis. *Fertil. Steril.* 30:444–447.

Pratt, R. M. 1984. Hormones, growth factors, and the receptors in normal and abnormal prenatal development. *Issues Rev. Teratol.* 2:189–217.

Pratt, R. M., Dencker, L., and Diewert, B. N. 1984. 2,3,7,8-Tetrachlorodibenzo-*p*-dioxin-induced cleft palate in the mouse. *Teratol. Carcinog. Mutagen.* 4:427–436.

Pratt, R. M., Kim, C. S., and Grove, R. I. 1984b. Role of glucocorticoids and epidermal growth factor in normal and abnormal palatal development. *Curr. Top. Dev. Biol.* 19:81–101.

Preminger, G. M., Koch, W. E., Fried, F. A., and Mandell, J. 1980. Utilization of the chick chorioallantoic membrane for in vitro growth of the embryonic murine kidney. *Am. J. Anat.* 159:17–24.

Rayburn, W., Wible-Kant, J., and Bledsoe, P. 1982. Changing trends in drug use during pregnancy. *J. Reprod. Med.* 27:569.

Redman, C. W. G. 1980. Treatment of hypertension in pregnancy. *Kid. Int.* 18:267.

Redman, C. W. G., and Ounsted, M. K. 1982. Safety for the child of drug treatment for hypertension in pregnancy. *Lancet* II:1237.

Rehan, N. E., Sobrero, A. J., and Fertig, J. W. 1975. The semen of fertile men: Statistical analysis of 1300 men. *Fertil. Steril.* 26:492.

Reilly, R. W., Thompson, J. A., Eielski, R. K., and Severson, C. D. 1967. Estradiol-induced wasting syndrome in neonatal mice. *J. Immunol.* 98:321–330.

Reinisch, J. 1977. Prenatal exposure of human fetuses to synthetic progestin and estrogen affects personality. *Nature (Lond.)* 266:561.

Reinisch, J. M., and Sanders, F. A. 1984. Prenatal gonadal steroidal influences on gender-related behavior. *Prog. Brain Res.* 61:407–416.

Rice, J. M. 1980. Incorporation of perinatal exposure to bioassays for carcinogenicity. In *Proceedings for Workshop on Methodology for Assessing Reproductive Hazards in the Work Place,* eds. P. F. Infante and M. F. Legator, pp. 247–260. Washington, D.C.: U.S. Department of Health and Human Services, publication 81-100.

Rice, J. M. 1984. Exposure to chemical carcinogens during pregnancy: Consequences for mother and conceptus. In *Human Trophoblast Neoplasms,* eds. R. A. Pattillo and R. O. Hussa, pp. 13–49. New York: Plenum.

Rice, J. M., Williams, G. M., Palmer, A. E., London, W. T., and Sly, D. L. 1981. Pathology of gestational choriocarcinoma induced in patas monkeys by ethylnitrosourea given during pregnancy. In *Placenta: Receptors, Pathology and Toxicology,* eds. R. K. Miller and H. A. Thiede, pp. 223–230. London: Saunders.

Rich, K. A., and de Kretser, D. M. 1983. Spermatogenesis and the Sertoli cell. In *The Pituitary and Testis: Clinical and Experimental Studies,* eds. D. M. de Kretser, H. G., Burger, and B. Hudson, pp. 84–105. New York: Springer-Verlag.

Roberts, D. W., and Chapman, J. R. 1981. Concepts essential to the assessment of toxicity to the developing immune system. In *Developmental Toxicology,* eds. C. A. Kimmel and J. Buelke-Sam, pp. 167–189. New York: Raven.

Rodier, P. M. 1978. Behavioral teratology. In *Handbook of Teratology,* vol. 4, pp. 397–428.

Rodier, P. M. 1980. Chronology of neuron development: Animal studies and the clinical implications. *Dev. Med. Child Neurol.* 22:525.

Rosenberg, M. J. 1984. Practical aspects of reproductive surveillance. In *Reproduction: The New Frontier in Occupational and Environmental Health Research,* eds. J. E. Lockey; G. K. Lemasters, and W. R. Keye, Jr., pp. 147–156. New York: Liss.

Rosengarten, H., and Friedhoff, A. J. 1979. Enduring changes in dopamine receptor cells of pups from drug administration to the pregnant and nursing rats. *Science* 203:1133–1135.

Rousseaux, C. G., Nicholson, S., and Schiefer, H. B. 1985. Fetal placental hemorrhage in pregnant CD-1 mice following one oral dose of T-2 toxin. *Can. J. Comp. Med.* 49:95–98.

Rowell, P. P. 1981. The effect of maternal cigarette smoking on the ability of human placental villae to concentrate alpha-aminoisobutyric acid in vitro. *Res. Comm. Subst. Abuse* 2:253–266.

Russell, L. 1977. Observation of rat Sertoli ectoplasmic ("junctional") specializations in their associations with germ cells of the rat testis. *Tissue Cell* 9:475–498.

Russell, L. B., Selby, P. B., von Halle, E., Sheridan, W., and Valcovic, L. 1981. The mouse specific-locus test with agents other than radiation: Interpretation of data and recommendations for future work. *Mutat. Res.* 86:329–354.

Russell, L. D. 1983. Normal testicular structure and methods of evaluation under experimental and disruptive conditions. In *Reproductive and Developmental Toxicity of Metals,* eds. T. W. Clarkson, G. F. Nordberg, and P. R. Sager, pp. 227–252. New York: Plenum.

Russell, W. L., Kelly, E. M., Hunsicker, P. R., Bangham, J. W., Maddux, S. C., and Phipps, E. L. 1979. Specific-locus test shows ethylnitrosourea to be the most potent mutagen in the mouse. *Proc. Natl. Acad. Sci. USA* 76:5818–5819.

Rustia, M., and Shubik, P. 1976. Prenatal induction of neurogenic tumors in hamsters by precursors of ethylurea and sodium nitrite. *J. NCI* 52:605–608.

Sager, P. R., Doherty, R. A., and Rodier, P. M. 1982. Effects of methyl mercury on developing mouse cerebral cortex. *Exp. Neurol.* 77:179.

Samawickarama, G., and Webb, W. 1979. Acute effects of cadmium during pregnancy and embryo fetal development in the rat. *Environ. Health Perspect.* 28:345–349.

Samawickarama, G., and Webb, W. 1981. The acute toxicity and teratogenicity of cadmium in the pregnant rat. *J. Appl. Toxicol.* 1:264–269.

Sandifer, S. H., Wilkins, R. T., Loadholt, C. B., Lane, L. G., and Eldridge, J. C. 1979. Spermatogenesis in agricultural workers exposed to dibromochloropropane (DBCP). *Bull. Environ. Contam. Toxicol.* 23:703–710.

Sastry, B. V. R., Olubadewo, J., Harbison, R., and Schmidt, D. 1977. *Arch Int. Pharmacol.* 229:23–36.

Saxen, L., and Repora, J. 1969. In *Genital Defects.* New York: Holt Rinehart and Winston.

Saxen, L. 1974. Twenty years of study of the etiology of congenital malformations in Finland. *Issues Rev. Teratology* 1:73–110.

Schilsky, R. L., Sherins, R. J., Hubbard, S. M., Wesley, M. N., Young, R. C., and DeVita, V. T. 1981. Long-term follow-up of ovarian function in women treated with MOPP chemotherapy for Hodgkin's disease. *Am. J.Med.* 71:552–556.

Schlumpf, M., Shoemaker, W. J., and Bloom, F. E. 1980. Innervation of embryonic rat cerebral cortex by catecholamine-containing fibers. *J. Comp. Neurol.* 192:361–376.

Schuler, R. L., Hardin, B. D., and Niemeier, R. W. 1982. *Drosophila* as a tool for the rapid assessment of chemicals for teratogenicity. *Teratog. Carcinog. Mutagen.* 2:293–301.

Schultz, T. W., Dumont, J. N., Clark, B. R., and Buchanan, M. V. 1982. Embryotoxic and teratogenic effects of aqueous extracts of tar from a coal gasification electrostatic precipitator. *Teratog. Carcinog. Mutagen.* 2:1–11.

Schwartz, D., and Mayaux, M. J. 1982. Female fecundatio as a function of age. *N. Engl. J. Med.* 307:404–406.

Schwartz, W. J. 1983. Early mammalian embryonic development. *Am. J. Ind. Med.* 4:51–61.

Sclarren, S. K., and Smith, D. W. 1978. Fetal alcohol syndrome. *N. Engl. J. Med.* 298:1063.

Scott, W. J., Jr. 1977. Cell duct in reduced proliferative rate. In *Handbook of Teratology,* eds. J. G. Wilson and F. C. Fraser, vol. 2, pp. 81–88. New York: Plenum.

Searle, A. G. 1977. The specific locus test in the mouse. In *Handbook of Mutagenicity Test Procedures,* eds. B. J. Kilbey, M. Legator, W. Nichols, and C.Ramel, pp. 311–324. New York: Elsevier Scientific.

Segal, S. J., ed. 1985. *Gossypol—A potential contraceptive for men.* New York: Plenum.

Setchell, B. P., and Waits, G. M. H. 1970. Changes in the permeability of the testicular capillaries and of the blood-testis barrier after injection of cadmium chloride in the rat. *J. Endocrinol.* 47:81–86.

Setchell, B. P., and Waits, g. M. H. 1975. The blood-testis barrier. In *Handbook of Physiology,* eds. D. W. Hamilton and R. O. Greep, section 7, vol. 5, pp. 143–172. Baltimore: Williams & Wilkins.

Sever, L. E., and Hessol, N. A. 1984. Overall design considerations in male and female occupational reproductive studies. In *Reproduction: The New Frontier in Occupational and Environmental Health Research,* eds. J. E. Lockey, g. K. Lemasteᵣ, and W. R. Keye, Jr., pp. 15–47. New York: Liss.

Shalet, S. M. 1980. Effects of cancer chemotherapy on gonadal function of patients. *Cancer Treat. Rev.* 7:141–152.

Shapiro, R. 1961. The effect of maternal ingestion of iophenoxic acid. *N. Engl. J. Med.* 264:378–381.

Sheehan, D. M., Branham, W. S., Medlock, K. L., Olsen, M. E., and Zehr, D. 1980. Estrogen plasma binding and regulation of development in the neonatal rat. *Teratology* 21:68A.

Shepard, T. 1980. *Catalog of Teratogenic Agents.* Baltimore: Johns Hopkins University Press.

Shepard, T. H., Fantel, A. G., Mirkes, P. E., Campbell, J. C., Faustman-Watts, E., Campbell, M., and Juchau, M. R. 1983. Teratology testing: I. Development and status of short-term prescreens. II. Biotransformation of teratogens as studied in whole embryo culture. In *Developmental Pharmacology,* eds. S. M. MacLeod, A. B. Okey, and S. P. Spielberg, pp. 147–164. New York: Liss.

Sher, J., Hailey, D., and Beard, R. 1972. The effects of diazepam on the fetus. *J. Obstet. Gynecol. Brit. Comm.* 79:635–638.

Shiromizu, K., and Mattison, D. R. 1982. Oocyte destruction by intraovarian injection of benzo(a)pyrene. In *Microsomes, Drug Oxidation, and Drug Toxicity,* eds. R. Sato and R. Kato, pp. 559–560. New York: Wiley-Intersciences.

Shoemaker, W. J., Baetge, G., Azad, R., Sapin, V., and Bloom, F. E. 1983. Effect of prenatal alcohol exposure on amine and peptide neurotransmitter systems. *Monogr. Neural. Sci.* 9:130–139.

Shum, S., Jensen, N. M., and Nebert, D. 1979. The murine Ah locus; Its utero toxicity and teratogenesis associated with genetic differences in benzo(a)pyrene metabolism. *Teratology* 20:365.

Simmons, R. D., Kellogg, C. K., and Miller, R. K. 1984a. Prenatal diazepam exposures in rats: Long-lasting, receptor-mediated effects on hypothalamic norepinephrine-containing neurons. *Brain Res.* 293:73–83.

Simmons, R. D., Miller, R. K., and Kellogg, C. K. 1984b. Prenatal exposure to diazepam alters central and peripheral responses to stress in adult rat offspring. *Brain Res.* 307:39–46.

Sims, P., and Grover, P. L. 1974. Hypoxides and polycyclic aromatic hydrocarbon metabolism in carcinogenesis. *Adv. Can. Res.* 20:165–274.

Siris, E. S., Leventhal, B. G., and Vaitukaitis, J. L. 1976. Effects of childhood leukemia and chemotherapy on puberty and reproductive functions in girls. *N. Engl. Med. J.* 294:1143–1146.

Smith, C. G. 1982. Drug effects on male sexual function. *Clin. Obstet. gynecol.* 25:525–531.

Smith, C. G. B., Beesch, N. F., Smith, R. G., and Beesch, P. K. 1979. Effects of tetrahydrocannabinol on the hypothalamic–pituitary axis in the ovariectomized rhesus monkey. *Fertil. Steril.* 31:335–339.

Smith, C. J. 1983. Reproductive toxicity: Hypothalamic–pituitary mechanisms. *Am. J. Ind. Med.* 4:107–112.

Snell, K. 1985. Biochemical disturbances of fetal development. *Biochem. Soc. Trans.* 13:73–75.

Song, B.-J., Gelboin, H. B., Park, S. S., Tsokos, J. C., and Friedman, F. K. 1985. Monoclonal antibody-directed radioimmunoassay detects cytochrome P450 in human placenta and lymphocytes. *Science* 228:490–492.

Spatz, M., and Laquer, G. 1967. Transplacental induction of tumors in Spraque-Dawley rats with crude cycad material. *J. NCI* 38:233–245.

Stave, U. 1978. *Perinatal Physiology.* New York: Plenum.

Steinberger, E., and Steinberger, A. 1975. Spermatogenic function of the testis. In *Handbook of Physiology,* eds. D. W. Hamilton and R. O. Greep, section 7, vol. 5, pp. 1–19. Baltimore: Williams & Wilkins.

Stern, R. S., Faranz, R., and Baum, C. 1984. Isotretinoin in pregnancy. *J. Am. Acad. Dermatol.* 10:851.

Stillman, R. J. 1982. In utero exposure to diethylstilbestrol. *Amer. J. Obstet. Gynecol.* 142:905–921.

Streissguth, A. P., Landesman-Dwyer, S., Martin, J. C., and Smith, D. W. 1980. Teratogenic effects of alcohol in humans and laboratory animals. *Science* 209:353–361.

Streissguth, A., Martin, D. C., Barr, H. M., Sandman, B. M., Kirchner, G. L., and Darby, B. L. 1984. Intrauterine alcohol and nicotine exposure: Attention and reaction time in 4-year-old children. *Dev. Psychol.* 20:533.

Sullivan, F. M. 1983. Behavioral teratology. Eleventh Conference of the European Teratology Society, Paris, pp. 29–31.

Suzuki, K., and Lee, I. P. 1981. Induction of aryl hydrocarbon hydroxylase and epoxide hydrolase in rat liver, kidney, testis, prostate glands, and stomach by a potent nematocide, 1,2-dibromo-3-chloropropane. *Toxicol. Appl. Pharmacol.* 58:151–155.

Tarlatzis, B. C., Sanyal, M. K., biggers, W. J., and Naftolin, F. 1984. Continuous culture of the postimplantation rat conceptus. *Biol. Reprod.* 31:415–426.

Tauber, P. F., Zaneveld, L. J. D., Propping, D., and Schumacher, G. F. B. 1975. Components of human sperm ejaculates. I. Spermatozoa, fructose, immunoglobins, albumin, lactoferrin, transferrin, and other plasma proteins. *J. Reprod. Fertil.* 43:249–267.

Taylor, A. N., Branch, B. J., and Kokka, N. 1982a. Effects of maternal ethanol consumption in rats on basal and rhythmic pituitary–adrenal function in neonatal offspring. *Psychoneuroendocrinology* 7:49–58.

Taylor, A. N., Branch, B. J., Kokka, N., and Poland, R. E. 1983. Neonatal and long-term neuroendocrine effects of fetal alcohol exposure. *Monogr. Neural. Sci.* 9:140–152.

Taylor, A. N., Branch, B. J., Liu, S. H., and Kokka, N. 1982b. Long-term effects of fetal ethanol exposure on pituitary–adrenal response to stress. *Pharmacol. Biochem. Behav.* 16:585–589.

Teramoto, S., Saito, R., Aoyama, H., and Shirasu, Y. 1980. Dominant lethal mutation induced in male rats by 1,2-dibromo-3-chloropropane (DBCP). *Mutat. Res.* 77:71–78.

Thomas, P. T., and Hindsall, r. D. 1979. The effect of perinatal exposure to tetrachlorodibenzo-o-dioxin on the immune response of young mice. *Drug. Chem. Toxicol.* 2:77–98.

Torkelson, T. R., Sadek, S. E., Rowe, V.K., Kodama, J. K., Anderson, H. H., Loquvam, G. S., and Hine, C. H. 1961. Toxicologic investigations of 1,2-dibromo-3-chloropropane. *Toxicol. Appl. Pharmacol.* 3:545–559.

Transler, D. G., and Fraser, F. C. 1977. Time-position relationships with particular reference to cleft lip and cleft palate. In *Handbook of Teratology,* eds. J. G. Wilson and F. C. Fraser, vol. 2, pp. 271–292.

Trapp, B. D., and Richelson, E. 1980. Usefulness for neurotoxicology of rotation-mediated aggregating cell cultures. In *Experimental and Clinical Neurotoxicology,* eds. P. S. Spencer and H. H. Schaumberg, pp. 803–819. Baltimore: Williams & Wilkins.

Trinder, E. 1979. Auditory fusion: A critical test with implication in differential diagnosis. *Br. J. Audiol.* 13:143–147.

Tsunoda, Y., and Chang, M. C. 1976. Fertilizing ability in vivo and in vitro of spermatozoa of rats and mice treated with a-chlorohydrin. *J. Reprod. Fertil.* 46:401–406.

Tuchmann-Duplessis, H., Auroux, M., and Haegel, P., eds. 1976. *Illustrated Human Embryology,* vol. 3. France: Masson and Company.

Tyler, M. S., and Pratt, R. M. 1980. Effect of epidermal growth factor on secondary palatal epithelium in vitro: Tissue isolation and recombination studies. *J. Embryol. Exp. Morphol.* 58:93–106.

Van der Veen, F., and Fox, H. 1982. The effects of cigarette smoking on the placenta: A light and electron microscopic study. *Placenta* 3:243–256.

Vorhees, C. V. 1983. Behavioral teratogenicity testing as a method of screening for hazards to human health: A methodological proposal. *Neurobehav. Toxicol. Teratol.* 5:469–474.

Vorhees, C. V., and Butcher, R. E. 1982. Behavioral teratogenicity. In *Developmental Toxicology,* ed. K. Snell, pp. 247–298. New York: Praeger.

Vos, J., and Moore, J. 1974. Suppression of cellular immunity in mice by maternal treatment with 2,3,7,8-tetrachlorodibenzo-p-dioxin. *Int. Arch Allergy Appl. Immunol.* 47:777–794.

Vreeburg, J. T. M., van Andel, M. V., Kort, W. J., and Westbroek, D. L. 1974. The effect of hemicastration on daily sperm output in the rat as measured by a new method. *J. Reprod. Fertil.* 41:355–359.

Waddell, W., and Marlowe, C. 1981. Transfer of drugs across the placenta. *Pharm. Therap.* 14:375–390.

Waller, D. P., Killinger, J. M., and Zaneveld, L. J. D. 1985. Physiology and toxicology of the male reproductive tract. In *Endocrine Toxicology,* eds. J. A. Thomas, K. S. Korach, and J. A. McLachlan, pp. 269–333. New York: Raven.

Warkany, J. 1976. Warfarin embryopathy. *Teratology* 14:205.

Warkany, J. 1978. Aminopterin and methotrexate: Folic acid deficiency. *Teratology* 17:353.

Warner, A. E., Guthrie, S. C., and Gilula, N. B. 1984. Antibodies to gap-junctional protein selectively disrupt junctional communication in the early amphibian embryo. *Nature (Lond.)* 311:127–131.

Ways, S. C., and Bern, H. A. 1979. Long-term effects of neonatal treatment with cortisol and/or estrogen in the female BALB/c mouse. *Proc. Soc. Exp. Biol. Med.* 160:94–98.

Webb, M. 1972. Protection by zinc against cadmium toxicity. *Biochem. Pharmacol.* 21:2767–2771.

Webb, P. D., Hole, N., McLaughlin, P. J., Stern, P. L., and Johnson, P. 1986. Biochemical and immunological aspects of the human trophoblast cell surface. *Trophoblast Res.,* in press.

Weir, B. J., and Rollands, I. W. 1977. Ovulation and atresia. In *The Ovary,* 2d ed., vol. 1, *General Aspects,* eds. S. Zucherman and B. J. Weir, pp. 265–302. New York: Academic.

Welch, R., Harrison, J., Gommi, B., Poppers, P., Finster, M., and Conney, A. 1969. Stimulatory effect of cigarette smoking and the hydroxylation of benzo(a)pyrene by enzymes in human placenta. *Clin. Pharm. Therap.* 10:100–110.

Whorton, D., Krauss, R.M., Marshall, S., and Milby, T. H. 1977. Infertility in male pesticide workers. *Lancet* 2:1259–1261.

Wide, M. 1983. Lead and development of the early embryo. In *Reproductive and Developmental Toxicity of Metals,* eds. T. Clarkson, G. Nordberg, and P. Sager, pp. 343–356. New York: Plenum.

Wier, P. J., and Miller, R. K. 1986. The pharmacokinetics of cadmium in the dually perfused human placenta. *Trophoblast Res.,* in press.

Wilcox, A. J. 1983. Surveillance of pregnancy loss and human populations. *Am. J. Ind. Med.* 4:285–291.

Wilk, A. L., Greenberg, J. H., Horigan, E. A., Pratt, R. M., and Martin, G. R. 1980. Detection of teratogenic compounds using differentiating embryonic cells in culture. *In Vitro* 16:269–276.

Willhite, C. 1981. Congenital malformations induced by laetrile. *Science* 215:513–515.

Willhite, C. 1982. Developmental toxicology of acetonitrile in the golden hamster. *Teratology* 27:313.

Williams, K. E. 1982. Biochemical mechanisms of teratogenesis. In *Developmental Toxicology,* ed. K. Snell, pp. 93–122. New York: Praeger.

Williams, K. E., Kidston, E. M., Beck, F., and Lloyd, J. B. 1975a. Quantitative studies in pinocytosis. I. Kinetics of uptake of ^{125}I polyvinyl pyrrolidone by rat yolk sac cultured in vitro. *J. Cell Biol.* 64:113–122.

Williams, K. E., Kidston, E. M., Beck, F., and Lloyd, J. B. 1975b. Quantitative studies of pinocytosis. II. Kinetics and protein uptake and digestion by rat yolk sac cultured in vitro. *J. Cell Biol.* 64:123–134.

Williams, K. E., Roberts, G. Kidston, M. E., Beck, F., and Lloyd, J. B. 1976. Inhibition of pinocytosis in rat yolk sac by trypan blue. *Teratology* 14:343–354.

Wilson, J. G. 1972. Environmental effects on development—Teratology. In *Pathophysiology of Gestation,* ed. N. F. Affli, vol. II, pp. 270–320. New York: Academic.

Wilson, J. g. 1977. Current status of teratology—General principles and mechanisms derived from animal studies. In *Handbook of Teratology,* eds. J. G. Wilson and F. C. Fraser, vol. 1, pp. 47–74. New York: Plenum.

Wilson, J. G. 1978. Survey of in vitro systems: Their potential use in teratogenicity screening. In *Handbook of Teratology,* eds. J. G. Wilson and F. C. Fraser, vol. 4, pp. 135–153. New York: Plenum.

Wilson, J. G., and Fraser, F. C., eds. 1977. *Handbook of Teratology,* vol. 1. New York: Plenum.

Wilson, J. G., and Warkany, J., eds. 1965. *Teratology Principles and Techniques.* Chicago: University of Chicago Press.

Witschi, E. 1962. Development of the rat. In *Growth Including Reproduction and Morphological Development,* eds. P. Altman and D. S. Dittmer, pp. 304–414. Washington, D.C.: Federal of American Societies for Experimental Biology.

Woodward, D. J., Hoffer, B. J., Siggins, G. R., and Bloom, F. E. 1972. The ontogenetic development of synpatic junctions, synaptic activation and responsiveness to neurotransmitter substances in rat cerebellar Perkinje cells. *Brain Res.* 34:73–97.

Wyrobek, A. J., Gordon, L. A., Burkhart, J. G., Francis, M. W., Kapp, R. W., Jr., Letz, G., Malling, H. V., Topham, J. C., and Whorton, M. D. 1983. An evaluation of human sperm as indicators of chemically induced alterations of spermatogenic function: A report of the U.S. Environmental Protection Agency Gene-Tox Program. *Mutat. Res.* 115:73–148.

Wyrobek, A. J., Watchmaker, G., and Gordon, L. 1984. An evaluation of sperm tests as indicators of germ-cell damage in men exposed to chemical or physical agents. *Prog. Clin. Biol. Res.* 160:385–405.

Yerusholmy, J. 1971. The relationship of parents' cigarette smoking to outcome of pregnancy. *Am. J. Epidemiol.* 93:143–158.

Young, M., Boyd, R., Longo, L., and Telgdy, G. 1981. *Placenta Transfer: Methods and Interpretations.* London: Saunders.

References Added in Proof

Brent, R. L., and Franklin, J. B. 1960. Uterine vascular clamping: New procedure for the study of congenital malformations. *Science* 132:89–91.

Brent, R. L., and Gorson, R. O. 1972. Radiation exposure in pregnancy. *Current Probl. Diagn. Radiol.* 2:1–48.

Bruce, N. W. 1972. Effects of temporary uterine ischaemia on the rat embryo at different maternal abdominal temperatures. *J. Reprod. Fertil.* 30:63–69.

Craig, J. M. 1966. Mechanism of serotonin induced abortion in rats. *Arch. Pathol. Lab. Med.* 81:257–263.

Franklin, J. B., and Brent, R. L. 1964. The effect of uterine vascular clamping on the developments of rat embryos three to fourteen days. *J. Morphol.* 115:273–290.

Honey, D. P., Robson, J. M., and Sullivan, F. M. 1967. Mechanism of inhibitory action of 5-hydroxytryptamine on placental functions. *Am. J. Obstet. Gynecol.* 99:250–259.

Lehtovista, P., and Forss, M. 1978. The acute effect of smoking on intervillous blood flow of the placenta. *Brit. J. Obstet. Gynecol.* 85:729–732.

Leist, K. H., and Graviler, J. 1974. Fetal pathology in rats following uterine-vessel clamping on day 14 of gestation. *Teratology* 10:55–67.

Rankin, J. H. 1978. Role of prostaglandins in the maintenance of placental circulation. In *Advances in Prostaglandins and Thromboxane Research,* eds. F. Coceani and P. M. Olley, pp. 261–269. New York: Raven Press.

Robson, J. M., and Sullivan, F. M. 1966. Analysis of actions of 5-hydroxytryptamine in pregnancy. *J. Physiol.* 184:717–732.

Slikker, W., Jr., Hill, D. E., and Young, J. P. 1982. Comparison of the transplacental pharmacokinetics of 17β-estradiol and diethylstilbestrol in the subhuman primate. *J. Pharm. Expt. Therap.* 221:173–182.

Chapter 8

Toxicity of Antineoplastic Drugs, with Special Reference to Teratogenesis, Carcinogenesis, and the Reproductive System

Charles L. Litterst

INTRODUCTION

The use of drugs in the clinical treatment of cancer has mushroomed in the past 15 years. During the late 1940s and throughout the 1950s, introduction of new drugs for this purpose occurred only sporadically and at a relatively slow rate. However, the mid to late 1960s saw a great surge in the introduction of new anticancer drugs, and there are now several dozen agents that are widely used clinically to treat various forms of human cancer, and several dozen other agents that are less widely used or whose use has been discontinued. Although the biological activity of some of these agents can be roughly grouped by chemical class (e.g., alkylating agents, antimetabolites, etc.), individual differences in structure, solubility, pharmacokinetics, metabolism, etc. make it difficult to adequately cover all drugs by such a generalization. Section II presents a capsular look at the relatively immediate toxic effects of nearly 30 standard, clinically useful anticancer drugs, as well as nearly a dozen of the most promising experimental agents (Table 1). Toxicity is mainly from what has been

The author wishes to thank Beverly Sisco, Laura Alpert, and Colleen Donnelly for their skillful typing of the manuscript. In addition, the assistance of the Investigation Drug Branch, National Cancer Institute, is gratefully acknowledged for their recommendations about the most promising investigational drugs.

Table 1 Drugs Discussed in Section II and Section III

Preferred name	Chemical name	Synonyms
Amsacrine	4'[9-Acridinylamino]-methansulfon-m-anisidine	AMSA
L-asparaginase	L-Asparagine amidohydrolase; an incompletely characterized enzyme with molecular weight 133,000 ± 5000	Elspar
5-Azacytidine	4-Amino-1-β-D-ribofuranosyl-s-triazin-2(1H)-one	
AZQ	2,5-Diaziridinyl-3,6-bis-(carboethoxyamino)-1,4-benzoquinone	Aziridinyl-benzoquinone
Bisantrene	9,10-Anthracenedicarboxaldehyde bis[(4,5-dihydro-1H-imidazole-2-yl) hydrazone]dihydrochloride	
Bleomycin	Mixture of several high-molecular-weight (>1255) polypeptides	
Busulfan	1,4-Butanediol, dimethanesulfonate	Myleran
Carboplatin	cis-Diammine-1,1-cyclobutane dicarboxylate platinum(II)	CBDCA; JM-8
Carmustine	1,3-Bis(2-chloroethyl)-1-nitrosourea	BCNU
Chlorambucil	4-[p-[Bis(2-chloroethyl)amino] phenyl]-butyric acid	Leukeran
Cisplatinum	cis-Diammine dichloroplatinum(II)	Cisplatin; Platinol; DDP
Cyclo-phosphamide	2-[Bis(2-chloroethyl)amino]-tetrahydro-2-H-1,3,2-oxazaphorine-2-oxide	Cytoxan; CTX; Endoxan
Cytarabine	1-β-D-Arabinofuranosylcytosine	Ara-C; cytosine arabinoside
Dacarbazine	5-(3,3-Dimethyl-1-triazenyl)-1H-imidazole-4-carboxamide	DTIC; imidazole carboxamide
Dactinomycin	Actinomycin[Thre-Val-Pro-Sar-Meval]; $C_{62}H_{86}N_{12}O_{16}$	Actinomycin D
Daunorubicin	(8S-cis)-8-Acetyl-10-[(3-amino-2,3,6-trideoxy-α-L-$lyxo$-hexapyranosyl)oxy]-7,8,9,10-tetrahydro-6,8,11-trihydroxy-1-methoxy-5,12-naphthacenedione	Daunomycin; rubidomycin
Deoxycoformycin	(R)-3-(2-Deoxy-β-D-erythropentofuranosyl)-3,6,7,8-tetrahydroimidazo(4,5-d)(1,3) diazepin-8-ol	Pentostatin
Doxorubicin	(8S-cis)-10-[(3-Amino-2,3,6-trideoxy-α-L-$lyxo$-hexopyranosyl)oxy]-7,8,9,10-tetra-hydro-6,8,11-trihydroxy-8-(hydroxyacetyl)-1-methoxy-5,12-naphthacenedione	Adriamycin
Etoposide	4-Demethyl-epipodophyllotoxin 9-(4,6-O-ethylidene-β-D-glucopyranoside)	VP-16
Fluorouracil	5-Fluor-2,4(1H,3H)-pyrimidinedione	5-FU
Hexamethyl-melamine	(1,3,5-Triazine-2,4,6-triyltrinitrilo) hexakis(methanol)	HMM
Isophosphamide	3-(2-Chloroethyl)-2-[(2-chloroethyl)amino] tetrahydro-2H-1,3,2–oxazaphosphorine 2-oxide	Ifosphamide

Table 1   Drugs Discussed in Section II and Section III (*Continued*)

Preferred name	Chemical name	Synonyms
Indicine N-oxide	(−)-$\alpha\beta$-Dihydroxy-α-isoproylbutyrate-1-methyl-1,2-dehydro-7β-hydroxy-8αpyrrolizidine N-oxide	
Lomustine	1-(2-Chloroethyl)-3-cyclohexyl-1-nitrosourea	CCNU
Mechlorethamine	2,2'-Dichloro-N-methyldiethylamine	Nitrogen mustard; HN$_2$; Mustargen
Melphalan	4-[Bis(2-chloroethyl)amino]-L-phenylalanine	Phenylalanine mustard; L-PAM; Alkeran; L-Sarcolysin
Mercaptopurine	6-Purinethiol	6-MP
Methotrexate	N-[p[[(2,4-Diamino-6-pteridinyl)methyl]methylamino]benzoyl] glutamic acid	MTX
Methyl GAG	2,2'-(1-Methyl-1,2-ethanediylidene)bis-[hydrazine carboximidamide]	Methylglyoxal bis(guanylhydrazone)
Mitomycin C	6-Amino-1,1a,2,8,8a,8b-hexahydro-8-(hydroxymethyl)-8a-methoxy-5-methylazirino(2',3':3,4)pyrrolo(1,2a)-indole-4,7-dine carbamate ester	Mutamycin
Mitoxantrone	1,4-Dihydroxy-5,8-bis[[2-[(2-hydroxyethyl)amino]ethyl]amino]-9,10-anthracenedione dihydrochloride	Dihydroxy-anthracinedione; DHAD
Procarbazine	N-Isopropyl-α-(2-methylhydrazino)-p-toluamide	Matulane; Natulan
Semustine	1-(2-Chloroethyl)-3-(4-methylcyclohexyl)-1-nitrosourea	Methyl-CCNU
Streptozotocin	2-Deoxy-2-(3-methyl-3-nitrosoureido)-D-glucopyranose	
Teniposide	4'-Demethylepipodophyllotoxin-9-(4,6,O,2-thenylidene-β-D-glucopyranoside)	VM-26
ThioTEPA	Tris-(1-aziridinyl)phosphine sulfide	Triethylene thiophosphoramide
Vinblastine	A high-molecular-weight antibiotic with formula $C_{46}H_{58}N_4O_9$	Velban
Vincristine	A high-molecular-weight antibiotic with formula $C_{46}H_{58}N_4O_{14}S$	Oncovin

observed in patients, but animal data are presented where relevant. Table 2 presents animal acute median lethality data for all of the agents discussed in the text. No attempt was made to include toxicity data on any of the numerous steroidal agents (e.g., prednisone, Tamoxifen, etc.) that are widely used. It was felt that this class of agents presented specific and unique toxicities and was a large enough group of generally utilized drugs to preclude its inclusion in this more restricted application.

In addition to the acute toxicity data presented in Section II, Section III presents toxicity data of a more chronic nature, and focuses on reproductive and carcinogenic effects (Table 3). This section is of necessity only an introduction to the areas and is

Table 2 Acute Median Lethal Doses for Antineoplastic Agents Discussed in the Text[a]

	Mouse LD50		Rat LD50	
Drug	**mg/kg**	**Reference**	**mg/kg**	**Reference**
Amsacrine	33.7 (iv)	Henry et al. (1980)		
L-Asparaginase	184–240	*Merck Index*, 9th ed.	36–46	*Merck Index*, 9th ed.
Azacytidine	116	Palm and Kensler (1971)		
AZQ	26.2–34.2	Unpublished[b]		
Bisantrene	225	Unpublished[b]		
Bleomycin	200	IARC (1981)		
	54	Houchens et al. (1977)		
Busulfan	116	Unpublished[b]	1.8	Scherf and Schmahl (1975)
			26	Hebborn et al. (1965)
			60	Murphy (1959)
Carboplatin	181	Bradner and Schurig (1981)	61	Unpublished[b]
Carmustine	32	Houchens et al. (1977)	30 (oral)	IARC (1981)
	42–56	Guarino et al. (1979)		
	19 (oral)	IARC (1981)		
Chlorambucil	64	Unpublished[b]	28	Hebborn et al. (1985)
			23–28	Chaube and Murphy (1968)
			24	Murphy (1959)
Cisplatinum	17.8	Schurig et al. (1980)	7.7	Ward and Fauvie (1976)
	15	Taniguchi and Baba (1982)		
Cyclophosphamide	159	Houchens et al. (1977)	160	IARC (1975)
	381–567	Unpublished[b]	182	Chaube et al. (1967)
	550	Chaube et al. (1967)	190	Scherf and Schmahl (1975)

(See footnotes on p. 315.)

Table 2 Acute Median Lethal Doses for Antineoplastic Agents Discussed in the Text[a] (Continued)

Drug	Mouse LD50 mg/kg	Reference	Rat LD50 mg/kg	Reference
Cytarabine	3800–4300 4407–4751	Guarino et al. (1979) Unpublished[b]		
Dacarbazine	1101 859–1400	Unpublished[b] Guarino et al. (1979)		
Dactinomycin	0.8 0.76	Houchens et al. (1977) Philips et al. (1960b)	0.4	Philips et al. (1960b)
Daunorubicin	7.6 5.6 8.0–9.2	Unpublished[b] IARC (1976) Guarino et al. (1979)		
Deoxycoformycin	100	Smyth et al. (1980)		
Doxorubicin	20.8 14.4 18–23	DiMarco et al. (1969) Houchens et al. (1977) Guarino et al. (1979)	12.6 (iv)	IARC (1976)
Etoposide	79–198	Unpublished[b]		
Fluorouracil	200 160 102–357	Harrison et al. (1978) Houghton et al. (1979) Guarino et al. (1979)	500	Scherf and Schmahl (1975)
Methyl GAG	157	Unpublished[b]		
Hexamethylmelamine	220	Philips and Thiersch (1950)	265	Philips and Thiersch (1950)
Isophosphamide	540	Greco et al. (1979)		
Indicine N-oxide	3700–4800	Unpublished[b]		
Lomustine	53–56	Thompson and Larson (1972)	70 (oral)	Thompson and Larson (1972)

Compound				
	5.5–4.5	Guarino et al. (1975)	1.1 (iv) 2	Merck Index, 9th ed. Murphy (1959)
Melphalan	23 20–29	Unpublished[b] Guarino et al. (1979)	18	Unpublished[b]
Mercaptopurine	240	Philips et al. (1956)	250 250	Philips et al. (1956) Scherf and Schmahl (1975)
Methotrexate	94	IARC (1981)	14 6–25	Scherf and Schmahl (1975) IARC (1981)
Mitomycin C	8.5 11–14 5–6	Philips et al. (1960a) Guarino et al. (1979) Hata (1978)	2.5 2.5 (iv) 3.0	Philips et al. (1960a) Hata (1978) Scherf and Schmahl (1975)
Mitoxantrone	9.7–11.3 (iv)	Henderson et al. (1982)	4.8–5.2 (iv)	Henderson et al. (1982)
Procarbazine	1320 (oral)	IARC (1981)	785 (oral) 350	Goldenthal (1971) Scherf and Schmahl (1975)
Semustine	38–73	Unpublished[b]	80	Unpublished[b]
Streptozotocin	264 (oral) 388	Evans et al. (1965) Unpublished[b]	138 (iv)	Merck Index, 9th ed.
Teniposide	80	Unpublished[b]		
ThioTEPA	27	Guarino et al. (1979)	8 15	Murphy (1959) Scherf and Schmahl (1975) (1975)
Vinblastine	3.6 5.6	Houchens et al. (1977) Nemeth et al. (1970)	2.2 2.0	Nemeth et al. (1970) Scherf and Schmahl (1975)
Vincristine	2.0–4.9 3.2 4.7	Guarino et al. (1979) Houchens et al. (1977) Nemeth et al. (1970)	1.2	Nemeth et al. (1970)

[a]Unless specifically noted, all values are for a single intraperitoneal injection to adult male animals, with observation times of either 14 or 30 days. Multiple values or ranges of values indicate different strains, different vehicles, multiple determinations, etc.

[b]Data from the files of the Toxicology Branch, National Cancer Institute, Bethesda, Md.

Table 3 Teratogenic and Carcinogenic Potential in Animals of Antineoplastic Drugs Discussed in the Text

Drug	Teratogenic[a]	Carcinogenic[b]
Amsacrine		?
L-Asparaginase	+ (Adamson and Fabro, 1968; Harbison, 1978)	?
Azacytidine	+ (Siefertova et al., 1968)	+ + (IARC, 1981)
AZQ		?
Bisantrene		?
Bleomycin		± (IARC, 1981; Harris, 1975)
Busulfan	+ (Karnofsky, 1967; Sieber and Adamson, 1975; Chaube and Murphy, 1968)	+ + (Dipaolo, 1969; Schmahl, 1975)
Carboplatin		?
Carmsutine	+ (Thompson et al., 1974)	+ (Weisburger, 1977; Schmahl and Habs, 1978, 1980)
Chlorambucil	+ (Sadler and Kochar, 1975; Karnofsky, 1967)	+ + + (Weisburger et al., 1975; (IARC, 1975)
Cisplatinum	+ (Lazar et al., 1979)	+ + (Leopold et al., 1979; IARC, 1981; Kempf and Ivankovic, 1986)
Cyclophosphamide	+ (Karnofsky, 1967; Sieber and Adamson, 1975; Chaube and Murphy, 1968)	+ + + (Weisburger et al., 1975; Schmahl, 1975; Schmahl and Habs, 1978, 1980)
Cytarabine	+ (Ritter et al., 1971)	0 (Weisburger, 1977)
Dacarbazine	+ (Thompson et al., 1975a)	+ + (IARC, 1981; Weisburger et al., 1975; Schmahl and Habs, 1978)
Dactinomycin	+ (Marquardt et al., 1976; Tuchmann-Duplessis et al., 1973; Karnofsky, 1967)	± (Svoboda et al., 1970; Weisburger et al., 1975)

Drug		
Daunorubicin	+ (Thompson et al., 1978)	+ + (Marquardt et al., 1976; Bertazolli et al., 1971; Philips et al., 1975; Weisburger, 1977)
Deoxycoformycin	?	?
Doxorubicin	+ (Thompson et al., 1978)	+ + (Marquardt et al., 1976; Bertazolli et al., 1971; Philips et al., 1975; Weisburger, 1977)
Etoposide	+ (Sieber et al., 1978)	?
Fluorouracil	+ (IARC, 1981; Sieber and Adamson, 1975; Chaube and Murphy, 1968)	O (IARC, 1981; Schmahl and Habs, 1980; Schmahl, 1975)
Methyl GAG	O (Chaube and Murphy, 1968)	?
Hexamethylmelamine	+	?
Isophosphamide	+ (Bus and Gibson, 1973)	+ (Sugimura et al., 1978; IARC, 1981)
Indicine N-oxide	?	?
Lomustine	+ (Thompson et al., 1975b)	+ (Weisburger, 1977)
Mechlorethamine	+ (Danforth and Center, 1954; Karnofsky, 1967; Sieber and Adamson, 1975)	+ + (Boyland and Horning, 1949; Shimkin et al., 1966; Heston, 1953; IARC, 1975)
Melphalan	+ (IARC, 1975)	+ + + (Weisburger et al., 1975; IARC, 1975)
Mercaptopurine	+ (IARC, 1981; Sieber and Adamson, 1975; Harbison, 1978; Chaube and Murphy, 1968)	± (Weisburger, 1977; Schmahl, 1975; Schmahl and Habs, 1978, 1980)
Methotrexate	+ (Milarsky and Gaynor, 1968; Sieber and Adamson, 1975; Harbison, 1978; Chaube and Murphy, 1968)	O (Weisburger, 1977; Schmahl, 1975; Schmahl and Habs, 1978, 1980)

(See footnotes on p. 318.)

Table 3 Teratogenic and Carcinogenic Potential in Animals of Antineoplastic Drugs Discussed in the Text (*Continued*)

Drug	Teratogenic[a]	Carcinogenic[b]
Mitomycin C	+ (Karnofsky, 1967)	+ + (Weisburger et al., 1975; Schmahl, 1975; Schmahl and Habs, 1978)
Mitoxantrone	?	?
Procarbazine	+ (Chaube and Murphy, 1969; Sieber and Adamson, 1975)	+ + (Weisburger et al., 1975; Adamson and Sieber, 1981; Schmahl and Habs, 1978)
Semustine	?	+ (Weisburger et al., 1977)
Streptozotocin	?	+ + (Weisburger et al., 1977)
Teniposide	+ (Sieber et al., 1978)	?
ThioTEPA	+ (IARC, 1975; Harbison, 1978)	+ + (Dipaolo, 1969; Adamson and Sieber, 1981; Schmahl, 1975)
Vinblastine	+ (Sieber et al., 1978; Karnofsky, 1967; Harbison, 1978; Sieber and Adamson, 1975)	+ (Weisburger, 1977; Schmahl, 1975; Schmahl and Habs, 1978)
Vincristine	+ (Sieber et al., 1978; Karnofsky, 1967; Harbison, 1978; Sieber and Adamson, 1975)	0 (Weisburger, 1977; Schmahl and Habs, 1978)

[a]Evaluation in either sex of any laboratory species. Includes fetal malformations, embryolethality and/or abortifacient abilities. + indicates definately established and ? indicates either untested or of equivocal standing due to conflicting or absent data.

[b]Rating: 0, 1 or more tests provide negative results; ±, equivocal or insufficient data; +, carcinogenic in only one species, strain, or sex; + +, carcinogenic in more than one species, strain, or sex, or by more than one route of administration; + + +, established human carcinogen; ?, unknown due to lack of data.

not meant to be an exhaustive compilation of numerous clinical experiences. One difficulty in preparing a review in these areas is that most antineoplastic drugs are used in combination regimens, making it difficult to ascribe specific effects to individual agents. No attempt has been made to include carcinogenic or reproductive toxicities of combinations of agents, and where specific drugs are mentioned in these sections, the reader can be certain that these instances are single drugs used without other drug therapy or radiotherapy.

ACUTE TOXIC EFFECTS

Standard Antineoplastic Drugs

Alkylating Agents   This class of antineoplastic drug is the prototype anticancer agent, whose mechanism of action is to transfer a reactive alkyl group onto cellular macromolecules.

The mechanism of action and clinical efficacy of *mechlorethamine* has been widely and most completely studied since the introduction of this agent into clinical medicine more than 40 years ago (Gilman and Philips, 1946). As with all alkylating agents, the major toxic side effects of mechlorethamine are nausea/vomiting and bone-marrow suppression. The former is universal and severe, beginning 3–6 h after dosing. Although symptoms usually have subsided by 18–24 h after onset, some patients have nausea and vomiting persist for up to 36 h. Some relief may be obtained by administration of systemic antiemetics. Bone-marrow suppression is characterized by decreases in all elements, with the leukocyte nadir occurring 10–14 days after drug administration. General recovery is by day 28. Management of this side effect is more difficult than with other alkylating agents developed later, because mechlorethamine is usually administered intravenously and thus marrow suppression is harder to control than with the newer, orally administered agents. Mechlorethamine is a highly irritating drug, related chemically to the vesicants utilized as chemical warfare agents. Consequently, mechlorethamine administration is characterized by numerous and often severe local reactions, which may be complicated by the highly acidic nature of the drug formulation. Thrombophlebitis is common within several days after administration and is characterized by a bluish-grey discoloration along the vein. Following extravasation, phlebitis, local pain, and inflammation will occur within hours and will be followed by necrosis and ulceration.

When mechlorethamine is utilized topically to treat mycosis fungoides and psoriasis, it causes two main cutaneous reactions. The first is a primary irritation presenting as erythema, pruritis, and burning. This irritation occurs within 2–3 weeks of commencing therapy and frequently resolves even with continued drug use. The second cutaneous reaction can be the dose-limiting toxicity for topical use and is a delayed allergic contact dermatitis, manifested mainly as pruritis but with eczematous dermatitis in some cases. Onset is 1–2 days after drug application. Sensitization occurs only after at least 2 weeks of exposure and may not occur until 12 months or more of therapy. Incidence may range from 28 to 68%. Alopecia is also a common side effect of mechlorethamine—and other alkylating agent—administration. The above reactions reflect the cytotoxic effect of these agents and are common in one degree or another to all alkylating agents. Ototoxicity also is relatively common, particularly when high doses of mechlorethamine are given by regional infusion, and is manifested as tinnitus, high-tone hearing loss, and other signs of eighth-nerve damage. Mechlorethamine also causes menstrual irregularities, which may lead to amenorrhea. In males, azoospermia is common. These effects may be reversible after discontinuation of the drug. Mechlorethamine is embryolethal and teratogenic in rodents by several routes of administration (DiPaolo, 1969; Adamson and Fabro, 1968). It produces various malignant tumors in animals (Boyland and Horning, 1949), but there is no strong evidence to implicate it as a human carcinogen.

Whereas mechlorethamine is the oldest alkylating agent still in widespread clinical use, *cyclophosphamide* (CTX) is the most widely used alkylating agent. Characteristic of the toxicity of this drug is a profound inhibition of the immune system, with depression of both humoral and cellular immune mechanisms. This side effect of CTX has been exploited by making CTX the drug of choice in several nonneoplastic diseases where immune suppression is a desired therapeutic effect, such as nephrotic syndrome and rheumatoid arthritis. CTX lacks the vesicant effect of mechlorethamine but causes a nearly universal nausea, vomiting, and anorexia, particularly when administered intravenously at high doses (60–120 mg/kg). Incidence is less (30–70%) at lower doses (30–40 mg/kg). Onset of nausea and vomiting is delayed about 6 h and can be expected to last 8–12 h. With long-term oral administration, nausea may persist and can be dose-limiting. Bone-marrow suppression, particularly leukopenia, is common and also may be dose-limiting. Thrombocytopenia and anemia also have been widely reported. Nadir of leukopenia is day 7–10, with recovery by day 18–27. Reversible alopecia occurs in 30–50% of patients. Large enough numbers of patients have received the drug over a use history of 15–20 years to reveal relatively uncommon drug-related side-effects. Among the most common are urinary bladder lesions, such as hemorrhagic cystitis and bladder fibrosis. These irritations arise apparently as a result of the excretion in the urine of a high percent of the drug as cytotoxic metabolites (Philips et al., 1961), including the carcinogen acrolein. Cystitis is seen clinically as polyuria, urgency and hematuria, which may persist after discontinuation of drug. A cyclophosphamide-induced pneumonitis has been reported in patients receiving long-term low-dose cyclophosphamide therapy, but not in patients receiving high-dose intermittent infusions. The pneumonitis is an alveolitis with fibroblast infiltration and ultimately the formation of an interstitial fibrosis. The incidence of death from this serious complication is near 40% of affected patients (Willson, 1978). Renal tubular necrosis resulting in renal failure also occurs, and this effect has also been related to the excretion of a toxic metabolite. Another manifestation of renal toxicity is a syndrome of inappropriate antidiuretic hormone secretion, which leads to water intoxication. This effect is of particular concern because patients are usually vigorously hydrated in an attempt to circumvent the hemorrhagic cystitis. Similarly to mechlorethamine, cyclophosphamide produces stomatitis, but ulceration is more common and more severe than with mechlorethamine. Hepatotoxicity with jaundice occurs rarely, and cardiac toxicity, particularly at very high doses (120–240 mg/kg), has been reported (O'Connel and Berenbau, 1974). The cardiac toxicity is a hemorrhagic cardiac necrosis, with electrocardiogram and X-ray evidence of myocardial damage (Slavin et al., 1975). There is also evidence that cyclophosphamide potentiates the cardiac toxicity of anthracyclines (Minow et al., 1975). Cyclophosphamide also produces a unique delayed dental toxicity in animals. As part of a generalized wasting syndrome frequently terminating in death, several authors have reported a variety of dental abnormalities (broken, absent, extranumerary, or extra long teeth), which begin appearing 130 days after a single ip dose (Vahlsing et al., 1975). Koppang et al. (1973) further characterized the abnormalities as being interrupted odotogenesis, with circulatory disturbances, dental constriction, and other tooth defects. Incidence was 76–100% depending on the dose between 75 and 100 mg/kg. As with mechlorethamine, amenorrhea is common and azoospermia also occurs, frequently with total testicular atrophy. Cyclophosphamide is teratogenic in several species, including rhesus monkeys, and also causes increased numbers of resorptions. It causes sterility in humans, and variously malformed children have been born to mothers who received CTX. CTX is carcinogenic in animals, causing lung and bladder tumors after oral or IV dosing, and it is a well established carcinogen in humans, causing not only acute nonlymphocytic leukemia but also bladder tumors.

Isophosphamide is an alkylating agent structurally similar to cyclophosphamide. It was developed for clinical use based on less animal toxicity and greater animal antitumor effect than was seen with cyclophosphamide. Initial trials in humans (Van Dyk et al., 1972) showed substantial toxicity when administered as a single high-dose bolus, however, with nausea/vomiting (94%), gross hematuria (55%), leukopenia (58%), and increased hepatic enzymes (31%). Subsequent studies (Schnitker et al., 1976; Costanzi et al., 1978) using a divided dose schedule (qd × 5) have eliminated the majority of the gross renal and urologic toxicities, but microhematuria detected by microscopic analysis is still detectable with an incidence of 15–40%. All toxicities are reversible and present no clinical difficulties. A small incidence of gross hematuria (10–14%) also is common, but is reversible within 3–5 days. Mild nausea/vomiting is still common in most series (Fossa and Talle, 1980; Costanzi et al., 1978) but nearly absent in others (Rodriguez, 1976). Major hematologic toxicity is leukopenia, with an incidence of 50–65% in most series. The leukopenia is severe enough to be associated with an occasional septic death. Increased liver serum enzymes also are still reported (22–26%), but the increases are mild and easily reversible. A low incidence of mental confusion is consistently reported (11–15%), mainly in patients over 60 years of age. Costanzi et al. (1978) compared a daily times 5 dosing schedule with a single bolus every 3 weeks and found the former schedule to produce a lower incidence and less severe hematuria than the latter. A more recent attempt by Fossa and Talle (1980) to circumvent the bladder toxicity utilized an intravenous antidote (sodium 2-mercaptosuccinate), which chemically combines with acrolein (Scheef et al., 1979). This study resulted in two toxic deaths with symptoms of both sepsis and renal involvement. Creatinine clearance decreased in all patients during the first 7 days of the study but resolved by 4 weeks. Leukopenia was severe ($< 1 \times 10^6$ cells/mm^3) in 54% of the patients and mild to moderate in another 27%. Severe nausea and vomiting occurred in all patients and lasted from 1 to 5 days. All patients reported lethargy and fatigue, and 45% suffered from hallucinations. Thrombophlebitis was frequent, and 45% suffered from hallucinations. Thrombophlebitis was frequent, and alopecia was universal. This side effect had been reported in other divided dose studies at up to 80% incidence. An interesting observation (Van Dyk et al., 1972) was that with single high doses, all patients who did not develop alopecia died within 19 days of the start of therapy with isophosphamide. Whether this was related to disease state or drug effects was not specified. Isophosphamide causes increased resorptions and growth retardation in fetal mice, as well as a large number and various kinds of fetal malformations. There are no data available on similar effects in humans. There is limited evidence to suggest that isophosphamide is mildly carcinogenic in mice.

There are four commonly utilized *nitrosourea* alkylating agents: carmustine, lomustine, semustine, and streptozotocin. The first three drugs are perhaps more widely recognized by their respective acronyms BCNU, CCNU, and methylCCNU, and because of similarities in toxicity they will be discussed together, and separately from streptozotocin. General toxicity of these three agents increases from methyl-CCNU to CCNU to BCNU, with BCNU the most toxic. Dose-limiting toxicity for CCNU, BCNU, and methylCCNU is myelosuppression, manifesting mainly as leukopenia and thrombocytopenia. Because of the ability of the nitrosoureas to inhibit stem-cell reproduction, bone-marrow effects are delayed both in onset and in recovery, and all elements are affected. In contrast to other toxicities, BCNU produces the most rapid marrow effects and recovery, with nadir of leukopenia at day 26–30 and recovery by day 35–50. In contrast, nadir of CCNU-induced myelosuppression is day 40–50 with recovery by day 60. MethylCCNU has a nadir of cell counts at day 25–60 with recovery prolonged until nearly day 90 after treatment. Severe anemia also may occur with prolonged nitrosourea therapy, although leukopenia and thrombocytopenia are more commonly encountered. Cumulative effects of overlapping treatment sequences are potentially life-threatening. Following subsequent doses, the nadir persists for a longer period of time, and equivalent doses produce a more profound decrease in cell counts. Thrombocytopenia is usually more severe, but leukopenia and anemia also are marked. These effects are delayed and prolonged, with a nadir occurring 3–5 weeks after treatment (thrombocytes) and 4–6 weeks after treatment (leucocytes), with nadirs lasting 1–2 weeks. Nausea and vomiting are very common (40–70%) following administration of these agents. The onset of nausea and vomiting is 2–4 h after dosing and may persist for 24 h. BCNU (carmustine) has the unique effect of producing a burning pain in the vein through which the drug is administered, even when no extravasation is apparent. Phlebitis is common. Stomatitis, mucositis, and alopecia are encountered with all three drugs, but at a relatively low incidence. Hepatotoxicity is relatively common (26% with BCNU and CCNU) and is usually reversible. Onset may be delayed for up to 120 days after treatment and is seen as transient, mild increases in serum parameters of liver function. Incidence can be up to 25%, but the elevations are transient and no serious sequelae develop. There are, however, isolated reports of death, with widespread hepatic necrosis, particularly with streptozotocin (Lokich et al., 1974). In addition, BCNU produces a central nervous system toxicity as well as optic neuritis, which may be related to the central effects. Of more recent and troubling concern is the occurrence of a relatively precipitous and delayed renal failure, which is not observed or predicted until several months to a year or more after treatment (Harmon et al., 1979). Fortunately the incidence has been low, because the outcome for involved patients has been discouraging.

Neurotoxicity has been reported in 9% (Ramirez et al., 1972) of patients following typical intravenous BCNU therapy. Symptoms are dizziness, loss of equilibrium, and ataxia. When BCNU is used intraarterially to treat patients with brain tumors, the incidence of facial pain and optical disfunction was 100%, with up to 30% of patients suffering focal seizures (Kaplan and Wiernik, 1982). Neurologic toxicity also was observed in dogs following intracarotid administration of BCNU and was manifested histologically as necrotizing arteriolitis of the internal carotids (DeWys and Fowler, 1973), which may be related to the burning sensation produced in veins of patients receiving the drug by traditional intravenous administration.

Both BCNU and CCNU produced evidence of mild renal toxicity in preclinical animal toxicity studies (Oliverio, 1973). This toxicity was manifested as delayed azotemia with histopathologic evidence of interstitial nephritis and acute tubular necrosis. In patients, CCNU has only a mild nephrotoxic potential, seen as mild azotemia in only a few instances. BCNU, however, is much more nephrotoxic, producing a 35% incidence of chronic renal failure in children. Incidences are lower in adults (18%), but pathology is similar, manifesting mainly as tubular atrophy and interstitial fibrosis with marked glomerular sclerosis. Of particular concern is the insidious onset of the renal failure. In patients receiving large cumulative doses (1500 mg/m^2) of nitrosoureas (mainly BCNU and methylCCNU) over a prolonged time course (1–2 years), gradually increasing azotemia is seen beginning 6–60 months after stopping drug treatment. The reason for this prolonged delay in onset is unknown. Semustine appears to present the greatest hazard from this delayed renal toxicity, but carmustine also produces a high incidence of the same effect (Weiss and Issell, 1982). BCNU (carmustine) produces a reversible infertility in male rats, with associated decreases in implantations and increased resorptions. It is a potent teratogen in rats. Administration of carmustine (BCNU) by several routes produces mainly lung tumors in rats. CCNU (lomustine) is teratogenic in rats. In rabbits, however, it produces an increase in resorptions but no fetal malformations (Thompson et al., 1975b). It is carcinogenic primarily in the rat, where both ip and iv administration lead to lung cancers.

Streptozotocin is the fourth nitrosourea in widespread clinical use, and its spectrum of toxic effects differs quantitatively and qualitatively from the first three discussed above. Myelosuppression is uncommon with streptozotocin, manifesting mainly as a mild anemia in a small percentage of patients. Dose-limiting toxicity is a serious and, in some series, nearly universal incidence of renal toxicity. Incidence of some evidence of renal dysfunction is about 65% in most studies (Broder and Carter, 1973), with serious toxicity being seen in up to 25% of patients. The renal effects can be fatal in greater than 10% of treated patients (Broder and Carter, 1973). The initial manifestation is proteinuria, and azotemia also may be seen. Serious toxicity is seen as a Fanconi-like syndrome with aminoaciduria, glucosuria, and tubular acidosis. Histologically, an interstitial nephritis and tubular atrophy are observed, consistent with the tubular effects mentioned above. Delayed but mild hepatotoxicity seen as transient elevations in serum enzymes is seen in about 15% of patients. Although hepatic necrosis has been observed at autopsy, the incidence is apparently very low. Myelosuppression is not common, but nausea and vomiting are universal, occurring 1–4 h after drug administration. Conventional antiemetics are of little help. In addition, diarrhea with abdominal cramps is seen occasionally (10% incidence).

Chlorambucil, melphalan, thioTEPA, and busulfan are all characterized as having relatively minor acute effects and relatively mild bone marrow suppression. *Chlorambucil* is one of the less toxic antineoplastic agents whose effects are characterized mainly by a delayed-onset myelosuppression. Although the leukopenia is mild to moderate, the white count will continue to drop for up to 10 days after cessation of drug. The nadir is day 14–28, with recovery usually by day 28–42. Mild gastointestinal disturbances are seen occasionally, particularly at higher doses. Dermatitis and hepatotoxicity may rarely be observed. Chlorambucil produces testicular atrophy and decreased sperm motility in mice and is strongly teratogenic (DiPaolo, 1969) and embryolethal in rats. Similarly, azoospermia with germinal-cell aplasia is common in humans treated with chlorambucil. It is carcinogenic in rats and mice and is considered to be a carcinogenic drug in humans by virtue of numerous studies documenting the appearance of acute nonlymphocytic leukemia in patients who received chlorambucil as a single agent for disease treatment.

Melphalan is a commonly used orally administered derivative of mechlorethamine with relatively little serious toxicity. Nausea and vomiting may occur at very high doses. Leukopenia with a nadir at 10–12 days persists for an uncharacteristically prolonged period and may not return to normal until 42–50 days after drug treatment. Melphalan is both embryolethal and teratogenic in rats and is carcinogenic in both rats and mice. In addition, it is well established as a carcinogen in humans.

The *thioTEPA* dose-limiting toxicity is leukopenia and thrombocytopenia, with the nadir at 7–10 days posttreatment and recovery by day 28. Nausea and vomiting are observed only occasionally and then at high doses. ThioTEPA is teratogenic in rodents and has been shown to be carcinogenic in rodents by several routes of administration (DiPaolo, 1969).

Busulfan is another alkylating agent whose toxicity has been exploited for therapeutic reasons. The major bone-marrow toxicity of busulfan is a selective granulocytopenia, and it has been used most widely to treat chronic granulocytic leukemia. Skin pigmentation resembling the melanosis of Addison's disease is common, particularly with long-term treatment. A relatively rare but well-established side effect of busulfan is the development of interstitial pulmonary fibrosis. Busulfan was the first antineoplastic agent to be associated with pulmonary toxicity characterized by a very delayed onset—more than 4 years of therapy and a total dose of at least 3 g of drug prior to the onset of symptoms are characteristic of most cases. The syndrome is characterized by the insidious onset, usually over the course of several months, of dyspnea and a nonproductive cough, and occasionally a low-grade fever. Chest X-rays may be normal or show diffuse infiltrates. Hypoxemia is present and a diffusion defect may be detected. Most patients die from progression of the disease, even if drug therapy is withdrawn. Survival averages only 5 months after diagnosis (Willson, 1978). Incidence of clinical signs and symptoms is reported to be 2.5–11.5%, and

12.5–42.5% of patients are reported to have histological abnormalities in the lung (atypical cells, interstitial edema) (Sostman et al., 1977). More recent estimates may be more accurate [4% and 12%, respectively (Ginsberg and Comis, 1982)]. Busulfan is also widely known for its reproductive effects, causing amenorrhea, sterility, impotence and gynecomastia in humans. In rodents it causes a persistent absence of germinal elements of the gonads (DiPaolo, 1969).

Finally, *dacarbazine* (DTIC) causes a mild bone-marrow suppression (leukopenia and thrombocytopenia), which may be delayed 2–4 weeks. The nadir is day 25–36, with recovery not occurring for 2 or more weeks. In addition, a moderate to severe nausea and vomiting occurs that has occasionally resulted in discontinuation of therapy. Incidence and severity of nausea and vomiting decrease during the last 2–3 days of the usual 5-day course of therapy. Of interest is the appearance of a flu-like hypersensitivity reaction occurring 5–7 days after drug administration and lasting 1–2 weeks. This syndrome is characterized by muscle pain, sinus congestion, headache, and malaise. Facial flushing and parasthesias also occur, which support the sensitizing nature of this drug. Thrombophlebitis with tissue necrosis is common following extravasation. Hepatotoxicity, manifested as increased serum bilirubin and transaminases, also occurs. Dacarbazine is teratogenic in rats and causes increased resorptions as well. It produces tumors in animals after administration via several routes of administration.

Antimetabolites This group of drugs substitutes for an obligate metabolic cofactor to block endogenous energy or nucleic acid synthesis.

One of the earliest antimetabolites to be developed was *5-fluorouracil* (FU), which has been in clinical use for almost 30 years. This drug demonstrates a well-established relation between incidence or severity of side effects and treatment schedule. This is particularly true with gastrointestinal side effects, such as diarrhea, anorexia, and nausea/vomiting. Stomatitis and diarrhea are early manifestations of toxicity and may be severe enough to indicate discontinuation of therapy. Systemic FU therapy leads to a high incidence (48–72%) of stomatitis, which begins with a dry mouth and a prominent oral burning sensation. Dysphagia is present after ulcers appear. Stomatitis is an indication to discontinue therapy. Alopecia also is common (20–57%). Another common cutaneous side effect is a seborrheic dermatitis, characterized by erythema and scaling. This has been exploited by using topical FU in the treatment of actinic keratosis. The effect is the same reaction described above, but is restricted to diseased tissue and does not affect the normal skin. This effect appears to be potentiated by sunlight, and residual redness and swelling may persist for several weeks, and will ultimately be followed by a period of hyperpigmentation lasting several months before all signs of the lesion disappear. Oral inflammation and diarrhea are usually mild but can proceed to ulceration in both the oropharynx and bowel. Bone-marrow suppression is mainly leukopenia and thrombocytopenia, and less often granulocytopenia. Nadir is on day 9–14 and recovery on day 16–24. There are also numerous dermatologic effects, such as alopecia, dermatitis (rash on extremities), extreme dryness, and sensitivity to sunlight. The photosensitization is characterized by erythema and pigmentation. Of particular interest following FU administration, particularly with intensive daily treatment schedules, is an acute cerebellar syndrome manifested by ataxia, nystagmus, dizziness, and slurred speech. The syndrome is reversible within 4–6 weeks after treatment is stopped. FU is embryolethal, teratogenic, and causes increased resorptions in several species, and it may cause growth retardation or resorptions in monkeys. There is no evidence for its carcinogenicity in either animals or humans (Schmahl, 1975; Schmahl and Habs, 1980; IARC, 1981).

One of the most widely studied antineoplastic drugs is *methotrexate* (MTX), particularly from a clinical pharmacology perspective, and it is one of the few drugs with a specific antidote for toxic effects. Toxicity from this drug is well correlated with blood levels, with toxicity becoming severe above plasma concentrations of 10^{-5} M at 24 h, 10^{-6} M at 48 hr, and at 10^{-7} M at 72 h after a 4-h infusion. At levels above these, leucovorin (N^5-formyl-tetrahydrofolic acid) may be administered every 6 h until blood levels decrease below 10^{-7} M. Generalized bone-marrow depression, with granulocyte and thrombocyte nadirs about day 10–12, is extremely common. Recovery is by day 21. Anemia becomes prevalent with chronic administration. The second site of major MTX toxicity is the lining of the alimentary tract, particularly the oropharynx and the intestinal tract. Oral mucositis predicts for more serious toxicity if drug administration is not immediately discontinued, and diarrhea and ulcerative stomatitis also are signs for immediate discontinuation of therapy. Methotrexate stomatitis (mouth ulcers) is manifested by ulceration of lips and buccal mucosa and the production of a viscous buccal secretion. The ulcers begin as small shallow painful white lesions with erythematous borders and evolve into frank ulcers. This side effect is controlled by leucovorin treatment but may appear 2–5 days after completion of the course of leucovorin. The relatively high incidence (25%) in nonrescued patients may be reduced to 10% or less with leucovorin rescue. Renal damage after MTX administration in very-high-dose protocols is frequent and is due to a physical crystallization of MTX out of tubular fluid and resulting physical damage to the tubule. This effect can be easily circumvented with maintenance of an adequate urine flow and maintenance of an alkaline urine pH. Continuous low-dose therapy with MTX produces hepatotoxicity, with cirrhosis and portal fibrosis (Menard et al., 1980). The fibrosis is rarely life-threatening or dose-limiting and is usually characterized by mild and transient increases in serum glutamic–oxaloacetic transferase (SGOT) and lactate dehydrogenase (LDH), which may resolve even with continued treatment. Occurrence of cirrhosis, however, is cause for greater concern, in part because onset and progress are poorly monitored by serum enzymology. Cirrhosis is usually cause for periodic biopsies (Coe and Bull, 1968). Incidence of portal fibrosis is 27–46%, and of cirrhosis approaches 20% (Dahl et al., 1971). Interestingly, high-dose infusions for short time periods produce only transient increases in serum enzymes, with none of the long-term complications associated with more chronic administration. Use of MTX as maintenance therapy, particularly in children, produces a pneumonitis characterized by interstitial pulmonary infiltrate with dyspnea, fever, and cyanosis. This toxicity is refractory to leucovoran rescue. Patients present with dyspnea and nonproductive cough. Various compromises of pulmonary function (hypoxia, diffusion defects) are common. Peripheral eosinophilia is present in half the cases. Radiographic examination shows a variety of basalar and mid-field infiltrates. Histologic alveolar damage

with interstitial infiltrates is seen, and progression to interstitial fibrosis and a granulomatous inflammatory response may occur. The syndrome appears reversible if drug
is withdrawn early, but death rate is greater than 10% of affected patients. Although
not encountered with routine systemic administration, three variations of neurologic
toxicity are observed when MTX is administered intrathecally. Acutely, meningeal
irritation and inflammation occur within 2–4 h after injection and last 2–3 days. The
syndrome is one of stiff neck, headache, and nausea/vomiting. The incidence varies
widely and may be as little as 10% or as great as 40–55%. Interestingly, the incidence
and severity of this effect decrease with concomitant cranial irradiation. A more
chronic result is the rapid (30 min–2 day) development of paralysis and leg pain,
lasting for as long as 2–5 months. The end result may be only partial recovery. This
effect has been attributed to a hypersensitivity reaction. Finally, patients may develop
a chronic disseminated necrotizing leukoencephalopathy characterized by demyelination, multifocal coagulation necrosis, astrocytic reaction without an inflammatory
cellular reaction, and little or no vascular changes. Intracerebral calcification also
may be detected. Incidence of leukoencephalopathy may be as high as 55%, but at
low doses a more realistic estimate would be 20% or less in most series. This syndrome begins insidiously in the first year after MTX therapy and is characterized by
confusion, ataxia, spasticity, tremors, and convulsions. Most patients live for years
with the affliction, but the leukoencephalopathy is usually ultimately fatal. Other less
serious side effects include nausea and vomiting, skin rashes, alopecia, and osteoporosis. MTX is strongly teratogenic and embryolethal in several species. It is similarly
associated with birth defects and increased numbers of spontaneous abortions in humans (Milarsky and Gaynor, 1968). A closely related analog, aminopterin, has been
used clinically as an abortifacient in humans. There is no evidence of carcinogenic
effects in animals (Schmahl and Habs, 1978; Weisburger, 1977), and its carcinogenic
activity in humans is questionable because only rare instances of neoplastic events
have occurred in patients who received only MTX as therapy.

In contrast to MTX, oral irritation and ulceration as well as significant nausea
and vomiting are uncommon with 6-mercaptopurine (6MP), a purine antagonist.
Nausea and vomiting when they occur are usually mild. Bone-marrow suppression is
common and usually seen as leukopenia (less commonly thrombocytopenia) occurring
on days 7–14 with recovery by day 21. This effect may be delayed in onset, and
blood counts may continue to fall after the drug has been discontinued. Hepatotoxicity characterized by jaundice is reported following 6MP administration (Einhorn and
Davidsohn, 1964) and this effect appears to be potentiated in the presence of adriamycin. Hepatotoxicity occurs relatively early (1–2 months) and at doses above 2 g/kg/
day and is seen as increases in serum transaminases. Incidence approaches 50% of
treated patients. Bilirubin is elevated, and icteric plasma is common (10–40% incidence). Serum enzyme abnormalities are reversible if drug is discontinued, but if not,
hepatic death can ensue (Burchenal et al., 1953). Histologically, cholestasis and hepatocyte necrosis are seen both in patients and animals (Philips et al., 1956; Green et
al., 1983). Renal toxicity is uncommon, is associated with very-high-dose 6MP therapy, and is characterized by hematuria secondary to crystals of 6MP forming in
tubules and collecting ducts. Administration of 6MP to female mice prior to mating

leads to sterility or infertility in female offspring. It is embryolethal and produces increased resorptions and terata in rats. It produces reversible oligospermia, and there is one report of a malformed infant born to a mother who had received mercaptopurine during pregnancy. Mercaptopurine appears to be a strong abortifacient, however, with 8 of 20 women who received mercaptopurine during the first trimester having spontaneous abortions (Nicholson, 1968). Although there is one report of the carcinogenicity of MP in animals (Weisburger, 1977), other laboratories have found MP to be noncarcinogenic (Sugimura et al., 1978; Schmahl and Habs, 1978, 1980), and the IARC found no evidence for its carcinogenicity in animals (IARC, 1981).

Cytarabine (Ara-C) is used primarily in myelogenous leukemia, mainly due to its immunosuppressive effects. Major toxicities are leukopenia and thrombocytopenia, with anemia occurring in roughly 15% of patients. Nadir of effect is day 12–14 with recovery by day 22–24. Nausea, vomiting, and diarrhea are common (25% incidence), with antiemetics offering little help. Thrombophlebitis is occasionally encountered. A mild reversible liver toxicity manifesting as an increase in serum enzymes has been reported in roughly 10% of patients. This is a serious complication due to the fact that the liver is the site of metabolic detoxication of Ara-C, and hepatic toxicity may delay detoxication of the drug and hence potentiate other toxicities. Ara-C also causes mild oral inflammation and ulceration, with a higher incidence in children (15%) than in adults (9%). When the drug is administered intrathecally to treat meningeal leukemia, arachnoiditis may occur. Interestingly, Ara-C has been implicated as a potentiating agent in toxicities more commonly encountered with other drugs. For example, the incidence of neurotoxicity following methotrexate/Ara-C combinations is greater than with methotrexate alone, whereas Ara-C only rarely produces this toxicity by itself. Finally, the development of pulmonary toxicity with severe pulmonary edema has been reported following Ara-C administration. Ara-C has been associated with pulmonary toxicity seen mainly as acute respiratory insufficiency with tachypnea, hypoxemia, and sudden onset of pulmonary infiltrates and frank edema. About one-third of patients who develop this toxicity experience the onset of symptoms during drug administration and 43% within a month after drug administration. Patients who received the drug shortly before death (<30 days) are most likely to experience the respiratory distress. Cytarabine produced dose-related fetal growth retardation and increased number of fetal malformations in rats but was not embryolethal (Ritter et al., 1971). Ara-C is not carcinogenic in animals (Weisburger, 1977).

Azacytidine is an analog of Ara-C with a nitrogen substitution in the pyrimidine ring. The spectrum of toxic effects are similar to Ara-C, but with a high incidence (70%) of severe nausea, vomiting, and diarrhea (50%), particularly following rapid iv injection. Up to 60% of patients also develop a fever for 1–4 h after drug treatment (McCredie et al., 1973). Hypotension also occurs, and the hematologic effects are mainly restricted to a selective neutropenia. Azacytidine is teratogenic and embryotoxic in mice only (Seifertova et al., 1968) and is mildly carcinogenic in mice (IARC, 1981).

Natural Products   Several of the most active antineoplastic agents are either plant extracts or products of bacterial fermentations and, although few in number, comprise a high percentage of usage in various experimental treatment protocols.

Dactinomycin was first isolated and utilized in the early 1940s and is still commonly used against a variety of solid tumors. Dose-limiting toxicity from this drug is myelosuppression presenting as leukopenia and thrombocytopenia, usually with a nadir occurring on day 14–21 followed by prompt recovery (day 21–28). Nausea and vomiting are severe and occur in most patients, beginning about 2–5 h after treatment and lasting for up to 24 h. Extravasation causes severe necrosis. Dactinomycin is immunosuppressive, but is not utilized for that purpose, as is cyclophosphamide. Stomatitis with ulceration is common, as are severe acne-like skin eruptions on the head, neck, and upper trunk. Dactinomycin causes a generalized increased pigmentation in face, neck, and upper trunk that may occur universally in a treated population. Reversible alopecia (50% incidence) appears 7–10 days after treatment begins and will affect eyebrows and lashes as well as scalp. Oral dactinomycin is one of only two commonly used antineoplastic agents that produce a highly characteristic dermal reaction referred to as radiation recall reaction. In areas of the skin that have previously been irradiated, a well-defined erythema and vesiculation will occur at a relatively high incidence (47–67%). The reaction occurs more commonly 2–3 months after irradiation but has been recorded in skin that had been irradiated 17 months prior to dactinomycin administration (Tan et al., 1959). Dactinomycin is teratogenic in rats and hamsters but produces embryolethality in the rabbit and mouse. It is carcinogenic in rodents, but no evidence has appeared to implicate it as a human carcinogen.

Doxorubicin and *daunorubicin* are anthracycline antibiotics that differ chemically by only a single hydroxyl group at the 14 position of the anthracycline ring. Although both have similar toxicities, the spectrum of antitumor activity of daunorubicin is mainly against leukemias, whereas doxorubicin is active against a variety of solid tumors. Nausea and vomiting are common (75%), as are anorexia and diarrhea. Alopecia is universal and affects not only the scalp but the axillary and pubic areas also. Severe necrosis occurs following extravasation. Leukopenia is the major hematologic toxicity (60–80%), but mild thrombocytopenia and anemia also may occur. Leukopenia nadir is day 10–14, with recovery by day 21–24. Stomatitis is severe and dose-dependent, particularly with doxorubicin, and hypersensitivity reactions (fever, urticaria, occasionally anaphylaxis) are not uncommon. Doxorubicin causes nearly universal alopecia, particularly of the facial hair, beginning 3–4 weeks after the first dose and progressing, even if the drug is stopped promptly. The hair loss persists several weeks after the drug is discontinued but hair will reappear fully in 2–5 months. Stomatitis at a relatively high incidence (71–100%) is the first sign of drug toxicity in about half of all patients. It is usually mild, but may be severe if preexisting liver disease is present. Intermittent dosing (once every third week) also has been found to decrease the incidence. It begins as a burning sensation and erythema of the oral mucosa, which becomes ulcerated in 1–3 days, usually on the sides of and below the tongue. The ulcers usually heal in 1–2 weeks. Doxorubicin is characterized by a mild radiation recall reaction similar to that described for dactinomycin. Perhaps the most troublesome toxic effect of these antibiotics is the occurrence of dose-dependent cardiac toxicities, often leading to a fatal congestive heart failure at high cumulative doses. Two forms of cardiotoxicity appear—an acute, early effect, and a delayed, later effect. The early effect is seen mainly as reversible electrocardiogram (ECG) changes occurring during the infusion and throughout the first 2–3 days following treatment. These early ECG changes are characteristically ST–T wave abnormalities, sinus tachycardia, and a low-voltage QRS complex. This effect is self-limiting and not life-threatening, and is not predictive of the late-onset cardiotoxicity. Incidence can be up to 40% of a treated population (Von Hoff et al., 1982). The second form of cardiotoxicity, occurring in both children and adults, is a dose-related, late-onset cardiomyopathy, seen mainly at cumulative doxorubicin doses above 550 mg/m^2 and presenting as classic congestive heart failure (CHF), with tachycardia, shortness of breath, distended neck veins, and other classic signs of CHF. Incidence of fatal outcome from this effect is near 60% in affected patients (Von Hoff et al., 1982). The overall incidence of CHF varies with total dose, but is about 9% in all patients. For patients receiving less than 550 mg/m^2, the incidence is less than 0.3%, while for patients receiving greater than 550 mg/m^2, the incidence is 30% (Von Hoff et al., 1982). Low weekly doses produce a lower incidence of CHF than do higher doses every 3 weeks. Very young children and very elderly adults have a greater risk of developing this toxic effect. Radiographic examination and serum enzyme assays have not been helpful in predicting or diagnosing this effect. Histopathologic evaluation shows a decrease in number of myocytes, with vacuolization and edema and an increased number of mitochondria. Daunorubicin manifests exactly the same cardiac toxicities as does doxorubicin, but the mortality is closer to 80% with this drug (Von Hoff et al., 1977). Early and transient electrocardiogram changes do not appear related to or to predict for the chronic effect. The lesion is well characterized (Von Hoff et al., 1982), but the mechanism whereby the lesion is produced is not yet understood. Daunorubicin and doxorubicin are both carcinogenic in rodents following a single administration (Marquardt et al., 1976). Daunorubicin produces mainly adenocarcinomas of the kidney and mammary gland, while doxorubicin produces mainly fibroadenomas (Bertazolli et al., 1971). Both drugs are potent teratogens in animals (Thompson et al., 1978).

Mitomycin C has been utilized for 25 years in chemotherapeutic regimens, primarily against solid tumors of the gastrointestinal tract, breast, and lung, in spite of the facts that it is one of the more acutely toxic of the antineoplastic drugs and that remissions resulting from the drug are unremarkable in duration (Crooke and Bradner, 1976). Major dose-limiting toxicity is myelosuppression, occurring in greater than two-thirds of patients. Myelosuppression is severe, with total marrow aplasia frequently reported. Anemia and leukopenia are most commonly reported, but thrombocytopenia also is common. Bone-marrow toxicity is dose-related, with toxicity rarely occurring below 50 mg total dose. Cumulative toxicity is common and frequently severe and life-threatening. The pancytopenia has a nadir between days 28 and 42 with recovery by day 56–60. Thrombocytopenia is first noted during week 5–6 of therapy, with leukopenia occurring subsequently, usually 1–2 weeks later. Leukopenia lasts 1–2 weeks, but thrombocytopenia will persist for 2–3 weeks. A common side effect that occurs in nearly all patients to some extent is a period of malaise and weight loss. Celulitis with necrosis and sloughing of skin occurs following extravasation. Nausea–vomiting and diarrhea with incidents of fever are reported in less than 20% of patients and are usually mild. Stomatitis and alopecia are reported to occur occasionally. Although cardiac and pulmonary toxicities are reported to occur following mitomycin C administration, the incidence is extremely low and the etiology is suspect. Thus, pulmonary toxicity is reported mainly in patients with preexisting pulmonary disease, and the cardiac toxicity appears to be a potentiation of cardiac toxicity resulting from treatment with well-established cardiotoxic drugs, such as doxorubicin. Renal toxicity, on the other hand, has been consistently related to mitomycin C treatment, such that, although occurring in only a small percentage of patients [10% (Hanna et al., 1981)], its relationship is well established. The syndrome is insidious in onset, often beginning several months after therapy. There are rapid elevations in BUN and creatinine, accompanied by proteinuria and occasionally hypertension. The histologic picture is one of glomerular sclerosis and primary renal vascular disease with death from renal insufficiency occurring within 3–9 months after onset of the renal complications. Although early estimates of renal effects were 1–2%, more recent studies suggest the incidence may be closer to 8–10%, with one study reporting a 6% incidence of renal death in patients with long-term treatment or who received very large total doses (Hanna et al., 1981). Tubular degeneration and interstitial fibrosis have been reported by some authors but reported to be absent by others. This difference may reflect differences in treatment regimen or total dose administered. Several patients receiving both mitomycin C and 5-fluorouracil were reported to have a microangiopathic hemolytic anemia with subsequent renal failure and death (Hanna et al., 1981). The etiology and mechanisms of action of this serious but infrequent renal effect are unknown. Mitomycin C is both teratogenic and carcinogenic in animals, but evidence of similar human effects is still too small for adequate evaluation.

Bleomycin is a mixture of several water-soluble antibiotics that has attracted attention because of its lack of myelosuppression. It also rarely causes gastrointestinal-tract toxicity. One of the most prevalent toxicities (greater than 50% incidence) is a hyperpigmentation and keratosis of the skin, particularly at joints. Urticaria, pruritis, and sclerosis occur, as well as other manifestations. Skin reactions are readily reversible upon discontinuation of the drug. A nearly universal side effect of bleomycin in all studies is a low incidence of stomatitis (15–38%). It is initially detected as erythema and local pain and progresses in 2–3 days to shallow necrotic ulcers, which heal in 3–4 days but which will recur immediately upon subsequent administration of the drug. Lips, lateral tongue surfaces, and buccal mucosa are most commonly affected. Patients with stomatitis always have other skin reactions, but other skin changes may occur without the stomatitis being present. Alopecia begins about 3 weeks after the start of drug therapy and is associated with only a partial loss of scalp hair in most cases. Another common (60% incidence) and much more transient effect is a high fever (103–104 °F) occurring 4–10 h after treatment and lasting for several days. A dose-dependent stomatitis also occurs, and the appearance of this effect often is predictive for the appearance of more serious toxicities. The most serious toxicity, however, is a dose-dependent pulmonary toxicity characterized histologically as a diffuse interstitial pulmonary fibrosis. Above 450 mg/m^2, incidence is 10% of patients, with a mortality of 10% of affected patients. The effect is insidious in onset and is manifested as progressive dyspnea and nonproductive cough. Bilateral rales and tachypnea are found on examination, and pulmonary function tests reveal hypoxia and a diffusion defect. Concomitant with respiratory symptoms, radiographic abnormalities can be found. Pulmonary function tests can frequently detect decreases in respiratory function before symptoms or radiographic effects are detected. The syndrome and the histopathologic changes are apparently nonspecific for bleomycin but are common to other drug-induced pulmonary toxicities as well. Nausea and vomiting may occur but are usually mild. There is a high incidence of fever and chills, usually during the first few hours after bleomycin administration. There is also an anaphylactic-like reaction with high fever, hypotension, and respiratory distress that leads to cardiovascular collapse. Fortunately, the incidence of this reaction is only about 1% of the total patient population. There is no evidence that bleomycin is embryotoxic in either humans or animals. Animal studies conducted to investigate the carcinogenicity of bleomycin were judged unevaluable due to deficiencies in the data (IARC, 1981). One author (Harris, 1975), however, reported bleomycin a carcinogen based on a personal communication, although no data were presented. There is no evidence to suggest that bleomycin is a human carcinogen.

Another natural product with no bone-marrow toxicity is L-asparaginase, an enzyme that hydrolyzes L-asparagine. Nausea, vomiting, anorexia, and fever are common. Not surprisingly, hypersensitivity reactions are observed in about 25% of patients, but only 10% experience an anaphylatic reaction. Some investigators feel the relatively low incidence of anaphylaxis is due in part to an immunosuppressive effect of the drug. The incidence of acute hypersensitivity reactions with L-asparaginase increases from 8% to 35% with repeated courses. Prior skin tests are unreliable predictors of these reactions, and there is an increased risk of reaction when returning to treatment after a period with no drug. Dose-limiting toxicity is hepatotoxicity, manifested as decreases in albumin, lipoproteins, and cholesterol, and increases in bilirubin, alkaline phosphatase, and transaminases. The lesion appears to be a fatty metamorphosis. The hepatotoxicity (decreases in clotting factors, proteins, and cholesterol) is apparently related to a generalized inhibition of protein synthesis produced by the drug and is readily reversible when the drug is discontinued. Another relatively unique effect is a defect in clotting ability, with decreases in fibrinogen and several clotting factors, and subsequent increases in prothrombin and partial thromboplastin times. Clinical occurrences of bleeding or hemorrhage are rare, however. Central nervous system toxicity is common with L-asparaginase therapy (30%) and is seen as lethargy, confusion, depression, and (rarely) seizures or coma. The incidence of central nervous system (CNS) toxicity is apparently dose-related only in children, whereas the severity of the CNS toxicity is dose-related in both children and adults. CNS toxicity is much more common in adults than in children, where occurrence is rare (Haskell, 1981). Mild electroencephalogram changes become normal when drug is discontinued. A relatively common (35% incidence) but mild and reversible renal toxicity is observed, and transient azotemia is the most common sign. Finally, the pancreas is a specific site of toxicity, most likely due to an inhibition of insulin synthesis caused by reduced levels of precursors (asparagine and glutamine). The result is usually seen as hypoglycemia, but may in severe cases be seen as hemorrhagic pancreatitis with elevated plasma amylase levels, severe hypoglycemia, and shock. Most signs and symptoms affect both adults and children receiving the drug, but the incidence of all side effects is routinely less in children than in adults. The one exception to this is the hypersensitivity reactions, where children appear to be more sensitive. In one series (Oettgen et al., 1970), the only reason for discontinuing therapy with L-asparaginase in children was severe hypersensitivity reactions (85%), but in adults only 17% of dose-limiting toxicity was due to similar reactions. Finally, much of the toxicity, particularly the sensitivity reactions, may be due to the bacterial source and preparation of L-asparaginase. Preparations from both *Escherichia coli* and *Erwinia carotovora* are used and have been found to be variously contaminated with a bacterial endotoxin that is responsible for fevers in patients. Other side effects also have been attributed to drug contaminations or formulations. L-Asparaginase has been found to increase resorptions and to produce fetal malformations in rabbits in a dose-dependent manner (Adamson and Fabro, 1968). There are no data to indicate L-asparaginase as a carcinogen in either animals or humans.

Two of the most intriguing drugs utilized in cancer chemotherapy are the vinca alkaloids *vinblastine* and *vincristine,* because these high-molecular-weight plant products differ structurally only slightly but have a dramatically different spectrum of toxic effects. The dose-limiting toxicity with vinblastine is bone-marrow suppression (mainly neutropenia), with a leukopenia nadir occurring on day 6–9 after treatment and recovery by day 21. Vincristine, on the other hand, is considered to have no significant bone-marrow suppression and is utilized as a combination agent in protocols with marrow-suppressive drugs. The vincristine effect on platelets is variable and may be either a mild thrombocytopenia (Steinherz et al., 1976) or, occasionally, thrombocytosis (Carbone et al., 1963). Interestingly, when studied in rats, this drug produced a variable increase or decrease in platelets depending on the dose (Robertson et al., 1970). The most significant difference in toxicity between the two drugs is related to effects on the central nervous system. The dose-limiting toxicity for vincristine is neurotoxicity, and although mild neurotoxicity sometimes occurs with vinblastine, the marrow-suppressive effects of this latter drug intervene before serious CNS effects are ever noted. The neurotoxicity is seen primarily as a peripheral nerve dysfunction with paresthesia of the hands and feet, various signs of motor weakness, neck and jaw pain, and sensory loss. All resolve within several weeks after the end of drug treatment. Toxic effects on the autonomic nervous system are frequently seen as colicky pain with constipation due to a decrease in gastrointestinal motility. Dysfunction of cranial nerves also is seen and manifests as facial palsies, ptosis, and vocal-cord paralysis. These nervous-system effects appear to be related to the ability of these drugs to inhibit microtubule formation in the neurons of central and peripheral nerves. Because of the ready reversibility of many of the early signs of vincristine neurotoxicity, the presence of these effects is frequently not adequate justification for discontinuation of drug treatment. Impaired hepatic function in patients has been shown to increase both incidence and severity of neurotoxicity from vincristine, but the vinca alkaloids usually are not hepatotoxic and the relationship between impaired liver function and neurotoxicity is unclear. Vincristine also produces hyponatremia with inappropriate secretion of antidiuretic hormone and elevated vasopressin levels. Hyperuricemia occurs with both vincristine and vinblastine due to the rapid breakdown of tumor tissue. Alopecia occurs with both drugs in about 20–45% of patients, but only vinblastine produces significant nausea, vomiting, diarrhea, or stomatitis. Both vinblastine and vincristine are teratogens in animals (Sieber et al., 1978), and vincristine is an abortifacient. Vinblastine causes growth retardation, increased resorptions, and various malformations when administered to pregnant mice, rats, or hamsters. There is no evidence of a similar effect in humans. Numerous animal studies have failed to establish with certainty that either vinblastine or vincristine is carcinogenic (Weisburger, 1977; Schmahl, 1975; Schmahl and Habs, 1978). However, one animal study has implicated vinblastine as a carcinogen (Weisburger, 1977), although the IARC found no evidence of carcinogenicity (IARC, 1981). There are two reports (Ezdinli et al., 1969; Swaim et al., 1971) of vincristine-associated secondary neoplasms in patients. In both cases, however, the patients had also received radiotherapy, so the association with vincristine is not unequivocal. Vincristine also has been implicated as a human carcinogen because one of the regimens in which vincristine is used (MOPP) in combination with other agents has been associated with second neoplasms in humans. The other agents in this regimen, however, include the recognized carcinogens procarbazine and mechlorethamine.

Miscellaneous Agents *Cisplatinum* is the first and at present only significant anticancer agent to be an inorganic molecule containing a heavy-metal atom. As might be expected with a heavy metal, the dose-limiting toxicity is to the kidney, with a proximal tubular dilatation and necrosis that proceeds to renal failure in a significant percentage of high-dose patients. The effect is dose-related and manifested as increased BUN and creatinine and decreased creatinine clearance. Low-molecular-weight proteinuria may also be present. Magnesium wasting is commonly seen and may be severe enough to produce tetany (Hayes et al., 1979). The renal effects are considered manageable with the use of extensive hydration and diuresis. Of greater practical consequence is severe nausea and vomiting, occurring in all patients beginning within an hour after administration and lasting from 4–6 h up to 24 h in some patients. The nausea and vomiting appear to be refractory to commonly used antiemetics. Hemorrhagic colitis is reported in various animal species, but this lesion has not been reported in patients. High-tone hearing loss is common when suitable parameters are evaluated, but functional hearing loss is rare and occurs only in newer ultra-high-dose protocols (Ozols et al., 1983). Cisplatinum is one of the few marrow-sparing anticancer drugs. Although most investigators consider cisplatinum to have little myelosuppressive effect, there is some evidence that it is mildly myelosuppressive. Hill et al. (1975), for example, in a series of previously untreated patients showed a 9% incidence of leukopenia defined as white blood cell (WBC) counts of less than 1000/mm^3. The incidence went up to 22% and 49% when leukopenia was defined as less than 2000 and less than 4000 cells/mm^3, respectively, indicating how important is the definition of clinical thresholds of toxicity. In other series where leukopenia was defined as less than 1000 cells/mm^3, a similar incidence has been reported (0–8%). Hemolytic anemia, however, has been reported. Peripheral neuropathy characterized by numbness and paresthesia is relatively common, and anaphylatic reactions occur occasionally. Cisplatinum is embryolethal in mice and causes growth retardation but no significant teratogenic effects. It is a mild carcinogen in mice and rats, with no evidence for embryotoxicity or carcinogenesis in humans.

Procarbazine dose-limiting toxicity is bone-marrow depression with leukopenia and thrombocytopenia. The nadir is day 25–36 with recovery by day 36–50. Nausea and vomiting are commonly encountered. One of its major uses is in treating brain tumors, because it crosses the blood–brain barrier more readily than most drugs. Therefore central nervous system toxicity is common and has led to its intravenous use being discontinued. Both altered levels of consciousness (8–13%) and a peripheral neuropathy were observed. The altered consciousness ranged from lethargy and sedation to depression and stupor, persisting for up to 72 h. Rarely, hallucinations and manic psychoses have occurred. Nonspecific slow-wave electroencephalogram changes have occurred in deeply lethargic or stuporous patients. Peripheral neurologic changes occur even with oral dosing (10–20%) and are characteristically paresthesias and decreased deep-tendon reflexes. Symptoms occur after several weeks of therapy and are readily reversible. Some patients report a diffuse aching pain in the proximal muscles, which may resolve even with continued therapy. All the neurotoxicity signs reverse after the drug is withdrawn. Various myalgias also may be encountered, and orthostatic hypotension occurs. Procarbazine is embryolethal and teratogenic in rodents. It is carcinogenic in rodents following ip, oral, or iv administration, and produces solid tumors in multiple tissues. It is associated with cancer in humans who have been treated with combination regimens containing procarbazine and have developed second malignancies as an apparent consequence.

Hexamethylmelamine (HMM) produces dose-limiting gastrointestinal (GI) toxicity, with severe nausea and vomiting occurring in greater than 50% of patients. Although the drug is usually administered orally, the GI effects are considered to be of central origin (Legha et al., 1976). Marrow depression with leukopenia (<2000 cells/mm^3) and thrombocytopenia (<75,000 cells/mm^3) occur in 20–40% of patients, with a nadir in week 3–4 and return to normal by week 6. Dose-limiting toxicity is frequently neurological, manifesting either as central or peripheral effects. Central effects are predominantly depression, insomnia, or dysphagia. Occasionally, hallucinations or petit mal-like seizures also may occur. A Parkinson-like syndrome, ataxia, and severe headache with nausea and vomiting also have been reported. Peripheral effects are mainly paresthesias, weakness, and decreased sensation. Most symptoms are mild, reversible, and occur after months of therapy. The incidence is apparently dose-dependent, with 13% reported at 150–225 mg/m^2/day for 21 days, and 28–50% at higher doses. Eczema-like skin rashes also occasionally are seen, but alopecia occurs rarely.

Promising Experimental Drugs

Amsacrine (AMSA) is one of the more promising new drugs currently undergoing late phase II and early phase III clinical trials. AMSA is formulated in dimethylacetamide and diluted for administration in lactic acid. A recent review (Issell, 1980) of AMSA attributed some of its human and animal toxicities, particularly phlebitis and neurotoxicity, to this unusual vehicle for administration. Major dose-limiting toxicity for AMSA has been hematologic, with leukopenia predominating. Anemia and thrombocytopenia also occur, but less frequently, and usually are less severe. Nadir of leukopenia is day 12, and recovery is complete by day 25. There is no evidence that the myelosuppression is cumulative. In early studies, phlebitis in the vein of injection was noted commonly, but this effect has been largely eliminated by further diluting the drug with 5% dextrose in water and using a longer infusion time. Other than the phlebitis, early studies uncovered no other serious or frequent nonhematologic toxicities, although nausea and vomiting, alopecia, and stomatitis were occasionally observed. More recent studies, however, have utilized substantially higher doses, particularly in the treatment of metastatic disease that was resistant to other therapies (Tannir et al., 1983). These high-dose studies have uncovered other toxicities and have found more serious and more frequent occurrences of the minor toxicities observed previously. Thus, in one series of 45 patients treated with total doses of up to 1000 mg/m^2, myelosuppression was severe, with platelet and red blood cell (RBC) transfusions required in all patients. Recovery was delayed until week 5 in some instances. Severe stomatitis characterized by painful ulceration and necrosis of the oropharyngeal mucosa was common (40%). Signs of hepatotoxicity also were common, with hyperbilirubinemia (50%) and increased serum alkaline phosphatase (37%) being the major clinical manifestations. One patient died of hepatotoxicity, presenting with jaundice, hyperbilirubinemia, and increased serum glutamic-oxaloacetic transferase (SGOT). Liver biopsy showed severe centrilobular necrosis and fatty degeneration. Marked alopecia was universal, but nausea and vomiting were mild, with only 4 patients exhibiting severe vomiting. In another series of 16 very-high-dose AMSA patients, mucositis was the dose-limiting toxicity within an incidence of 40%, and myelosuppression was severe enough to be associated with 25% incidence of septicemia and 25 incidents of unexplained fever that were attributed to neutropenia (Tannir et al., 1983). In this series, nausea and vomiting were universal and several cases of diarrhea were recorded. Alopecia was not mentioned. In addition to the phlebitis mentioned above, several early studies mentioned cardiac toxicity or neurologic toxicity that were not reported in later studies. Phlebitis may still occur, but the incidence is very low due to slower infusion rate and dilution in 5% dextrose prior to administration. Legha et al. (1979) reported several patients that experienced grand mal seizures with normal EEG, brain scans, and cerebrospinal fluid (CSF) examinations during AMSA infusions. These seizures have subsequently been attributed to the dimethylacetamide vehicle (Issell, 1980). AMSA-induced seizures immediately prior to death also have been observed in preclinical animal toxicity studies in both mice and dogs at doses of vehicle that were totally nontoxic when administered alone (Henry et al., 1980). Myelosuppression also was predicted by these animal toxicity studies, as was the hepatotoxicity that was reported above. Vehicle-induced hepatotoxicity also was noted in the animal studies (Henry et al., 1980), however.

The major dose limiting toxicity of the podophyllotoxin derivative *etoposide* (VP-16) is leukopenia. Thrombocytopenia may also occur, but it is less common and less severe. No cumulative effects on the bone marrow have been observed. Nausea and vomiting are common and may occur in up to 50% of patients. Onset is immediately following the infusion. When etoposide is administered orally, nausea and vomiting are severe enough to become dose-limiting. Reversible alopecia, sometimes resulting in complete loss of hair, is nearly universal with etoposide, occurring in greater than 90% of patients in some series (Jungi and Senn, 1975). Fever and chills have regularly been associated with etoposide administration. When short infusion times have been used for iv administration, hypotension has been observed. Oral administration has been associated with stomatitis. The etoposide analog *teniposide* (VM-26) exhibits much the same spectrum of effects as does etoposide, except for a more common occurrence of anaphylactic responses, presenting with fever and cardiovascular and respiratory collapse. The incidence of teniposide-induced hypotension is also much higher than with etoposide, and teniposide is associated with a severe, prolonged abdominal pain following intraperitioneal administration. One author attributes this to the vehicle (Rozencweig et al., 1977), but these drugs are reported to cause a unique prolonged death in rodents treated intraperitioneally (Stahelin, 1976). The deaths take place between 30 and 50 days after single ip administration of otherwise innocuous doses and are characterized by ascites, severe inflammation, and fibrosis of the peritoneal cavity. Whether this is vehicle-related has not been proven, but the abdominal pain in patients could be related to the late-developing peritonitis observed in animals. A similar late death syndrome characterized by peritoneal fibrosis and ascites has been reported following the ip administration of adriamycin in rats (Litterst et al., 1982), and cyclophosphamide-induced late deaths (day 44–60) in rodents, characterized by decreased spleen and thymus weights and leukopenia, also have been reported (Stenram and Nordlinder, 1968).

A unique and interesting new drug is *2-deoxycoformycin*, an inhibitor of adenosine deaminase. It was originally developed to potentiate the activity of antineoplastic drugs whose activity was metabolically terminated by adenosine deaminase (e.g., Ara-A, Ara-C). Deoxycoformycin, however, was found to have antitumor activity of its own. The drug is a potent immunosuppressant, with early studies producing a mean 80% decrease in lymphocyte count beginning 48 h after initial dosing in 94% of the patients (Smyth et al., 1980). Subsequent work has confirmed the lymphopenia, with an incidence up to 100% (Poplack et al., 1981). The nadir begins at day 5 and persists for 10–12 days before returning to normal by day 14. Dose-limiting toxicity may be either central nervous system (CNS), renal, or hepatic, depending on patient population or dose regimen. CNS toxicity appears in all series that have been published and ranges to an incidence of 60%. Signs and symptoms are most commonly lethargy, confusion, and somnolence, beginning several days after initiation of therapy and persisting for up to 3 weeks (Major et al., 1981a). However, a severe, terminal encephalopathy with coma and seizures also occurs. The lethargy is accompanied by a generalized slowing of electrical activity on the electroencephalogram

(Major et al., 1981b). Acute renal failure (ARF) has been associated with deoxycoformycin administration in as high as 50% of patients (Karnofsky, 1982). Other series report only isolated patients experiencing ARF, while still others report only elevated creatinine levels. Some authors attribute the renal failure to hyperuricemia (Smyth et al., 1980), and more recent series with relatively low incidences of serious renal toxicity have included routine alopurinol administration concomitant with the deoxycoformycin (Poplack et al., 1981; Smyth et al., 1980). Hepatotoxicity is characterized by generally mild increases in serum hepatic enzymes in about one-third of all treated patients. Occasional patients, however, have died of hepatic complications with SGOT values of 2900 and lactate dehydrogenase (LDH) values of 4900 (Poplack et al., 1981) and a histologic pattern of centrilobular fatty degeneration. A mild conjuctivitis is routinely reported at an incidence of 19–33%. The conjuctivitis resolves spontaneously within the first 1–2 weeks after drug is withdrawn. Finally, there are reports of pulmonary involvement, with pulmonary infiltrates or bronchitis (33–75%). Diarrhea has been reported (35%), as have isolated instances of leukopenia, anemia, and thrombocytopenia. Some studies have found hematologic parameters difficult to evaluate due to the underlying disease effects in the patients (Poplack et al., 1981). There appears to be no cumulative toxicity, and all signs and symptoms except those that ultimately will be fatal resolve within 2–3 weeks after discontinuing the drug. Grever et al. (1983) have wisely cautioned that the acute effects listed above do not address the possible long-term consequences that may ensue due to the severe immunosuppression, and investigators should be alert to these insidious hazards.

Mitoxantrone (dihydroxyanthracenedione) is a synthetic anthroquinone that shares structural similarities with doxorubicin and daunorubicin; it was developed specifically in an attempt to avoid the dose-limiting cardiotoxicity of those drugs. It is very active in animal tumors and when compared with an equitoxic (bone marrow) dose of adriamycin demonstrated neither clinical (Henderson et al., 1982) nor histologic (Sparano et al., 1982) signs of cardiotoxicity. Toxicity of mitoxantrone in dogs was restricted to leukopenia and anemia, both of which occurred in a predictable fashion 6 days after dosing and were reversible before the next cycle of drug (schedule: once every 3 weeks). In addition, emesis, skin sores, and lethargy were reported. In spite of the lack of cardiac toxicity in animal tests, at least three separate studies have detected a small (10%) incidence of cardiac toxicity during early phase I testing (Schell et al., 1982; Wynert et al., 1982; Yap et al., 1981b). Both the acute ECG changes and more chronic congestive heart failure (CHF), as discussed with anthracyclines, have been noted. Schell et al. (1982) reported 4 cases of CHF appearing in 31 patients, but all 4 had received prior adriamycin, and Yap et al. (1981b) noted 2 cases of CHF in 23 patients. In their daily × 5 dosing schedule, Wynert et al. (1982) noted a 25% incidence of minor ECG changes, most of which were ST–T wave changes. In another series, no cardiac effects were observed (Von Hoff et al., 1980; Alberts et al., 1980; Stewart-Harris and Smith, 1982). Large studies will be required to establish the true incidence and potential severity of these effects in patients and whether mitoxantrone causes CHF in non-adriamycin-treated patients.

Other signs and symptoms of toxicity are encouragingly mild and infrequent. Myelosuppression is characterized mainly by leukopenia and granulocytopenia. The nadir differs among the various studies, with one report of a nadir by day 10 and return to normal by day 21 (Wynert et al., 1982), and another report of a nadir at day 20–21 and recovery by day 28–35 (Stewart et al., 1982). Neutropenia occurs less frequently but has been associated with several incidents of sepsis (Stewart-Harris and Smith, 1982). Mild alopecia has been reported with an incidence of 12–50%, although Von Hoff et al. (1980) reported no alopecia in their study. Nausea and vomiting are usually infrequent and mild when they occur, but Stewart-Harris and Smith (1982) reported that up to 35% of their population reported mild and transient nausea and 21% suffered a short duration of mild vomiting. That same series had a 12% incidence of uncharacterized parasthesias. Extravasation has been reported to have occurred with no local tissue reaction (Wynert et al., 1982).

Indicine N-*oxide* is a pyrrolizidine alkaloid that is undergoing clinical trials against a number of solid tumors and refractory leukemias. Expected toxicity from this compound, based on historical records of injections of the plant source of the drug in both human and animals, would predict hepatotoxicity. Preclinical animal toxicity studies bore out this prediction when dogs and monkeys had increases in serum transaminases and bilirubin. Early clinical tests showed myelosuppression to be the dose-limiting toxicity, with predominantly leukopenia, although thrombocytopenia also occurred. Leukopenia has been implicated in several cases of sepsis (Nichols et al., 1981), and in one series (Nichols et al., 1981) platelet transfusions were required in 50% of the patients at doses above 3 g/m^2/day and there were deaths related to severe thrombocytopenia. Nadir of cell counts was on day 18–19, with recovery by day 25 (day 34 for thrombocytes). Bone-marrow toxicity appeared cumulative by virtue of the fact that at intermediate doses (≤ 2.7 g/m^2/day) decreases in blood counts did not occur until day 3 or 4. Anemia occurred in 27% of patients but mostly at lower or intermediate doses. Hepatotoxicity has been observed occasionally (7–13%) and is characterized by mild increases in serum transaminases that peak about day 19 and return to normal within 2 weeks (Ohnuma et al., 1982; Kovach et al., 1979). Some authors have reported acute hepatotoxicity with jaundice (Letendre, 1981). Transient increases in creatinine, indicative of mild renal toxicity, occurred more frequently (20%). Subsequent studies have confirmed the mild hepatoxicity (13%), characterized by increases in bilirubin and transaminases.

Methyl GAG was originally developed in the late 1950s and tested for clinical activity in the early 1960s. Although it demonstrated excellent activity against several human solid tumors, the toxicity was so great as to preclude any significant clinical use. The most serious effect was a mucositis that appeared to be specific for methyl GAG by affecting the esophagus and pharynx most severely. In the middle 1970s the exceptional therapeutic advantage gained from methyl GAG prompted a reinvestigation of its use, with much more promising results. Whereas the original 1960s dosing schedule was a daily intravenous infusion at doses of 3–15 mg/kg, Knight et al. (1979) subsequently administered methyl GAG as an infusion once weekly at 250 or 500 mg/m^2 and confirmed earlier indications of lower toxicity. In this series of 90 evaluable cases, fully 74% suffered no reported toxic effects of drug administration. Nausea and vomiting were observed in 16%, and serious mucositis occurred in 19% of the patients and contributed to 1 drug-induced death. Knight et al. also reported that all toxicities appeared to be cumulative, with greater incidence and severity with higher numbers of courses of therapy. Several other subsequent phase II studies (Yap et al., 1981a; Knight et al., 1982) have confirmed the bone-marrow-sparing effect of methyl GAG, with incidences of mild anemia (38%) and mild thrombocytopenia (19%) reported. Other studies report no myelosuppression (Zeffren et al., 1981). Two studies have reported dose-limiting toxicity to be a syndrome of severe weakness, fatigue, and lethargy appearing after 2-4 courses of therapy in 25-63% of patients (Zeffren et al., 1981; Kelsen et al., 1982). Another common and troublesome side effect is a severe pain and weakness in the lower extremeties, reported at 17-19%. Several studies report neuralgias or myopathy or thrombophlebitis, which might be the same syndrome but more specifically defined. Knight et al. in their original publication (Knight et al., 1979) reported the syndrome of lethargy and weakness in 3 of their 90 cases. Nausea and vomiting are commonly reported at various incidences (16-65%), but all episodes are mild. Diarrhea also is commonly reported (20-35%). Mucositis affecting the pharynx or esophagus is still reported at a relatively high incidence (20-37%). Nearly every series studied reports the toxicity to be cumulative, with various signs and symptoms not appearing until after three to six courses of therapy and then reappearing even after therapy had been interrupted to allow the symptom to disappear. This increasing sensitivity may be related to the excessive toxicity observed in the original daily × 5 dosing schedule. Methyl GAG has been found to be nonteratogenic in mice (Chaube and Murphy, 1968).

Aziridinylbenzoquinone (AZQ) was synthesized in order to combine optimum water solubility to allow easy formulation and optimum lipid solubility to allow for penetration into the central nervous system. It was found to be active against CNS tumors and intracranial leukemias in animals (Driscoll et al., 1979) and thus has been tested against malignant brain tumors in humans. Major dose-limiting toxicity is myelosuppression, with leukopenia and thrombocytopenia. Less than 20% of the leukopenic events are severe. In a phase I study where various increasing doses were administered, Schilsky et al. (1982) observed a maximum myelosuppression at 17.5 mg/m^2 (76%) but less severe and less common (44%) effects at doses above that. Anemia also was relatively common (29%), although no incidents of bleeding or petechia were recorded. The nadir of the myelosuppression was between days 15 and 18 with recovery common by day 29-34. Nausea appearing 3-4 h after dosing was present (10-17%), but severe vomiting occurred in only a few cases. Another phase I study reported severe myelosuppression, but no nausea/vomiting or alopecia (Griffin et al., 1982). One phase II study reported constipation (19%) and occasional occurrences of stomatitis and alopecia (Creagan et al., 1982).

Bisantrene is a guanido-substituted anthracene that is being developed, along with mitoxantrene, as a second-generation anthracycline in an attempt to avoid the dose-limiting cardiotoxicity of daunorubicin and doxorubicin. This drug has recently completed phase I clinical trials, and several early phase II results also have been published (Perry et al., 1982; Ahmed et al., 1983). Hematologic toxicity is primarily a mild leukopenia, with 56-64% of patients treated experiencing nadir counts of less than 3000 cells/mm^3. The nadir is on day 9, with recovery by day 19-24. Thrombocytopenia occurs much less frequently (16%) and is very mild. The most serious dose-limiting nonhematologic toxicity is severe thrombophlebitis, occurring in the limb of the infusion. Phlebitis occurs consistently in about one-third of all patients regardless of the study. This syndrome begins with a burning sensation and erythemia along the vein and limb, occurring within several hours after the infusion. There is severe limb swelling, which has persisted for 3–4 months (Scher et al., 1982). Reports of necrosis following extravasation have been variable, with one report of necrosis and ulceration (Von Hoff et al., 1981) and another with no necrosis reported following immediate and aggressive treatment (Spiegel et al., 1982). There is one report of a delayed thrombophlebitis occurring 2–7 days after infusion in 38% of the patients treated at doses above 60 mg/m^2 daily × 5 (Yap et al., 1982). This persisted for 3–4 weeks and progressed to ulceration in 1 patient. Another toxic reaction of some concern is characterized by elevated body temperature with associated chills. In one series, 20% of the patients had body temperatures of greater than 104° (Ahmed et al., 1983). A syndrome of fatigue and malaise lasting 2–3 days after treatment also has been reported in several series at relatively high frequency (30–56%). This occurs usually after the second of three treatments and becomes worse after the third treatment. Mild nausea and vomiting are commonly reported (21–41%) and last 2–4 h. In every series, even in the phase II trials, there are some patients (20%) who experience no side effects of treatment. Toxicity does not appear to be cumulative except for the malaise mentioned above. There is no evidence of cardiotoxicity either in patients or in special animal studies designed to compare bisantrene with doxorubicin (Von Hoff et al., 1981).

In an attempt to circumvent the dose-limiting renal toxicity and severe nausea and vomiting of cisplatinum, several analogs of cisplatinum have been synthesized and tested for their efficacy and toxicity in animals. Phase I and early Phase II studies have been completed for several of these analogs (Lee et al., 1983) and the most promising candidate for further trials is *carboplatin* (Calvert et al., 1983). Dose-limiting toxicity is myelosuppression, with thrombocytopenia predominating. Leukopenia also occurs. At very high doses during a phase I study (Calvert et al., 1982), 80% of all patients experienced platelet decreases to less than 100×10^6 cells/ml, with a nadir 3 weeks after treatment and recovery by day 28–32. The nadir of the leukopenia was 34–38 days after treatment. Very high doses (520 mg/m^2) cause mild anemia characterized by decreasing hemoglobin. In early phase II studies, 39% of patients treated at 300 mg/m^2 every month for 5 months required blood transfusions. Renal toxicity was mild, occurred mainly at higher doses (320, 520 mg/m^2), and was characterized by twofold to fivefold increases in various urinary enzymes, but changes in [^{151}Cr]EDTA clearance occurred only in patients with preexisting renal impairment (Evans et al., 1983). The enzymuria occurred 7–9 days after treatment and returned to normal by day 10–12. Nausea and vomiting appearing 6–12 h after treatment occurred commonly at all doses above 80 mg/kg (80% incidence) and generally resolved within 1 day. Mild paresthesias were reported rarely (8%), but there was a progression of preexisting peripheral neuropathy in patients who had previously received cisplatinum.

LONG-TERM TOXIC EFFECTS

Effects on the Reproductive System

The effect of antineoplastic drugs on gonadal function might be expected because of the ability of these drugs to affect rapidly dividing cells. Indeed, chemicals from nearly every class of antineoplastic drug have been implicated as gonadotoxins in human males (Chapman, 1983), with a preponderance of agents falling into the alkylator category. Interestingly, fewer total agents have been shown to affect reproductive status in females than in males (Chapman, 1983). Drugs most commonly associated with gonadal toxicity are mainly alkylating agents. Busulfan, chlorambucil, and cyclophosphamide have been routinely and widely implicated in sexual dysfunction in both males and females. There is one report of a vinblastine affect on female reproduction. Vinblastine, vincristine, doxorubicin, cytarabine, methotrexate, and procarbazine have been shown to be toxic mainly in males. In addition, there are several drugs that have demonstrated gonadal toxicity of one kind or another in male animals but are not toxic in the human male. Although it is possible that an appropriate patient population or group size has not as yet been studied to uncover such effects, these agents (lomustine, 5-FU, bleomycin, thioTEPA) are used to treat acute leukemia, and this patient population is generally found to have normal fertility and sexual function. Furthermore, it is widely recognized that any cytotoxic drugs that cause gonadal toxicity as single agents cause similar effects but at much lower total doses when used in combination regimens. Most of the above-mentioned agents that do not cause toxicity in human males are utilized in combination regimens where sensitivity might be expected to be very high. The reason for this apparent resistance of human testes is unknown. Effects of these same drugs on reproductive function in female animals have not been addressed.

Common signs and symptoms of gonadal toxicity in the male are oligospermia, azoospermia, decreased sperm motility, and germ-cell aplasia. Less commonly, abnormal serum and urinary gonadotropin levels and alterations in sperm morphology are observed. The effects of methotrexate on fertility are relatively unique among the gonadotoxic antineoplastics, because methotrexate apparently does not alter sperm production by an effect on the germinal layer, but rather affects mature sperm cells, producing reversible abnormalities in motility, count, or morphology (Chapman, 1983). Furthermore, these effects appear to be reversible within 70-90 days after therapy, as might be expected if the effect was not on the germinal layer. The symptoms of drug-induced ovarian failure are symptoms of menopause, with amenorrhea, postmenopausal plasma levels of estrogens and gonadotropins, decreased libido, hot flashes, and irritability. These symptoms are more severe in younger women. There is some evidence that male infertility (primarily azoospermia) may be at least partially reversible if doses are low or if patients are studied over a long enough time period (Buchanan et al., 1975; Sussman and Leonard, 1980). A similar effect in females, particularly in middle-aged women, is not common. It may be that the sensitivity of the gonad to these drugs and the ability of the male to partially reverse may be related to the finite number of germinal cells in the ovary and their decreasing number with progressing age, compared with the potential ability of male germinal epithelium to regenerate and repopulate the testes after cytotoxic insult. Reversibility of ovarian failure may depend on the site and mechanism of action of the cytotoxic agent. If these drugs actually cause a depletion in the number of primary follicles in the ovary, then recovery is less likely to occur than if the effect is merely to impair the normal maturation process of the follicles. Definitive histological studies to answer this question have not yet been conducted. Although not as commonly observed with men as with women, loss of libido and impotence do occur, frequently related to drug-induced decreases in general activity. Usually, however, males exhibit no significant decrease in libido or performance, even though sperm counts may be zero. Females on the other hand manifest a significant decrease in libido and performance, which is consistent with the premature menopause produced by the ovarian failure induced by the cytotoxic drug. In males, testosterone production by Leydig and Sertoli cells of the testes appears to be little affected by drug treatment (Roeser et al., 1978), and only the tubular epithelium, which is responsible for production of mature sperm cells, appears affected. This has been assumed from normal libido and potency, normal testosterone blood levels, but azoospermia. Recently, however, several papers have raised the question of Leydig-cell involvement, and the probability is now accepted that Leydig cells may be histologically altered even though no functional changes (e.g., decreased testosterone production) occur [see discussion in Schilsky and Erlichman (1982)]. A similar conclusion may be drawn from the fact that several antineoplastic drugs are reported to cause gynecomastia (busulfan, vincristine, MOPP regimen), and it can be argued that this is a clinical manifestation of Leydig-cell malfunction. However, definitive work still needs to be done to establish the involvement of these cells in cytotoxic drug toxicity.

Perhaps the greatest factor contributing to sensitivity of patients to gonadal toxicity of antineoplastic agents (except for agent specificity) is the age of the patient. It has traditionally been thought that the prepubertal (e.g., childhood) gonad was relatively resistant to the effects of cytotoxic agents. This is generally true for the female, but some results suggest that the prepubertal testes may be more sensitive to cytotoxic drugs than has generally been thought (Schilsky and Erlichman, 1982). An excellent discussion of this problem is presented by Shalet (1980). In women, gonadal dysfunction seen as ovarian failure is also age-dependent in adults. Women in their early twenties are most resistent to irreversible, total ovarian failure, and as age increases toward the normal menopausal age, risk of irreversible ovarian failure increases. This relationship was dramatically demonstrated by Koyama et al. (1977), who showed that the cumulative dose of cyclophosphamide necessary to induce amenorrhea was 5.2 g, 9.3 g, and 20.4 g in patients whose ages were 40–49 years, 30–39 years, and 20–29 years, respectively.

The influence of the patient's disease on fertility and on gonadal toxicity of antineoplastic drugs has been addressed by some authors, and the results are interesting but inconclusive. For example, there is evidence that serious disease states in general lead to azoospermia or oligospermia, even without the added complication of cytotoxic drug therapy. Destruction of spermatogonia has occurred in childhood leukemia patients who died early in their disease and had therefore received little drug therapy. This suggests that testicular function may be an early casualty of the disease. However, fertility in leukemia patients has never been seriously questioned, and Chapman et al. (1981) showed 100% infertility in adult males after only two courses of MVPP therapy, indicating how soon after drug treatment gonadal damage can be produced. Other studies have suggested that men with Hodgkin's disease showed a decrease in libido prior to receiving chemotherapy (Chapman et al., 1981). Whether this indicates an effect of disease on endocrine function of the testes or merely a generalized decrease in activity level of the cancer patient has not yet been established.

Chronic renal failure is known to be associated with oligospermia, with testicular biopsies showing exactly the same lesions as have been described for patients receiving chlorambucil and cyclophosphamide (Phadke et al., 1970). An interesting result (Roeser et al., 1978) demonstrated a recovery of spermatogenesis in patients with non-Hodgkin's lymphoma after a 34-month follow-up but no similar recovery in patients with Hodgkin's disease after a 52-month follow-up. Whether this differential recovery of testicular function is related to the disease or to differences in the drug regimens is questionable.

It has also been established that there is a threshold dose below which drug-induced infertility may be reversible, or below which incidence may be less than at higher doses. With chlorambucil, azoospermia was always present a doses above 25 mg/kg. Cyclophosphamide produced universal azoospermia at cumulative doses above 18 g when the drug was taken orally. Of interest, however, is that the incidence and reversibility of azoospermia at similar doses when cyclophosphamide was administered intravenously are not firmly established. Irreversible changes in fertility were noted in early trials of mechlorethamine at cumulative doses above 400 mg (Spitz, 1948). It has been difficult to draw conclusions regarding the reversibility of gonadal damage. Most data from single-drug regimens suggest a good potential for recovery of sexual function, particularly in males. Thus when 26 men who had received cyclophosphamide therapy were evaluated for testicular function 15–49 months after completing their therapy, 12 were found to have fully normal sperm counts (Buchanan et al., 1975). When combination regimens are evaluated, however, recovery of spermatogenesis is much less favorable. In large populations of patients treated with MOPP or MVPP, both of which contain more than one agent that by itself is known to cause azoospermia, total infertility lasts at least a full year after cessation of therapy; more than 90% of treated men are infertile after 2 years (Whitehead et al., 1982); and at 4 years after treatment, more than 80% were still infertile (Roeser et al., 1978). There is evidence of reversibility of chlorambucil infertility at low doses (Richter et al., 1970), and azoospermia in men treated with drug combinations also has been shown to be slowly reversible within a 3-year time period. Adriamycin, cyclophosphamide, and cytarabine have produced results in mouse testes that suggest a reversible effect, and the inhibition of DNA synthesis in mouse testes was shown to be slowly reversible for cyclophosphamide, lomustine, thioTEPA, chlorambucil, and busulfan, but with almost no recovery by procarbazine (Lu and Meistrich, 1979). These animal results suggest that a single injection may lead to a nonpermanent effect on testicular function. Unfortunately, most standard chemotherapeutic protocols utilize multiple doses over very prolonged time courses, and this may serve to depress testicular function so severely that practical recovery is unlikely. Reversibility has been reported for methotrexate in psoriasis patients, as discussed above, and in leukemia patients receiving cyclophosphamide or Ara-C. Six of 8 women who received cyclophosphamide for less than 9 months experienced typical cyclophosphamide-induced ovarian failure but had a return of normal and regular menses after therapy (Kumar et al., 1972). This contrasts with only 10% incidence of reversal for patients with an average of 18 months of therapy with cyclophosphamide (Uldall et al., 1972).

Effects on the Developing Fetus

Because the primary target of nearly all cytotoxic antineoplastic agents is the rapidly dividing cell, the toxicity of these agents to the developing fetus and on the progress of fetal development is not surprising. A very large number of antineoplastic drugs have been shown to produce some form of fetal toxicity in animals (Harbison, 1978; Chaube and Murphy, 1968), and in humans the same potential for fetal effects is present, but fortunately the documented incidence of chemotherapy-induced human fetal toxicity is reassuringly low. Fetal intoxication can be classified as either effects on fetal growth and maturation, which would be seen in humans as spontaneous abortions or preterm births, or malformations of the fetus. Both kinds of effects have been observed with antineoplastic drug therapy, particularly when administered during the first trimester of pregnancy. In animals this toxicity can include a decrease in the number of viable young, a decrease in the fertility index of the young, various kinds and incidences of malformation in offspring, or an increase in the incidence of resorptions. In animals a variety of defects in both fetal growth and normal development are observed with any teratogenic agents. Many of these, such as decreased litter size and missing tails, have little relevance to humans. In addition, it has been shown that the middle trimester is the most sensitive time for fetal toxicity to occur in animal tests (Sokal and Lessman, 1972). This has led Sokal and Lessman (1972) to conclude that animal tests are of little value in predicting for teratologic potential in humans. Support is provided for this argument when the apparent insensitivity of the human fetus to cytotoxic drug-induced abnormalities is considered. Although this may be true for specific kinds of abnormalities, the potential to affect fetal growth and development predicted by animal tests cannot be ignored. Even in humans, Nicholson (1968) found that the type of malformation could not be predicted by knowing the drug that was administered, and even frequency has been difficult to estimate. Both of these parameters are difficult to define because of the very small number of cases to study.

Furthermore, although obvious macroscopic effects of antineoplastic drugs on the fetus can easily be evaluated and catalogued, effects on genetic material in the fetus are less easily or readily studied. Thus the recent flurry of interest in vaginal adenocarcinoma in women whose mothers were exposed to diethylstilbesterol during a critical stage in fetal development should caution us against optimistically precluding teratogenicity of a drug based merely on initial observations. Later development of cancer, immune deficiency, learning disability, or other similar effects may not be detectable for many years.

The consensus of numerous authors is that when administered during the second and third trimester of pregnancy, even those agents that are highly teratogenic in animals or have demonstrated teratogenic activity during the first trimester of human pregnancy offer little teratogenic hazard. When used during the first trimester, busulfan, chlorambucil, cyclophosphamide, 6-mercaptopurine, and methotrexate all have been associated with incidents of fetal malformations. Other agents (mechlorethamine, procarbazine, 5-fluorouracil, vinblastine) have been given to women during the first trimester and have produced no teratogenic effects. Reports on other commonly used newer agents are very sparse, possibly because increased awareness of the potential hazard has led to fewer of these agents being administered to women of child-bearing age, and more emphatic cautions are being voiced about becoming pregnant while on antineoplastic drug therapy. In addition, there are reported instances where the administration of these suspected teratogens has been associated with delivery of apparently normal infants (chlorambucil, busulfan, 6-mercaptopurine).

Chlorambucil is mildly teratogenic, producing retinal damage in one instance (Rugh and Skaredoff, 1965) and renal abnormalities in another instance (Shotten and Monie, 1963). In the later case, the mother also had received mechlorethamine and radiation during the pregnancy.

Busulfan has been strongly implicated as a teratogen in an instance where other agents also were given during pregnancy (Diamond et al., 1960). However, because a normal infant was conceived and delivered previously while the mother was on the same multiple-drug regimen minus only busulfan, that drug was assumed to be the cause of the defects. The infant was stunted, had multiple malformations, including ovarian aplasia, and died at 10 weeks of age.

Cyclophosphamide (CTX) has been associated with birth of a stunted infant with multiple soft-tissue and skeletal malformations (Greenberg and Tanaka, 1964). Although the mother had received mechlorethamine prior to CTX, CTX was the only drug administered around the time of conception and during the first weeks of pregnancy. A second incident was a spontaneously delivered dead fetus with no toes and a single coronary artery (Toledo et al., 1971). This mother also was exposed to diagnostic X-irradiation to the uterus, however. In this case, CTX was administered intravenously during the first trimester with oral maintenance therapy during the remainder of gestation.

One of the most potent teratogenic agents in humans is an analog of methotrexate, aminopterin, which is no longer used as a chemotherapeutic agent. This drug is reported to cause in excess of 50% serious malformations, including hydrocephalus, cleft palate, and meningomyelocele (Finkbeiner, 1974). When given during the first trimester, aminopterin also is a potent abortefacient and has been used therapeutically in that capacity. When administered in multiple, small doses during early pregnancy, it causes 80–85% incidence of abortion. Although incidents of MTX administration during the first trimester are few, it should be assumed that MTX has a similar teratogenic potential, because incidents of MTX-related malformations have been reported. Another patient treated with MTX also received actinomycin D and vinblastine and delivered a term infant with encephalopathy, anemia, and a urinary-tract infection (Hutchinson et al., 1968). In six additional patients receiving MTX, three during the first trimester, neither abortions nor fetal malformations were reported (Stutzman and Sokal, 1968). Furthermore, in a 10-year follow-up of 100 women who received MTX, there have been 30 successful pregnancies with no evidence of fetal malformations (Karnofsky, 1967).

Because many of these drugs have been demonstrated to cross the placenta, systemic toxicity from the drug might be expected to occur in the fetus. Incidents of this, however, are low enough to be labeled as curiosities, with only several examples reported in the literature. One reason for this may be the wide variations in neonatal examination techniques, with some physicians being thankful enough for a normal delivery and apparently healthy infant that complete blood studies are not conducted. In one instance 5-fluorouracil treatment during pregnancy was associated with reversible "neonatal drug intoxication" (Stadler and Knowles, 1971), and there is another report of an infant with slight leukopenia being delivered to a mother suffering from severe thrombocytopenia and anemia following treatment with triethylenemelamine for 11 weeks prior to delivery (Nicholson, 1968). Although not usually discussed as possible systemic drug toxicities, widespread reports of stunting and decreased birth weights (Barber, 1981; Ross, 1976; Nicholson, 1968) in infants born to mothers who have received chemotherapy may be additional examples of such toxicities. There are also anecdotal observations of hematopoetic depression in neonates attributable to systemic drug toxicity of transplacental antineoplastic drugs (Barber, 1981). It is also recognized that treatment with multiple agents may be more hazardous to the developing fetus than treatment with single agents. In addition to obvious fetal malformations, some drugs, such as chlorambucil and mechlorethamine, have produced spontaneous abortions (Stutzman and Sokal, 1968), and although 6-mercaptopurine has been only rarely associated with fetal malformation, it is routinely associated with premature births, including infant deaths (Finkbeiner, 1974). Other agents also have become associated with increased incidence of spontaneous abortions, but case studies are small and many patients also had radiation or multiple-drug therapy.

Much of the early literature in this area is concerned with drugs that are no longer used and therefore will not be discussed. The reader is referred to appropriate reviews for more details on these drugs (Chaube and Murphy, 1968; Sokal and Lessman, 1972).

Development of Second Malignancies

The possible risk to patients of cancer produced by antineoplastic drugs was recognized almost as early as chemotherapy first began to be used in cancer treatment (Shimkin, 1954). However, it has only been the past decade that clinicians, statisticians, epidemiologists, and other scientists have seriously begun to address this question. The field is fraught with uncertainty and debate, and this brief review will attempt only to synthesize the numerous difficulties and present the most widely accepted conclusions.

One of the most significant questions addressed by investigators in this areas was on the influence of the primary disease on the appearance of a secondary neoplasm. This question was first addressed because the earliest diseases in which drug-induced secondary neoplasms were noted were malignancies of the lymphoreticular and hematopoietic systems, where it was first suggested that the high incidence of acute leukemias in patients with lymphomas or Hodgkin's disease might be related to drug treatment. The concern, however, was that the appearance of leukemia was merely a progression of the natural history of the lymphoma itself and not causally related to therapy. It is argued that both the primary and secondary neoplasms are diseases of the same system and thus might be manifestations of the same disease origins but with spread to newer sites or actual change of disease form. This latter event has been reported consistently for the transition of Hodgkin's disease to various forms of leukemia (Chan and McBride, 1972; Newman et al., 1970). Another disease that has traditionally had a small incidence of leukemia associated with it is polycythemia vera (PV), where as early as the turn of the century an association between the two diseases was noted. Even now, investigators in this area recognize a small incidence of leukemia as part of the natural history of PV (Berk et al., 1981). The influence that drug therapy has on the acute leukemia incidence may be merely to prolong survival of patients so that the later effect—that is, the leukemia—can be observed. Prior to the widespread use of alkylating agents in the treatment of lymphoma, survival rates for these patients were less than 12 months, but with the advent of single- and multiple-drug treatment regimens, survival increased to greater than 48 months (Costa et al., 1973), thus possibly allowing latent leukemia to be observed. Recently, however, large studies of patients with nonlymphatic cancers have been conducted and published that suggest a drug-therapy-related incidence of second tumors.

Another clinical situation in which the appearance of secondary neoplasms has been noted following drug therapy is renal transplants and other situations where strongly immunosuppressive drugs are administered. Because most antineoplastic agents are at least mildly immunosuppressive, and some of the agents most closely linked to secondary neoplasms (e.g., cyclophosphamide) are strongly so, it is further argued that the drug serves only to predispose patients to second tumors by virtue of its suppression of normal immune function. This would allow latent oncogenic viruses to be expressed or might serve as a promotor for initiators that are already present but suppressed by the active immune system. This has been proposed as a mechanism for the involvement of antimetabolites in the carcinogenic process. These drugs have routinely been found to be not carcinogenic by themselves (see Table 3), but some authors (Harris, 1975) have proposed them as promotors or cocarcinogens.

Frequently, the time between diagnosis of the first cancer and diagnosis of the second is dramatically different in "spontaneous" second malignancies as opposed to "therapy-related" cancers. Appearance of drug-related tumors is an average of 4–6 years after commencing chemotherapy, while spontaneous second tumors may occur simultaneously with the original disease or very shortly after onset of drug treatment (Rosner and Grunwald, 1975).

Furthermore, it is recognized that the presence of cancer frequently predisposes the cancer patient to the development of additional primary neoplasms. Thus, colon, breast, and head–neck cancer patients are at greater risk of developing disease-related second tumors (as distinct from metastatic disease) than are patients with other types of cancers (Rosner et al., 1978). Hodgkin's disease or myeloma patients, for example, occasionally present with simultaneous leukemias (Rosner and Grunwald, 1975). However, it is argued that the leukemia observed in cases of simultaneous development is not the same acute leukemia that is observed in suspected cases of drug-induced cancers. This difference is discussed in detail later. It has been estimated that the occurrence of a second primary tumor in a patient who already has cancer is 2–11% of cases and that these second malignancies may be due to chance, genetic predisposition, or to a common carcinogenic stimulus (Penn, 1982).

A second area of importance is the type of tumor that develops in patients following chemotherapy. Far and away the most common type is an acute leukemia (AL), most generally fitting the criteria for nonlymphocytic (acute nonlymphocytic leukemia, ANLL), although the characteristics are quite variable and heterogeneous. Characteristic in most cases, however, is the appearance of a preleukemic state characterized by the often insidious onset of pancytopenia, which may be dominated by anemia, thrombocytopenia, or leukopenia. Kyle (1982) reports that discontinuation of therapy at this stage rarely prevents the subsequent development of the ANLL. Death ensues rapidly, often within days, and certainly within weeks (Auclerc et al., 1979), and may even precede the actual onset of the leukemia. The ANLL is completely refractory to chemotherapy. This characteristic acute leukemia is observed in patients with Hodgkin's disease, multiple myeloma, non-Hodgkin's lymphoma and other diseases of the hematopoietic/lymphoreticular systems.

Risk of contracting this—and other—second malignancies is very difficult to calculate but may be anywhere from 5- to 10-fold greater for a series of Hodgkin's-disease patients (cited in Kyle, 1982) to greater than 100-fold greater for some multiple-myeloma patients (Gonzalez et al., 1977). One reason for the difficulty in calculating the actual risk of contracting secondary malignancies for those patients receiving a given drug is that the risk increases for those patients with longer survival times. Thus, Kyle (1982) showed the risk to increase from 2.8% to 10.1% at survival times of 5 years and 10 years, respectively, for multiple-myeloma patients. A second reason is that the control population to which the drug-exposed patient is compared is extremely important. Thus, the risk of contracting a second malignancy is greater when drug-treated patients are compared with a naive, age-matched normal population than when compared with a diseased, but not drug-treated, population. The risk will change again when compared with cohorts treated with radiation or other drugs or drug combinations. The appropriate control group is frequently not cited in references that report risk of developing drug-induced neoplasms.

The average time between onset of chemotherapy and development of ANLL in all non-Hodgkin's lymphoma patients ranges from 40 months in one series (Cascioto and Scott, 1979) to 60 months in another (Kyle, 1982). In most cases, evidence of the primary disease for which the chemotherapy had originally been given was absent. In Hodgkin's-disease patients the onset of AL was 53 months to 6 years (Kyle, 1982).

In many cancers chemotherapy is accompanied by radiotherapy, particularly in Hodgkin's disease. The presence of this leukemogenic treatment modality further complicates the evaluation of drug therapy as carcinogenic. In a series of multiple-myeloma patients summarized by Kyle (1982), radiation did not increase the incidence of acute leukemia (AL) over that seen in drug-only treated patients, and in a series of Hodgkin's-disease patients, no incidence of AL was detected in 236 patients who received only radiotherapy, while 3.5% of patients treated with chemotherapy and radiotherapy developed AL (Valagussa et al., 1980). It is, therefore, generally held that although radiation may not itself induce AL in cancer patients, there is some evidence that the interaction of chemotherapy and radiotherapy may in some cases increase the incidence of drug-associated secondary malignancies (Toland et al., 1978). One unique finding, however, is that dactinomycin therapy actually decreased the incidence of radiation-induced secondary malignancies in childhood cancers (D'Angio et al., 1976).

Non-Hodgkin's lymphoma (NHL) also has been observed in patients receiving drug therapy and has been related to therapy-induced cancer. NHL developed at a median time of 94 months after drug therapy in Hodgkin's disease patients. The incidence of this posttherapy malignancy is counted in tens of cases, rather than in the hundreds as is the case for acute leukemia. Incidence of various solid tumors following chemotherapy for multiple myeloma is usually not increased.

The development of solid tumors as secondary malignancies is less likely than the development of leukemia, but it does occur, particularly in patients with lymphoma, where sarcomas were the most prevalent tumor in a large series reported by Arsenau et al. (1977). In addition, cyclophosphamide use is associated with an increased incidence of lymphomas with primary sites in the brain (Schilsky and Erlichman, 1982), and the induction of bladder tumors in patients undergoing therapy with cyclophosphamide is well established and is the only case where carcinogenesis data in animals with respect to site and type of malignancy is similar to human data (Wall and Clauson, 1975).

It is extremely difficult to ascribe carcinogenic activity to individual drugs used to treat cancer, because the trend is increasingly toward multiple-drug regimens. Thus, the popular MOPP regimen for treatment of Hodgkin's disease contains mechlorethamine, vincristine, prednisone, and procarbazine. This regimen is one that is commonly implicated in therapy-associated secondary tumors. At least two of the agents (mechlorethamine and procarbazine) have been shown to be carcinogenic in animals and to be probably carcinogenic in humans. Which, if any, individual agent may be responsible for the carcinogenic effects of this regimen in humans is therefore difficult to determine with any certainty. This is a single example, and the discipline contains many other similar examples.

In general, alkylating agents are present in most therapeutic regimens that have been associated with therapy-related second neoplasms, and these agents, as a class, are generally considered to be probably carcinogenic in humans. The highly reactive nature of these chemicals and the large number of instances of carcinogenesis in animals (Sieber and Adamson, 1975; Weisburger, 1977; Schmahl and Habs, 1978, 1980) lend support to the concept of their carcinogenicity. In spite of the prevalence of multiple-drug regimens, there are several drugs whose use as single agents has been followed by the appearance of second cancers so frequently that that carcino-genic activity in humans can be ascribed to them with some certainty.

Several authors have adopted the wise policy of referring to the relative carcino-genic potential of a drug based on available data rather than merely dogmatically saying it is carcinogenic or not. Thus, the antimetabolites (MTX, 5-FU) are "unlikely to be" or are "apparently not" carcinogenic in humans, while cyclophosphamide and melphalan are carcinogenic in humans. Using this relative scheme, the following drugs have been found to produce cancer in humans: cyclophosphamide, melphalan, and chlorambucil. The following agents are "probably" carcinogenic in humans but data are still insufficient to allow further comment: busulfan, dacarbazine, procarba-zine, lomustine, and thioTEPA. Several drugs can be listed as probably not, or un-likely to be, carcinogenic in humans: vinblastine, 6-mercaptopurine, 5-fluorouracil, and methotrexate. In addition, there are numerous drugs that have never been studied for their relationship to second (or primary) tumors in humans. It is tempting to assume that if a drug is not listed above, it is noncarcinogenic in humans, but such an assumption would be unwarranted. Several antineoplastic drugs are known to be carcinogenic in animals (see Table 3) under various conditions of dose, regimen, and route, or to be mutagenic in any of a large number of potential in vitro or in vivo assay systems: daunorubicin, doxorubicin, cisplatinum, carmustine, mechlore-thamine, and vincristine. These agents obviously have a strong potential of being carcinogenic in humans.

Chlorambucil is one of the agents to which human carcinogenicity can reasonably be assigned. In the cases reviewed by the IARC in 1981 (IARC, 1981), at least 35 cases of second malignancies directly attributable to chlorambucil were recorded. These were patients with both malignant and nonmalignant diseases who had received chlorambucil as the only therapy. With only a few exceptions, all of the secondary malignancies were acute nonlymphocytic leukemia (ANLL). In addition, there were nearly 3000 other case histories of patients who had developed second cancers after receiving chlorambucil in addition to either radiation or other drugs. At that time, IARC concluded chlorambucil had only "probable" carcinogenic ability in humans. Subsequently, convincing evidence for the leukemogenic potential of chlorambucil was published by the Polycythemia Vera Study Group (Berk et al., 1981). In their study of the incidence of acute leukemia in polycythemia vera (PV) patients treated only with chlorambucil, they found 16 cases of ANLL in 141 patients treated with the drug and only 1 case of ANLL in 134 patients treated by phlebotomy alone. Interest-ingly, the incidence of ANLL in chlorambucil-treated patients was even greater than in those patients receiving radiotherapy with phosphorus-32 (9/156). The Study Group concluded that the risk of developing ANLL with chlorambucil was so great that they no longer recommend its use in this disease. Additionally, 12 cases of ANLL have been diagnosed from among 1400 ovarian cancer patients (Greene et al., 1982). Of these 12, 2 received chlorambucil as their only therapy. In addition, chlorambucil has been shown to be a potent carcinogen in animals (Weisburger et al., 1975).

The second antineoplastic drug with proven carcinogenic activity in humans as evaluated by the IARC is melphalan. This drug, like chlorambucil, is also an alkylating agent. Melphalan was recognized (IARC, 1979) as being carcinogenic in humans based on its strongly carcinogenic ability in rodents and on the numerous reported instances of acute nonlymphocytic leukemia (ANLL) in patients receiving melphalan for long periods of time. In one early study, Rosner and Grunwald (1974) reported four cases of ANLL in multiple-myeloma patients who had received only melphalan therapy for their disease. The mean interval from diagnosis of the myeloma to diagnosis of leukemia was 49 months. Eight other myeloma patients who received melphalan and developed ANLL were also treated with either radiation or other chemotherapeutic agents. In a more recent study that also supports the IARC finding, Green et al. (1983) reported the incidence of ANLL appearing in ovarian cancer patients who were treated with alkylating agents. Seven patients out of 12 who acquired ANLL were treated only with melphalan. The other five patients received various combinations of melphalan with radiation or other cytotoxic drugs. Melphalan is a potent carcinogen in animals, causing lung tumors after intraperitoneal administration and skin tumors after dermal application.

The third anticancer drug that is carcinogenic in humans is cyclophosphamide. At least 20 cases of malignancies have occurred in patients receiving cyclophosphamide for nonmalignant diseases (e.g., glomerulonephritis and rhematoid arthritis), and 23 cases of second malignancies have occurred in cancer patients receiving only cyclophosphamide as therapy. Of all 43 undisputed cases, 17 were ANLL and an additional 14 were bladder cancers. The bladder cancer likely arises as a result of the metabolic decomposition of cyclophosphamide into acrolein, a known carcinogen, and the excretion of acrolein via the urine (Alarcon and Meienhofer, 1971). In addition, one of the toxic effects of systemic cyclophosphamide therapy is hemorraghic cystitis due to bladder irritation caused by the metabolic decomposition products of cyclophosphamide. The occurrence of bladder tumors is one of the few occasions where animal carcinogenesis data correlate well with human data, because both carcinomas and papillomas of the urinary bladder were reported when cyclophosphamide was given orally on a qd × 5 schedule to rats. In addition, the rat study detected a significant increase in tumor incidence at doses that, when extrapolated to human use, were lower than those used clinically to treat cancer (Schmahl and Habs, 1979).

Other antineoplastic agents could easily be considered human carcinogens based on small numbers of case histories where a second neoplasm developed after exposure of the patient to a single drug, combined with a strong carcinogenic response in animal tests. Thus, thioTEPA has been implicated as the only agent administered to several patients who developed acute leukemia (Rosner et al., 1978; Belpomme et al., 1974), and this drug is carcinogenic in animals (IARC, 1975). Busulfan is another agent that is strongly carcinogenic in animals (IARC, 1974) and that has been the only drug administered to small number of patients who subsequently developed second malignancies (Youness et al., 1978). Busulfan is further implicated because its dihydroxy analog, treosulfan, is considered carcinogenic in humans (IARC, 1981). Finally, Schmahl and Habs (1980) concluded that streptozotocin, nitrosoureas, and procarbazine were all "definitely or likely" carcinogens in humans. These and other similar agents are best classified as "probably" carcinogenic in humans until larger patient populations developing secondary tumors can be studied. Schmahl et al.

(1982) have recently reviewed the association between many of these "probable" agents and second human neoplasms.

REFERENCES

Adamson, R. H., and Fabro, S. 1968. Embryotoxic effects of L-asparaginase. *Nature (Lond.)* 218:1164–1165.

Adamson, R., and Sieber, S. 1981. Chemically-induced leukemia in humans. *Environ. Health Perspect.* 39:93–103.

Ahmed, T., Kemeny, N. E., Michaelson, R. A., and Harper, H. D. 1983. Phase II trial of bisantrene in advanced colorectal cancer. *Cancer Treat. Rep.* 67:307–308.

Alarcon, R. A., and Meienhofer, J. 1971. Formation of the cytotoxic aldehyde acrolein during in vitro degradation of cyclohosphamide. *Nature (New Biol.)* 233:250–252.

Alberts, D. S., Griffith, K. S., Goodman, G. E., Herman, T. S., and Murray, E. 1980. Phase I clinical trial of mitoxantrone: A new anthracenedione anticancer drug. *Cancer Chemother. Pharmacol.* 5:11–15.

Arseneau, J. C., Canellos, G. P., Johnson, R., and DeVita, V. 1977. Risk of new cancer in patients with Hodgkin's disease. *Cancer* 40:1912–1916.

Auclerc, G., Jacquillat, G., Auclerc, M., Weil, M., and Bernard, J. 1979. Posttherapeutic acute leukemia. *Cancer* 44:2017–2025.

Barber, H. 1981. Fetal and neonatal effects of cytotoxic agents. *Obstet. Gynecol.* 58:(Suppl. 5):41S–47S.

Belpomme, D., Carde, P., Oldham, R., Mathe, G., Jacquillat, C., Chelloul, M., Weil, M., Auclerc, G., Weisgerber, C., Tanzer, T., and Bernard, J. 1974. Malignancies possibly secondary to anticancer therapy. *Recent Results Cancer Res.* 49:115–123.

Berk, P. D., Goldberg, J. D., Silverstein, M. N., Weinfield, A., Donovan, P. D., Ellis, J. T., Landow, S. A., Laszlo, J., Najean, Y., Pisciotta, A. V., and Wasserman, L. R. 1981. Increased incidence of acute leukemia in polycythemia vera associated with chlorambucil therapy. *N. Engl. J. Med.* 304:441–447.

Bertazolli, C., Chieli, T., and Solcia, E. 1971. Different incidence of breast carcinomas or fibroadenomas in daunomycin or adriamycin treated rats. *Experientia* 27:1209–1210.

Boyland, E., and Horning, E. S. 1949. Induction of tumors with nitrogen mustards. *Br. J. Cancer* 3:118–123.

Bradner, W. T., and Schurig, J. 1981. Toxicology screening in small animals. *Cancer Treat. Rev.* 8:93–102.

Border, L. E., and Carter, S. K. 1973. Pancreatic islet cell carcinoma, II: Results of therapy with streptozotocin in 52 patients. *Ann. Int. Med.* 79:108–118.

Buchanan, J. D., Fairley, K. F., and Barrie, J. 1975. Return of spermatogenesis after stopping cyclophosphamide therapy. *Lancet* ii:156–157.

Burchenal, J., Murphy, M., Ellison, R. Sykes, M., Tan, T., Leone, L., Karnofsky, D., Graver, L., Dargeon, H., and Rhoads, C. 1953. Clinical evaluation of a new antimetabolite, 6-mercaptopurine, in the treatment of leukemia and allied diseases. *Blood* 8:965–999.

Bus, J. S., and Gibson, J. E. 1973. Teratogenicity and neonatal toxicity of ifosfamide in mice. *Proc. Soc. Exp. Biol. Med.* 143:965–970.

Calvert, A., Harland, S., Newell, D., Siddik, A., Jones, A., McElwain, T., Raju, S., Wiltshaw, E., Smith, I., Baker, F., Peckham, M., and Harrap, K. 1982. Early clinical studies with *cis*-Diammine-1,1-cyclobutane dicarboxylate platinum II. *Cancer Chemother. Pharmacol.* 9:140–147.

Calvert, A. H., Harland, S. J., Harrap, K. R., Wiltshaw, E., and Smith, I. E. 1983. JM-8 Development and clinical projects. In *Platinum Coordination Complexes in Cancer Chemotherapy*, eds. M. Hacker, E. Douple, and I. Krakoff, pp. 240–252. Boston: Nijhoff.

Carbone, P. P.., Bono, V., Frei, E., and Brindley, C. O. 1963. Clinical studies with vincristine. *Blood* 21:640–647.

Casciato, D. A., and Scott, J. L. 1979. Acute leukemia following prolonged cytotoxic agent therapy. *Medicine* 58:32–47.

Chan, B. W., and McBride, J. A. 1972. Hodgkin's disease and leukemia. *Can. Med. Assoc. J.* 106:558–561.

Chapman, R. M. 1983. Gonadal injury resulting from chemotherapy. *Am. J. Ind. Med.* 4:149–161.

Chapman, R. M., Sutcliffe, S. B., and Malpas, J. S. 1981. Male gonadal function in Hodgkin's disease: A prospective study. *J. Am. Med. Assoc.* 245:1323–1328.

Chaube, S., and Murphy, M. 1968. The teratogenic effects of the recent drugs active in cancer chemotherapy. *Adv. Teratol.* 3:181–219.

Chaube, S., and Murphy, M. L. 1969. Fetal malformations produced in rats by procarbazine. *Teratology* 2:23–32.

Chaube, S., Kury, G., and Murphy, M. L. 1967. Teratogenic effects of cyclophosphamide in the rat. *Cancer Chemother. Reports* 51:363–379.

Coe, R., and Bull, F. 1968. Cirrhosis associated with methotrexate treatment of psoriasis. *J. Am. Med. Assoc.* 206:1515–1520.

Costa, G., Engle, R. L., and Schilling, A. 1973. Melphalan and prednisone: Effective combination for treatment of multiple myeloma. *Am. J. Med.* 54:589–599.

Costanzi, J., Gagliano, R., Loukas, D., Panettiere, F., and Hokanson, J. 1978. Ifosfamide in the treatment of recurrent or disseminated lung cancer. *Cancer* 41:1715–1719.

Creagan, E. T., Schutt, A. J., Ahmann, D. L., and Green, S. J. 1982. Phase II study of an aziridinylbenzoquinone (AZQ) in disseminated malignant melanoma. *Cancer Treat. Reports* 66:2089–2090.

Crooke, S., and Bradner, W. 1976. Mitomycin C: A review. *Cancer Treat. Rev.* 3:121–139.

Dahl, M. G., Gregory, M. M., and Schever, P. J. 1971. Liver damage due to methotrexate in patients with psoriasis. *Br. Med. J.* 1:625–630.

Danforth, C. H., and Center, E. 1954. Nitrogen mustard as a teratogenic agent in the mouse. *Proc. Soc. Exp. Biol. Med.* 86:705–707.

D'Angio, G. J., Meadows A., Mike, V., Harris, C., Evans, A., Jaffe, N., Newton, W., Schweisguth, O., Sutow, W., and Morris-Jones, P. 1976. Decreased risk of radiation associated second malignant neoplasms in actinomycin D treated patients. *Cancer* 37:1177–1185.

DeWys, W. D., and Fowler, E. H. 1973. Report of vasculitis and blindness after intracarotid injection of 1,3-bis(2-chloroethyl)-1-nitrosourea (BCNU) in dogs. *Cancer Chemother. Rep.* 57:33–40.

Diamond, I., Anderson, M. M., and McCreadie, S. R. 1960. Transplacental transmission of busulfan (myleran) in a mother with leukemia. *Pediatrics* 25:85–90.

DiMarco, A., Gaetani, M., and Scarpinato, B. 1969. Adriamycin—A new antibiotic with antitumor activity. *Cancer Chemother. Rep. (Part I)* 53:33–37.

DiPaolo, J. A. 1969. Teratogenic agents: Mammalian test systems and chemicals. *Ann. NY Acad. Sci.* 163:801–812.

Driscoll, J. S., Dudeck, L., and Congelton, G. 1979. Potential CNS antitumor agents. VI, Aziridinylbenzoquinone III. *J. Pharm. Sci.* 68:185–188.

Einhorn, M., and Davidsohn, I. 1964. Hepatotoxicity of mercaptopurine. *J. Am. Med. Assoc.* 88:802–806.

Evans, B. D., Raju, K. S., Calvert, A. H., Harland, S. J., and Wiltshaw, E. 1983. JM 8 (*cis*diammine 1,1-cyclobutane dicarboxylate platinum II): A new platinum analogue active in the treatment of advanced ovarian carcinoma. *Cancer Treat. Rep.* 67:997–1005.

Evans, F., Gerritsen, G., Mann, K., and Owen, S. 1965. Antitumor and hyperglycemic activity of streptozotocin (NSC-37917) and its cofactor, U-15,774. *Cancer Chemother. Rep.* 48:1–6.

Ezdinli, E. Z., Sokal, J., Aungst, C., Kim, U., and Sandberg, A. 1969. Myeloid leukemia in Hodgkin's disease: Chromosomal abnormalities. *Ann. Int. Med.* 71:1097–1104.

Finkbeiner, J. A. 1974. Antineoplastic chemotherapy in pregnancy. In *Surgical Disease in Pregnancy,* eds. H. R. Barber and E. A. Graber, pp. 711–718. Philadelphia: Saunders.

Fossa, S., and Talle, K. 1980. Treatment of metastatic renal cancer with ifosfamide and mesnum with and without irradiation. *Cancer Treat. Rep.* 64:1103–1108.

Gilman, A., and Philips, F. S. 1946. The biological actions and therapeutic applications of 2-chloroethyl amines and sulfides. *Science* 103:409–414.

Ginsberg, S. J., and Comis, R. L. 1982. Pulmonary toxicity of antineoplastic agents. *Semin. Oncol.* 9:34–51.

Goldenthal, E. I. 1971. Compilation of LD50 values in newborn and adult animals. *Toxicol. Appl. Pharmacol.* 18:185–207.

Gonzalez, E., Trujillo, J. M., and Alexanian, R. 1977. Acute leukemia in multiple myeloma. *Ann. Int. Med.* 86:449–443.

Greco, C., Corsi, A., Caputo, M., Cavallari, A., and Calabresi, F. 1979. Cyclophosphamide and iphosphamide against Lewis lung carcinoma: Evaluation of toxic and therapeutic effects. *Tumori* 65:169–180.

Green, D., Williams, P., Simpon, L., Blumenson, L., and Murphy, G. 1983. Evaluation of the chronic hepatic toxicity of 6-mercaptopurine in the Wistar rat. *Oncology* 40:138–142.

Greenberg, L. H., and Tanaka, K. R. 1964. Congenital anomalies probably induced by cyclophosphamide. *J. Am. Med. Assoc.* 188:423–426.

Greene, M. H., Boice, J. D., Greer, B. E., Blessing, J. A., and Dembo, A. J. 1982. Acute nonlymphocytic leukemia after therapy with alkylating agents for ovarian cancer. A study of five randomized clinical trials. *N. Engl. J. Med.* 307:1416–1421.

Grever, M., Bisaccia, E., Scarborough, D., Metz, E., and Neidhart, J. 1983. Investigation of 2'-deoxycoformycin in the treatment of cutaneous T-cell lymphoma. *Blood* 61:279–282.

Griffin, J., Newman, R., McCormack, J., and Krakoff, I. 1982. Clinical and clinical pharmacologic studies of aziridinylbenzoquinone. *Cancer Treat. Rep.* 66:1321–1325.

Guarino, A., Rozencweig, M., Kline, I., Penta, J., Venditti, J., Llyod, H., Holzworth, A., and Muggia, F. 1979. Adequacies and inadequacies in assessing murine toxicity data with antineoplastic agents. *Cancer Res.* 39:2204–2210.

Hanna, W. T., Kraus, S., Regester, R. F., and Murphy, W. M. 1981. Renal disease after mitomycin C therapy. *Cancer* 118:2583–2588.

Harbison, R. D. 1978. Chemical-biological reactions common to teratogenesis and mutagenesis. *Environ. Health Perspect.* 24:87–100.

Harmon, W., Cohen, H., Sahneeberger, and Grupe, W. 1979. Chronic renal failure in children treated with methyl CCNU. *N. Engl. J. Med.* 300:1200–1203.

Harris, C. C. 1975. Immunosuppressive anticancer drugs in man: Their oncogenic potential. *Radiology* 114:163–166.

Harrison, S. D., Denine, E. P., and Peckham, J. C. 1978. Qualitative and quantitative toxicity of single and sequential sublethal doses of 5-fluorouracil in BDF mice. *Cancer Treat. Rep.* 62:533–545.

Haskell, C. 1981. L-Asparaginase: Human toxicology and single agent activity in nonleukemic neoplasms. *Cancer Treat. Rep.* 65:57–59.

Hata, T. 1978. Approaches to improved anticancer activity with mitomycins. In *Advances in Cancer Chemotherapy,* eds. S. Carter et al., pp. 83–93. Baltimore: University Park Press.

Hayes, F. A., Green, A. A., Senzer, N., and Pratt, C. B. 1979. Tetany: A complication of cisdichlorodiammine platinum therapy. *Cancer Treat. Rep.* 63:547–548.

Hebborn, P., Mishra, L. C., Dalton, C., and Williams, J. P. 1965. Dental lesions in rats induced by radiomimetic agents. *Arch. Pathol.* 80:110–115.

Henderson, B., Dougherty, W., James, V., Tilley, L., and Noble, J. 1982. Safety assessment of a new anticancer compound, mitoxantrone, in beagle dogs: Comparison with doxorubicin. 1. Clinical observations. *Cancer Treat. Rep.* 66:1139–1249.

Henry, M., Port, C., and Levine, B. S. 1980. Preclinical toxicologic evaluation of 4-(9-acridinylamino) methanesulfon-M-anisidide (AMSA) in mice, dogs, and monkeys. *Cancer Treat. Rep.* 64:855–860.

Heston, W. 1953. Occurrence of tumors in mice injected subcutaneously with sulfur mustard and nitrogen mustard. *J. Natl. Cancer Inst.* 14:131–140.

Hill, J. M., Loeb, E., Maclellan, A., Hill, N. O., Khan, A., and King, J. J. 1975. Clinical studies of platinum coordination compounds in the treatment of various malignant diseases. *Cancer Chemother. Rep.* 59:647–659.

Houchens, D. P., Johnson, R. K., Gaston, M. R., and Goldin, A. 1977. Toxicity of cancer chemotherapeutic agents in athymic (nude) mice. *Cancer Treat. Rep.* 61:103–104.

Houghton, J. A., Houghton, P. J., and Wooten, R. S. 1979. Mechanism of induction of gastrointestinal toxicity in the mouse by 5-fluorouracil, 5-fluorouridine and 5-fluoro-2-deoxyuridine. *Cancer Res.* 39:2406–2413.

Hutchinson, J. R., Peterson, E. P., and Zimmermann, E. A. 1968. Coexisting metastatic choriocarcinoma and normal pregnancy. Therapy during gestation with maternal remission and fetal survival. *Obstet. Gynecol.* 31:331–336.

IARC. 1974. *IARC Monogr. Eval. Carcinog. Risk Chem. Hum.* 4: *Some Aromatic Amines, Hydrazine and Related Substances,* N-*Nitroso Compounds and Miscellaneous Alkylating Agents.* International Agency for Research in Cancer, Lyon, France.

IARC. 1975. *IARC Monogr. Eval. Carcinog. Risk Chem. Hum.* 9: *Some Aziridines,* N-, S-, *and* O-*Mustards and Selenium.* International Agency for Research on Cancer, Lyon, France.

IARC. 1976. *IARC Monogr. Eval. Carcinog. Risk Chem. Hum.* 10: *Some Naturally Occurring Substances.* International Agency for Research on Cancer, Lyon, France.

IARC. 1979. *IARC Monogr. Eval. Carcinog. Risk Chem. Hum.* Suppl. 1: *Chemical and Industrial Procedures Associated with Cancer in Humans,* pp. 4–13. International Agency for Research on Cancer, Lyon, France.

IARC. 1981. *IARC Monogr. Eval. Carcinog. Risk Chem. Hum.* 26: *Some Antineoplastic and Immunosuppressive Agents.* International Agency for Research on Cancer, Lyon, France.

Issell, B. 1980. Amsacrine (AMSA). *Cancer Treat. Rev.* 7:73–83.

Jungi, W. F., and Senn, H. J. 1975. Clinical study of the new podophyllotoxin derivative, 4'-demethylepipodophyllotoxin 9-(4,6-O-ethylidene-β-D-glucopyranoside) (NSC-141540; VP-16-213) in solid tumors in man. *Cancer Chemother. Rep.* 59:737–742.

Kanofsky, J. R., Roth, D. G., Smyth, J. F., Baron, J. M., Sweet, D. L., and Ultman, J. E. 1982. Treatment of lymphoid malignancies with 2'-deoxycoformycin. *Am. J. Clin. Oncol.* 5:179–183.

Kaplan, R. S., Wiernik. P. H. 1982. Neurotoxicity of antineoplastic drugs. *Semin. Oncol.* 9:103–130.

Karnofsky, D. A. 1967. Late effects of immunosuppressive anticancer drugs. *Fed. Proc.* 26:925–932.

Kelsen, D., Chapman, R., Bains, M., Hellan, R., Dukeman, M., and Golbey, R. 1982. Phase II study of methyl-GAG in the treatment of esophageal carcinoma. *Cancer Treat. Rep.* 66:1427–1429.

Kempf, S. R., and Ivankovic, S. 1986. Carcinogenic effect of cisplatin in BD IX rats. *J. Cancer Res. Clin. Oncol.* III:133–136.

Knight, W., Livingston, R., Fabian, C., and Costanzi, J. 1979. Phase I–II trial of methyl-GAG: A Southwest Oncology Group pilot study. *Cancer Treat. Rep.* 63:1933–1957.

Knight, W., Loesch, D. M., Leichman, L. P., Fabian, C., and O'Bryan, R. M. 1982. Methyl-GAG in advanced colon cancer: A phase II trial of the Southwest Oncology Group. *Cancer Treat. Rep.* 66:2099–2100.

Koppang, H. S. 1973. Histomorphometric investigation on the effect of cyclophosphamide on dentinogenesis of rat incisor. *Scand. J. Dent. Res.* 81:383–396.

Kovach, J., Ames, M., Powis, G., Moertel, C., Hahn, R., and Creagan, E. 1979. Toxicity and pharmacokinetics of a pyrrolizidine alkaloid, indicine N-oxide, in humans. *Cancer Res.* 39:4540–4544.

Koyama, H., Wada, T., Nishizawa, Y., Iwanaga, T., Aoki, Y., Teresawa, T., Kosaki, G., Yamamoto, T., and Wada, A. 1977. Cyclophosphamide-induced ovarian failure and its therapeutic significance in patients with breast cancer. *Cancer* 39:1403–1409.

Kumar, R., McEvoy, J., Biggart, J., and McGeown, M. 1972. Cyclophosphamide and reproductive function. *Lancet* i:1212–1214.

Kyle, R. 1982. Second malignancies associated with chemotherapeutic agents. *Semin. Oncol.* 9:131–141.

Lazar, R, Conran, P. C., and Damjanov, I. 1979. Embryotoxicity and teratogenicity of cis-diammine dichloroplatinum. *Experientia* 35:647–648.

Lee, F., Conetta, R., Issell, T., and Lenz, L. 1983. New platinum complexes in clinical trials. *Cancer Treat. Rev.* 10:39–51.

Legha, S. S., Slavik, M., and Carter, S. K. 1976. Hexamethylmelamine: An evaluation of its role in the therapy of cancer. *Cancer* 38:27–35.

Legha, S., Latreilla, J., McCredie, K., and Bodey, G. 1979. Neurologic and cardiac rhythm abnormalities associated with 4-(9-acridinylamino) methanesulfon-M-anisidide (AMSA) therapy. *Cancer Treat. Rep.* 63:2001–2003.

Leopold, W. R., Miller, E. C., and Miller, J. A. 1979. Carcinogenicity of antitumor cis-platinum (II) coordination complexes in the mouse and rat. *Cancer Res.* 39:913–918.

Letendre, L., Smithson, W., Gilchrist, G., Burgert, E., Hoagland, C., Ames, M., Powis, G., Phil, D., and Kovach, J. 1981. Activity of indicine N-oxide in refractory acute leukemia. *Cancer* 47:437–441.

Litterst, C., Collins, J., Lowe, M., Arnold, S., Powell, D., and Guarino, A. 1982. Local and systemic toxicity resulting from large-volume ip administration of doxorubicin in the rat. *Cancer Treat. Rep.* 66:157–161.

Lokich, J., Drum, D., and Kaplan, W. 1974. Hepatic toxicity of nitrosourea analogues. *Clin. Pharmacol. Ther.* 16:363–367.

Lu, C., and Meistrick, M. 1979. Cytotoxic effects of chemotherapeutic drugs on mouse testis cells. *Cancer Res.* 39:3575–3582.

Major, P., Agarwal, R., and Kufe, D. 1981a. Clinical pharmacology of deoxycoformycin. *Blood* 58:91–96.

Major, P., Agarwal, R., and Kufe, D. 1981b. Deoxycoformycin: Neurological toxicity. *Cancer Chemother. Pharmacol.* 5:193–196.

Marquardt, H., Philips, F., and Sternberg, S. 1976. Tumorigenicity in vivo and induction of malignant transformation and mutagenesis in cell cultures by adriamycin and daunomycin. *Cancer Res.* 36:2065–1069.

McCredie, K. B., Bodey, G. P., Burgess, M. A., Gutterman, J. U., Rodriquez, V., Sullivan, M. P., and Freireich, E. J. 1973. Treatment of acute leukemia with 5-azacytidine. *Cancer Chemother. Rep.* 57:319–323.

Menard, D. B., Gisselbrecht, C., Marty, M., Reyes, F., and Dhumeaux, D. 1980. Antineoplastic agents and the liver. *Gastroenterology* 78:142–164.

Merck Index, 1976. Merck & Co., Inc. Rahway, N.J. 9th Edition.

Milarsky, A., and Gaynor, M. 1968. Methotrexate induced congenital malformations. *J. Pediatr.* 72:790–795.

Minow, R. A., Benjamin, R. S., and Gottlieb, J. A. 1975. Adriamycin cardiomyopathy. An overview with determination of risk factors. *Cancer Chemother. Rep. (Part 3)* 6:195–201.

Murphy, M. L. 1959. Comparison of teratogenic effects of 5 polyfunctional alkylating agents on the rat fetus. *Pediatrics* 23:231–244.

Nemeth, L., Somfi, S., Gal, F., and Kellner, B. 1970. Comparative studies concerning the tumor inhibition and toxicology of vinblastine and vincristine. *Neoplasma* 17:345–347.

Newman, D. R., Maldonado, J. E., Harrison, E. C., Kiely, J. M., and Linman, J. W. 1970. Myelomonocytic leukemia in Hodgkin's disease. *Cancer* 25:128–133.

Nichols, W., Moertel, C., Rubin, J., Schutt, A., and Britell, J. 1981. Phase II trial of indicine *N*-oxide (INDI) in patients with advance colorectal carcinoma. *Cancer Treat. Rep.* 65:337–339.

Nicholson, H. O. 1968. Cytotoxic drugs in pregnancy. Review of reported cases. *J. Obstet. Gynecol. Br. Commonw.* 73:307–312.

O'Connell, T. X., and Berenbaum, M. D. 1974. Cardiac and pulmonary effects of high doses of cyclophosphamide and isophosphamide. *Cancer Res.* 34:1586–1591.

Oettgen, H., Stephenson, P., Schwartz, M., Leeper, R., Tallae, L., Tan, C., Clarkson, B., Golbey, R., Krakoff, I., Karnofsky, D., Murphy, M., and Burchenal, J. 1970. Toxicity of *E. coli* L-asparaginase in man. *Cancer* 25:253–278.

Ohnuma, T., Sridhar, K., Ratner, L., and Holland, J. 1982. Phase I study of indicine *N*-oxide in patients with advanced cancer. *Cancer Treat. Rep.* 66:1509–1575.

Oliverio, V. T. 1973. Toxicology and pharmacology of the nitrosoureas. *Cancer Chemother. Rep. (Part 3)* 4:13–20.

Ozols, R. F., Deisseroth, A. B., Javadpour, N., Barlock, A., Messerschmidt, G. L., and Young, R. C. 1983. Treatment of poor prognosis nonseminomatous testicular cancer with a "high dose" platinum combination chemotherapy regimen. *Cancer* 51:1803–1807.

Palm, P. E., and Kensler, C. J. 1971. Toxicology of a new pyrimidine antimetabolite, 5-azacytidine, in mice, hamsters and dogs. *Toxicol. Appl. Pharmacol.* 19:382–383.

Penn, I. 1982. Second neoplasms following radiotherapy or chemotherapy for cancer. *Am. J. Clin. Oncol.* 5:83–96.

Perry, M. C., Forastiere, A. A., Richards, F., Weiss, R. B., and Anbar, D. 1982. Phase II trial of bisantrene in advanced colorectal cancer: A cancer and leukemia Group B study. *Cancer Treat. Rep.* 66:1997–1998.

Phadke, A., MacKinnon, K., and Dossetor, J. 1970. Male fertility in uremia: Restoration by renal allografts. *Can. Med. Assoc. J.* 102:607–608.

Philips, F. S., and Thiersch, J. B. 1950. Nitrogen mustard-like actions of 2,4,6-tris(ethylenimino)-S-triazene and other bis(ethylenimines). *J. Pharmacol. Exp. Ther.* 100:398–407.

Philips, F. S., Schwartz, H. S., and Sternberg, S. F. 1960a. Pharmacology of mitomycin C. I. Toxicity and pathologic effects. *Cancer Res.* 20:1354–1361.

Philips, F., Schwartz, H., Sternberg, S., and Tan, C. 1960b. The toxicity of actinomycin D. *Ann. N.Y. Acad. Sci.* 89:348–360.

Philips, F. S., Sternberg, S. S., Coronin, A. P., and Vidal, P. M. 1961. Cyclophosphamide and urinary bladder toxicity. *Cancer Res.* 21:1577–1589.

Philips, F. S., Sternberg, S. S., Hamilton, L., and Clark, D. A. 1956. Toxic effects of 6-mercaptopurine and related compounds. *Ann. N.Y. Acad. Sci.* 54:283–296.

Philips, F. S., Gilladoga, A., Marquardt, H., Sternberg, S., and Vidal, P. M. 1975. Some observations on the toxicity of adriamycin. *Cancer Chemother. Rep. (Part 3)* 6:177–181.

Poplack, D., Sallan, S., Rivera, G., Holcenberg, J., Murphy, S., Blatt, J., Lipton, J., Venner, P., Glaubiger, D., Ungerleider, R., and Johns, D. 1981. Phase I study of 2'-deoxycoformycin in acute lymphoblastic leukemia. *Cancer Res.* 41:3343–3346.

Ramirez, F., Wilson, W., Grage, T., and Hill, G. 1972. Phase II evaluation of 1,3-bis(2-chloroethyl)-1-nitrosourea (BCNU) in patients with solid tumors. *Cancer Chemother. Rep.* 56:787–790.

Richter, P., Calamera, J. C., Morgenfeld, M. C., Kierszenbaum, A. L., Lavieri, J. C., and Mancini, R. E. 1970. Effect of chlorambucil on spermatogenesis in the human with malignant lymphoma. *Cancer* 23:1026–1030.

Ritter, E. J., Scott, W. J., and Wilson, J. G. 1971. Teratogenesis and inhibition of DNA synthesis induced in rat embryo by cytosine arabinoside. *Teratology* 4:7–14.

Robertson, J. H., Crozier, E. H., and Woodend, B. E. 1970. Effect of vincristine on platelet counts in rats. *Br. J. Hematol.* 19:331–337.

Rodriguez, G, Bodey, E., Freireich, K., McCredie, E., McKelvey, E., and Tashima, G. 1976. Reduction of ifosfamide toxicity using dose fractionation. *Cancer Res.* 36:2945–2948.

Roeser, H., Stocks, A., and Smith, A. 1978. Testicular damage due to cytotoxic drugs and recovery after cessation of therapy. *Aust. N.Z. J. Med.* 8:250–254.

Rosner, F., Carey, R. W., and Zarrabi, M. H. 1978. Breast cancer and acute leukemia: Report of 24 cases and review of the literature. *Am. J. Hematol.* 4:157–172.

Rosner, F., and Grunwald, H. (for acute Leukemia Group B), 1974. Multiple myeloma terminating in acute leukemia. Report of 12 cases and review of the literature. *Am. J. Med.* 57:927–939.

Rosner, F., and Grunwald, H. 1975. Hodgkin's disease and acute leukemia. Report of eight cases and review of the literature. *Am. J. Med.* 58:339–353.

Ross, G. 1976. Congenital anomalies among children born of mothers receiving chemotherapy for gestational trophoblastic neoplasms. *Cancer* 37:1043–1047.

Rozencweig, M., von Hoff, D., Henney, J., and Muggia, F. 1977. VM 26 and VP 16-213: A comparative analysis. *Cancer* 40:334–342.

Rugh, R., and Skaredoff, L. 1965. Radiation and radiometric chlorambucil and the fetal retina. *Arch. Ophthal.* 74:382–393.

Sadler, T. W., and Kochhar, D. M. 1975. Teratogenic effects of chlorambucil on *in vivo* and *in vitro* organogenesis in mice. *Teratology* 12:71–78.

Scheef, W., Klein, H., Brock, N., Burkert, H., Gunther, U., Hoeferjanker, H., Mitrenga, D., Schnitker, J., and Voigtmann, R. 1979. Controlled clinical studies with an antidote against the urotoxicity of oxazaphosphorines: Preliminary results. *Cancer Treat. Rep.* 63:501–505.

Schell, F. C., Yap. H.-Y., Blumenschein, G., Valdeviesco, M., and Bodey, G. 1982. Potential cardiotoxicity with mitoxantrone. *Cancer Treat. Rep.* 66:1641–1642.

Scher, H., Schwartz, S., Yagoda, A., Watson, R., and Faye, L. 1982. Phase II trial of bisantrene for advance hypernephroma. *Cancer Treat. Rep.* 66:1653–1655.

Scherf, H. R., and Schmahl, D. 1975. Experimental investigations on immunodepressive properties of carcinogenic substances in male Sprague Dawley rats. *Recent Results Cancer Res.* 52:76–87.

Schilsky, R. L., and Erlichman, C. 1982. Late complications of chemotherapy: Infertility and carcinogenesis. In *Pharmacological Principles of Cancer Treatment,* ed. B. Chabner, pp. 109–131. Philadelphia: Saunders.

Schilsky, R., Kelley, J., Ihde, D., Howser, D., Cordes, R., and Young, R. 1982. Phase I trial and pharmacokinetics of aziridinylbenzoquinone (NSC 182986) in humans. *Cancer Res.* 42:1582–1586.

Schmahl, D. 1975. Experimental investigations with anticancer drugs for carcinogenicity with special reference to immuno depression. *Recent Results Cancer Res.* 52:18–78.

Schmahl, D., and Habs, M. 1978. Experimental carcinogenesis of antitumor drugs. *Cancer Treat. Rev.* 5:175–184.

Schmahl, D., and Habs, M. 1979. Carcinogenic action of low-dose cyclophosphamide given orally to Sprague-Dawley rats in a life-time experiment. *Int. J. Cancer* 23:706–712.

Schmahl, D., and Habs, M. 1980. Drug-induced cancer. *Curr. Top. Pathol.* 69:333–369.

Schmahl, D., Habs, M., Corenz, M., and Wagner, I. 1982. Occurrence of second tumors in man after anticancer drug treatment. *Cancer Treat. Reviews* 9:167–194.

Schnitker, J., Brock, N., Burkert, H., and Fichtner, E. 1976. Evaluation of a cooperative clinical study of the cytostatic agent ifosfamide. *Arzneim.—Forsch.* 26:1783–1792.

Schurig, J. E., Bradner, W. T., Huftalen, J. B., Doyle, G. J., and Gylys, J. A. 1980. Toxic side effects of platinum analogs. In *Cisplatin: Current Status and New Developments,* eds. A. W. Prestayko, S. T. Crooke, and S. K. Carter, pp. 227–236. New York: Academic.

Seifertova, M., Vesely, J., and Sorm, F. 1968. Effects of 5-azacytidine on developing mouse embryo. *Experientia* 24:487–488.

Shalet, S. 1980. Effects of cancer chemotherapy on gonadal function of patients. *Cancer Treat. Rev.* 7:141–152.

Shimkin, M. B. 1954. Pulmonary tumor induction in mice with chemical agents used in the clinical management of lymphomas. *Cancer* 7:410–413.

Shimkin, M. B., Weisburger, J., Weisburger, E., Gubareff, N., and Suntzeff, V. 1966. Bioassay of 29 alkylating chemicals by the pulmonary tumor response in strain A mice. *J. Natl. Cancer Inst.* 36:915–935.

Shotten, D., and Monie, I. W. 1963. Possible teratogenic effects of chlorambucil on the human fetus. *J. Am. Med. Assoc.* 186:74–75.

Sieber, S., and Adamson, R. 1975. Toxicity of antineoplastic agents in man: Chromosomal aberrations, antifertility effects, congenital malformations and carcinogenic potential. *Adv. Cancer* 22:57–155.

Sieber, S. M., Whang-Peng, J., Botkin, C., and Knutsen, T. 1978. Teratogenic and carcinogenic effects of some plant-derived antitumor agents (vincristine, colchicine, maytansine, VP-16, VM-26) in mice. *Teratology* 18:31–46.

Slavin, R. E., Millan, J.C., and Mullins, G. M. 1975. Pathology of high dose intermittent cyclophosphamide therapy. *Hum. Pathol.* 6:693–709.

Smyth, J., Paine, R., Jackman, A., Harrap, K., Chassin, M., Adamson, R., and Johns, D. 1980. The clinical pharmacology of the adenosine deaminase inhibitor 2'-deoxycoformycin. *Cancer Chemother. Pharmacol.* 5:93–101.

Sokal, J., and Lessmann, E. 1972. Effects of cancer chemotherapeutic agents on the human fetus. 172:1765–1771.

Sostman, H. D., Mathay, R. A., and Putman, C. E. 1977. Cytotoxic drug-induced lung disease. *Am. J. Med.* 62:608–615.

Sparano, B. M., Gordon, G., Hall, C., Iatropoulos, M. J., and Noble, J. F. 1982. Safety assessment of a new anticancer compound mitoxantrone in beagle dogs: Comparison with doxorubicin II histologic and ultrastructural pathology. *Cancer Treat. Rep.* 66:1145–1158.

Spiegel, R., Blum, R., Levin, M., Pinto, C., Wernz, J., Speyer, F., Hoffman, K., and Muggia, F. 1982. Phase I clinical trial of 9,10-anthracene dicarboxaldehyde (bisantrene) administered in a five-day schedule. *Cancer Res.* 42:354–358.

Spitz, S. 1948. Histological effects of nitrogen mustards on human tumors and tissues. *Cancer* 1:383–398.

Stadler, H. E., and Knowles, J. 1971. Fluorouracil in pregnancy. *JAMA* 217:214–215.

Stahelin, H. 1976. Delayed toxicity of epipodophyllotoxin derivatives (VM 26 and VP-16-213), due to a local effect. *Eur. J. Cancer* 12:925–931.

Steinherz, P. G., Miller, D. R., Hilgartner, M. W., and Schmalzer, E. A. 1976. Platelet dysfunction in vincristine treated patients. *Br. J. Hematol.* 32:439–450.

Stenram, U., and Nordlinder, H. 1968. Delayed deaths in rats treated with cyclophosphamide. *Nature (Lond).* 219:1154–1155.

Stewart, J., McCormack, J., and Krakoff, I. 1982. Clinical and clinical pharmacologic studies of Mitoxantrone. *Cancer Treat. Rep.* 66:1327–1331.

Stewart-Harris, R. C., Smith, I. E. 1982. Mitoxantrone: A phase II study in the treatment of patients with advanced breast carcinoma and other solid tumors. *Cancer Chemother. Pharmacol.* 8:179–182.

Stutzman, L., and Sokal, J. 1968. Use of anticancer drugs during pregnancy. *Clin. Obstet. Gynecol.* 11:416–427.

Sugimura, T., Umezawa, K., Matsushima, T., Sawamura, M., Seino, Y., Yahagi, T., and Nagao, M. 1978. Mutagenicity of cancer drugs—Prediction of the risks of a second tumor and use of the mutation test for monitoring improvement of drugs. In *Advances in Cancer Chemotherapy*, eds. S. Carter et al., pp. 283–296. Baltimore: University Park.

Sussman, S., and Leonard, J. M. 1980. Psoriasis, methotrexate and oligospermia. *Arch. Dermatol.* 116:215–217.

Svoboda, D., Reddy, J., and Harris, C. 1970. Invasive tumors induced in rats with actinomycin D. *Cancer Res.* 30:2271–2279.

Swaim, W., Windschitt, H., Doscherholmen, A., Bankole, R., and Bates, H. 1971. Chronic myelogenous leukemia in Hodgkin's disease: Immunofluorescence of cells. *Cancer* 27:569–573.

Tan, C., Dargeon, H., and Burchanel, J. 1959. Effects of Actinomycin D on cancer in childhood. *Pediatrics* 24:544–561.

Taniguchi, S., and Baba, T., 1982. "Two route chemotherapy" using cisdiammine platinum and its antidote, sodium thiosulfate, for peritoneally disseminated cancer in rats. *Gann* 73:475–479.

Tannir, N., Spitzer, G., Schell, F., Legha, S., Zander, A., and Blumenschein, G. 1983. Phase II study of high dose amsacrine (AMSA) and autologous bone marrow transplantation in patients with refractory metastatic breast cancer. *Cancer Treat. Rep.* 67:599–600.

Thompson, D. J., Mollello, J., Strebing, R. J., Dyke, I. L., and Robinson, V. B. 1974. Reproduction and teratologic studies with oncolytic agents in the rat and rabbit. I. BCNU. *Toxicol. Appl. Pharmacol.* 30:422–439.

Thompson, D. J., Mollello, J., Strebing, R. J., and Dyke, I. L. 1975a. Reproduction and teratologic studies with oncolytic agents in the rat and rabbit II. DTIC. *Toxicol. Appl. Pharmacol.* 33:281–290.

Thompson, D. J., Mollello, J. A., Strebing, R. J., and Dyke, I. L. 1975b. Reproductive and teratologic studies with 1-(2-chloroethyl)-3-cyclohexyl-1-nitrosourea (CCNU) in the rat and rabbit. *Toxicol. Appl. Pharmacol.* 34:456–466.

Thompson, D. J., Mollello, J., Strebing, R., and Dyke, I. L. 1978. Teratogenesis of adriamycin and daunomycin in the rat and rabbit. *Teratology* 17:151–157.

Thompson, G. R., and Larson, R. E. 1972. A toxicologic comparison of the potency and activity of 1,3-bis(2-chloroethyl)-1-nitrosourea (BCNU) and 1-(2-chloroethyl)-3-cyclohexyl-1-nitrosourea (CCNU) in mice and rats. *Toxicol. Appl. Pharmacol.* 21:405–413.

Toland, D. M., Coltman, C. A., and Moon, T. E. 1978. Second malignancies complicating Hodgkin's disease. *Cancer Clin. Trials* 1:27–33.

Toledo, T. M., Harper, R. C., and Moser, R. H. 1971. Fetal effects during cyclophosphamide and irradiation therapy. *Ann. Int. Med.* 74:87–91.

Tuchmann-Duplessis, H., Hiss, D., Mottot, G., and Rosner, I. 1973. Embryotoxic and teratogenic effect of actinomycin D in the Syrian hamster. *Toxicology* 1:131–133.

Uldall, P., Kerr, D., and Tacchi, D. 1972. Sterility and cyclophosphamide. *Lancet* i:693–694.

Vahlsing, H. L., Feringa, E. R., Britten, A. G., and Kinning, W. K. 1975. Dental abnormalities in rat after a single dose of cyclophosphamide. *Cancer Res.* 35:2199–2202.

Valagussa, P., Santoro, A., and Kenda, R. 1980. Second malignancies in Hodgkin's disease: A complication of certain forms of treatment. *Br. Med. J.* 280:216–219.

Van Dyk, J., Falkson, H., Merwe, A., and Falkson, G. 1972. Unexpected toxicity in patients treated with Iphosphamide. *Cancer Res.* 32:921–924.

Von Hoff, D., Rozencweig, M., Layard, M., Slavik, M., and Muggia, F. 1977. Daunomycin-induced cardiotoxicity in children and adults: A review of 110 cases. *Am. J. Med.* 62:200–208.

Von Hoff, D. D., Pollard, E., Kuhn, J., Murray, E., and Coltman, C. . 1980. Phase I clinical investigation of 1,4-dihydroxy-5,8-bis{{2[(2-hydroxyethyl)amino]ethyl}amino}}9,10-anthracene dione dihydrochloride (NSC-301739), a new anthracenedione. *Cancer Res.* 40:1516–1518.

Von Hoff, D., Myers, J., Kuha, J., Sandback, J., Pocelinko, R., Clark, G., and Coltman, C. 1981. Phase I clinical investigation of 9,10-anthracendicarboxaldehyde bis[4,5-dihydro-1*H*-imidazol-2-yl)hydrazone] dihydrochloride (CL216,942). *Cancer Res.* 41:3118–3121.

Von Hoff, D. D., Rozencweig, M., and Piccart, M. 1982. Cardiotoxicity of anticancer agents. *Semin. Oncol.* 9:23–33.

Wall, R. L., and Clausen, K. P. 1975. Carcinoma of the urinary bladder in patients receiving cyclophosphamide. *N. Engl. J. Med.* 293:217–273.

Ward, J. M., and Fauvie, K. A. 1976. Nephrotoxic effects of *cis*-diamminedichloroplatinum(II) in male F-344 rats. *Toxicol. Appl. Pharmacol.* 38:535–547.

Weisburger, E. 1977. Bioassay program for carcinogenic hazards of cancer chemotherapeutic agents. *Cancer* 40:1935–1949.

Weisburger, J. H., Griswold, D. P., Prejean, J. D., Casey, A. E., Wood, H. B., and Weisburger, E. K. 1975. Carcinogenic properties of some of the principal drugs used in clinical cancer chemotherapy. *Recent Results Cancer Res.* 52:1–16.

Weiss, R. B., and Issell, B. F. 1982. The nitrosoureas: Carmustine (BCNU) and lomustine (CCNU). *Cancer Treat. Rev.* 9:313–330.

Whitehead, E., Shalet, S. M., Blackledge, G., Todd, I., Crowther, D., and Beardwell, C. B. 1982. Effects of Hodgkin's disease and combination chemotherapy on gonadal function in the adult male. *Cancer* 49:418–422.

Willson, J. K. 1978. Pulmonary toxicity of antineoplastic drugs. *Cancer Treat. Rep.* 62:2003–2008.

Wynert, W., Harvey, H., Lipton, A., Schweitzer, J., and White, D. 1982. Phase I study of a 5-day schedule of mitoxantrone (dihydroxyanthracenedione). *Cancer Treat. Rep.* 66:1303–1306.

Yap, H.-Y., Blumenschein, G., Schell, F., and Bodey, G. 1981. Phase II evaluation of methyl-GAG in patients with refractory metastatic breast cancer. *Cancer Treat. Rep.* 65:465–467.

Yap, H.-Y., Blumenschein, G. R., Schell, F. C., Buzdar, A. U., Valdevieso, M., and Bodey, G. P. 1981b. Dihydroxyanthracenedione: A promising new drug in the treatment of metastatic breast cancer. *Ann. Int. Med.* 95:694–697.

Yap, B., Yap, H., Blumenschein, G., Bedikan, A., Pocelinko, R., and Bodey, G. 1982. Phase I clinical evaluation of 9,10-anthracenedicarboxyaldehyde [bis(4,5-dihydro-1*H*-imidazol-2-yl)hydrazone]dihydrochloride (Bisantrene). *Cancer Treat. Rep.* 66:1517–1520.

Youness, E., Dosik, G., Benjamin, R. S., and Trujillo, J. M. 1978. Acute myelomonocytic leukemia following a chemotherapeutic regimen for metastatic sarcoma. *Cancer Treat. Rep.* 62:1513–1516.

Zeffren, J., Yagodo, A., Watson, R. C., Natale, R. B., Blumenreich, M. S., Chapman, R., and Howard, J. 1981. Phase II trial of methyl-GAG in advanced renal cancer. *Cancer Treat. Rep.* 65:525–527.

Chapter 9

Toxicology of Insecticides, Rodenticides, Herbicides, and Fungicides

William F. Durham

INTRODUCTION

Humans have long viewed insects, rodents, weeds, and other unwanted organisms as intruders and sought means for their control. Early use of chemical insecticides dates back to use of the arsenical Paris green, an imported dye, to combat the invasion of the potato fields of Mississippi by the Colorado potato beetle, *Leptinotarsa decemlineata*. The result was so satisfactory that orchardists soon adopted Paris green to aid in their fight against the codling moth whose larvae mine apples and pears.

The era of modern synthetic pesticides only began, however, during World War II with the introduction of chlorophenothane (DDT) and 2,4-dichlorophenoxyacetic acid (2,4-D). DDT was first used in this country by the military for delousing as a preventative of typhus fever. Subsequent use was to kill the mosquito to combat malaria.

CHLORINATED HYDROCARBON INSECTICIDES

Among the pesticides in the chlorinated hydrocarbon group are DDT [1,1,1-trichloro-2,2-bis(p-chlorophenyl) ethane], benzene hexachloride (BHC), 1,2,3,4,5,6-hexachlorocyclohexane (lindane γ-isomer of BHC), toxaphene (chlorinated camphene), and the cyclodiene compounds aldrine, dieldrin, endrin, chlordane, and heptachlor. Dieldrin, the epoxide of aldrin, is a mammalian metabolite of aldrin, but is also an effective insecticide.

DDT is the prototype compound for the chlorinated hydrocarbon insecticides [see Hayes (1982) for background information]. DDT was first synthesized in 1874, but its effectiveness as an insecticide was not noted until 1939. This discovery by Dr. Paul Mueller, a Swiss chemist, earned him a Nobel prize in 1948. During World War II, the United States began producing large quantities of DDT for control of vector-borne diseases, such as typhus and malaria, to which our troops were exposed. After 1945, agricultural, public health, and household usage of DDT became widespread. By 1959, annual usage was approximately 80 million pounds, with about 80% of this used on cotton and additional large quantities used on peanuts and soybeans. The popularity of DDT was due to its reasonable cost, effectiveness, persistence, and versatility. Some of the characteristics of DDT that contributed to its early popularity, particularly its persistence, later became the basis for public concern over possible hazards involved in DDT use. Although some warnings against such hazards were raised earlier, it was the publication of Rachel Carson's book *Silent Spring* in 1962 that stimulated widespread public concern over use of the chemical. Following consideration by four government committees and an extensive legal hearing process, the U.S. Environmental Protection Agency (EPA) cancelled the remaining crop uses of DDT in the United States effective December 31, 1972. This decision was based on findings of persistence, transport, biomagnification, toxicological effects on lower life forms, and on the absence of benefits of DDT relative to the availability of effective and less environmentally harmful substitutes. Later agency actions have cancelled or restricted the use of other compounds in this group, including aldrin/dieldrin, endrin, heptochlor, and toxaphene.

The chlorinated hydrocarbon insecticides and many of their metabolites are stored in adipose tissue in exposed animals, including humans. This fact is not surprising in view of the known solubility of these compounds in fats and fat solvents and their practical insolubility in water. However, the quantitative differences in storage among these compounds do not parallel the differences in their solubility in fat. For example, in studies with rats, it was noted that the equilibrium storage levels of BHC isomers following dietary intake were unrelated to the in vitro solubility of the compounds in rat fat, with the exception that solubility was a limiting factor.

It is a fundamental axiom in pharmacology that all compounds approach a steady state of storage in which the daily dosage (exposure) and the daily excretion are approximately equal. For a given compound and species, there will be a different plateau level of storage for each dosage. In general, doubling the dosage will double the storage, but in some instances storage may not increase quite as rapidly as dosage. The major factor governing storage is exposure or dosage. Also important is the increased biotransformation (resulting in decreased storage) from induction of liver microsomal enzyme activity. This enzyme activity may be induced by exposure to other pesticides, chemicals, or drugs. Other factors that may influence storage are species, sex, age, nutritional status, disease, and the integrity of organs, especially the liver and kidneys.

DDT storage in humans has been studied carefully. In early studies of such storage, DDT-derived material was found at a concentration of about 7 ppm in the fat of a man with occupational exposure for 4 years and a history of eating DDT-treated foods. The first general survey for DDT was carried out by Laug and his colleagues in California in 1950. They demonstrated DDT residues ranging from 0 to 34 ppm (mean, 5.3 ppm) in the fat of 75 persons with no special occupational exposure. Later surveys using the improved methodology of gas–liquid chromatography have shown the presence in fat and blood from the general population of the United States and other countries of DDT isomers and metabolites (o,p-DDT, p,p'-DDE, o,p'-DDE, p,p'-DDD, o,p'-DDD) and other chlorinated hydrocarbon insecticides (BHC, dieldrin, and heptachlor epoxide). Storage levels of DDT in the United States general population have declined significantly since its use was cancelled in 1972.

The acute and subchronic toxicity of DDT to humans as well as its kinetics have been studied in human volunteers. A total of 90 men received daily oral doses of DDT at 0, 3.5, or 35 mg/man for periods up to 2 years. These doses were chosen as being about 20 and 200 times, respectively, the ordinary dietary level of DDT. The highest dose chosen was about one-fifth of that estimated to cause transient mild sickness, based on animal experiments and on the smallest single acute dose known to produce mild illness in humans. No clinical effect associated with DDT dosage was detected by the men themselves or by careful physical examination and laboratory testing. The kinetics study shows that about 1 year was required for the men to reach equilibrium of DDT storage. The loss of DDT from body fat storage was found to be quite slow.

Some of the chlorinated hydrocarbon insecticides produce characteristic histologic changes in the livers of rodents at relatively low dosage levels. These effects were first reported for DDT by Laug et al. in 1950. The changes in the parenchymal cells of the liver consisted of an increased deposition of fat, margination of cytoplasmic granules, hypertrophy of the cells, and—most characteristic—the formation of complex, lypoid, cytoplasmic inclusion bodies termed "lipospheres" by Ortega et al. (1956). Other chlorinated hydrocarbons pesticides known to produce similar changes include chlordane, dieldrin, lindane, and toxaphene, along with the narcotic sedative phenobarbital. Later, similar microscopic changes in the rat liver were found generally to be associated with compounds inducing hepatic microsomal enzyme activity and an increase in smooth endoplasmic reticulum in the liver cell. At sufficient dosage levels and times, these changes in susceptible species can progress to tumor formation.

In carcinogenesis bioassays carried out through the program of the National Cancer Institute, p,p'-DDE, chlordecone (Kepone), chlordane, heptachor, toxaphene, and aldrin were found to produce liver tumors in mice and/or rats.

The principal, if not the exclusive, action of DDT and the other chlorinated hydrocarbons insecticides is on the central nervous system. The exact nature of this action is unknown. In animals, the earliest apparent effect of DDT poisoning is abnormal susceptibility to fear, with violent reaction to stimuli that normally would go unnoticed. There is definite motor unrest and an increased frequency of spontaneous movements. A fine tremor appears and becomes constant, interfering with normal activity. As the nervous-system involvement progresses, there are attacks of epileptiform tonoclonic convulsions.

Diagnosis and Treatment of Poisoning

Exposure to the chlorinated hydrocarbon pesticides can be determined by measurement of levels of these materials or their metabolites in blood or adipose tissue. In certain instances, excretion of biotransformation products can also be monitored in urine. For example, DDA excretion serves as a good indicator of exposure to DDT.

Treatment of poisoning is primarily directed toward control of convulsions and other nervous system involvement. Barbiturates (pentobarbital or phenobarbital) are recommended both for promoting increased biotransformation and for sedation. Diazepam should also be an effective sedative. Calcium gluconate is reported to control convulsions caused by some chlorinated hydrocarbon insecticides. Cholestyramie has been found useful in promoting the intestinal excretion of chlordecone (Kepone).

The chlorinated hydrocarbon insecticide chlordecone was responsible for an outbreak of industrial poisoning in Hopewell, Va., in 1975. Kepone has had little U.S. pesticidal use, but the compound served as a raw material for preparation of Kelevan, a pesticide used primarily for control of banana-borer weevils in Central and South America. In Hopewell, Kepone was produced in a makeshift plant in a renovated gasoline service station. Industrial hygiene in the plant was poor. Seventy-six of 133 persons (57%) who worked in the Kepone plant developed illness characterized by nervousness, tremor, weight loss, opsoclonus, pleuritis, and joint jaws and oligospermia. Illness incidence rates for production workers (64%) were significantly higher than for nonproduction personnel. The mean blood Kepone level for workers with illness was 2.53 ppm, and for those not showing symptoms, 0.60 ppm. Detectible levels of Kepone were found in the blood in 40 of 214 community residents tested. Significant levels of Kepone were also found in the air and water in this area and in fish and shellfish from the James River, resulting in restrictions on the fishing industry.

ORGANIC PHOSPHORUS COMPOUNDS

The organic phosphorus compounds currently constitute the most widely used chemical type of pesticides for insect control. Also, the relatively high acute toxicity of many of these compounds and their predominant role among the newer synthetic pesticides in the etiology of human poisoning cases makes them of concern to the toxicologist.

Early work leading to the development of the organic phosphorus compounds as insecticides was carried out by Dr. Gerhard Schrader working in Germany for I. G. Farben Industrie in the 1930s [see Hayes (1982) for details]. Among other compounds, he synthesized and studied parathion, which came on the U.S. market in 1947.

Since some organic phosphorus compounds are alkylating agents, there has been concern over possible mutagenic and carcinogenic effects from these materials. Some OP insecticides have shown genotoxic effects in in vitro tests (e.g., acephate, demeton, monocrotophas, trichlorfos, and dichloros). However, there does not seem to be evidence for a mutagenic effect from in vivo studies, and National Cancer Institute

(NCI) carcinogenic bioassays were negative for dichlorvos (Witherup et al., 1976) and for methyl parathion, malathion, and diazinon, equivocal for parathion for the production of adrenal cortical tumors in rats, and positive for tetrachlorvinphos for liver tumors in mice. Tetrachlorvinphos contains organochlorine and gives the hepatocarcinogenic response typical of chlorinated hydrocarbon compounds.

The prototype compound for insecticidal use among the organic phosphorus (OP) group is parathion (O,O-diethyl O-p-nitrophenyl phosporothioate). There are a large number of other OP compounds now in use as pesticides. Some of the other representative compounds are malathion [S-[1,2-bis(ethocycarbonyl)ethyl]O,O-dimethyl phosphorithioate], dichlorvos (DDVP, 2,2-dichlorovinyl dimethyl phosphate), EPN (O-ethyl 9-p-nitrophenyl phenylphosphonothioate), diazinon [O,O-diethyl O-(2-isopropyl-4-methyl-6-pyrimidyl) phosphorothioate], and azinphosmethyl [guthion, O,O-dimethyl s[4-oxo-1,2,3-benzothriazine-3(4H)-ylmethyl phosphordithioate]].

Potentiation

The production of an effect by a combination of two agents greater than would be expected on the basis of simple additive effect is known as *potentiation*.

Various combinations of the organic phosphorus pesticides have been shown to potentiate each other. Potentiation among these compounds was first shown to occur for malathion plus EPN (Frawley et al., 1957). The maximum synergistic effect (88–134 times) has been observed with malathion plus triorthocresyl phosphate (TOCP). The mechanism by which potentiation occurs has been elucidated and appears to involve the interference of one compound with the metabolism of the second. Thus, EPN apparently interferes with the degradation of malathion or its more toxic metabolite malaoxon. The potentiation of malathion toxicity by TOCP is very probably attributable to a similar inhibition.

Moeller and Rider (1962) gave repeated oral doses of EPN and malathion in combination to volunteers and concluded that no effect occurred at or near these dose levels. On this basis there would seem to be no danger from residues of potentiating compounds in food, provided that the individual tolerance levels are not excluded (DuBois, 1961).

Toxicity and Mechanism of Action

The organic phosphorus group of pesticides includes compounds with a wide range of acute toxicity. Since these compounds are esters of phosphoric acid, they tend to be hydrolyzed relatively easily and, in general, do not persist in the environment in the way that the chlorinated hydrocarbon compounds do.

These compounds owe their pharmacologic effect primarily, if not entirely, to their ability to inhibit the enzyme cholinesterase, with a resultant overstimulation of the parasympathetic nervous system by the excess acetylcholine that accumulates. A small abnormal accumulation of acetylcholine at the synapse or myoneural junction produces an abnormal increase in function (e.g., fasciculation of muscle), while greater accumulation rapidly produces a decrease in function (e.g., paralysis). It has been suggested that certain direct effects of the anticholinesterase organic phosphorus compounds do not depend on inhibition of cholinesterase. Foremost among these effects is delayed neurotoxicity.

Absorption of the organic phosphorus anticholinesterases may occur through the lungs, gastrointestinal tract, or skin. Absorption of these materials is more rapid and more complete through the former two routes than through the latter. Respiratory exposure may be of predominant importance wherever there is a sufficient concentration of vapor or of aerosol fine enough to inhale. However, in agricultural and public health usage, workers' contamination is predominantly on their skin. The oral route of exposure occurs in accidental poisoning (particularly of children), in murder, and in suicide.

Although many of the organophosphate compounds have a high acute toxicity, agricultural residues of these materials on food have not been a problem, due to their rapid breakdown and the fact that they are not stored in the animal body. Direct contamination of food by concentrated formulations of these insecticides during shipment has been the cause of several outbreaks of poisoning in other countries.

Organophosphate poisoning may vary in severity, in rapidity of onset, in duration, and in range, depending on the route and the magnitude of exposure. Minor exposure to a vapor or aerosol of a direct inhibitor of cholinesterase may produce local effects on the eye or respiratory system through local absorption and without systemic effects. The optic effects consist of miosis, a sensation of pressure in or behind the eye, headache, and conjunctival hyperemia. Unilateral manifestation of these optic effects has been implicated in visual difficulties experienced by pilots applying these materials. The local effects on the respiratory tract may involve increased secretion, a feeling of tightness in the chest, and occasionally wheezing. Localized massive dermal exposure can lead to muscular fasciculation and sweating confined to the area of absorption.

Systemic effects may follow absorption by any route. If there has been adequate exposure to a vapor or aerosol, the local respiratory effects already described will appear, but they will be rapidly followed by more systemic manifestations. The muscarine-like effects are usually first to appear. They include anorexia, nausea, sweating, epigastric and substernal tightness (probably due to cardiospasm), heartburn, belching, and tightness in the chest. The sequence of symptoms varies somewhat with the route of exposure—gastrointestinal effects usually being earliest after ingestion; sweating, and at times muscular fasciculations, after dermal exposure; and respiratory effects after inhalation. More severe exposure by whatever route produces abdominal cramps, increased peristalsis, vomiting, diarrhea, salivation, lacrimation, profuse sweating, pallor, and dyspnea. In some subjects there is audible wheezing. More severe signs and symptoms include involuntary defecation and urination, excessive bronchial secretions, and (according to some authors) pulmonary edema.

Nicotine-like effects appear usually after the muscarine-like effects have reached moderate severity. These include muscle twitching, fasciculations, and cramps. At about the same time, there appear increased fatigability and mild, generalized weakness, which is increased by exertion. Extensive exposure produces severe weakness, including weakness of the muscles of respiration. There may be a mild or moderate elevation of blood pressure.

The effects on the central nervous system include tension, anxiety, restlessness, giddiness, and emotional lability. Late effects include insomnia, excessive dreaming, and occasionally nightmares. Greater exposure produces headache, tremor, drowsiness, difficulty in concentration, slowness of recall, and confusion. Lethal or near-lethal doses produce ataxia, slurring of words, multiple repetition of the last syllable of words, coma, areflexia, Cheyne–Stokes breathing, and finally, respiratory arrest.

The cause of death may usually be attributed to interference with respiration. Animal experiments have proved that the anticholinesterase organophosphate compounds interfere with respiration in at least four ways, including bronchoconstriction, excessive respiratory secretion, failure of the muscles of respiration, and depression of the respiratory center.

Delayed Neurotoxicity

Delayed neurotoxic effects in humans poisoned with tri-o-cresylphosphate (TOCP) were recognized in the 1920s and 1930s. An estimated 20,000 cases of peripheral neuropathy occurred in the United States in those prohibition days from drinking Jamaica ginger that had been adulterated with TOCP. The illness was referred to as "ginger paralysis" or "ginger jake." The characteristic clinical sign was bilateral and symmetrical placid paralysis of the distal muscles, predominantly of the lower extremities, occurring some 7–10 days following ingestion. Although some of these victims recovered fairly promptly and all showed some improvement with time, some remained affected for life. Histological study of central and peripheral nerve tissue from animal experiments has shown extensive disruption of the myelin sheath, suggesting a process of demyelination as the primary mechanisms leading to ataxia. A second large incident of TOCP neurotoxicity occurred in Morocco in 1959 as a result of ingestion of lubricating oil containing TOCP, which had been mixed with olive oil for human consumption.

Although fortunately not in epidemic form, delayed neurotoxicity has been caused in humans by some organophosphate insecticides. In 1951, a group of three chemical-plant workers who were engaged in pilot-plant production of the experimental insecticide mipafox (bis-isopropyl-aminofluorophosphine oxide) developed acute cholinergic signs and symptoms that responded to atropine. After apparent full recovery from the acute illness, two of these workers gradually developed weakness in the legs over a 2- to 3-week period. Another outbreak of polyneuropathy occurred in chemical-plant workers in Texas who were engaged in the manufacture of leptophos. However, the etiology of these cases is not clear, since these workers had also had exposure to the known neurotoxin n-hexane. The other pesticides reported to have caused delayed neuropathy in humans are DEF and trichlorofon.

Since recognition of the association between the organophosphate compounds and delayed neurotoxicity, testing for this effect has been required for new, chemically related substances prior to their commercial use as pesticides. The best experimental animal for the OP-induced delayed neurotoxic illness in humans is the chicken. Normal laboratory animal species, including the rat, mouse, rabbit, and hamster are refractory. All of the OP compounds known to have caused polyneuropathy in humans have tested positively in chickens. A number of other OP compounds of varying structures have also been found to produce this effect in chickens. However, the compounds differ with regard to reversibility of the illness and, as with other modalities of toxicity, with regard to minimum effective dosage.

In considering structure–activity relationships, there appears to be no rationale that accounts for the diversity of OP structures producing this effect. However, Abou-Donia (1979) has pointed out that phenylphosphonothioate esters are almost uniformly neurotoxic. This group includes leptophos and EPN, among others.

The biochemical mechanism involved in delayed neurotoxicity seems to involve the enzyme neurotoxic esterase (NTE). Johnson (1975) and his colleagues and other workers have shown an excellent correlation for a wide variety of OP compounds and species between inhibition of NTE activity and occurrence of delayed neurotoxicity. Johnson believes that, in order for clinical polyneuropathy to occur, approximately 70–80% of the NTE must be inactivated through an irreversible or "aged" reaction.

A recent study has suggested that a ChE-inhibiting, phosphorus-containing impurity may be at least partly responsible for the neurotoxic effect produced by n-hexane.

Diagnosis and Treatment of Poisoning

Significant exposure to an organic phosphorus pesticide can be determined by measurement of blood cholinesterase level. Although both the general esterase of plasma and the acetylcholinesterase of erythrocytes are inhibited by OP exposure, the latter enzyme level generally correlates more closely with clinical status. Also, exposure to these compounds can be determined by the measurement of urinary alkylphosphate or phenolic metabolites. The most widely used metabolite exposure test procedures measures excretion of p-nitrophenol and is applicable to those OP compounds that, on hydrolysis, form p-nitrophenol or one of its congeners. Although applicable to a restricted group of compounds, this test has proved to be a more sensitive measure of OP absorption than is cholinesterase inhibition.

There are two types of antidotes available for treatment of OP poisoning:

1 Atropine serves as a pharmacologic antagonist to the accumulated acetylcholine. Atropine is an effective antidote to the muscarinic effects of acetylcholine and thus relieves many of the symptoms of OP poisoning, reduces heart block, and dries secretions of the respiratory tract. However, atropine does not block the nicotinic action of acetylcholine and thus does not protect against muscular weakness. The effective dose of atropine for treatment of OP poisoning is greater than that needed for other purposes, but the poisoned patient has an increased tolerance for atropine.

2 Oximes serve as specific biochemical antidotes by reversal of formation of the enzyme–inhibitor complex. The most widely used oxime for this purpose is 2-pyridine aldoxime methochloride (2-PAM or pralidoxime chloride). 2-PAM is most effectively used in combination with atropine, since the two antidotes are potentiative in combination.

CARBAMATE COMPOUNDS

The carbamate insecticides are synthetic derivatives of carbamic acid (NH_2COOH). These compounds are homologs of physostigmine (or eserine), the principal alkaloid of the plant *Physostigma venenosum* (calabar bean). Physostigmine was known to be an inhibitor of cholinesterase, and both it and other, later, synthetic carbamates have had pharmaceutical use in treatment of glaucoma, paralytic ileus, and myasthenia gravis.

Acute and Chronic Toxicity

The primary pharmacologic action of both the medicinal and the insecticidal carbamates is inhibition of cholinesterase. The important difference between the mechanism of toxic action of carbamates and that of organophosphates is that the cholinesterase inhibition by carbamates is apparently reversible.

The mammalian toxicity of insecticidal carbamates varies over a broad range. Carbaryl (Sevin, 1-naphthyl-*N*-methylcarbamate), the most widely used carbamate insecticide, has a relatively low acute oral toxicity (LD50 of 630 mg/kg to rats), while aldicarb [Temik, 2-methyl-2-(methylthio)propionaldehyde *O*-M-(methylcabamoyl)oxime] is highly toxic (acute oral LD50 to rats 1 mg/kg). Other carbamates in use as insecticides include propoxur (Baygon, *o*-isopropoxyphenyl methyl carbamate), carbofuran (Furadan, 2,3-dihyoro-2,2-dimethyl-7-benzofuranyl methylcarbamate), and methomyl [Lannate, methyl *N*-(methylcarbamoyl)-oxythioacetimidate].

The acute signs and symptoms of carbamate insecticide poisoning can be referred to local accumulation of acetylcholine and thus are parasympathomimetic in nature. They differ from the manifestations of organic phosphorus poisoning primarily in their brevity. However, unlike organophosphates, carbamates do not seem to produce delayed neurotoxicity. The carbamate insecticides do not seem to have mutagenic or carcinogenic activity, although urethane (ethyl carbamate) readily induces pulmonary tumors in mice. However, nitrosocarbaryl (formed by reaction between nitrous acid and carbaryl) is carcinogenic to rats. (Carbaryl has been reported to cause teratologic effects in dogs at dosage levels as low as 6.25 mg/kg · day during gestation. Effects on reproduction either have not been seen in other species or occur at much higher dosage levels. The difference between species in this regard is thought to be due to differences in metabolism of the compound. Although metabolism of carbaryl to 1-naphthol is a major metabolic pathway in most species studied, including humans, the dog differs in this regard) (Weil et al., 1972).

Diagnosis and Treatment of Poisoning

Just as in the case of the OP compounds, exposure to the carbamates can be detected from determination of blood cholinesterase level. However, since the carbamate-cholinesterase complex is less stable than its OP congener, care must be taken in the measurement procedure chosen, lest the added substrate, dilution, or other factors dissociate the inhibited enzyme complex. Also, time is a factor in this dissociation, so the determination must be done without delay. There is also the possibility of using urinary excretion levels of the phenolic metabolites for diagnostic purposes. For example, exposure to carbaryl can be detected in the basis of α-naphthol excretion levels.

Atropine sulfate is the recommended antidote for poisoning by cholinesterase-inhibiting carbamate insecticides. The effectiveness of oximes in the treatment of carbamate poisoning seems to vary between compounds. Therapeutic efficacy is never very great and, for some carbamates, such as carbaryl, oxime treatment is harmful. The mechanism for the aggravation of carbaryl poisoning is unknown, although it has been postulated that the formation of a cholinesterase-inhibitory carbamyl oxime product through a 2-PAM/carbaryl reaction may occur. However, isolation of such a product has not been possible.

Metabolism

There are two related but mechanistically different processes for carbamate metabolism in biological systems. The carbamate ester linkage is hydrolyzed in both processes, liberating the phenolic or enolic moiety. The reactions are as follows:

$$
RO-\overset{\overset{O}{\|}}{C}NHCH_3 \begin{cases} \xrightarrow{Esterase} ROH + CH_3NH\overset{\overset{O}{\|}}{C}_2\diagdown OH & (1) \\[2em] \longrightarrow [RO\overset{\overset{O}{\|}}{C}NHCH_2OH] + ROH + CO_2 + NH_2 + HCHO & (2) \end{cases}
$$

Reaction 1 involves direct enzymic hydrolysis of the carbamate ester linkage, while reaction 2 involves hydrolysis after prior oxidation of the carbamate moiety.

BOTANICAL INSECTICIDES

Nicotine

Nicotine was first used as an insecticide in 1763. The pure alkaloid was isolated in 1828 by Posselt and Reimmans and synthesized in 1904 by Posselt and Rotschy. The alkaloids nornicotine and anabasine are structurally similar to nicotine and are also used as insecticides.

Nicotine is quite toxic orally and can also be absorbed dermally. The acute oral LD50 of nicotine sulfate for rats is 83 mg/kg; the dermal value is 285 mg/kg (Gaines, 1969). The onset of symptoms of acute nicotine poisoning is rapid, and death may occur within a few minutes. Due to its alkalinity, the free alkaloid has a local caustic action in the mouth and stomach. In serious poisoning cases, respiratory failure and circulatory collapse occur. Death results from respiratory failure due to paralysis of the muscles of respiration. In therapy, primary attention should be focused on support of the respiration.

Rotenone

Rotenone is obtained by extraction from roots of the plants *Derris elliptica* from Malaya and the East Indies and *Lonchocarpus* species from South America. The toxic prinicples of these plants include a number of other related compounds in addition to rotenone. These plants have been used as fish poisons for many centuries, and the extracted rotenone is very toxic to fish. Rotenone exhibits a considerable degree of selective toxicity, with high toxicity for insects and low toxicity to mammals. Acute poisoning with rotenone is rare in humans, and rotenone preparations have been used topically to treat scabies, head lice, and other ectoparasites because of their relative safety. Rotenone is an irritant and produces local effects of conjunctivitis and dermatitis, along with pharyngitis, rhinitis, and severe pulmonary irritation following respiratory exposure. Following ingestion, gastrointestinal irritation occurs with manifestations of epigastric pain, abdominal cramps, nausea, and vomiting.

Rotenone acts as a respiratory enzyme inhibitor, acting between NAD^+ and coenzyme Q and blocking mitochondrial respiration. Since oxidative phosphorylation is coupled with the respiratory chain, ATP is not produced (Haley, 1978). The induction of mammary tumors in rats given rotenone intraperitoneally at a dosage of 1.7 mg/kg·day for 42 days has been reported.

Pyrethrum

Pyrethrum is found in the flowers of *Chrysanthemum cinerariaefolium,* which are supplied primarily from Kenya. Pyrethrum powders were first used around 1800, and by 1851 their use was worldwide. There are six known insecticidally active compounds in pyrethrum. These compounds are esters made up of different combinations of two acids and three alcohols.

Pyrethrum has a low toxicity to mammals. The acute oral LD50 to rats is about 1500 mg/kg. Pyrethrum is fast-acting toward insects and is commonly used in fly sprays and other household insecticides. The commercial formulations commonly contain piperonyl butoxide, sesamin, or other synergists.

The primary toxic effect of pyrethrum in mammals is on the central nervous system. However, injury to humans from pyrethrum has more frequently resulted from the allegenic properties of the material rather than its direct toxicity (Hayes, 1982). Thus, contact dermatitis is the most common clinical manifestation of exposure and occurs more frequently in individuals who are sensitive to ragweed pollen. Pyrethrum, particularly in combination with piperonyl butoxide, produces characteristic microscopic changes in the rat liver cell (enlargement, margination, and cytoplasmic inclusions) similar to those produced by DDT. These changes are indicative of liver microsomal enzyme induction.

BIORATIONAL PESTICIDES

Concern over the real and potential adverse effects of chemical pesticides has led to much interest in the use of biological materials to control pests. Some natural plant materials (pyrethrum, rotenone, nicotine) were among the earliest pesticides and have already been discussed. The biorational pesticides include microorganisms (bacteria, viruses, and fungi) and biochemicals (compounds that modify insects or other pests with regard to growth development, reproduction, or behavior, and including pheromones, kairomones, allomones, juvenile hormones, neuropeptides, endysones, and sex attractants). These "natural" materials provide greater species specificity than do chemical pesticides and thus offer hope for decreased effect on beneficial species as well as for overcoming acquired resistance to chemical controls in some pests. Biorational pesticides play an important role in integrated pest management (IPM) programs as a means of reducing dependence on chemical pesticides.

Approximately 1500 naturally occurring microorganisms or microbial by-products that are pathogenic to insects have been identified as potentially useful insecticidal agents. The biochemical agents seem to have received less and more recent attention, although a number of these materials have been registered, beginning in 1973 with a house-fly pheromone.

As in the case of chemical pesticides, manufacturers must provide efficacy and human and environmental safety data to secure EPA registration for biological pesticides. However, the required tests are somewhat different for biological than for chemical pesticides. Safety testing for the biologicals places emphasis on reproducibility of the organism in human and other mammalian test systems. Unfortunately, the great specificity of most microbial insect pathogens limits their control usefulness to a narrow host range and thus also limits their commercial attractiveness. The application of genetic engineering to microbial insect pathogens holds promise to develop strains with greater insecticidal effectiveness and other improved control characteristics.

Bacterial Insecticides

Bacillus thuringiensis was the first insect microbial preparation to achieve registration and widespread usage. This material is registered for control of lipidopteran larvae on field crops, trees, ornamentals, home vegetable gardens, and stored grains and grain products. The primary insecticidal activity of the spore-forming bacterium *B. thuringiensis* resides in a parasporal glycoprotein crystal that is synthesized and crystallized within the parent cell.

Viral Insecticides

A number of insect baculoviruses have been registered for use as insecticides. The viruses of the baculovirus subgroup NPV (nuclear polyhedrosis virus) and GV (granulosis virus) are occluded in proteinaceous crystals, thus providing shelf-life and environmental stability and formulation compatability with other chemicals. For pesticidal use, the occluded viruses are sprayed on foliage; susceptible insects are affected after consuming the treated foliage.

Fungal Insecticides

Although many species of fungi can affect insects, fungal insecticides have undergone little commercial development to date. However, *Hirsutella thompsonii* is used for the control of the citrus rust mite and *Nomurea rileyi* for cabbage looper and velvet bean caterpillar.

RODENTICIDES

Rats and mice are harmful both from the standpoint of damaging food supplies, including stored products, as well as growing crops, and from the standpoint of spreading human diseases. Rodents are hosts for vectors of a number of human diseases, including plague, endemic rickettsiosis, leishmaniasis, spirochetosis, tularemia, leptospirosis, tick-borne encephalitis, and listeriosis (Hayes, 1982).

Inorganic Rodenticides

A number of inorganic compounds have seen popular use as rodenticides in the past. However, these materials have relatively high hazards for people and domestic animals due to their high toxicity and lack of selectivity.

Zinc phosphide has been used for many years as a rodenticide and is effective against all species of rats and mice. The safety of this compound for humans and domestic animals derives from the emetic action of the zinc moiety in animals that can vomit. The toxicity to rodents of zinc phosphide is fully accounted for by the toxicity of the phosphine produced by its reaction with gastric hydrochloric acid (Hayes, 1982).

Thallium sulfate was introduced for use as an insecticide in this country around 1930. Thallium had early drug use for the prevention of night sweats in tuberculosis, in which connection it was observed that treated patients suffered a rapid and complete loss of hair. Thallium acetate was used as a depilatory in the treatment of ringworm of the scalp in children. In the period between 1935 and 1955, 778 persons were reported to have been poisoned by thallium salts, of whom 46 (6%) died of thallitoxicosis.

Thallium salts are quite toxic to rats, with an acute oral LD50 of 35 mg/kg. The toxic actions resemble those of arsenic in many respects. Signs of acute poisoning become evident within 12–24 h after ingestion of a toxic dose and can be referred to the gastrointestinal tract (irritation), nervous system (acute ascending paralysis and psychic disturbances), and circulatory system. The acute cardiovascular effects of thallium may be the result of ability of thallium ions to substitute for potassium ions, particularly in potassium-activated ATPase.

Other inorganic materials with historical and possibly some current use as rodenticides include elemental (white) phosphorus, barium carbonate, and arsenic trioxide.

Red Squill

Red squill is a dark-red powder prepared from the bulb *Urginea maritima*, which grows around the Mediterranean coast. The toxic action of red squill depends on the presence of two cardiac glycosides, scillaren A and scillaren B. These glycosides exert an action on the heart similar to that of digitalis. The most important property of red squill from a safety standpoint is its natural emetic action, which causes vomiting in humans and most other animals. The acute oral LD50 of red squill is 500 mg/kg for rats. Symptoms produced in humans from ingestion of a toxic dose of red squill include abdominal pain and vomiting, ventricular irregularities, and convulsions.

α-Naphthylthiourea (ANTU)

ANTU was developed during World War II as an effective control agent for the Norway rat. It is not effective with all rat strains. Many other animal species, including the monkey, are resistant. Use experience has shown low hazard to humans. In the original field trials in 1360 blocks in Baltimore with potential exposure for some 500,000 workers and residents, no compound-related human illnesses or fatalities were noted over the 3-year test period. However, even susceptible rats develop a resistance or shyness toward baits containing ANTU. As a result, the use of this material has declined, and it has little use today.

In addition to Norway rats, dogs are also susceptible to ANTU poisoning. Death in these two species is due to pulmonary edema.

Sodium Fluorocetate (Compound 1080) and Fluoroacetamide (Compound 1081)

Sodium fluoroacetate is a white powder that is soluble in water. It is usually formulated with a black dye so that the formulated material does not appear edible. This compound is highly toxic not only to rodents (acute oral LD50 of 3–7 mg/kg in rats) but also to domestic animals and humans. The use of these compounds is restricted to pest-control operators.

Sir Rudolph Peters carried out early studies on the toxicity and mode of action of fluoracetate and coined the term "lethal synthesis" to describe its conversion in vivo into a toxic entity. In vivo, as a part of the Krebs cycle, the fluorine-substituted acetate condenses with oxaloacetate to form fluorocitrate. The fluorocitrate inhibits the enzyme aconitase, preventing the conversion of citrate to isocitrate, blocking the Krebs cycle, and inhibiting oxidative energy metabolism.

Clinically, nausea and apprehension usually begin about 2 h after ingestion. Epileptiform convulsions follow and eventually lead to severe depression. Pulsus alternans may occur, followed by ventricular fibrillation and death. Treatment consists of providing additional acetate ion for the Krebs cycle. Both ethyl alcohol and monoacetin have proven to be effective antidotes in animal studies.

Fluoroacetamide resembles fluoreacetate in mode of action, but has a longer latent period and somewhat lower toxicity. Specific therapy utilizing acetamide was effective in fluoroacetamide-treated rats.

Pyriminil

Pyriminil (Vacor) is a substituted urea compound that kills rats by nicotinamide antagonism. This compound is effective against warfarin-resistant strains of rats, and, since it may be effective in a single dose, the problem of avoidance behavior is eliminated.

However, ingestion of pyriminil by accident or with suicidal intent has resulted in a number of deaths from ketoacidosis, pneumonitis, gastrointestinal-tract perforations, and cardiac arrhythmias. Survivors almost invariably develop diabetic mellitus and a peripheral neuropathy characterized by marked postural hypertension, ileus, and urinary retention. Since pyriminil is a substituted urea, it is structurally related to the well-known diabetogenic compound alloxan. All of these compounds seem to exert their diabetogenic effect through destruction of the insulin-secreting B-cells of the pancreas. Nicotinamide has been shown to be effective in reversing pyriminil toxicity in rats. However, several human cases indicate that nicotinamide does not prevent diabetes or neurologic deterioration.

Pyriminil was withdrawn from the U.S. market in 1979.

HERBICIDES

There is a wide range of chemical compound types in use as herbicides. Prior to World War II, mainly inorganic compounds were used for this purpose. However, these compounds are not very selective in their action and tend to persist in the soil. Some inorganic compounds, such as sodium arsenite and sodium chlorate, are still used. Many of the newer synthetic herbicides are quite specific and selective in their action, so that they can be used to control weeds in growing crops or lawns. Weed seedlings are more easily killed than the mature forms, and recognition of this principle has led to the development of "preemergence" and "postemergence" herbicides.

In general, the herbicides present less of a toxic hazard to humans and domestic animals than do the compounds used as insecticides. However, some herbicides, such as paraquat, do present a high degree of acute hazard, and others, such as 2,4,5-T and silvex, possess toxic potential based on contaminants. Two organic phosphorus cholinesterase-inhibiting compounds (DEF and merphos) used as defoliants in cotton fields can cause delayed neuropathy (see above).

Chlorophenoxy Acids

The chlorophenoxy acid-type herbicides include 2,4-D (2,4-dichlorophenoxyacetic acid), 2,4,5-T (2,4,5-trichlorophenoxyacetic acid), and silvex [2-(2,4,5-trichlorphenoxy) propionic acid]. These compounds are formulated for weed control in the form of various salts and esters to produce material of low volatility in order to minimize the risk of harm to useful plants growing near treated fields. Compounds in this class exert their toxic action on plants by acting as growth hormones. They apparently have no hormonal action in animals.

The acute oral toxicities of 2,4,-D and 2,4,5-T are low, with LD50 values in the range of 300–700 mg/kg for most species, with the exception of the dog, which seems to be more sensitive. Poisoned animals display a disinclinnation to move and develop myotonia with rigidity of the skeletal muscles and ataxia. The acute toxicity in humans is also low. One report cites a self-experiment in which a man consumed 500 mg 2,4-D daily for 21 days with no noticeable effects (Assouly, 1951). In a clinical trial against disseminated coccidioidomycosis, patients were given multiple intravenous doses of 2,4-D (Seaburg, 1983). A dosage of 2000 mg was without effect, but 3600 mg produced coma, muscle fibrillation, hyporeflexia, and urinary inconsistence. These effects disappeared within a 48-h period. The production of myotonia, as seen with 2,4-D poisoning, seems to be a general property of the phenoxy acids.

The overriding toxicologic concern relative to 2,4,5-T and silvex relates to their contamination with 2,3,7,8-TCDD (2,3,7,8-tetrachlorodibenzo-p-dioxin), 2,3,7,8-TCDD is formed during the synthesis of 2,4,5-T or silvex by condensation of two molecules of 2,4,5-trichlorophenol. 2,3,7,8-TCDD has not been found in 2,4-D nor would it be expected, since the starting material for 2,4-D synthesis is 2,4-dichlorophenol. Dimerization of 2,4-chlorophenol should yield a dichlorodibenzo-p-dioxin, which is much less toxic than the 2,3,7,8-TCDD.

2,4,5-T has been used extensively on rangelands, pastures, rice and nursery crops. In the 1960s, when the military began to apply herbicides in Vietnam as the best means of defoliating forest areas to remove cover used as a concealment by the enemy, a 50–50 mixture of the n-butyl esters of 2,4,-D and 2,4,5-T, known as Agent Orange, was the most significant formulation used. Some Vietnam veteran groups and others have attributed a variety of illnesses suffered by these veterans to their exposure to dioxin as a result of this Agent Orange usage. A number of epidemiology studies are now underway to look for any health problems that could be associated with military service in Southeast Asia. Dioxin contamination problems have also occurred closer to home. Waste oil from a chemical plant that produced 2,4,5-T and later hexachlorophene was used to spray horse arenas and other sites in eastern Missouri, most notably the town of Times Beach.

2,3,7,8-TCDD is one of the most toxic substances known. In the most susceptible species—the guinea pig—the acute oral LD50 is 0.6 mg/kg. There are large variations in sensitivity between species, with the rat and monkey being intermediate and the hamster least susceptible. One characteristic of acute lethal 2,3,7,8-TCDD poisoning is the protracted time between exposure and death. During this period, the animals lose weight, and thymic atrophy is seen at autopsy. Hepatotoxic effects, including fatty degeneration and porphyria, also occur in some species. Dioxin is a potent inducer of a number of liver microsomal and other enzymes, particularly aryl hydrocarbon hydroxylase. 2,4,5-T containing 2,3,7,8-TCDD produces cleft palate and other teratologic effects in mice and rats. However, 2,3,7,8-TCDD contamination does not seem to be the only factor, and some teratologic activity seems to be due to 2,4,5-T itself, to other contaminants, or to a 2,4,5-T/2,3,7,8-TCDD interaction (Courtney, 1977). 2,3,7,8-TCDD alters the immune response and decreases immunocompetence in exposed animals. In carcinogenesis bioassay, 2,3,7,8-TCDD has been found to induce dose-related increases in liver and thyroid tumors in rats and mice. In studies in Sweden of workers exposed to phenoxyacetic acid herbicides in forestry or agriculture, Hardell and his coworkers (1979) found an increased risk of developing soft-tissue sarcoma associated with exposure.

Triazines and Triazoles

These cyclic nitrogen compounds have a low order of acute toxicity. The major toxicologic concern with these materials is the carcinogenic effect of the triazole compound amitrole (3-amino-1,2,4-triazole).

The triazine herbicides include atrazine (2-chloro-4-ethylamino-6-isopropylamine-s-triazine) and simazine [2-chloro-4,6-bis(ethylamino)-s-triazine]. The rat oral LD50 values range from 1750 mg/kg for simazine to 5000 mg/kg for atrazine. Neither compound was tumorigenic to mice given oral exposures for 18 months at the maximum tolerated doses.

Although amitrole is chemically related to the triazine compounds, it has some toxicologic differences from them. In animal experiments, amitrole has shown a low acute toxicity with no toxicity at the highest single oral and dermal dosages they tested (4080 and 2500 mg/kg, respectively). Amitrole does have an antithyroid action. The mechanism in this effect seems to be through inhibition of thyroid peroxidase. This enzyme converts iodide to an oxidized form, which iodinates the tyrosine. Thus, inhibition of thyroid peroxidase produces a decrease in thyroid hormone levels. This condition, in turn, stimulates the pituitary gland to produce an excess of thyrotropic hormone, causing hyperplasia of the thyroid gland. Amitrole, along with other antithyroid compounds, can induce thyroid tumors. Tumors in other sites, including the liver and pituitary gland, have been reported in some studies, usually at dosages above that required for production of thyroid tumors. The use of amitrole in cranberry bogs resulted in illegal residues on cranberries being detected near Thanksgiving in 1959. There are presently no tolerances for this compound on food products in the United States.

Carbamate Herbicides

The carbamate herbicides differ from the carbamate insecticides in having little or no anticholinesterase activity. This group of carbamates, thiocarbamates, and dithiocarbamates has a generally low order of acute toxicity. Propham (isopropyl-N-phenylcarbamate) has an acute LD50 of 1000 mg/kg in the rat. Although some related compounds, such as ethyl carbamate (urethane), have been shown to be tumorigenic, both propham and chloropropham did not cause a significant increase in tumors in mice after oral administration for 18 months at the highest tolerated level.

Bipyridyl Compounds

The bipyridyl herbicide paraquat has caused many deaths following accidental or deliberate ingestion of the concentrated formulation of the material. In 1977, it was reported that there had been 564 deaths throughout the world from this compound (Harley et al., 1977). Dermal or respiratory absorption due to occupational exposure seems to have produced poisoning only rarely and usually after failure to follow label instructions (Hayes, 1982).

The clinical course of paraquat poisoning consists of two stages. The first or destructive phase lasts from 2 to 7 days. During this time, there is disintegration of the alveolar epithelium, producing dyspnea and showing diffuse opacities over the lung fields in chest X-rays. There is often a temporary oliguric renal failure. This phase is seldom fatal unless a large dose of paraquat has been taken. The second or proliferative phase lasts from 1 to 4 weeks and is characterized by a diffuse proliferation of fibroblastic tissue into the alveolar spaces, finally completely obliterating the alveolar architecture. Clinically, the patient experiences severe dyspnea and cyanosis. Death usually occurs from respiratory failure. Thus, the clinical cause of paraquat intoxication is often protracted and there is no known antidote. Treatment consists in removing the paraquat from the gastrointestinal tract with an adsorbent, such as bentonite or Fuller's Earth and from the blood with forced diuresis and/or hemodailysis. Immunosuppressive and cytotoxic drugs also appear to be helpful. Oxygen therapy is not recommended since oxygen seems to potentiate the toxicity of paraquat (Hayes, 1982).

FUNGICIDES

Fungicides, like insecticides and especially herbicides, are comprised of a heterogenous group of compounds, many of which are chemically unrelated. Although many of these materials have a low order of mammalian toxicity, several fungicides are of toxicologic concern and interest.

Dithiocarbamate Fungicides

The chemical structures involved here are the dimethyldithiocarbamates (such as ferbam, thiram, and ziram) and the ethylenebisdithiocarbamates (such as maneb, nabam, and zineb). In addition to the two basically different dithiocarbamate structures, a number of different metal moieties (zinc, manganese, iron, and sodium) occur in these compounds. The compounds have had widespread use in agriculture. They have a relative low order of acute toxicity, with acute rat oral LD50 values in the range of several hundred milligrams to several grams per kilogram. The most sensitive measure of toxic effect of the dithiocarbamate fungicides is the antithyroid action. The ethylenebisdithiocarbamate series of compounds, but not the dimethyldithiocarbamates, have been reported to be carcinogenic, due apparently to the metabolism of the former compounds to ethylenethiourea, a known thyroid carcinogen.

Another toxic property of the dithiocarbamate group is potentiation of alcohol.

The dithiocarbamate fungicide thiram is the methyl analog of disulfiram (Antabuse), a compound that is used therapeutically to produce an adverse reaction and induce aversion to alcohol. In one reported case, a woman experienced dermatitis particularly on her face every Sunday night after her bath. Bathing on weeks days had no such effect. Further investigation found that she was using a thiram-containing soap daily and that she drank cocktails "only on Sunday."

Hexachlorobenzene

As the name implies, hexachlorobenzene is a substituted benzene and should not be confused with the insecticide benzene hexachloride, which is a cyclic alkane derivative (hexachlorocyclohexane). Although the acute toxicity of HCB is low, repeated doses even at low levels can produce poisoning. Hexachloroenzene is avidly stored in adipose tissues in exposed animals. Its presence has been reported in human fat. As with other chlorinated hydrocarbons, the primary toxic effect of hexachlorobenzene is one the nervous system, although the liver is also affected after repeated doses.

An epidemic of hexachlorobenzene poisoning occurred in Turkey in the 1950s due to the consumption of treated wheat that was intended for use as seed. Some 5000 cases of porphyria cutanea tarda occurred. In addition to disturbance in porphyrin metabolism, clinical manifestations of photosensitization, hypertricphosis, hepatomegaly, weight loss, and enlargement of the thyroid gland and lymph nodes were reported.

Hexachlorobenzene is known to occur as a contaminant in other pesticides (Dacthal and PCNB) and may be responsible for or contribute to their toxicity.

Phthalimide Derivatives

Captan and folpet have a low order of both acute and chronic oral toxicity to laboratory animals. In the rat, acute oral LD50 values reported by various investigators are in the order of several grams per kilogram. The structural similarity of captan to thalidomide has prompted study of captan as a possible teratogen.

In reviewing the work of Boyd and his coworkers on the effect of severe dietary protein restriction on the toxicity of various pesticides to rats, Hayes (1975) has pointed out the disproportionate increase produced in the toxicity of captan. No mechanism has been proposed for this effect.

Captan and folpet exhibited extensive genotoxic activity in short-term bioassays for gene or point mutations and primary DNA damage and repair. Captan also produced tumors of the duodenum when fed to male rats at dietary levels of 8000 or 16,000 ppm (about 350 or 700 mg/kg) for 80 weeks.

REFERENCES

Abou-Donia, M. D. 1979. Delayed neurotoxicity of phenylphosphonothionate esters. *Science* 205:713–714.

Assouly, M. 1951. Descherbant selectifs et substances de croissance pergu technique. Effet pathologique sur l'homme au cour de la fabrication de l'ester de 2,4-D. *Arch. Mal. Prof. Med. Trav. Secur. Soc.* 12:26–30.

Courtney, K. D. 1977. Prenatal effects of herbicides. Evaluation by the prenatal development index. *Arch. Environ. Contam. Toxicol.* 6:33–46.

DuBois, K. P. 1961. Potentiation of the toxicity of organophosphorus compounds. *Adv. Pest Control Res.* 4:117–151.

Frawley, J. P., Fugart, H. N. Hagan, E. C., Blake, J. R., and Fitzhugh, O. G. 1957. Marked potentiation in mammalian toxicity from simultaneous administration of two anticholines-terase compounds. *J. Pharmacol. Exp. Ther.* 121:96–106.

Gaines, T. B. 1969. Acute toxicity of pesticides. *Toxicol. Appl. Pharmacol.* 4:515–524.

Haley, T. J. 1978. A review of the literature of rotenone. *J. Environ. Pathol. Toxicol.*, 1:315–337.

Haley, T. J. 1979. A review of the toxicology of paraquat. *Clin. Toxicol.* 14:1–46.

Harley, J. B., Grinspan, S., and Root, R. K. 1977. Paraquat suicide in a young woman: Results of therapy directed against the superoxide radical. *Yale J. Biol. Med.* 50:481–488.

Hayes, W. J., Jr. 1975. *Toxicology of Pesticides.* Baltimore: Williams & Wilkins.

Hayes, W. J., Jr. 1982. *Pesticides Studied in Man..* Baltimore: Williams & Wilkins.

Johnson, M. K. 1975. The delayed neuropathy caused by some organophosphorus esters: Mechanism and challenge. *CRC Crit. Rev. Toxicol.* 3:289–316.

Laug, E. P., Nelson, A. A., Fitzhugh, O. G., and Kunze, F. M. 1950. Liver cell alteration and DDT storage in the fat of the rat induced by dietary levels of 1 to 50 oom DDT. *J. Pharmacol. Exp. Ther.* 98:268–273.

Moeller, H. C., and Rider, J. A. 1962. Plasma and red cell cholinesterase activity as indications of the threshold of the incipient toxicity of ethyl-*p*-nitrophenyl thionobenzene phosphonate (EPN) and malathion in human beings. *Toxicol. Appl. Pharmacol.* 4:123–130.

Ortega, P., Hayes, W. J., Jr., Durham, W. F., and Mattison, A. 1956. *DDT in the diet of the rat.* Public Health Monograph, No. 43, PHS 484.

Seaburg, J. H. 1983. Toxicity of 2,4-dichlorophenoxyacetic acid for man and dog. *Arch. Environ. Health* 7:202–209.

Weil, C. S., Woodside, M. D., Carpenter, C. P., and Smythe, H. F., Jhr. 1972. Current status of tests of carbaryl for reproductive and tertatogenic effects. *Toxicol. Appl. Pharmacol.* 21:390–404.

Witherup, S., Jolley, W. J., Stemmer, K., and Pfitzer, E. S. 1976. Chronic studies with 2,2-dichlorovinyl dimethyl phosphate (DDVP) in dogs and rats including observations on rat reproduction. *Toxicol. Appl. Pharmacol.* 19:377.

Chapter 10

Mechanisms of Metal-Induced Cell Injury

Peter L. Goering

Prakash Mistry

Bruce A. Fowler

INTRODUCTION

Cellular injury from toxic metals may occur by a number of diverse molecular mechanisms and at many levels of biological organization within a given target organ or cell population. Direct changes in the activities of key biomolecules or biochemical pathways are always a major component of any toxic process produced by metals. Membrane localization of sensitive biochemical processes within a particular organelle system (i.e., the mitochondrion) may also play an important role in a toxic process. In this case, metal-induced membrane damage is associated with subsequent loss of biochemical function for those processes or molecules that require membrane integrity for normal activity. Distinguishing between direct and secondary toxic effects is a major challenge confronting the toxicologist concerned with understanding mechanisms of metal-induced cell injury.

This review delineates some current mechanisms of metal-induced cell damage at both the molecular and organelle level. Particular emphasis is given to factors known to influence susceptibility to a given metal. We believe that this approach provides an integrated assessment of the known ways in which metals produce toxicity for a given organ, cell type, organelle, or specific group of molecules. In addition, this chapter also examines known interactive factors, such as developmental stage of the organism, physiological status, sex, nutritional status, concomitant exposure to other toxicants, dose regimen, etc., that have been shown to be capable of influencing metal-induced toxicity at a number of biological levels with respect to both the nature and site of toxicity. A review of these data should give the reader some basic insights into not only the mechanisms of metal-induced injury but also how these mechanisms may be influenced by interactive factors.

PHYSIOLOGICAL FACTORS IN METAL TOXICITY

While the primary focus of the present chapter is to examine biochemical mechanisms of metal-induced cell injury, it is clear that physiological factors such as gradients (electrochemical, osmotic), transport systems in specific cell membranes, and primary physiological function of a particular organ may profoundly influence which cells in a given organ are damaged. A complete discussion of these physiological parameters is outside the scope of this chapter, but such factors should be taken into consideration when evaluating data from in vivo experimental studies from the viewpoint of metal pharmacokinetics and cell-specific effects.

ROLES OF SUBCELLULAR ORGANELLE SYSTEMS IN MECHANISMS OF METAL TOXICITY

Cell Membrane

In order for a toxic metal species to enter a cell, some interaction with the plasma membrane is required. For some chemical species of metals/metalloids, such as methylmercury, cadmium–metallothionein, or arsenate, movement across the membrane may be facilitated, respectively, by lipophilicity, by transport of the metal bound to a protein that is absorbed via endocytosis, and by chemical similarity to an essential and readily absorbed nutrient (e.g., phosphate). Other metals, such as lead, appear to enter cells via either passive diffusion or binding to the membrane with subsequent endocytosis (Victery et al., 1984). While the possibility for membrane dysfunction from the above metals does exist, there is presently little direct experimental evidence that such effects do occur, and hence, these agents are regarded as being primarily intracellular toxicants under both acute and chronic exposure conditions (Fowler, 1972a,b; Fowler et al., 1974, 1975, 1979; Fowler and Woods, 1977a; Woods and Fowler, 1977b; Squibb et al., 1979, 1982, 1984; Squibb and Fowler, 1984; Brown et al., 1976). On the other hand, strong oxidizing agents such as inorganic mercury (Hg^{2+}) and chromate (Cr^{6+}) are known to produce marked ultrastructural and biochemical effects on cell membranes (Gritzka and Trump, 1968; Ganote et al., 1975; Evan and Dail, 1974; Kempson et al., 1977; Foulkes, 1983) following acute administration.

Chronic in vivo exposure studies (Madsen and Christensen, 1978; Carmichael and Fowler, 1979) utilizing Hg^{2+}, however, have demonstrated little evidence of membrane effects, suggesting that the rate at which a metal arrives at the membrane may be important in determining both the nature and site of action. In summary, the extent to which measurable toxic changes occur in the cell membrane is a function of the chemical form of the metal administered, the dose regimen employed, and whether a sensitive "indicator" of membrane dysfunction is available.

It should also be pointed out that most biological membranes are capable of compensatory or adaptive changes in response to toxic metals under chronic exposure conditions in vivo. These responses may involve changes in membrane protein synthesis patterns (Levander et al., 1980) or altered relationships to organelles such as the mitochondria, which produce ATP for a number of membrane functions. The major point to be emphasized is that the inherent dynamic and integrated nature of biological membranes at the tissue, cell, organelle, and molecular levels of organization increases the difficulty of developing a comprehensive mechanistic approach to metal-induced cell injury involving this essential cellular component.

Mitochondria

The mitochondrion is a major intracellular target for the toxicity of many metals. The susceptibility of this organelle appears to stem from a number of factors, such as rapid mitochondrial membrane transport of many essential and toxic substances, high metabolic activity, and sensitivity of essential mitochondrial processes to disruption. Metal-induced mitochondrial damage may occur either directly or secondarily to altered mitochondrial biogenesis or physical swelling. Evaluation of the integrated and complex relationships that exist between mitochondrial structure and function appears to be of central importance in understanding mechanisms of metal toxicity in this organelle.

In discussing these relationships, it should first be noted that the mitochondrion is divided into four major physical compartments: outer membrane, intermembrane space, inner membrane, and matrix. Each of these compartments contain specific metabolic processes and enzyme activities (Fowler et al., 1982a) and hence shows differential sensitivities to metal-induced toxicity. The mitochondrial membranes, in particular, seem to be highly sensitive to perturbation by a number of metals and metalloids. Exposure to a number of agents in vivo, including arsenate (Brown et al., 1976; Fowler and Woods, 1979; Fowler et al., 1979), methylmercury (Fowler et al., 1975; Fowler and Woods, 1977a,b), and lead (Goyer, 1968; Goyer and Krall, 1969; Goyer and Rhyne, 1975; Fowler et al., 1980), has clearly demonstrated disturbances of mitochondrial membrane marker enzyme activities and respiratory function associated with marked in situ alterations in membrane ultrastructure, such as mitochondrial swelling (Fig. 1). In particular, mitochondrial respiration supported by NAD-linked substrates (pyruvate/malate, glutamate, and α-ketoglutarate) has been found to be more sensitive to metal inhibition than respiration supported by succinate. The molecular mechanism for this selective substrate effect has usually been attributed to reaction of agents like trivalent arsenic with the dithiol-containing lipoic acid cofactor of the dehydrogenase complex involved in metabolizing these substrates (Ulmer and Vallee, 1969; Squibb and Fowler, 1983). However, other studies (Matlib and Srere, 1976) have shown that phosphate-induced physical swelling of mitochondria will

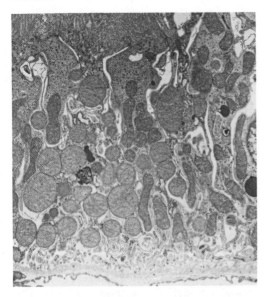

Figure 1 Electron micrograph of rat renal proximal tubule cell following prolonged oral exposure to lead, demonstrating in situ mitochondrial swelling, × 5670.

produce similar inhibitory effects on NAD-linked respiration, suggesting that perturbation of mitochondrial structure disrupts an obligatory relationship between the dehydrogenase complex for these substrates, which is located in the mitochondrial matrix, and the electron transport chain of the inner membrane. Succinate dehydrogenase, which is associated with the inner membrane and hence located in the same intramitocondrial compartment as the electron transport chain, is not influenced directly by mitochondrial swelling. The point here is to emphasize that our interpretation of the mechanism(s) of metal-induced toxicity for this organelle is highly dependent on understanding the relationships between mitochondrial structure, localization of specific biochemical processes (e.g., enzymes) within that structure, and overall function.

Mitochondria also participate in a number of interorganelle processes involving heme biosynthesis and the metabolism of products generated in other cellular organelles such as the endoplasmic reticulum (Fig. 2). The effects of various metals on mitochondrial heme biosynthesis pathway enzymes will be discussed at length in a subsequent section, but it is worth noting at this point the relatively unstudied area of interorganelle interactions and the influence of metals on these processes with respect to cell injury.

Mitochondrial–microsomal interactions have been studied by a number of investigators (Axelrod, 1956; Bachman and Golberg, 1970; Cinti and Schenkman, 1972; Cinti et al., 1972, 1976; Denk et al., 1976; Moldeus et al., 1973; Schenkman et al., 1973; Fowler et al., 1982b) with respect to the influence of mitochondria and mitochondrial NAD-dependent aldehyde dehydrogenase on the measurement of toxic aldehydes generated by microsomal oxidative dealkylation reactions (Fig. 2). These

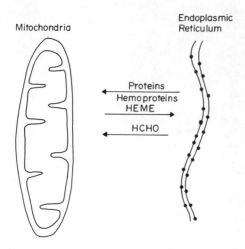

Figure 2 Diagram showing interactions between mitochondria and the endoplasmic reticulum with respect to heme utilization and aldehyde metabolism.

toxic aldehydes may be metabolized by mitochondrial NAD-dependent dehydrogenase if the proper experimental conditions are met (Fowler et al., 1982b). The metabolic activity of this dehydrogenase is regulated by mitochondrial NAD levels or NAD/NADH ratios, which are in turn controlled by NAD-linked substrate respiration. Prolonged oral exposure of rats to arsenate (As^{5+}) has been shown to selectively inhibit NAD-linked substrate respiration of liver mitochondria with concomitant increases in mitochondrial NAD/NADH ratios (Fowler et al., 1979). This, in turn, has been found to markedly increase the endogenous activity of mitochondrial aldehyde dehydrogenase and accelerate mitochondrial metabolism of formaldehyde generated by microsomal oxidative dealkylation of aminopyrine (Fowler et al., 1982b). The importance of this concept rests with the fact that cells are integrated structures and that perturbations of one organelle may produce "ripple" effects in the overall function of other systems.

Lysosomes

Many metals accumulate within lysosomes and influence the biochemical function of this organelle system. Mercury, administered in the form of methylmercury (Fowler et al., 1974, 1975) or Hg^{2+} (Madsen and Christensen, 1978), has been found to be present in kidney proximal-tubule cell lysosomes and to affect the activities of a number of specific lysosomal marker enzymes. Cadmium administered as cadmium–metallothionein (CdMT) also accumulates within renal proximal-tubule cell lysosomes (Fowler and Nordberg, 1978; Squibb et al., 1979) with subsequent degradation of the CdMT complex to release Cd^{2+} (Cain and Holt, 1983; Squibb et al., 1984). The free Cd^{2+} ions inhibit lysosomal proteolytic function (Squibb et al., 1982, 1984; Squibb and Fowler, 1984), which results in cell injury (Fig. 3). Thus, the lysosome system has a central role in regulating the cellular toxicity of this metal in a target cell population, and the mechanism of cadmium-induced tubular-cell injury is mediated by its inhibitory effects on normal lysosomal function.

The normal structure and function of the cellular lysosomal system may also be indirectly affected by metals due to lysosomal autophagy of other metal-damaged organelles. For example, accumulation of indium and iron within hepatocyte autophagic lysosomes following acute administration of indium chloride (In^{3+}) primarily damages the structure of the endoplasmic reticulum (Fowler et al., 1983), with concomitant induction of microsomal heme oxygenase (see section on heme metabolism). In this case, it appears that both these metals accumulate in the lysosomes following autophagy of the endoplasmic reticulum membranes, leading to subsequent alterations in both lysosomal volume density and marker-enzyme activities.

Endoplasmic Reticulum (Microsomes)

The acute administration of many metals, including cobalt (Woods and Carver, 1977), cadmium (Krasny and Holbrook, 1977; Pence et al., 1977; Schnell et al., 1979; Maines and Kappas, 1977a), tin (Kappas and Maines, 1976), indium (Woods et al., 1979; Fowler et al., 1983), and methylmercury (Lucier et al., 1973; Fowler et al., 1975), produces marked inhibition of a number of both cytochrome P-450 and noncytochrome P-450 enzyme activities. One study (Fowler et al., 1983), which combined ultrastructural/biochemical analyses of the endoplasmic reticulum, indicated that indium produced a marked disruption of the endoplasmic reticulum structure, which was associated with alteration of microsomal enzyme activities. Therefore, the

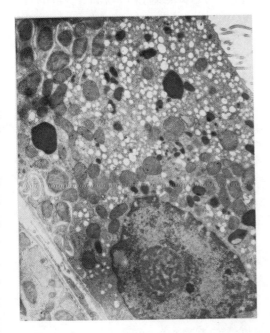

Figure 3 Electron micrograph of a renal proximal-tubule cell from a rat given a single intraperitoneal injection of cadmium–metallothionein, showing marked proliferation of pinocytotic vesicles and small electron dense lysosomes, ×7385.

integral association between the structure of this organelle system and biochemical manifestations of toxicity cannot be overstated. Evaluating both types of parameters is necessary so that one may discern whether a particular biochemical change produced by exposure to a given metal is a specific effect or occurs as part of a more general toxic process involving metal-induced perturbations in the structure of an organelle system like the endoplasmic reticulum with subsequent changes in a host of biochemical processes localized in this structure.

Nucleus

The intranuclear movement of metals and metalloids, such as arsenate (Soronsen et al., 1982), lead (Goyer et al., 1970; Moore et al., 1973; Fowler et al., 1980), bismuth (Fowler and Goyer, 1975), and mercury–selenium (Carmichael and Fowler, 1979), has been demonstrated in a number of biological systems. The effects of these metals, which produce intranuclear inclusion bodies, on nuclear function have been relatively unstudied with the notable exception of lead. Early studies by Choie and Richter (1972a,b; 1974a,b) showed that in vivo exposure of rats or mice to acute or chronic doses of lead resulted in marked stimulation of DNA/RNA and protein synthesis in renal proximal tubule cells and concomitant formation of intranuclear inclusion bodies (Fig. 4). These structures have been demonstrated by a number of investigators (Goyer et al., 1970; Moore et al., 1973; Fowler et al., 1980) to contain the highest intracellular concentrations of lead once the process of formation is initiated. In addition, in vivo lead exposure is also associated with karyomegaly of proximal

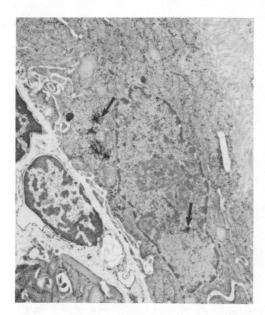

Figure 4 Electron micrograph of a renal proximal-tubule cell from a lead-injected rat, showing both nuclear and cytoplasmic inclusion bodies (arrows), × 5670.

tubule cells even at dose levels below which inclusion bodies are observed (Fowler et al., 1980). Data from these studies indicate that the intranuclear movement of lead produces marked biochemical changes in both nuclear structure and functional activity of renal proximal-tubule cells, which may be responsible for the 40–50% incidence of renal adenocarcinoma observed in rodents following chronic high-dose exposure (IARC, 1980; Task Force on Metals and Carcinogenesis, 1981).

Studies with metals such as methylmercury (Brubaker et al., 1973) and cadmium administered as cadmium–metallothionein (Squibb et al., 1982) have shown that these agents, under acute exposure conditions, produce marked inhibitory effects on nucleic acid synthesis in kidneys of rats. Such data suggest that the mechanism(s) of metal-induced changes in nuclear activity are varied and complex and probably depend not only on the dose and metal administered but also on the molecular species of metal transported into the nucleus (see section on high-affinity metal-binding proteins).

CHEMICAL REACTIONS OF METALS WITH BIOMOLECULES

Metal Interaction with Biological Ligands at the Chemical Level

In discussing mechanisms of metal toxicity, it is important to note that most toxic metals/metalloids (arsenic, cadmium, indium, platinum, tin, chromium, mercury, lead, bismuth, thallium) are soft Lewis acids (i.e., capable of accepting an electron from a soft Lewis base such as sulfur). Only a few of the known toxic metals are hard Lewis acids (e.g., beryllium and aluminum) that react with hard Lewis bases such as oxygen (Williams, 1984). The importance of this concept is that on a chemical basis most of the major toxic metals will preferentially react with SH group(s) of biological molecules, with less opportunity for interactions with other potential electron donors such as COOH or $H_2PO_4^{-2}$, provided these groups are not present in great excess relative to available SH groups (Kägi and Hapke, 1984; Fowler et al., 1984). Such a basic chemical view is consistent with numerous reports in the literature (Voegtlin et al., 1931; Webb, 1966; Woods et al., 1984; Squibb and Fowler, 1983) that indicate that much of the metabolic inhibition associated with these agents does indeed appear to stem from their interaction with SH groups of biological molecules. It should be noted, however, that most of these studies were performed under in vitro conditions and that other potentially competing high-affinity binding compartments (e.g., metallothionein) were usually not present. Therefore, caution must be exercised in extrapolating these results to the in vivo situation. The importance of understanding metal–metal competition for a particular binding site or competition among different binding sites for the same metal cannot be overstated, since intracellular metal-binding patterns usually appear to play a central role in metal toxicity. The known and possible roles played by high-affinity metal-binding proteins, inclusion bodies, and mineral concretions in mediating the bioavailability of toxic metals to sensitive biochemical processes will be considered in a subsequent section.

Mechanisms of Metal Inhibition
of Specific Enzyme Activities by Direct Action

Historically, the oldest and most well-known direct action of a toxic metal/metalloid is that of trivalent arsenic binding to the vicinal thiol groups of lipoic acid, which is an essential cofactor of the pyruvate dehydrogenase complex. Reaction of arsenic with this cofactor forms a stable intermediate (Fig. 5) that inactivates the complex (Peters, 1955; Massey et al., 1962). A more complete review of metal interactions with SH groups of enzymes has been given elsewhere (Webb, 1966; Squibb and Fowler, 1983).

Another type of direct inhibitory mechanism may involve displacement of an essential metal cofactor from an enzyme by a toxic metal competing for the same binding site. An example of this would be the well-known lead-induced inhibition of the zinc-dependent enzyme δ-aminolevulinic acid dehydratase (ALAD). In this case, lead displaces zinc from its SH-mediated binding site, thereby producing an inhibitory effect (Finelli et al., 1975; Tsukamoto et al., 1980). The kinetics of lead inhibition of ALAD appear to be primarily noncompetitive (i.e., decreased V_{max}); however, the K_m of the enzyme for its substrate decreases slightly, indicating a "mixed" type of inhibition pattern (Weissberg and Voytek, 1974; also see section on metal interaction with heme metabolism for details).

In general, a large number of in vitro studies have shown that, as predicted on a chemical basis, the reaction of metals acting as soft Lewis acids with SH groups of various enzymes may be invoked to adequately explain observed patterns of enzyme inhibition (Webb, 1966). Extrapolation of these data to the in vivo situation may provide a simple explanation for the cellular toxicity of many metals if a host of potential intrinsic and extrinsic interactive factors are not taken into consideration. Subsequent sections of this chapter will review the known effects of various metals on several sensitive metabolic systems and examine possible direct and indirect mechanisms of toxicity for each metabolic process in relation to interactive factors that may mediate the observed effects.

BIOLOGICAL ROLES OF HIGH-AFFINITY
METAL-BINDING PROTEINS

In recent years, it has become increasingly evident that the toxic potential of metals such as cadmium, mercury, and lead is highly dependent on their intracellular bioavailability, which appears to be regulated to a degree by binding to high-affinity

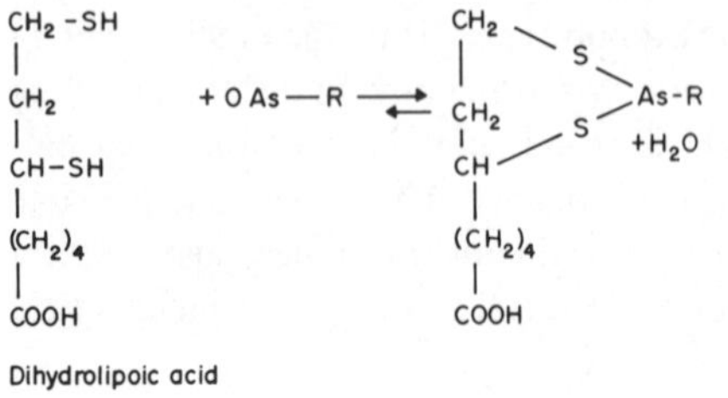

Figure 5 Diagrammatic representation of trivalent arsenic interaction with the dihydrolipoic acid cofactor of the pyruvate dehydrogenase complex, illustrating stable ring formation; OAs, organic arsenic. *(From Fowler, 1977.)*

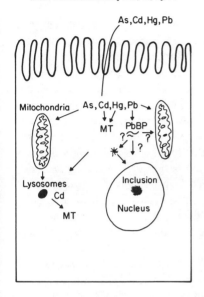

Known Intracellular Binding of As, Cd, Hg, Pb

Figure 6 Diagrammatic representation of the known intracellular binding patterns of cadmium and lead in a renal proximal-tubule cell, showing the multiple binding ligands; MT, metallothionein; PbBP, lead-binding proteins.

cytosolic proteins (Fowler et al., 1984; Nordberg, 1984; Nordberg and Kojima, 1979; Oskarsson et al., 1982; Squibb et al., 1979), intranuclear inclusion bodies (Fowler et al., 1980, 1984; Moore et al., 1973), or lysosomes (Fowler et al., 1980; Fowler and Nordberg, 1978; Squibb and Fowler, 1984; Squibb et al., 1982). These intracellular "sinks" appear to be at least partially capable of sequestering toxic metals away from sensitive organelles or metabolic sites until their capacity is exceeded by either the administered or accumulated dose of a given metal. It should be noted that there are also a number of interactive factors that appear capable of influencing the capacity of these storage sites. Nutritional status of the organism and the presence or absence of other essential metals may greatly alter the distribution of metals within intracellular compartments. A schematic representation of known cadmium- and lead-binding sites in an idealized kidney proximal tubule cell is presented in Fig. 6. The major point of the figure is that the known intracellular binding sites of these two metals appear to be different, although previously described in vivo interactive effects between these two elements (Mahaffey and Fowler, 1977; Mahaffey et al., 1981) may also occur as described below.

The present review of this area is focused on briefly examining the known characteristics and apparent roles played by several high-affinity metal-binding proteins in mediating the intracellular bioavailability and hence toxic potential of metals such as cadmium and lead in biological systems. It is hoped that by using these two important toxic metals as examples, some general insights into the regulatory roles of high-affinity biological ligands for metals will be illustrated. At this stage in our knowledge of intracellular metal partitioning, it is also of particular importance to put forward new hypotheses that will aid in expanding our understanding of the relationships between binding of metals to high-affinity bioligands and cellular injury.

Metallothionein

Metallothionein (MT) is a low-molecular weight (approximately 7000 daltons) protein that has been extensively studied in mammals and is also known to exist in a number of nonmammalian species. The general structural and chemical characteristics of MT are given in Table 1 and have been extensively described elsewhere (Nordberg and Kojima, 1979). From the perspective of regulating the intracellular bioavailability of cadmium, zinc, mercury, silver, bismuth and copper, MT appears to mediate the intracellular toxicity of these metals through several mechanisms. For example, in vivo exposure to cadmium in mammals via the lungs or gastrointestinal tract results in transport of cadmium in the blood on high-molecular-weight proteins with extensive uptake of cadmium in the liver (Nordberg, 1984; Nordberg and Kojima, 1979) and subsequent hepatic induction of MT. Depending on the dose administered or duration of exposure, cadmium has been subsequently found in the circulation bound to MT (Garvey and Chang, 1981; Nordberg, 1984). An important aspect of this observation from a toxicological perspective concerns the highly efficient uptake of cadmium–MT by kidney proximal-tubule cells following glomerular filtration (Cain and Holt, 1983; Cherian and Shaikh, 1975; Cherian et al., 1976; Garvey and Chang, 1981; Nordberg et al., 1975; Squibb and Fowler, 1984; Squibb et al., 1982). Depending on the concentration of cadmium or cadmium–MT administered, proximal-tubule cell damage and low-molecular-weight tubular proteinuria develop following lysosomal degradation of the cadmium–MT complex to yield non-thionein-bound cadmium prior to induction of renal MT (Fig. 7). Thus, transport of cadmium bound to MT in the circulation plays a key role in mediating the nephrotoxicity of this metal. Intracellular MT production also appears to be an important biochemical mechanism for mediating the intracellular bioavailability/toxicity of cadmium, and there are several well-documented examples of this function described below.

Role of Metallothionein in Mediating Effects of Cadmium on the Hepatic Microsomal Mixed-Function Oxidase System   Numerous studies have shown that

Table 1   Mammalian Metallothionein

Characteristic	Description
Molecular weight	6800
Structure	>95% Random
Cysteine content	30%
Aromatic amino acids	None
Metal-binding capacity	7 g-atom metal/mol
Metal-binding clusters	(A) 4 metals
	(B) 3 metals
SH:metal ratio	4:1
Metals bound	Cd, Zn, Hg, Ag, Bi, Cu
Polymorphic forms	Yes
K_d for Cd	$\sim 10^{-16}\ M$

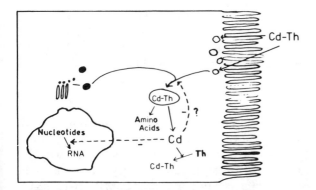

Figure 7 Diagrammatic representation of overall Cd–thionein (CdMT) metabolism in renal proximal-tubule cells, showing lysosomal degradation of absorbed CdMT with release of Cd^{2+} followed by stimulation of renal metallothionein synthesis and/or binding to the native renal metallothionein pool.

acute parenteral administration of cadmium decreases hepatic microsomal cytochrome P-450 content and markedly inhibits associated mixed-function oxidase enzyme activities (Drummond and Kappas, 1980; Krasny and Holbrook, 1977; Lui and Lucier, 1981; Maines and Kappas, 1977b; Pence et al., 1977; Roberts and Schnell, 1982a,b; Schnell et al., 1979). Administration of high oral doses of cadmium for prolonged periods does not produce this phenomenon, since most (70–90%) of the hepatic cadmium is bound to MT (Schnell et al., 1979). Recent in vitro studies (Roberts and Schnell, 1982a) have demonstrated that cadmium ion (Cd^{2+}) is quite effective but that cadmium bound to MT is relatively ineffective at inhibiting cytochrome P-450-mediated microsomal enzyme activities. It should also be noted with respect to this particular toxic endpoint that other in vivo studies (Roberts and Schnell, 1982b) have shown that while cadmium binding to MT appears to play a role in the observed tolerance, other factors, such as changes in P-450 turnover or synthetic patterns, also appear to be operating. For metals, such as indium, that do not induce MT (Fig. 8) but produce similar effects on microsomal P-450 function, this

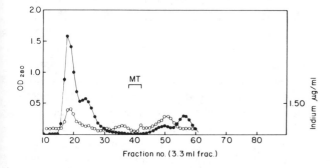

Figure 8 Sephadex G-75 chromatogram of rat liver cytosol 16 h following injection with indium ($InCl_3$, 40 mg/kg). Note the absence of metallothionein binding.

protein does not appear to mediate the observed effects, and lysosomal sequestration may be a more important mechanism (Fowler et al., 1983). Recent studies (Lui and Lucier, 1981) have shown that hormonal factors involving the pituitary also play a role in the susceptibility of the hepatic P-450 system to inhibition by cadmium. Thus, factors other than MT are important in mediating the deleterious effects of cadmium on this intracellular system.

Effects of Protein Turnover on Cadmium Binding to Metallothionein Studies by a number of authors (Nordberg and Kojima, 1979) have shown that MT turns over in a manner similar to other cytosolic proteins. The half-lives of cadmium–MT, ZnMT, and apothionein have been calculated to be about 3.5 days, 17 h, and 6 h, respectively. Thus, the presence of cadmium on this protein gives MT a considerably longer intracelllular half-life in comparison with other metals.

One important aspect of cadmium–MT turnover is that under long-term exposure conditions (6 months), cadmium redistributes into other cellular compartments of the kidney but not the liver (Ridlington et al., 1981). The turnover of MT hence appears to have a marked impact on its ability to bind cadmium and regulate the intracellular bioavailability of cadmium in a major target tissue in vivo.

Summary of Metallothionein Function with Respect to Cellular Injury It is clear that mammalian MT plays a significant role in mediating both the transport and the toxicity of metals such as cadmium. On an intracellular basis, this protein is capable of protecting sensitive metabolic processes from cadmium ion providing it is present in sufficient quantities. Other factors, such as dose administered, hormonal status, protein synthetic patterns, zinc status (Petering et al., 1984), and turnover of MT, are important parameters that can influence the extent to which this molecule is able to regulate the intracellular bioavailability of cadmium and other toxic metal ions.

Cytosolic Lead-Binding Components

Recent studies (Oskarsson et al., 1982; Mistry et al., 1983) have demonstrated that target tissues (kidney, brain), but not other organs (liver, lung), possess high-affinity cytosolic lead-binding components that appear to play a major role in the initial intracellular binding of lead. Two cytosolic lead-binding components (PbBP) with molecular masses of approximately 63,000 and 11,500 daltons have been identified and partially purified (Fig. 9). Saturation analysis of these two binding components has shown that they each possess a dissociation constant (K_d) for lead of approximately 10^{-8} M (Mistry et al., 1984). In vitro dissociation studies with other cations have shown that metals such as cadmium and zinc readily displace most of the lead from these molecules. The importance of this phenomenon rests with the potential role of these components in mediating the previously reported (Mahaffey and Fowler, 1977; Mahaffey et al., 1981) in vivo interaction between lead and cadmium in kidneys of rodents concomitantly exposed to these elements. Rats exposed to both lead and cadmium exhibited a 60% reduction in total renal lead, complete abolition of intranuclear inclusion-body formation, and a marked increase in the urinary excretion of uroporphyrin and coporporphyrin relative to rats exposed to lead alone (Fig. 10).

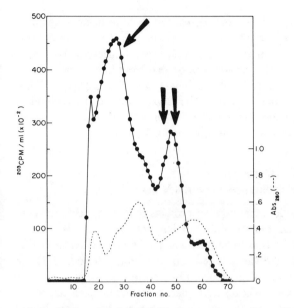

Figure 9 Sephadex G-200 column chromatography profile of rat kidney cytosol, showing lead-binding peaks at 63,000 (arrow) and 11,500 (double arrow) daltons.

These data indicate that total tissue concentrations of lead are probably less meaningful in multielement exposure situations than is an understanding of the intracellular binding characteristics/bioavailability of elements such as lead in target tissues and cells. Concomitant exposure to two metals that compete for the same molecular binding site(s) may result in a quantitative decrease in the total tissue burden of a given metal but may actually increase its intracellular bioavailability to sensitive biochemical systems such as the heme biosynthetic pathway (Woods and Fowler, 1982).

The roles of the cytosolic lead-binding components described above in formation of cytoplasmic or intranuclear lead inclusion bodies are presently unknown. Chemically, these molecules are not of the same size or isoelectric point as proteins recov-

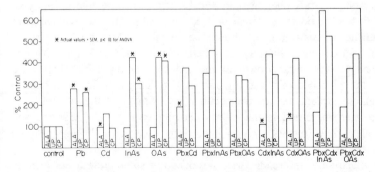

Figure 10 Effects of concomitant exposures to lead × cadmium × arsenic on urinary porphyrin excretion patterns, showing distinctive patterns for each regimen: ALA, δ-aminolevulinic acid; UP, uroporphyrin; CP, coproporphyrin. (From Fowler and Mahaffey, 1978.)

ered from isolated lead intracellular inclusion bodies, which have been reported to possess apparent molecular masses of 27,000 (Moore et al., 1973) and 32,000 (Shelton and Egle, 1982) daltons. On the other hand, these molecules have been shown to enhance the cell-free nuclear translocation of lead from kidney cytosol and appear to act as "receptors" for this metal in the kidney (Mistry et al., 1984). Further research is needed to determine if one or both of the isolated cytosolic lead-binding components are involved in inclusion body formation or whether these molecules actually compete against the nuclear inclusion proteins for lead.

Biological Roles of High-Affinity Cytosolic Cadmium- and Lead-Binding Proteins—An Overall View

Cells possess high-affinity cytosolic metal-binding proteins that are capable of regulating the uptake and intracellular bioavailability/toxicity of many metals such as cadmium and lead. These proteins appear to be of two general types: (1) those such as MT whose synthesis is regulated by divalent metal cations, and (2) those such as the tissue-specific lead-binding components that appear to be normal constituents of cells and bind metals due to the presence of vacant or displaceable binding sites capable of accepting exogenous toxic metals with formation of stable bonding arrangements (Nordberg and Kojima, 1979; Fowler et al., 1984). Therefore, there appears to be competition between these different molecular binding sites for metal cations, such that those sites with higher affinities/binding stabilities outcompete those with lower affinities/stabilities. Depending on a number of factors such as protein turnover, redistribution of metals into "sinks" with greater stability (i.e., lead intranuclear inclusion bodies), and interactive effects between metals, the more effective binding ligands, which usually possess multidentate SH-mediate binding sites, will outcompete other intracellular ligands and thereby mediate the intracellular bioavailability and toxicity of metals. Furthermore, there appears to be competition among high-affinity binding ligands for the same metals. Thus, while most of the intracellular burden of cadmium will be bound to MT, there is always a small fraction (non–MT-bound cadmium) distributed among proteins such as PbBP that have lower affinities for cadmium than MT but higher affinities than other intracellular ligands. The importance of understanding this phenomenon and further evaluating the capacity of these molecules to bind toxic metals such as lead and cadmium rests with a more complete mechanistic understanding of the extent to which these binding ligands regulate the intracellular bioavailability of metals. In addition to explaining the clearly documented in vivo interaction between lead and cadmium in kidney on a molecular basis, the presence of these high-affinity molecules in the kidney also provides a reasonable explanation for the peculiar insensitivity of the cytosolic enzyme δ-ALAD to lead inhibition in the kidney (Fowler et al., 1980; Goering and Fowler, 1984) unless other metals such as indium are concomitantly administered (Woods and Fowler, 1982).

In the above discussion, the reader was introduced to some current but general concepts of how metals produce cell injury on chemical, biochemical, and organelle system levels and how the toxicity of metals is mediated by high-affinity metal-binding proteins in target organs such as kidney and liver. It is important to extend this discussion to highly sensitive metabolic systems that may be at particular risk for toxicity, in order to give the reader an understanding of how these concepts work in practice. The heme biosynthetic/degradation pathway, due to its well-known sensitivity to metals, and the endocrine/reproductive systems will be used as examples, since exposure to metals has been associated with impairment of heme metabolism and endocrine/reproductive function in both humans and experimental animals. A discussion of the specific toxic effects of various metals on these systems will provide the reader with a further understanding of the multiplicity of mechanisms involved in metal toxicity in systems where a number of biological factors are operating.

MECHANISMS OF METAL–INDUCED TOXICITY TO SPECIFIC AND HIGHLY SENSITIVE METABOLIC SYSTEMS

Heme Biosynthetic/Degradation Pathway

The heme biosynthetic/degradative pathway is particularly sensitive to alteration by metals. The inhibition of heme synthesis is of serious consequence, since heme is required by a number of cellular processes. The formation of the microsomal hemoprotein cytochrome P-450 would be compromised, resulting in a reduced capacity to biotransform xenobiotics as well as endogenous compounds. Reduction in synthesis of mitochondrial cytochrome oxidase, another heme-requiring protein, drastically affects cellular respiration and energy production. The synthesis and functional activity of other hemoproteins, such as hemoglobin, catalase, and tryptophan pyrrolase, would also be markedly affected.

Heme biosynthesis (Fig. 11) takes place in two cellular compartments, the mitochondrion and cytoplasm, and involves the formation of a number of pyrrole interme-

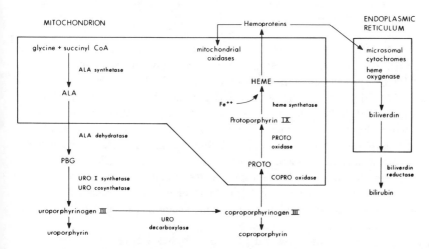

Figure 11 The heme biosynthetic/degradation pathway, showing mitochondrial, endoplasmic reticulum, and cytosolic components.

diates. The initial reaction of the pathway, which occurs in the mitochondrion, involves the combination of a tricarboxylic acid cycle intermediate, succinate (as succinyl CoA), and the amino acid glycine. This reaction is catalyzed by δ-aminolevulinic acid synthetase and requires the cofactor pyridoxal 5'-phosphate. This step is rate-limiting in heme synthesis under normal physiological conditions. The product of this reaction is δ-aminolevulinic acid (ALA), which moves out of the mitochondrion into the cytoplasm. The second step of the pathway involves the condensation of 2 mol ALA to form the monopyrole, porphobilinogen, catalyzed by ALA dehydratase (porphobilinogen synthetase). In the next step, 4 mol porphobilinogen combine to form the tetrapyrrole, uroporphyrinogen III, by the action of uroporphyrinogen I synthetase (porphobilinogen deaminase) and uroporphyrinogen III cosynthetase. Following a series of decarboxylation reactions involving the uroporphyrinogen pyrrole rings and catalyzed by uroporphyrinogen decarboxylase, coproporphyrinogen III is formed. This intermediate enters the mitochondrion, where it is decarboxylated by coproporphyrinogen oxidase to form protoporphyrinogen IX, which is subsequently oxidized by protoporphyrinogen oxidase to protoporphyrin IX. The final step of the pathway is catalyzed by heme synthetase (ferrochelatase), which inserts ferrous iron into protoporphyrin to form heme. Heme exerts negative feedback control over the rate-limiting step of the pathway, the ALA synthetase reaction. The mechanism of this feedback control involves repression of the synthesis of ALA synthetase, rather than inhibition of the preformed enzyme (Maines and Kappas, 1977a).

The degradation of heme to its excretory form, bilirubin, consists of two primary steps. The first step results in the oxidation of heme to form the open-chain tetrapyrrole ring, with loss of iron by the action of heme oxygenase, which is located in the endoplasmic reticulum (Fig. 11). The product of this reaction, biliverdin, is reduced by the action of bilverdin reductase, located in the cytoplasm, to form bilirubin. Bilirubin can undergo a phase II conjugation reaction via glucuronidation for excretion as bilirubin glucuronide.

δ-Aminolevulinic Acid Synthetase (ALAS) The synthesis and activity of ALAS, which catalyzes the rate-limiting step of the heme biosynthetic pathway, is regulated by end-product inhibition, that is, heme (Granick, 1966; Whiting and Granick, 1976). Metal regulation of ALAS is presently believed to result from the direct interaction of ALAS with metals that mimic the previously known inhibitory action of heme. Regulation of this enzyme hence does not necessarily involve an intact metal–porphyrin chelate. Evidence for this mechanism includes the fact that metals that are incapable of forming a heme in vivo, such as nickel and platinum inhibit ALAS production to the same extent as those that are capable of forming a metalloporphyrin heme complex (e.g., iron and cobalt). The mechanism of metal repression of ALAS involves inhibition of enzyme synthesis rather than inhibition of preformed enzyme activity (Maines and Kappas, 1977a,b).

In animal studies, acute injection of lead increases ALAS activity in kidney, while liver ALAS activity is reduced under both acute (parenteral) and chronic (drinking water) exposure (Silbergeld et al., 1982). In contrast, chronic parenteral administration of lead (24 weeks) increases ALAS activity in the liver. In the kidney, parenteral injection of lead causes a progressive increase in ALAS activity, while chronic exposure via drinking water decreases ALAS activity in kidney (Meredith and Moore, 1979; Fowler et al., 1980). The lack of ALAS induction in kidney under chronic exposure conditions may be due to decreased mitochondrial protein synthesis or inhibition of the enzyme to a degree that any inductive effect was not apparent.

Cobalt displays biphasic effects on heme biosynthesis in the liver. Initially, cobalt inhibits the synthesis of ALAS, probably via direct binding of ionic metal to an enzyme regulatory site. Several hours after injection, a moderate increase in ALAS formation occurs, due to derepression of enzyme synthesis resulting from cellular heme depletion following cobalt induction of heme oxygenase, the first enzyme in the heme degradation pathway (Maines et al., 1976). Cadmium, indium, and thallium administered parenterally also elicit a time-dependent biphasic action on ALAS activity in liver, characterized by an initial decrease followed by a rebound increase in activity (Yoshida et al., 1979; Woods et al., 1979, 1984).

Chronic oral methylmercury exposure increases ALAS activity in rat kidney. This effect is associated with increased urinary excretion of porphyrins, despite the absence of overt renal toxicity as assessed by standard function tests (Fowler and Woods, 1977a; Woods and Fowler, 1977a). In contrast, manganese inhibits ALAS activity in brain and liver; however, unlike most organs (e.g., liver), an increase in heme oxygenase activity is not observed. This effect may be due to an undefined compensatory mechanism or buffering capacity within the brain to maintain homeostasis (Maines, 1980).

Prolonged oral exposure to arsenate via drinking water results in depression of ALAS activity in certain species; however, this effect is not observed with arsenate in vitro. These in vivo changes probably result from a gradual perturbation of the mitochondrial membrane structure following arsenic accumulation in the target organ (Woods and Fowler, 1978).

δ-Aminolevulinic Acid Dehydratase (ALAD)   Inhibition of ALAD is a very early and sensitive indicator of lead exposure in various species, including humans (Roels et al., 1975; Finelli et al., 1975; Stuik, 1974; Cools et al., 1976). The activity of ALAD is inhibited by lead both in vitro and in vivo in a variety of tissues, including blood (erythrocytes), liver, kidney, brain, and bone marrow (Millar et al., 1970; Weissberg and Voytek, 1974; Buchet et al., 1976; Davis and Avram, 1978; Dresner et al., 1982; Silbergeld et al., 1982). Liver ALAD is more sensitive than kidney ALAD to inhibition by lead both in vivo (Fowler et al., 1980) and in vitro (Goering and Fowler, 1984). Brain ALAD in developing rats is particularly sensitive to inhibition by lead (Millar et al., 1970; Gerber et al., 1978), most likely attributable to an underdeveloped blood–brain barrier.

Human studies reveal that there is an inverse relationship between blood lead levels and enzyme activity, with a blood lead threshold of 15–20 μg/dl (Hernberg and Nikkanen, 1970; Granick et al., 1973; Lauwerys et al., 1974; Roels et al., 1975). This inverse correlation was also observed between blood lead concentration and hepatic and erthyrocyte ALAD activity in lead workers whose blood lead values ranged from 12 to 56 $\mu g/dl$ (Secchi et al., 1974). Chronic exposure of humans to alkyl lead can also affect heme synthesis. Chronic sniffing of leaded gasoline among children resulted in a 70% decrease in mean ALAD activity (Boeckx et al., 1977). In contrast, an increase in erythrocyte ALAD activity was evident in rats and human workers exposed to lead (Fujita et al., 1981, 1982), likely due to compensatory ALAD synthesis in bone-marrow cells.

ALAD is an allosteric enzyme consisting of eight subunits, each containing one zinc atom and eight sulfhydryl groups (Wilson et al., 1972; Wu et al., 1974). Lead is believed to inactivate ALAD by replacing zinc in a stoichiometric manner (Tsukamoto et al., 1980). On the other hand, the inhibition of ALAD by lead can be reversed by addition of zinc and reducing agents, such as glutathione and dithiothreitol (Abdulla and Haeger-Aronsen, 1971; Finelli et al., 1975; Mitchell et al., 1977). Glutathione removes lead from sulfur groups on the enzyme and may reduce oxidized sulfur groups; zinc may displace Pb from the enzyme active site.

Activity of ALAD may also be regulated by high-affinity lead-binding proteins in kidney and brain (Oskarsson et al., 1982; Goering and Fowler, 1984) (see section on metal-binding proteins). The renal lead-binding proteins presumably chelate lead and remove it from ALAD in kidney; this may explain the relative insensitivity of renal ALAD to lead inhibition compared to liver ALAD (Goering and Fowler, 1984).

Of the three heavy metals, lead, mercury, and cadmium, only lead inhibits human erythrocyte ALAD in vivo (Lauwerys and Buchet, 1973; Lauwerys et al., 1973). The lack of inhibition by cadmium and mercury in vivo could be attributable to circulating metallothionein, which acts to chelate these metals and subsequently protects ALAD.

The response of human erythrocyte ALAD activity to cadmium and zinc in vitro is biphasic, with low concentrations of either metal activating the enzyme, with eventual inhibition at higher concentrations. Cadmium, like zinc, reverses lead-induced inhibition of ALAD and is a more potent activator of ALAD than is zinc. On the other hand, cadmium inhibition of ALAD, unlike that caused by lead, cannot be reversed by zinc (Davis and Avram, 1978). Other metals showing a similar biphasic response include mercury, aluminum, copper, and zinc (Meredith et al., 1974; Davis and Avram, 1980; Mitchell et al., 1977). The group IIIA trace metal indium inhibits both renal and hepatic ALAD in vitro; however, indium inhibits only renal ALAD in vivo. This tissue-specific effect is due to the preferential accumulation of indium by the kidney proximal-tubule cell with selective localization in the cytosol. Zinc reverses the indium-induced inhibition of renal ALAD in vitro and in vivo, suggesting that indium acts by binding with sulfhydryl groups on the enzyme (Woods and Fowler, 1982).

Uroporphyrinogen I Synthetase (UROS) The activity of UROS, the third enzyme in the heme biosynthetic pathway, is increased in liver following exposure to arsenate, and this effect is species-specific; enzyme activity is elevated in mouse but not rat liver. The mechanism of this increase is unknown (Woods and Fowler, 1978). The enzyme is also susceptible to inhibition by mercury and silver. Inhibition is prevented by sulfhydryl reagents, which implies that the mechanism of inhibition involves metal-binding to enzyme sulfhydryl group(s) (Bogarad, 1963). Rat and human erythrocyte UROS is sensitive to the inhibitory effect of lead in vitro; however, hepatic enzyme activity is relatively insensitive (Piper and Tephly, 1974).

Uroporphyrinogen Decarboxylase (UROD) Hepatic UROD, which catalyzes the stepwise decarboxylation of uroporphyringen to coproporphyrinogen, is also susceptible to inhibition by trace metals in vitro, including cadmium, cobalt, and mercury. The inhibition of enzyme activity is reversed in the presence of sulfhydryl reducing agents, which suggests that the mechanism of metal inhibition involves the binding of metal to the sulfhydryl group(s) of the enzyme, a mechanism similar to that proposed for ALAD inhibition by metals. Interestingly, in contrast to its effect on ALAD activity, lead does not inhibit UROD in vitro, despite its propensity to bind sulfhydryl groups. A reasonable explanation for these differences is that the ALAD active site possesses a dithiol while the UROD active site contains a monothiol, which is known to be less chemically reactive with lead (Ulmer and Vallee, 1969). Elevated concentrations of uroporphyrin in urine of animals exposed to mercury and arsenic for prolonged periods suggest that UROD may also be inhibited by trace metals in vivo (Woods et al., 1981).

Coproporphyrinogen Oxidase Essentially, very limited data exist describing the effects of metals on the penultimate step in the heme biosynthetic pathway, the conversion of coproporphyrinogen III into protoporphyrinogen via coproporphyrinogen oxidase. Chronic exposure to methylmercury results in a marked increase in urinary coproporphyrin, which suggests inhibition of coproporphyrinogen oxidase activity by this organometal (Woods and Fowler, 1977a).

Heme Synthetase Heme synthetase (ferrochelatase) catalyzes the final step in the heme biosynthetic pathway by inserting ferrous iron into the protoporphyrin tetrapyrrole ring. Chronic exposure of rats to lead results in significant inhibition of heme synthetase in the kidney (Fowler et al., 1980). The renal enzyme is also inhibited in vitro at lead concentrations of 10^{-4}–10^{-5} M (Gibson and Goldberg, 1970). Indirect evidence suggests that in humans lead exposure decreases heme formation in erythrocytes, kidney, and liver. Accumulation of zinc protoporphyrin, indicative of heme synthetase inhibition, in erythrocytes occurs in lead-exposed children and adult workers (Piomelli et al., 1982; Roels et al., 1975). Formation of the heme-containing protein cytochrome P-450 and P-450-mediated xenobiotic biotransformation decreases in humans exposed to lead (Alvares et al., 1975; Meredith et al., 1977; Mahaffey et al., 1982).

Alterations in heme synthetase activity occur after exposure to other metals. Heme synthetase activity in rat kidney is inhibited after chronic methylmercury exposure (Fowler and Woods, 1977a). Chronic exposure to pentavalent arsenic also depresses enzyme activity in rat liver. This effect occurs prior to and independent of any compromise in hepatic mitochondrial or microsomal hemoprotein function, such as cytochrome oxidase and mixed-function oxidase activities (Woods and Fowler, 1977b). Thus, the early changes in heme synthetase and ALAS activities induced by arsenate with resultant characteristic urinary porphyrin excretion patterns may be utilized in the clinical analysis of pretoxic exposure to this element in human populations. In addition to inhibition of heme synthetase, the decrease in heme formation from protoporphyrin following exposure to metals may result, at least in part, from the impaired mitochondrial transport of iron. Since metal exposure disrupts mitochondrial structure (swelling) and function (decreased respiration), the ability of the heme synthetase to utilize iron may be compromised.

Heme Oxygenase Metals not only affect various steps in heme synthesis but also alter the rate of heme degradation. As a general rule, most metals enhance heme degradation by induction of the microsomal enzyme heme oxygenase, which catalyzes the conversion of heme to biliverdin. The consequences of the induction of heme oxygenase activity by metals are associated with cellular effects of toxicological significance, including reductions in microsomal heme and cytochrome P-450 levels, impairment of cytochromes P-450- and P-448-dependent mixed-function oxidase activities, and depletion of mitochondrial respiratory cytochromes (Maines and Kappas, 1977a). Thus, cellular respiration, as well as the ability to metabolize endogenous compounds and xenobiotics, would be compromised.

Induction of heme oxygenase activity following a single injection of metals is rapid and persists for 3–4 days. All metals examined, including chromium, manganese, ferric and ferrous iron, cobalt, nickel, copper, tin, cadmium, indium, mercury, thallium, lead, platinum, silver, and selenium, induce heme oxygenase in the liver (Maines and Kappas, 1977a; Woods et al., 1979, 1984; Eaton et al., 1980). Various metals also induce heme oxygenase in other tissues, such as kidney, lung, intestinal mucosa, and skin. The extent of induction is tissue-specific with respect to the inducing metal. For example, cobalt and cadmium are the most potent inducers of heme oxygenase activity in the liver. In contrast, nickel, tin, and platinum induce the enzyme to the highest extent in kidney, while in the heart, mercury is the most potent inducer. The inducing effects of metals are not observed in vitro; thus, the action of metals is probably exerted at the regulatory site for the synthesis of the enzyme (Maines and Kappas, 1977a). Protein-synthesis inhibitors block metal induction of heme oxygenase, indicating that increased enzyme activity following metal treatment is a result of de novo synthesis of heme oxygenase and does not result from metal action on the preformed enzyme (Maines and Sinclair, 1977).

The induction of heme oxygenase by metals may be altered by interactions with various other metals. Manganese and zinc are potent inhibitors of tin- and nickel-mediated induction of renal heme oxygenase when blocking ions are administered prior to or simultaneously with inducer ions. On the other hand, zinc attenuates the induction of hepatic heme oxygenase by cobalt, cadmium, and nickel (Drummond and Kappas, 1979). These blocking ions lose their effect (within minutes) when administered subsequent to the inducing ions. This indicates that the inducing ions rapidly distribute to the regulatory site(s) to initiate enzyme induction.

In addition to metal–metal interactions, induction of heme oxygenase activity by metals can be affected by interactions with metal-chelating constituents such as metallothionein or reduced glutathione. Since zinc induces formation of metallothionein, a thiol-rich protein that readily sequesters a subsequent dose of cadmium, the blocking effect of zinc on cadmium-mediated induction of heme oxygenase may be explained by sequestration of cadmium by metallothionein (Drummond and Kappas, 1980). Likewise, a relationship exists between the cellular concentration of thiol groups and the ability of metals to induce heme oxygenase, such that the action of metals possessing a high-affinity for thiol groups (e.g., cadmium and cobalt) is blocked when such metals are complexed with reduced glutathione or thiol-containing amino acids. Conversely, depletion of glutathione with diethyl maleate augments the inducing effect of cobalt on heme oxygenase (Maines and Kappas, 1976).

Several metals, specifically those of group IIIA, have unique effects on heme metabolism and cellular heme-dependent functions. Indium causes the rapid induction of heme oxygenase and a concomitant initial inhibition and subsequent rebound increase in ALAS activity (Woods et al., 1979). This response pattern is also typically observed with most other metals (Maines and Kappas, 1977a). These effects are associated with degradation of microsomal heme content and a decline in cytochrome P-450 content and P-450-mediated biotransformation of xenobiotics. The action of indium is unique, however, in that the metal fails to alter mitochondrial hemoprotein function (i.e., respiratory cytochromes) as compared with other metals such as cobalt and nickel, which deplete mitochondrial, as well as microsomal, heme content (Woods et al., 1979).

Thallium, another group IIIA transition element, also causes induction of heme oxygenase and transient inhibition of ALAS with a concomitant reduction in P-450-mediated mixed-function oxidase activity. These changes occur independently of effects on microsomal heme or cytochrome P-450 content, both of which are unaffected; however, thallium-induced impairment of microsomal cytochrome P-450 oxidative capacity appears to be mediated through inhibition of NADPH-cytochrome c (P-450) reductase, a flavoprotein component of the microsomal P-450 system. This effect of thallium is unique in that the mechanism of metal inhibition of microsomal P-450 oxidative activity has been largely attributed to perturbation of heme biosynthesis and depletion of cellular heme. The mechanism of thallium inhibition of NADPH-cytochrome c (P-450) reductase has been attributed to its properties as a flavoprotein antagonist and/or sulfhydryl inhibitor (Woods et al., 1984).

While the usual response of heme oxygenase to metals is induction of activity, a novel response of heme oxygenase in the testis to cadmium has been described. Cadmium, a potent inducer of heme oxygenase in liver, causes a marked depression of enzyme activity in rat testes (Maines et al., 1982). A comparison of this effect in Leydig and Sertoli cell populations reveals that inhibition occurs to a higher degree in the Leydig cells, which constitute the primary site of heme and hemoprotein biosynthetic activities in testes. The cadmium-mediated inhibition of heme oxygenase activity in testes does not result from a direct action of the metal on the enzyme or from a decreased total microsomal protein content, but is postulated to involve the known capacity of cadmium to decrease blood glucose levels by altering carbohydrate and cyclic AMP metabolism (Maines, 1984).

Heme Metabolism and Biological Indicators of Metal Exposure A primary goal in the clinical assessment of metal exposure is the establishment of sensitive biological indicators that detect low-level exposure to metals and reflect cellular dys-function prior to the onset of overt toxicity. The development of metal-specific bio-logical response profiles based on an understanding of the subcellular mechanisms of metal toxicity is essential to achieve this goal. Measurement of circulating or excreted metabolites from affected organelle systems may afford a relatively specific estima-tion of the in vivo toxic effects. Circulating and urinary excretion patterns of oxidized heme pathway intermediates, the porphyrins, have been utilized as relatively sensitive indicators of exposure to various metals, primarily lead, and will be discussed below.

Lead exposure in laboratory animals and humans increases the levels of circulat-ing and urinary ALA, the initial heme pathway intermediate, due to inhibition of ALAD and an increase in ALAS activity. Urinary ALA has been employed as an index of lead exposure, primarily in occupational situations. The health significance of inhibition of ALAD by lead with accumulation of ALA is not well understood. Elevated levels of circulating or tissue ALA have been linked to several neurotoxic effects, including paralysis, behavioral changes, blockade of neuromuscular transmis-sion, and inhibition of sodium-potassium-dependent ATPase and membrane ion trans-port (Moore et al., 1980).

While alterations in circulating and urinary porphyrin patterns provide useful estimates of exposure to lead, a possible link exists between lead-induced perturba-tions in heme biosynthesis and lead neurotoxicity, including effects on both brain neurochemistry and behavior. The potential relationship between porphyrinopathic mechanisms and lead neurotoxicity can be explained by (1) similarities between symptoms of lead neurotoxicity and hereditary disorders of heme synthesis, that is, acute porphyrias, which include vomiting, paralysis, peripheral neuropathies, demye-lination and seizures, and (2) increases in urinary ALA, which characterize both conditions. ALA readily crosses the blood–brain barrier and is also formed within the brain following lead inhibition of brain ALAD. Both ALA in vitro and lead in vivo interfere with the release of neurotramsitter γ-aminobutyric acid in the central ner-vous system (CNS) (Brennan and Cantrill, 1979; Silbergeld et al., 1982). High levels of ALA also impair voluntary movement in laboratory animals (Moore and Meredith, 1976). Thus, in addition to the direct neurotoxic effects, lead-induced porphyrin-opathy may contribute to neurotoxicity by altering heme biosynthesis.

Exposure to lead also results in the elevation and accumulation of protoporphyrin IX in erythrocytes. Accumulation of this heme pathway intermediate is due to the inability of heme synthetase to insert ferrous iron into the tetrapyrrole porphyrin ring to form heme and/or impaired iron transport into the mitochondrion. Following expo-sure to lead, zinc ion is placed into the porphyrin ring to the exclusion of iron to form zinc protoporphyrin. Elevation of zinc protoporphyrin has been correlated with the concentration of lead in blood and has been a reliable indicator of lead exposure in children and lead workers. Increases in urinary coproporphyrin levels are also typical of lead exposure, due to the inhibition of coproporphyrinogen oxidase.

While most studied in the case of lead, porphyrin response profiles are being developed for exposure to other metals at doses that produce no signs of overt toxic-ity. Chronic exposure to methylmercury causes a unique urinary porphyrin excretion pattern characterized by elevated coproporphyrin and uroporphyrin levels with coproporphyrin predominant (Woods and Fowler, 1977a). Low doses of cadmium alone in the diet do not alter the urinary excretion of ALA, uroporphyrin, or coproporphyrin. Low-level exposure to inorganic or organic arsenic produces no changes in ALA excretion but markedly increases the urinary excretion of uroporphyrin due to activation of UROS, with a smaller increase in coproporphyrin excretion (Woods and Fowler, 1977b; Woods and Fowler, 1978; Mahaffey et al., 1981).

While knowledge of porphyrin patterns is useful for assessment of exposure to metals, environmental exposure of humans to toxic metals frequently involves multiple exposures to several different metals. Thus, the ability to discern the effects of low-level exposure to these metals can be obscured by interactions between metals that alter the usual biological responses to exposure for a given metal (Fig. 10). Concomitant administration of cadmium and lead to rats results in a decrease in the elevated urinary ALA concentration typically observed following exposure to lead alone, elevates uroporphyrin, but does not alter the lead effect on coproporphyrin levels. Exposure to a combination of lead and arsenic produces no change in lead-induced increases in ALA excretion, produces an additive effect on coproporphyrin excretion, and does not alter the arsenic effect on uroporphyrin excretion, indicating that this latter effect is rather specific for arsenic. Concomitant exposure to all three metals produces no change in ALA excretion patterns and elevates coproporphyrin levels, which are accompanied by additive effects on uroporphyrin excretion. Thus, while the urinary excretion of ALA, coproporphyrin, and uroporphyrin is elevated following exposure to lead, concomitant exposure to cadmium and/or arsenic markedly alters the magnitude of these changes. Of the three heme pathway intermediates, ALA appears to be the most specific for lead exposure, since changes in uroporphyrin and coproporphyrin levels are also observed with arsenic (Mahaffey et al., 1981).

Effects of Metals on Endocrine and Reproductive Function

The effects of metals on endocrine and reproductive function are areas that have received far less attention than heme metabolism, but it is clear from the available literature that these systems are highly sensitive to metal-induced perturbation. This section examines the known effects of metals on endocrine/reproductive function with respect to both sensitivity and inherent complexity of the mechanisms involved. Such a review will provide the reader with a concise perspective on this important area of research.

Hypothalamo–Pituitary–Gonad Axis It is well known that male and female reproductive organs are under complex neuroendocrine and hormonal control. Metals could affect the reproductive system by altering any of these processes, either directly in the reproductive organs or indirectly through interference with the hypothalamus–pituitary regulatory system.

Although the exact mechanism(s) by which the hypothalamus and pituitary glands regulate reproductive function in both male and female is uncertain, the release of two gonadotropins, follicle-stimulating hormone (FSH) and leuteinizing hormone (LH), from the pituitary is known to play an important role. The release of these two hormones is regulated by the gonadotropin-releasing hormone (GnRH) secreted by the hypothalamus (Pohl and Knobil, 1982). Metals may interfere with the synthesis, release, transport, metabolism, or binding of these hormones to their receptors. Both animal and human studies, however, reveal little information on such effects. Lancranjan et al. (1975) reported no difference in urinary gonadotropin levels in battery-factory workers exposed to toxic levels of lead (mean blood lead of 74.5 μg/dl) versus those exposed to very low levels (mean blood lead of 23 μg/dl). Similar results were reported by Molinini et al. (1981) from their study on moderately exposed battery-factory workers. Sandstead et al. (1970a), however, observed increased urinary levels of gonadotropin in lead-intoxicated mean, and Braunstein et al. (1978) found lower serum LH levels after stimulation with GnRH in lead-exposed workers compared with controls. This suggests that high-level lead exposure in humans may alter hypothalamic–pituitary function, causing a defect in the reproductive system.

Animal studies have shown that adverse effects of lead on hypothalamic–pituitary function occur mainly in immature rodents. Lead intoxication in neonatal rats interferes with normal pituitary function, particularly in relation to storage and release of FSH. The prepubertal surge in serum FSH at day 15 is significantly reduced in lead-intoxicated female rats. Male rats showed no change in serum FSH compared with controls, despite a significant increase in pituitary FSH levels (Petrusz et al., 1979). Furthermore, perpubertal exposure to lead was reported to reduce FSH binding to testicular receptors (Wiebe et al., 1982); thus, alterations in gonadal response to FSH or LH brought about by changes in receptor–hormone interaction may augment the effect of metals on hypothalamo–pituitary function. Cadmium and mercury are known to accumulate in the pituitary, and it has been suggested that they may also affect reproductive function by altering gonadotropin dynamics (Berlin and Ullberg, 1963; Lamperti and Printz, 1974; Lamperti and Niewenhuis, 1976; Der et al., 1977). Thus, metal-induced changes in neuroendocrine function may alter gonadal development and subsequent function, with these effects being more pronounced if exposure occurs at an early age.

Metals acting directly on the gonads and accessory organs can also interfere with reproductive function in both males and females by affecting a number of processes such as gametogenesis, implantation of fertilized ovum, and maintenance of pregnancy. Although the precise mechanisms are unknown, alterations in hormonal regulation of these organs can provide possible mechanisms for these effects. For example, lead exposure in utero and during lactation has been reported to significantly reduce the prepubertal surge of androgens, testosterone, and 5α-dihydrotestosterone in the Sertoli cells of rat testes (Wiebe et al., 1982). Since this surge is thought to be important in spermatogenesis (Ahmad et al., 1973), it was suggested that early exposure to lead may impede gametogenesis. The reduction in steroidogenesis was attributed to direct inhibition of the enzymes involved and/or to a reduced gonadotropin stimulus caused by decreased binding of FSH to testicular receptors.

Injury to the testes is considered to be pathognomonic for acute cadmium exposure. This injury occurs at a dose that is not toxic to other organs (Parizek and Zahor, 1956; Gunn et al., 1961). Exposure to cadmium causes vascular-bed damage and interstitial edema in the testis, leading to hemorrhage, reduced androgen production by the Leydig cells, necrosis of the Sertoli cells, inhibition of spermatogenesis, and eventually testicular atrophy (Meek, 1959; Parizek, 1960; Gunn et al., 1963). These changes are observed in rats, susceptible strains of mice, and many other scrotal mammalian species; however, the testes of nonscrotal mammals (e.g., hedgehog and shrew) and the gonads of birds are not affected by cadmium (Samarawickrama, 1979). The testes of newborn rats are also not damaged by cadmium (Wong and Klaassen, 1980).

Cadmium produces testicular injury only after acute exposure but not after chronic exposure (Kotsonis and Klaassen, 1977, 1978). Induction of what was previously thought to be a metallothionein-like protein by low chronic doses of cadmium or zinc provided a mechanism to explain the protection of testes from damage (Parizek, 1957; Ito and Sawauchi, 1966; Nordberg, 1971). However, more recent application of rigorous characterization criteria, including amino acid analysis, indicates that the cadmium/zinc-binding protein in rat testis cytosol cannot be classified as a metallothionein (Waalkes et al., 1984a,b).

Lead also accumulates in the testes of adult animals and is associated with testicular degeneration, inhibition of spermatogenesis, and Leydig-cell atrophy (Timms and Schulz, 1966; Chowdhury et al., 1984). Since cholesterol and ascorbate are essential for spermatogenesis, low testicular ascorbate levels and nonutilization of cholesterol for testosterone synthesis in Leydig cells may account for the inhibition of spermatogenesis (Chowdhury et al., 1984). Lead accumulation has also been associated with impaired Leydig-cell function and decreased serum testosterone levels in humans (Braunstein, 1978).

Both cadmium and lead have been reported to reduce weights of gonads and accessory sex organs in males (Khare et al., 1978; Saksena et al., 1977; Laskey et al., 1984). Since these organs are dependent on androgens for growth (Liao et al., 1973), some of the weight loss may be due to reduced steroid levels, while some may be attributed to inhibition of steroid binding to its cytosolic receptor (Donovan et al., 1980) and/or alteration in the configuration of the steroid–receptor complex (Liao et al., 1973) by these metals.

Pre- and postnatal exposure to lead and cadmium have been suggested to alter ovarian function and reduce estrogen production, leading to changes in normal pubertal progression in females (Vermande-Van Eck and Meigs, 1960; Parizek et al., 1968; Hilderbrand et al., 1973; Der et al., 1977; Grant et al., 1980). Whether this is due to direct inhibition of the estrogen-synthesizing enzymes in the ovary or to changes in the hypothalamic–pituitary–ovarian axis is not known.

Exposure of adult females to lead and cadmium also affects ovarian–uterine function, causing interference with implantation and development of the embryo (Nordström et al., 1978; Rom, 1976; Hilderbrand et al., 1973; Der et al., 1974; Jacquet et al., 1976; Wide and Nilsson, 1977; Giavini et al., 1980). Furthermore, administration of progesterone and administration of estradiol were reported to reverse the adverse effects of lead on implantation in mice (Wide, 1980; Jacquet, 1978). However, conflicting results have been reported concerning the effects of lead on serum concentrations of progesterone and estradiol in these animals (Jacquet et al., 1977; Wide and Wide, 1980; Leonard et al., 1983). Recent studies showing inhibition of steroid binding to endometrial and myometrial cytosolic receptors by various metals, including lead and cadmium, may provide a possible mechanism of action (Young et al., 1977; Sanborn et al., 1971; Kontula et al., 1974; Wide and Wide, 1980). Furthermore, changes in relative receptor concentration for the two steroids may also play a role in metal-induced inhibition of implantation (Wide and Wide, 1980).

The placenta of rodents and humans and the fetal membranes, including both amnion and chorion, of humans contain a metallothionein-like protein (Lafont et al., 1976; Waalkes et al., 1984b). Levels of this protein can be increased upon exposure to cadmium or zinc (Lucis et al., 1972; Wolkowski, 1974; Waalkes et al., 1984b). While only speculative, metallothionein-like proteins could function in transport and/or homeostasis of zinc and copper between maternal and fetal tissues. Furthermore, since levels of these proteins can be increased experimentally in human reproductive tissues by cadmium (Waalkes et al., 1984b) and since cadmium accumulates in placentae of smoking women while fetal cord blood levels of the metal are not altered (Kuhnert et al., 1982), placental metallothionein-like proteins could act as a barrier by sequestering low levels of cadmium, preventing exposure of the fetus to this potentially teratogenic metal (Waalkes et al., 1984b).

From these studies it appears that metal-induced alterations in hormonal homeostasis in reproductive organs can greatly influence reproductive function in both males and females. The majority of these reports, however, have been on the effects of high-level metal exposure, and further studies are needed to evaluate the effects of prolonged low-level exposure.

The Renin–Angiotensin System and Hypertension The relationship between long-term lead and cadmium exposure and hypertension is controversial, with conflicting results generated from both human (Belknap, 1936; Cramer and Dahlberg, 1966; Wedeen et al., 1975; Lilis et al., 1968; Beevers et al., 1976; Perry and Schroeder, 1955; Thind, 1972; Morgan, 1976; Lewis et al., 1972) and animal studies (Perry et al., 1979; Schroeder, 1964; Ohanian and Iwai, 1979; Porter et al., 1974). In this section, only the effects of metals on the renin–angiotensin system (RAS) and their role in hypertension are discussed.

The RAS plays an important role in the regulation of arterial blood pressure [for details on the mechanism of action of this system, see Peach (1977)]. Briefly, renin, a proteolytic enzyme, is secreted into the bloodstream by the kidneys and catalyzes the initial regulatory step in the formation of angiotensin II (AII) and angiotensin III. These two peptides exert a number of effects on various tissues, the end result of which is an increase in arterial blood pressure. The AII stimulates aldosterone secretion from the adrenal gland, which increases sodium retention and also results in an elevation of blood pressure. Thus, chemicals that produce alterations in renin secretion—that is, metals—may result in changes in blood pressure.

Clinical studies on lead-intoxicated patients have produced conflicting results as to the effects of lead on the RAS, with some showing decreased plasma renin activity (PRA) (McAllister et al., 1971; Sandstead et al., 1970b) while others exhibit no change (Campbell et al., 1979). In contrast to human studies, acute parenteral administration of lead to rats and dogs (Goldman et al., 1981; Mouw et al., 1978) and long-term chronic exposure of rats [500 ppm Pb in drinking water (Fleischer et al., 1980)] were associated with an increase in PRA. The studies in dogs (Goldman et al., 1981) suggested that the increase in PRA was due to an inhibition of hepatic renin clearance. In addition, these authors observed that despite the large increase in PRA, blood levels of AII did not increase with lead treatment, suggesting that lead inhibited AII converting enzyme or increased AII clearance. More recent studies (Keiser et al., 1983) in rats chronically exposed to lead (500 and 1000 ppm in drinking water) showed a biphasic increase in PRA, with only the lower dose showing an increase in activity. Furthermore, this increase in PRA was due to an increase in renin secretion rather than inhibition of renin clearance. The high-dose animals were observed to have low plasma AII/PRA ratios despite normal levels of PRA, suggesting inhibition of formation or clearance of AII.

Victery et al. (1982a) reported a dose-dependent effect of lead on development of hypertension in male but not female rats. Exposure to 100 ppm lead in utero and continued through lactation and weaning elevated blood pressure in males, while males and females exposed to 500 ppm were normotensive. PRA was significantly reduced in the 100-ppm-exposed male rats and normal in the 500-ppm treatment groups. Victery et al. argued that since hypertension was associated with reduced PRA and AII levels, the RAS was probably not directly involved in the hypertensive response. Further in utero exposure studies in rats (Victery et al., 1982b) at lower exposure levels (5 and 25 ppm) showed a significant reduction in basal renal renin concentrations in both treatment groups and a significant reduction in PRA at the 25-ppm level at 5 months. A subsequent study (Victery et al., 1983) using the same in utero exposure regimen, but in which treatment was terminated at 1 month of age, showed significantly elevated PRA values in all lead-exposed groups (5, 25, 100 and 500 ppm). Renal renin concentrations were also increased in the 100- and 500-ppm groups. The increase in PRA after short-term, low-dose exposure to lead suggests that the general human population may be at risk for development of hypertension due to low-level lead exposure.

The studies discussed above suggest that exposures to lead, including low levels, produce significant changes in the RAS. The direction and magnitude of these changes appear to be mediated by a number of factors, including exposure level, duration of exposure, age, and sex, as well as dietary sodium content. However, the mild hypertension produced by low chronic lead exposure does not appear to be sustained by the RAS. Furthermore, a recent study (Webb et al., 1981) suggests that lead-induced hypertension in rats may be associated with changes in the vascular responsiveness to α-adrenergic agents.

The increase in PRA observed in rats following low-level exposure to cadmium is also thought not to play a role in cadmium-induced hypertension (Perry and Erlanger, 1975). One possible mechanism for the hypertensive effect of cadmium is its direct action on some vascular beds, resulting in vasoconstriction (Perry et al., 1967). A recent review on the cadmium/hypertension debate is presented by Templeton and Cherian (1983).

Vitamin D Metabolism and Parathyroid Function Both vitamin D and parathyroid hormone play an important role in a complex system regulating calcium homeostasis. Thus, metal-induced interference with vitamin D metabolism and/or parathyroid-gland function will seriously affect calcium homeostasis.

Lead intoxication decreases plasma 1,25-dihydroxyvitamin D [2,25(OH)$_2$D$_3$] levels in a number of species, and this effect is more pronounced under calcium- and phosphorus-deficient diets (Rosen et al., 1980; Smith et al., 1981; Edelstein et al., 1984). The decrease appears to be related to interference with the renal conversion of 25-hydroxyvitamin D to 1,25(OH)$_2$D$_3$ (Smith et al., 1981; Edelstein et al., 1984). Furthermore, lead ingestion has been shown to completely block the intestinal calcium transport response to 1,25(OH)$_2$D$_3$ in rats fed low-calcium diets and to partially block this response in rats fed high-calcium diets (Smith et al., 1981). The mechanism of lead-induced inhibition of intestinal calcium transport in response to the active form of vitamin D is unknown; it may be a general toxic effect of lead on the gastrointestinal epithelium, or a specific effect on the vitamin D system, such as reduced 1,25(OH)$_2$D$_3$ receptor levels, which in turn would inhibit synthesis of the calcium-transport component.

Vitamin D and its metabolites have been reported to increase lead absorption in both the duodenum and the distal portion of the small intestine (Smith et al., 1978; Mahaffey et al., 1979; Edelstein et al., 1984). The mechanism by which this increased lead absorption occurs is unknown, but it is thought to involve the vitamin D-regulated calcium binding protein in the duodenum (Edelstein et al., 1984). Thus, the lead-induced decrease in conversion of vitamin D to its active 1,25(OH)$_2$D$_3$ metabolite may have a beneficial effect in preventing further toxicity by reducing lead absorption.

Exposure to cadmium is also known to alter calcium homeostasis; in fact, perturbation of calcium metabolism, induced by long-term cadmium exposure, along with low dietary intake of calcium, vitamin D, and protein, is thought to play a role in the etiology of an osteomalacia-type syndrome in Japan known as itai-itai disease (Tsuchiya, 1978). Due to the complex nature of the system regulating calcium homeostasis, the exact mechanism(s) responsible for the cadmium-induced alterations in calcium metabolism is (are) currently unknown; however, disturbances in vitamin D transport and/or metabolism, in addition to changes in parathyroid-gland function, may be important (Jones and Fowler, 1980). Vitamin D-binding protein (known as Gc-globulin) has been demonstrated in urine of patients with itai-itai disease (Teranishi et al., 1983), suggesting an alteration in vitamin D homeostasis. Cadmium has also been shown to inhibit 1-hydroxylation of vitamin D in vitro (Suda et al., 1974; Kimura et al., 1974); however, this effect is prevented following induction of CdMT, suggesting that interference with formation of 1,25(OH)$_2$D$_3$ in kidney following in vivo exposure to cadmium does not occur. The high-affinity lead-binding protein in kidney cytosol (Oskarsson et al., 1982; Mistry et al., 1984) may also regulate lead-induced inhibition of 1,25(OH)$_2$D$_3$ formation.

REFERENCES

Abdulla, M., and Haeger-Aronsen, B. 1971. ALA-Dehydratase activity by zinc. *Enzyme* 12:708–710.

Ahmad, N., Halfmeyer, G. C., and Eik-Nes, K. B. 1973. Maintenance of spermatogenesis in rats with intratesticular implants containing testosterone or dihydrotestosterone (DHT). *Biol. Reprod.* 8:411–419.

Alvares, A. P., Kapelner, S., Sassa, S., and Kappas, A. 1975. Drug metabolism in normal children, lead-poisoned children, and normal adults. *Clin. Pharmacol. Ther.* 17:179–183.

Axelrod, J. 1956. The enzymatic N-demethylation of narcotic drugs. *J. Pharmacol. Exp. Ther.* 117:322–330.

Bachman, E., and Golberg, L. 1970. Aspects of the determination of biphenyl hydroxylase activity in liver homogenates. II. Sex and species differences in the effect of mitochondria. *Exp. Mol. Pathol.* 13:269–280.

Beevers, D. G., Erskine, E., Robertson, M., Beattie, A. D., Goldberg, A., Campbell, B. C., Moore, M. R., and Hawthorne, V. M. 1976. Blood-lead and hypertension. *Lancet* 2(7975):1–3.

Belknap, E. L. 1936. Clinical studies on lead absorption in the human. III. Blood pressure observations. *J. Ind.Hyg.* 18:380–390.

Berlin, M., and Ullberg, S. 1963. The fate of Cd^{109} in the mouse. An autoradiographic study after a single intravenous injection of $CD^{109}Cl_2$. *Arch. Environ. Health* 1:686–693.

Boeckx, R. L., Posti, B., and Coodin, F. J. 1977. Gasoline sniffing and tetraethyl lead poisoning in children. *Pediatrics* 60:140–145.

Bogorad, L. 1963. Enzymatic mechanisms in porphyrin synthesis: Possible enzymatic blocks in porphyrias. *Ann. N.Y. Acad. Sci.* 104:676–688.

Braunstein, G. D., Dahlgren, J., and Loriaux, D. L. 1978. Hypogonadism in chronically lead-poisoned men. *Infertility* 1:33–51.

Brennan, M. S. W., and Cantrill, R. C. 1979. δ-Aminolaevulinic acid is a potent agonist for GABA autoreceptors. *Nature (Lond.)* 280:514–515.

Brown, M. M., Rhyne, B. C., Goyer, R. A., and Fowler, B. A. 1976. The intracellular effects of chronic arsenic administration on renal proximal tubule cells. *J. Toxicol. Environ. Health* 1:507–516.

Brubaker, P. E., Klein, R., Herman, S. P., Lucier, G. W., Alexander, L. T., and Long, M. D. 1973. DNA, RNA, and protein synthesis in the brain, liver and kidneys of asymptomatic methyl mercury treated rats. *Exp. Mol. Pathol.* 18:263–280.

Buchet, J.-P., Roels, H., Hubermont, G., and Lauwerys, R. 1976. Effect of lead on some parameters of the heme biosynthetic pathway in rat tissues in vivo. *Toxicology* 6:21–34.

Cain, K., and Holt, D. E. 1983. Studies of cadmium-thionein induced nephropathy: Time course of cadmium-thionein uptake and degradation. *Chem. Biol. Interact.* 43:223–237.

Campbell, B. C., Beattie, A. D., Elliott, M. L., Goldberg, A., Moore, M. R., Beevers, D. G., and Tree, M. 1979. Occupational lead exposure and renin release. *Arch. Environ. Health* 34:439–443.

Carmichael, N. G., and Fowler, B. A. 1979. Effects of separate and combined chronic mercuric chloride and sodium selenate administration in rats: Histological, ultrastructural and X-ray microanalytical studies of liver and kidney. *J. Environ. Pathol. Toxicol.* 3:399–412.

Cherian, M. G., and Shaikh, Z. A. 1975. Metabolism of intravenously injected cadmium-binding protein. *Biochem. Biophys. Res. Commun.* 65:863–869.

Cherian, M. G., Goyer, R. A., and Delaquerriere-Richardson, L. 1976. Cadmium-metallothionein-induced nephrotoxicity. *Toxicol. Appl. Pharmacol.* 38:399–408.

Choie, D. D., and Richter, G. W. 1972a. Cell proliferation in rat kidney induced by lead acetate and effects of uninephrectomy on the proliferation. *Am. J. Pathol.* 66:265–275.

Choie, D. D., and Richter, G. W. 1972b. Cell proliferation in rat kidneys after prolonged treatment with lead. *Am. J. Pathol.* 68:359–370.

Choie, D. D., and Richter, G. W. 1974a. Cell proliferation in mouse kidney induced by lead. I. Synthesis of deoxyribonucleic acid. *Lab. Invest.* 30:647–651.

Choie, D. D., and Richter, G. W. 1974b. Cell proliferation in mouse kidney induced by lead. II. Synthesis of ribonucleic acid and protein. *Lab. Invest.* 30:652–656.

Chowdhury, A. R., Dewan, A., and Gandhi, D. N. 1984. Toxic effect of lead on the testes of rat. *BioMed. Biochim. Acta* 43:95–100.

Cinti, D. L., and Schenkman, J. B. 1972. Hepatic organelle interaction. I. Spectral investigation during drug biotransformation. *Mol. Pharmacol.* 8:327–338.

Cinti, D. L., Ritchie, A., and Schenkman, J. B. 1972. Hepatic organelle interaction. II. Effect of tricarboxylic acid cycle intermediates on *N*-demethylation and hydroxylation reactions in rat liver. *Mol. Pharmacol.* 8:338–344.

Cinti, D. L., Keyes, S. R., Lemelin, M. A., Denk, H., and Schenkman, J. B. 1976. Biochemical properties of rat liver mitochondrial aldehyde dehydrogenase with respect to oxidation of formaldehyde. *J. Biol. Chem.* 251:1571–1577.

Cools, A., Salle, H. J. A., Verberk, M. M., and Zielhuis, R. L. 1976. Biochemical response of male volunteers ingesting inorganic lead for 49 days. *Int. Arch. Ocucp. Environ. Health* 38:129–139.

Cramer, K., and Dahlberg, L. 1966. Incidence of hypertension among lead workers. *Br. J. Ind. Med.* 23:101–104.

Davis, J. R., and Avram, M. J. 1978. A comparison of the stimulatory effects of cadmium and zinc on normal and lead-inhibited human erythrocytic aminolevulinic acid dehydratase activity in vitro. *Toxicol. Appl. Pharmacol.* 44:181–190.

Davis, J. R., and Avram, M. J. 1980. Correlation of the physicochemical properties of metal ions with their activation and inhibition of human erythrocytic aminolevulinic acid dehydratase (ALAD) in vitro. *Toxicol. Appl. Pharmacol.* 55:281–290.

Denk, H., Moldeus, P. W., Schulz, R. A., Schenkman, J. B., Keyes, S. R., and Cinti, D. L. 1976. Hepatic organelle interaction. IV. Mechanism of succinate enhancement of formaldehyde accumulation from endoplasmic reticulum *N*-dealkylations. *J. Cell Biol.* 69:589–598.

Der, R., Fahim, Z., Hilderbrand, D., and Fahim, M. 1974. Combined effect of lead and low protein diet on growth, sexual development and metabolism in female rats. *Res. Commun. Chem. Pathol. Pharmacol.* 1:723–738.

Der, R., Fahim, Z., Yousef, M., and Fahim, M. 1977. Effects of cadmium on growth, sexual development and metabolism in female rats. *Res. Commun. Chem. Pathol. Pharmacol.* 16:485–505.

Donovan, M. P., Schenin, L. G., and Thomas, J. A. 1980. Inhibition of androgen–receptor interaction in mouse prostate gland cytosol by divalent metal ions. *Mol. Pharmacol.* 17:156–162.

Dresner, D. L., Ibrahim, N. G., Mascarenhas, B. R., and Levere, R. D. 1982. Modulation of bone marrow heme and protein synthesis by trace elements. *Environ. Res.* 28:55–66.

Drummond, G. S., and Kappas, A. 1979. Manganese and zinc blockade of enzyme induction: Studies with microsomal heme oxygenase. *Proc. Natl. Acad. Sci. USA* 76:5331–5336.

Drummond, G. S., and Kappas, A. 1980. Metal ion interactions in the control of haem oxygenase induction in liver and kidney. *Biochem. J.* 192:637–648.

Eaton, D. L., Stacey, N. H., Wong, K.-L., and Klaassen, C. D. 1980. Dose-response effects of various metal ions on rat liver metallothionein, glutathione, heme oxygenase, and cytochrome P-450. *Toxicol. Appl. Pharmacol.* 55:393–402.

Edelstein, S., Fullmer, C. S., and Wasserman, R. M. 1984. Gastrointestinal absorption of lead in chicks: Involvement of the cholecalciferol endocrine system. *J. Nutr.* in press.

Evan, A. P., and Dail, W. G., Jr. 1974. The effects of sodium chromate on the proximal tubules of the rat kidney: Fine structural damage and lysozymuria. *Lab. Invest.* 30:704–715.

Finelli, V. N., Klauder, D. S., Karaffa, M. A., and Petering, H. G. 1975. Interaction of zinc and lead on δ-aminolevulinate dehydratase. *Biochem. Biophys. Res. Commun.* 65:303–311.

Fleischer, N., Mouw, D. R., and Vander, A.J. 1980. Chronic effects of lead on renin and renal sodium excretion. *J. Lab. Clin. Med.* 95:759–770.

Foulkes, E. C. 1983. Tubular sites of action of heavy metals, and the nature of their inhibition of amino acid reabsorption. *Fed. Proc.* 42:2965–2968.

Fowler, B. A. 1972a. Morphologic effects of dieldrin and methylmercuric chloride on pars recta segments of rat kidney proximal tubules. *Am. J. Pathol.* 69:163–174.

Fowler, B. A. 1972b. Ultrastructure evidence for nephropathy induced by long-term exposure to small amounts of methyl mercury. *Science* 175:780–784.

Fowler, B. A. 1977. Toxicology of environment arsenic. In *Toxicology of Trace Elements*, eds. R. A. Goyer and M. A. Mehlman, pp. 79–122. New York: Halstead.

Fowler, B. A., and Goyer, R. A. 1975. Bismuth localization within nuclear inclusions by X-ray microanalysis: Effects of accelerating voltage. *J. Histochem. Cytochem.* 23:722–726.

Fowler, B. A., and Mahaffey, K. R. 1978. Interactions among lead, cadmium, and arsenic in relation to porphyrin excretion patterns. *Environ. Health Perspect.* 25:87–90.

Fowler, B. A., and Nordberg, G. F. 1978. The renal toxicity of cadmium metallothionein: Morphometric and X-ray microanalytical studies. *Toxicol. Appl. Pharmacol.* 46:609–624.

Fowler, B. A., and Woods, J. S. 1977a. Ultrastructural and biochemical changes in renal mitochondria during chronic oral methyl mercury exposure. *Exp. Mol. Pharmacol.* 27:403–412.

Fowler, B. A., and Woods, J. S. 1977b. The transplacental toxicity of methyl mercury to fetal rat liver mitochondria: Morphometric and biochemical studies. *Lab. Invest.* 36:122–130.

Fowler, B. A., and Woods, J. S. 1979. The effects of prolonged oral arsenate exposure on liver mitochondria of mice: Morphometric and biochemical studies. *Toxicol. Appl. Pharmacol.* 50:177–187.

Fowler, B. A., Brown, H. W., Lucier, G. W., and Beard, M. E. 1974. Mercury uptake by renal lysosomes of rats ingesting methyl mercury hydroxide: Ultrastructural observations and energy-dispersive X-ray analysis. *Arch. Pathol.* 98:297–301.

Fowler, B. A., Brown, H. W., Lucier, G. W., and Krigman, M. R. 1975. The effects of chronic oral methyl mercury exposure on the lysosome system of rat kidney. Morphometric and biochemical studies. *Lab. Invest.* 32:313–322.

Fowler, B. A., Woods, J. S., and Schiller, C. M. 1979. Studies of hepatic mitochondrial structure and function: Morphometric and biochemical evaluation of in vivo perturbation by arsenate. *Lab. Invest.* 41:313–320.

Fowler, B. A., Kimmel, C. A., Woods, J. S., McConnell, E. E., and Grant, L. D. 1980. Chronic low level lead toxicity in the rat. III. An integrated toxicological assessment with special reference to the kidney. *Toxicol. Appl. Pharmacol.* 56:59–77.

Fowler, B. A., Lucier, G. W., and Hayes, A. W. 1982a. Organelles as tools in toxicology. In *Principles and Methods of Toxicology,* ed. A. W. Hayes, pp. 635–658. New York: Raven.

Fowler, B. A., Woods, J. S., Squibb, K. S., and Davidian, N. M. 1982b. Alteration of hepatic mitochondrial aldehyde dehydrogenase activity by sodium arsenate: The relationship to mitochondrial–microsomal oxidative interactions. *Exp. Mol. Pharmacol.* 37:351–357.

Fowler, B. A., Kardish, R., and Woods, J. S. 1983. Alteration of hepatic microsomal structure and function by acute indium administration: Ultrastructural, morphometric and biochemical studies. *Lab. Invest.* 48:471–478.

Fowler, B. A., Abel, J., Elinder, C.-G., Hapke, H.-J., Kägi, J. H. R., Kleiminger, J., Kojima, Y., Schoot-Uiterkamp, A. J. M., Silbergeld, E. K., Silver, S., Summer, K. H., and Williams, R. J. P. 1984. Structure, mechanism and toxicity. In *Changing Metal Cycles and Human Health,* ed. J. Nriagu, pp. 391–404. New York: Springer-Verlag, Dahlem Workshop Reports.

Fujita, H., Orii, Y., and Sano, S. 1981. Evidence of increased synthesis of δ-aminolevulinic acid dehydratase in experimental lead-poisoned rats. *Biochim. Biophys. Acta* 678:39–50.

Fujita, H., Sato, K., and Sano, S. 1982. Increase in the amount of erythrocyte δ-aminolevulinic acid dehydratase in workers with moderate lead exposure. *Int. Arch. Occup. Environ. Health* 50:287–297.

Ganote, C. E., Reimer, K. A., and Jennings, R. B. 1975. Acute mercuric chloride nephrotoxicity: An electron microscopic and metabolic study. *Lab. Invest.* 31:633–647.

Garvey, J. S., and Chang, C. C. 1981. Detection of circulating metallothionein in rats injected with zinc or cadmium. *Science* 214:805–807.

Gerber, G. B., Maes, J., Gilliavod, N., and Casale, G. 1978. Brain biochemistry of infant mice and rats exposed to lead. *Toxicol. Lett.* 2:51–63.

Giavini, E., Prati, M., and Vismara, C. 1980. Effects of cadmium, lead, and copper on rat preimplantation embryos. *Bull. Environ. Contam. Toxicol.* 25:702–705.

Gibson, S. L. M., and Goldberg, A. 1970. Defects of haem synthesis in mammalian tissues in experimental lead poisoning and experimental porphyria. *Clin. Sci.* 38:63–72.

Goering, P. L., and Fowler, B. A. 1984. Regulation of lead inhibition of δ-aminolevulinic acid dehydratase by a low-molecular weight, high affinity renal lead-binding protein. *J. Pharmacol. Exp. Ther.* 231:66–71.

Goldman, J. M., Vander, A. J., Mouw, D. R., Keiser, J., and Nicholls, M. G. 1981. Multiple short-term effects of lead on the renin–angiotensin system. *J. Lab. Clin. Med.* 97:251–263.

Goyer, R. A. 1968. The renal tubule in lead poisoning. I. Mitochondrial swelling and aminoaciduria. *Lab. Invest.* 19:71–77.

Goyer, R. A., and Krall, R. 1969. Ultrastructural transformation in mitochondria isolated from kidneys of normal and lead intoxicated rats. *J. Cell Biol.* 41:393–400.

Goyer, R. A., and Rhyne, B. C. 1975. Toxic changes in mitochondrial membranes and mitochondrial function. In *Pathobiology of Cell Membranes I,* eds. B. F. Trump and A. U. Arstila, pp. 383–428. New York: Academic.

Goyer, R. A., Leonard, D. L., Morre, J. F., Rhyne, B., and Krigman, M. R. 1970. Lead dosage and the role of the intranuclear inclusion body. *Arch. Environ. Health* 20:705–711.

Granick, S. 1966. The induction in vitro of the synthesis of δ-aminolevulinic acid synthetase in chemical porphyria: A response to certain drugs, sex hormones, and foreign chemicals. *J. Biol. Chem.* 241:1359–1375.

Granick, J. L., Sassa, S., Granick, S., Levere, R. D., and Kappas, A. 1973. Studies in lead poisoning. II. Correlation between the ratio of activated and inactivated δ-aminolevulinic acid dehydratase of whole blood and the blood lead level. *Biochem. Med.* 8:149–159.

Grant, L. D., Kimmel, C. A., West, G. L., Martinez-Vargas, C. M., and Howard, J. L. 1980. Chronic low-level lead toxicity in the rat. II. Effects of postnatal physical and behavioral development. *Toxicol. Appl. Pharmacol.* 56:42–58.

Gritzka, T. L., and Trump, B. F. 1968. Renal tubular lesions caused by mercuric chloride. Electron microscopic observations: Degeneration of the pars recta. *Am. J. Pathol.* 52:1225–1277.

Gunn, S. A., Gould, T. C., and Anderson, W. A. 1961. Zinc protection against cadmium injury to rat testis. *Arch. Pathol.* 71:274–282.

Gunn, S. A., Gould, T. C., and Anderson, W. A. 1963. The selective injurious response of testicular and epididymal blood vessels to cadmium and its prevention by zinc. *Am. J. Pathol.* 42:685–702.

Hernberg, S., and Nikkanen, J. 1970. Enzyme inhibition by lead under normal urban conditions. *Lancet* 1(7637):63–64.

Hilderbrand, D. C., Der, R., Griffin, W. T., and Fahim, M. S. 1973. Effects of lead acetate on reproduction. *Am. J. Obstet. Gynecol.* 115:1058–1065.

IARC. 1980. Some metals and metallic compounds. *IARC Monogr. Eval. Carcinog. Risk Chem. Hum.* 23:39–141. World Health Organization, Lyon, France.

Ito, T., and Sawauchi, K. 1966. Inhibitory effects on cadmium-induced testicular damage by pretreatment with smaller cadmium dose. *Okajimas Folia Anat. Jpn.* 42:107–117.

Jacquet, P. 1978. Influence de la progesterone et de l'oestradiol exogene sur les processe de l'implantation embryonnaire chez la souris femelle intoxiqu]e par le plomb. *C.R. Soc. Biol.* 172:1037–1040.

Jacquet, P., Leonard, A., and Gerber, G. B. 1976. Action of lead on the early divisions of the mouse embryo. *Toxicology* 6:129–132.

Jacquet, P., Gerber, G. B., Leonard, A., and Maes, J. 1977. Plasma hormone levels in normal and lead-treated pregnant mice. *Experientia* 33:1375–1377.

Jones, H. S., and Fowler, B. A. 1980. Biological interactions of cadmium with calcium. *Ann. N.Y. Acad. Sci.* 355:309–318.

Kägi, J. H. R., and Hapke, H.-J. 1984. Biochemical interactions of mercury, cadmium, and lead. In *Changing Metal Cycles and Human Health,* ed. J. O. Nriagu, pp. 237–250. New York: Spring-Verlag, Dahlem Workshop Reports.

Kappas, A., and Maines, M. D. 1976. Tin: A potent inducer of heme oxygenase in kidney. *Science* 192:60–62.

Keiser, J. A., Vander, A. J., and Germain, C. L. 1983. Clearance of renin in unanesthetized rats: Effects of chronic lead exposure. *Toxicol. Appl. Pharmacol.* 69:127–137.

Kempson, S. A., Ellis, B. G., and Price, R. G. 1977. Changes in rat renal cortex, isolated plasma membranes and urinary enzymes following the injection of mercury chloride. *Chem. Biol. Interact.* 18:217–234.

Khare, N., Der, R., Ross, G., and Fahim, M. 1978. Prostatic cellular changes after injection of cadmium and lead into rat prostate. *Res. Commun. Chem. Pathol. Pharmacol.* 20:351–365.

Kimura, M., Otaki, N., Yoshiki, S., Kuzuki, M., Horiuchi, N., and Suda, T. 1974. The isolation of metallothionein and its protective role in cadmium poisoning. *Arch. Biochem. Biophys.* 165:340–348.

Kontula, K., Janne, O., Luukkainen, T., and Vihko, R. 1974. Progesterone-binding protein in human myometrium. Influence of metal ions on binding. *J. Clin. Endocrinol. Metab.* 38:500–503.

Kotsonis, F. N., and Klaassen, C. D. 1977. Toxicity and distribution of cadmium administered to rats at sublethal doses. *Toxicol. Appl. Pharmacol.* 41:667–680.

Kotsonis, F. N., and Klaassen, C. D. 1978. The relationship of metallothionein to the toxicity of cadmium after prolonged oral administration to rats. *Toxicol. Appl. Pharmacol.* 45:39–54.

Krasny, H. R., and Holbrook, D. J., Jr. 1977. Effects of cadmium on microsomal hemoproteins and heme oxygenase in rat liver. *Mol. Pharmacol.* 13:759–765.

Kuhnert, P. M., Kuhnert, B. R., Bottoms, S. F., and Erhard, B. S. 1982. Cadmium levels in maternal blood, fetal cord blood, and placental tissues of pregnant women who smoke. *Am. J. Obstet. Gynecol.* 142:1021–1025.

Lafont, J., Rouanet, J., Besancon, P., and Moretti, J. 1976. Existence d'une metallothionein dans le placenta. *C.R. Acad. Sci. Paris* 283:417–420.

Lamperti, A. A., and Niewenhuis, R. 1976. The effects of mercury on the structure and function of the hypothalamo–pituitary axis of the hamster. *Cell Tissue Res.* 170:315–324.

Lamperti, A. A., and Printz, R. H. 1974. Localization, accumulation, and toxic effects of mercuric chloride on the reproductive axis of the female hamster. *Biol. Reprod.* 11:180–186.

Lancranjan, I., Popeseu, H. I., Gavanescu, O., Klepsch, I., and Serbanescu, M. 1975. Reproductive ability of workmen occupationally exposed to lead. *Arch. Environ. Health* 30:396–401.

Laskey, J. W., Rehnberg, G. L., Laws, S. C., and Hein, J. F. 1984. Reproductive effects of low acute doses of cadmium chloride in adult male rats. *Toxicol. Appl. Pharmacol.* 73:250–255.

Lauwerys, R. R., and Buchet, J. P. 1973. Occupational exposure to mercury vapors and biological action. *Arch. Environ. Health* 27:65–68.

Lauwerys, R. R., Buchet, J. P., and Roels, H. A. 1973. Comparative study of effect of inorganic lead and cadmium on blood δ-aminolevulinate dehydratase in man. *Br. J. Ind. Med.* 30:359–364.

Lauwerys, R., Buchet, J. P., Roels, H. A., and Materne, D. 1974. Relationship between urinary δ-aminolevulinic acid excretion and the inhibition of red cell δ-aminolevulinate dehydratase by lead. *Clin. Toxicol.* 7:383–388.

Leonard, A., Gerber, G. B., and Jacquet, P. 1983. Effect of lead on reproductive capacity and development of mammals. In *Reproductive and Developmental Toxicity of Metals,* eds. T. W. Clarkson, G. F. Nordberg, and P. R. Sager, pp. 357–368. New York: Plenum.

Levander, O. A., Welsh, S. O., and Morris, V. C. 1980. Erythrocyte deformability as affected by vitamin E deficiency and lead toxicity. *Ann. N.Y. Acad. Sci.* 355:227–239.

Lewis, G. P., Jusko, W. J., and Coughlin, L. L. 1972. Cadmium accumulation in man: Influence of smoking, occupation, alcoholic habit, and disease. *J. Chronic Dis.* 25:717–726.

Liao, S., Tymoczko, J. L., Castaneda, E., and Liang, T. 1973. Androgen receptors and androgen-dependent initiation of protein synthesis in the prostate. *Vit. Horm.* 33:297–317.

Lilis, R., Gaurilescu, N., Nestorescu, B., Dumitrio, C., and Roventa, A. 1968. Nephropathy in chronic lead poisoning. *Br. J. Ind. Med.* 25:196–202.

Lucier, G. W., Matthews, H. B., Brubaker, P. E., Klein, R., and McDaniel, O. S. 1973. Effects of methyl mercury on microsomal mixed-function oxidase components of rodents. *Mol. Pharmacol.* 9:237–246.

Lucis, O. H., Lucis, R., and Shaikh, Z. A. 1972. Cadmium and zinc in pregnancy and lactation. *Arch. Environ. Health* 25:14–22.

Lui, E. M. K., and Lucier, G. W. 1981. Hypophyseal regulation of cadmium-induced depression of the hepatic monooxygenase system in the rat. *Mol. Pharmacol.* 20:165–172.

Madsen, K. M., and Christensen, E. I. 1978. Effects of mercury on lysosomal protein digestion in the kidney proximal tubule. *Lab. Invest.* 38:165–174.

Mahaffey, K. R., and Fowler, B. A. 1977. Effects of concurrent administration of dietary lead, cadmium, and arsenic in the rat. *Environ. Health Perspect.* 19:165–171.

Mahaffey, K. R., Smith, C., Tanaka, Y., and DeLuca, H. F. 1979. Stimulation of gastrointestinal lead absorption by 1,25-dihydroxyvitamin D-3. *Fed. Proc.* 38:384.

Mahaffey, K. R., Capar, S. G., Gladen, B. C., and Fowler, B.A. 1981. Concurrent exposure to lead, cadmium, and arsenic. *J. Lab. Clin. Med.* 98:463–481.

Mahaffey, K. R., Rosen, J. F., Chesney, R. W., Peeler, J. T., Smith, C. M., and De Luca, H. F. 1982. Association between age, blood lead concentration, and serum 1,25-dihydroxycholecalciferol levels in children. *Am. J. Clin. Nutr.* 35:1327–1331.

Maines, M.D. 1980. Regional distribution of the enzymes of heme biosynthesis and the inhibition of 5-aminolaevulinate synthase by manganese in the rat brain. *Biochem. J.* 190:315–321.

Maines, M. D. 1984. Characterization of heme oxygenase activity in Leydig and Sertoli cells of the rat testes: Differential distribution of activity and response to cadmium. *Biochem. Pharmacol.* 33:1493–1502.

Maines, M. D., and Kappas, A. 1976. Studies on the mechanism of induction of haem oxygenase by cobalt and other metal ions. *Biochem. J.* 154:125–131.

Maines, M. D., and Kappas, A. 1977a. Metals as regulators of heme metabolism. *Science* 198:1215–1221.

Maines, M. D., and Kappas, A. 1977b. Regulation of heme pathway enzymes and cellular glutathione content by metals that do not chelate with tetrapyrroles: Blockade of metal effects by thiols. *Proc. Natl. Acad. Sci. USA* 74:1875–1878.

Maines, M. D., and Sinclair, P. 1977. Cobalt regulation of heme synthesis and degradation in avian embryo liver cell culture. *J. Biol. Chem.* 252:219–223.

Maines, M. D., Janousek, V., Tomio, J. M., and Kappas, A. 1976. Cobalt inhibition of synthesis and induction of δ-aminolevulinate synthase in liver. *Proc. Natl. Acad. Sci. USA* 73:1499–1503.

Maines, M. D., Chung, A.-S., and Kutty, R. K. 1982. The inhibition of testicular heme oxygenase activity by cadmium: A novel cellular response. *J. Biol. Chem.* 257:14116–14121.

Massey, V., Hofmann, T., and Palmer, G. 1962. The relation of function and structure in lipoyl dehydrogenase. *J. Biol. Chem.* 237:3820–3828.

Matlib, M. A., and Srere, P. A. 1976. Oxidative properties of swollen rat liver mitochondria. *Arch. Biochem. Biophys.* 174:705–712.

McAllister, R. G., Jr., Michelakis, A. M., and Sandstead, H. H. 1971. Plasma renin activity in chronic plumbism: Effects of treatment. *Arch. Intern. Med.* 127:919–923.

Meek, E. S. 1959. Cellular changes induced by cadmium in mouse testis and liver. *Br. J. Exp. Pathol.* 40:503–506.

Meredith, P. A., and Moore, M. R. 1979. The influence of lead on haem biosynthesis and biodegradation in the rat. *Biochem. Soc. Trans.* 7:637–639.

Meredith, P. A., Moore, M. R., and Goldberg, A. 1974. The effects of aluminum, lead and zinc on δ-aminolaevulinic acid dehydratase. *Biochem. Soc. Trans.* 2:1243–1246.

Meredith, P. A., Campbell, B. C., Moore, M. R., and Goldberg, A. 1977. The effects of industrial lead poisoning on cytochrome P-450 mediated phenazone (antipyrine) hydroxylation. *Eur. J. Clin. Pharmacol.* 12:235–239.

Millar, J. A., Cummings, R. L. C., Battistini, V., Carswell, F., and Goldberg, A. 1970. Lead and δ-aminolaevulinic acid dehydratase levels in mentally retarded children and lead-poisoned suckling rats. *Lancet* 2(7675):695–698.

Mistry, P., Megginson, M., and Fowler, B. A. 1983. Characterization of partially purified lead-binding components from rat kidney cytosol. *Fed. Proc.* 42:2267.

Mistry, P., Lucier, G. W., and Fowler, B. A. 1984. High affinity lead binding proteins in rat kidney cytosol mediate cell-free nuclear translocation of lead. *J. Pharmacol. Exp. Ther.* 232:462–469.

Mitchell, R. A., Drake, J. E., Wittlin, L. A., and Rejent, T. A. 1977. Erythrocyte porphobilinogen synthase (delta-aminolaevulinate dehydratase) activity: A reliable and quantitative indicator of lead exposure in humans. *Clin. Chem.* 23:105–111.

Moldeus, P. W., Cha, Y. N., Cinti, D. L., Schenkman, J. B. 1973. Heaptic organelle interaction. III. Mitochondrial modification of microsomal drug metabolism. *J. Biol. Chem.* 248:8574–8584.

Molinini, R., Assennato, G., Altamura, M., Gagliano Candel, R., Gagliard, T., and Paci, C. 1981. Lead effects on male fertility in battery workers. Proceedings of the 10th International Congress on Occupational Health, September 25–October 1, Cairo.

Moore, M. R., and Meredith, P. A. 1976. The association of delta-aminolevulinic acid with the neurological and behavioural effects of lead exposure. In *Trace Substances in Environmental Health—X: Proc. University of Missouri 10th Annual Conference on Trace Substances in Environmental Health,* ed. D. D. Hemphill, pp. 363–371. Columbia, Mo.: University of Missouri.

Moore, J. F., Goyer, R. A., and Wilson, M. 1973. Lead-induced inclusion bodies: Solubility, amino acid content and relationship to residual acidic nuclear proteins. *Lab. Invest.* 29:488–494.

Moore, M. R., Meredith, P. A., and Goldberg, A., 1980. Lead and heme biosynthesis. In *Lead Toxicity,* eds. R. L. Singhal and J. A. Thomas, pp. 79–117. Baltimore-Munich: Urban and Schwarzenberg.

Morgan, W. D. 1976. Blood cadmium and hypertension. *Lancet* 2:1361.

Mouw, D. R., Vander, A. J., Cox, J., and Fleischer, M. 1978. Acute effects of lead on renal electrolyte excretion and plasma renin activity. *Toxicol. Appl. Pharmacol.* 46:435–447.

Nordberg, G. F. 1971. Effects of acute and chronic cadmium exposure on the testicles of mice with special reference to the possible protective effects of metallothionein. *Environ. Physiol. Biochem.* 1:171–187.

Nordberg, G. F., Goyer, R., and Nordberg, M. 1975. Comparative toxicity of cadmium-metallothionein and cadmium chloride on mouse kidney. *Arch. Pathol.* 99:192–197.

Nordberg, M. 1984. General aspects of cadmium: Transport, uptake and metabolism by the kidney. *Environ. Health Perspect.* 54:13–20.

Nordberg, M., and Kojima, Y. 1979. Metallothionein and other low molecular weight metal-binding proteins. In *Metallothionein, Experientia* Suppl. 34, eds. J. H. R. Kägi and M. Nordberg, pp. 41–116. Basel: Birkhauser.

Nordström, S., Beckman, L., and Nordenson, I. 1978. Occupational and environmental risks in and around a smelter in northern Sweden. III. Frequencies of spontaneous abortion. *Hereditas* 88:51–54.

Ohanian, E. V., and Iwai, J. 1979. Effects of cadmium ingestion in rats with opposite genetic predisposition to hypertension. *Environ. Health Perspect.* 28:261–266.

Oskarsson, A., Squibb, K. S., and Fowler, B. A. 1982. Intracellular binding of lead in the kidney: Partial isolation and characterization of postmitochondrial supernatant lead-binding components. *Biochem. Biophys. Res. Commun.* 104:290–298.

Parizek, J., and Zahor, Z. 1956. Effect of cadmium salts on testicular tissue. *Nature (Lond.)* 177:1036–1037.

Parizek, J. 1957. The destructive effect of cadmium ion on testicular tissue and its prevention by zinc. *J. Endocrinol.* 15:56–63.

Parizek, J. 1960. Sterilization of the male by cadmium salts. *J. Reprod. Fertil.* 1:294–309.

Parizek, J., Oskadolova, I., Bemes, I., and Pitha, J. 1968. The effect of a subcutaneous injection of cadmium salts on the ovaries of adult rat in persistent oestros. *J. Reprod. Fertil.* 17:559–562.

Peach, M. J. 1977. Renin-angiotensin system: Biochemistry and mechanisms of action. *Physicol. Rev.* 57:313–370.

Pence, D. H., Miya, T. S., and Schnell, R. C. 1977. Cadmium alteration of hexobarbital action: Sex related differences in the rat. *Toxicol. Appl. Pharmacol.* 39:89–96.

Perry, M. M., Jr., and Erlanger, M. 1975. Mechanism of cadmium induced hypertension. In *Trace Substances in Environmental Health,* ed. D. D. Hemphill, pp. 339–348. Columbia, Mo.: University of Missouri.

Perry, H. J., Jr., and Schroeder, H. A. 1955. Concentration of trace metals in urine of treated and untreated hypertensive subjects. *J. Lab. Clin. Med.* 46:936.

Perry, H. M., Erlanger, M., and Perry, E. F. 1979. Increase in the systolic pressure of rats chronically fed cadmium. *Environ. Health Perspect.* 28:251–260.

Perry, H. M., Erlanger, M. W., Yunice, A., and Perry, E. F. 1967. Mechanisms of the acute hypertensive effect of intra-arterial cadmium and mercury in anesthetized rats. *J. Lab. Clin. Med.* 70:963–972.

Petering, D. H., Loftsgaarden, J., Schneider, J., and Fowler, B. 1984. Metabolism of cadmium, zinc and copper in the rat kidney: The role of metallothionein and other binding sites. *Environ. Health Perspect.* 54:73–81.

Peters, R. A. 1955. Biochemistry of some toxic agents. I. Present state of knowledge of biochemical lesions induced by trivalent arsenic poisoning. *Bull. Johns Hopkins Hosp.* 97:1–20.

Petrusz, P., Weaver, C. M., Grant, L. D., Mushak, P., and Krigman, M. R. 1979. Lead poisoning and reproduction: Effects on pituitary and serum gonadotropins in neonatal rats. *Environ. Res.* 19:383–391.

Piomelli, S., Seaman, C., Zullow, D., Curran, A., and Davidow, B. 1982. Threshold for lead damage to heme synthesis in urban children. *Proc. Natl. Acad. Sci. USA* 79:3335–3339.

Piper, W. N., and Tephly, T. R. 1974. Differential inhibition of erythrocyte and hepatic uroporphyrinogen I synthetase activity by lead. *Life Sci.* 14:873–876.

Pohl, C. R., and Knobil, E. 1982. The role of the central nervous system in the control of ovarian function in higher primates. *Annu. Rev. Physiol.* 44:583–593.

Porter, M. C., Miya, T. S., and Bousquet, W. F. 1974. Cadmium: Inability to induced hypertension in the rat. *Toxicol. Appl. Pharmacol.* 27:692–696.

Ridlington, J. W., Winge, D. R., and Fowler, B. A. 1981. Long-term turnover and stability of cadmium-metallothionein following an initial low dose in rats. *Biochim. Biophys. Acta* 673:177–183.

Roberts, S. A., and Schnell, R. C. 1982a. Cadmium inhibition of in vitro hepatic oxidative drug metabolism in the rat: Comparison between ionic cadmium and cadmium-thionein. *Res. Commun. Chem. Pathol. Pharmacol.* 35:349–352.

Roberts, S. A., and Schnell, R. C. 1982b. Cadmium-induced inhibition of hepatic drug oxidation in the rat: Time dependency of tolerance development and metallothionein synthesis. *Toxicol. Appl. Pharmacol.* 64:42–51.

Roels, H. A., Buchet, J. P., Lauwerys, R. R., and Sonnet, J. 1975. Comparison of in vivo effect of inorganic lead and cadmium on glutathione reductase system and δ-aminolevulinate dehydratase in human erythrocytes. *Br. J. Ind. Med.* 32:181–192.

Rom, W. N. 1976. Effects of lead on the female and reproduction: A review. *Mt. Sinai J. Med.* 43:542–552.

Rosen, J. F., Chesney, R. W., Hamstra, A., DeLuca, H. F., and Mahaffey, K. R. 1980. Reduction in 1,25-dihydroxyvitamin D in children with increased lead absorption. *N. Engl. J. Med.* 20:1125–1131.

Saksena, S. K., Dahlgren, L., Lav, I. F., and Chang, M. C. 1977. Reproductive and endocrinological features of male rats after treatment with cadmium chloride. *Biol. Reprod.* 16:609–613.

Samarawickrama, G. P. 1979. Biological effects of cadmium in mammals. In *The Chemistry, Biochemistry and Biology of Cadmium,* ed. M. Webb, pp. 341–421. New York: Elsevier/North Holland.

Sanborn, B. M., Rao, B. R., and Korenman, S. G. 1971. Interaction of 17β-estradiol and its specific uterine receptor. Evidence for complex kinetic and equilibrium behavior. *Biochemistry* 10:4955–4961.

Sandstead, H. H., Orth, D. N., Abe, K., and Stiel, J. 1970a. Lead intoxication: Effects on pituitary and adrenal function in man. *Clin. Res.* 18:76.

Sandstead, H. H., Michelakis, A. M., and Temple, T. E. 1970b. Lead intoxication: Its effects on the renin-aldosterone response to sodium deprivation. *Arch. Environ. Health* 20:356–363.

Schenkman, J. B., Cinti, D. L., and Moldeus, P. 1973. The mitochondrial role in hepatic cell mixed-function oxidations. *Ann. N.Y. Acad. Sci.* 212:420–427.

Schnell, R. C., Means, J. R., Roiberts, S. A., and Pence, D. H. 1979. Studies on cadmium-induced inhibition of hepatic microsomal drug biotransformation in the rat. *Environ. Health Perspect.* 28:273–279.

Schroeder, H. A. 1964. Cadmium hypertension in rats. *Am. J. Physiol.* 207:62–66.

Secchi, G. C., Erba, L., Cambiaghi, G. 1974. Delta-aminolevulinic acid dehydratase activity of erythrocytes and liver tissue in man: Relationship to lead exposure. *Arch. Environ. Health* 28: 130–132.

Shelton, K. R., and Egle, P. M. 1982. The proteins of lead-induced intranuclear inclusion bodies. *J. Biol. Chem.* 257:11802–11807.

Silbergeld, E. K., Hruska, R. E., Bradley, D., Lamon, J. M., and Frykholm, B. C. 1982. Neurotoxic aspects of porphyrinopathies: Lead and succinylacetone. *Environ. Res.* 29:459–471.

Smith, C. M., DeLuca, H. F., Tanaka, Y., and Mahaffey, K. R. 1978. Stimulation of lead absorption by vitamin D administration. *J. Nutr.* 108:843–847.

Smith, C. M., DeLuca, H. F., Tanaka, Y., and Mahaffey, K. R. 1981. Effect of lead ingestion on functions of vitamin D and its metabolites. *J. Nutr.* 111:1321–1329.

Sorensen, E. M. B., Smith, N. K. R., and Ramirez-Mitchell, R. 1982. Electron probe X-ray microanalysis of arsenic inclusions in fish. *Arch. Environ. Contam. Toxicol.* 11:469–473.

Squibb, K. S., and Fowler, B. A. 1983. Biochemical mechanisms of arsenical toxicity. In *Biological and Environmental Effects of Arsenic,* ed. B. A. Fowler, pp. 233–270. New York: Elsevier/North Holland.

Squibb, K. S., and Fowler, B. A. 1984. Intracellular metabolism and effects of circulating cadmium-metallothionein in the kidney. *Environ. Health Perspect.* 54:31–35.

Squibb, K. S., Ridlington, J. W., Carmichael, N. G., and Fowler, B. A. 1979. Early cellular effects of circulating cadmium-thionein on kidney proximal tubules. *Environ. Health Perspect.* 28:287–296.

Squibb, K. S., Pritchard, J. B., and Fowler, B. A. 1982. The renal metabolism and toxicity of metallothionein. In *Biological Roles of Metallothionein. Proc. USA–Japan Workshop on Metallothionein,* ed. E. C. Foulkes, pp. 181–192. New York: Elsevier/North Holland.

Squibb, K. S., Pritchard, J. B., and Fowler, B. A. 1984. Cadmium-metallothionein nephropathy: Relationships between ultrastructural/biochemical alterations and intracellular cadmium binding. *J. Pharmacol. Exp. Ther.* 229:311–321.

Stuik, E. 1974. Biological response of male and female volunteers to inorganic lead. *Int. Arch. ArbeitsMed.* 33:83–97.

Suda, T., Horiuchi, N., Ogata, E., Ezawa, I., Otaki, N., and Kimura, M. 1974. Prevention by metallothionein of cadmium-induced inhibition of vitamin D activation reaction in kidney. *FEBS Lett.* 42:23–26.

Task Force on Metals and Carcinogens. Sidney Belman (Ed.). 1981. *Environ. Health Perspect.* 40:11–20.

Templeton, D. M., and Cherian, M. G. 1963. Cadmium and hypertension. *Trends Pharmacol. Sci.* 4:501–503.

Teranishi, H., Kasuya, M., Aoshima, K., Kato, T., and Migita, S. 1983. Demonstration of vitamin D-binding protein (Gc-globulin) in the urine of itai-itai disease patients. *Toxicol. Lett.* 15:7–12.

Thind, G. S. 1972. Role of cadmium in human and experimental hypertension. *J. Air. Pollut. Control Assoc.* 22:267–270.

Timms, F., and Schulz, G. 1966. Hoden und schwermetalle. (Testicles and heavy metals). *Histochemie* 1:15–21.

Tsuchiya, K. 1978. Epidemiological studies. In *Cadmium Studies in Japan—A Review,* ed. K. Tsuchiya, pp. 133–367. New York: Elsevier/North Holland.

Tsukamoto, I., Yoshinaga, T., and Sano, S. 1980. Zinc and cysteine residues in the active site of bovine liver δ-aminolevulinic acid dehydratase. *Int. J. Biochem.* 12:751–756.

Ulmer, D. D., and Vallee, B. L. 1969. Effects of lead on biochemical systems. In *Trace Substances in Environmental Health—II, Proc. University of Missouri's 2d Annual Conference on Trace Substances in Environmental Health,* ed. D. D. Hemphill, pp. 7–27. Columbia, Mo.: University of Missouri–Columbia.

Vermande-Van Eck, G. I., and Meigs, J.W. 1960. Changes in the ovary of the rhesus monkey after chronic lead intoxication. *Fertil. Steril.* 11:223–234.

Victery, W., Vander, A. J., Shulak, J. M., Schoeps, P., and Julius, S. 1982a. Lead, hypertension, and the renin-angiotensin system in rats. *J. Lab. Clin. Med.* 99:354–362.

Victery, W., Vander, A. J., Markel, H., Katzman, L., Shulak, J. M., and Germain, C. 1982b. Lead exposure begun in in utero decreases renin and angiotensin II in adult rats (41398). *Proc. Soc. Exp. Biol. Med.* 170:63–67.

Victery, W., Vander, A. J., Schoeps, P., and Germain, C. 1983. Plasma renin is increased in young rats exposed to lead in utero and during nursing (41517). *Proc. Soc. Exp. Biol. Med.* 172:1–7.

Victery, W., Miller, C. R., and Fowler, B. A. 1984. Lead accumulation by rat renal brush border membrane vesicles. *J. Pharmacol. Exp. Ther.* 231:589–596.

Voegtlin, C., Rosenthal, S. M., and Johnson, J. M. 1931. The influence of arsenicals and crystalline glutathione on the oxygen consumption of tissues. *Public Health Rep.* 46:339–354.

Waalkes, M. P., Chernoff, S. B., and Klaassen, C. D. 1984a. Cadmium-binding proteins of rat testes. Characterization of a low-molecular mass protein that lacks identity with metallothionein. *Biochem. J.* 220:811–818.

Waalkes, M. P., Poisner, A. M., Wood, G. W., and Klaassen, C. D. 1984b. Metallothionein-like proteins in human placenta and fetal membranes. *Toxicol. Appl. Pharmacol.* 74:179–184.

Webb, J. L. 1966. In *Enzyme and Metabolic Inhibitors,* vol. 3, pp. 595–793. New York: Academic.

Webb, R. C., Winquist, R. J., Victery., W., and Vander, A. J. 1981. In vivo and in vitro effects of lead on vascular reactivity in rats. *Am. J. Physiol.* 24:H211–H216.

Wedeen, R. P., Maesaka, J. K., Weiner, B., Lipat, G. I., Lyons, M. M., Vitale, L. F., and Joselow, M. M. 1975. Occupational lead nephropathy. *Am. J. Med.* 59:630–641.

Weissberg, J. B., and Voytek, P. E. 1974. Liver and red-cell porphobilinogen synthase in the adult and fetal guinea pig. *Biochim. Biophys. Acta* 364:304–319.

Whiting, M. J., and Granick, S. 1976. δ-Aminolevulinic acid synthase from chick embryo liver mitochondria. II. Immunochemical correlation between synthesis and activity in induction and repression. *J. Biol. Chem.* 251:1346–1353.

Wide, M. 1980. Interference of lead with implantation in the mouse: Effect of exogenous oestradiol and progesterone. *Teratology* 21:187–191.

Wide, M., and Nilsson, O. 1977. Differential susceptibility of the embryo to inorganic lead during periimplantation in the mouse. *Teratology* 16:273–276.

Wide, M., and Wide, L. 1980. Estradiol receptor activity in uteri if pregnant mice given lead before implantation. *Fertil. Steril.* 34:503–508.

Wiebe, J. P., Barr, K. J., and Buckingham, K. D. 1982. Lead administration during pregnancy and lactation affects steroidogenesis and hormone receptors in testes of offspring. *J. Toxicol. Environ. Health* 10:653–666.

Williams, R. J. P. 1984. Structural aspects of metal toxicity. In *Changing Metal Cycles and Human Health*, ed. J. O. Nriagu, pp. 251–263. New York: Springer-Verlag.

Wilson, E. L., Buger, P. E., and Dowdle, E.B. 1972. Beef-liver δ-aminolevulinic acid dehydratase. *Eur. J. Biochem.* 29:563–571.

Wolkowski, R. M. 1974. Differential cadmium-induced embryotoxicity in two inbred mouse strains. I. Analysis of inheritance of the response to cadmium and the presence of cadmium in fetal and placental tissues. *Teratology* 10:243–262.

Wong, K. L., and Klaassen, C. D. 1980. Age difference in the susceptibility to cadmium induced testicular damage in rats. *Toxicol. Appl. Pharmacol.* 55:456–466.

Woods, J. S., and Carver, G. T. 1977. Action of cobalt chloride on the biosynthesis, degradation and utilization of heme in fetal rat liver. *Drug. Metab. Dispos.* 5:487–492.

Woods, J. S., and Fowler, B. A. 1977a. Renal porphyria during chronic methyl mercury exposure. *J. Lab. Clin.Med.* 90:266–272.

Woods, J. S., and Fowler, B. A. 1977b. Effects of chronic arsenic exposure on hematopoietic function in adult mammalian liver. *Environ. Health Perspect.* 19:209–213.

Woods, J. S., and Fowler, B. A. 1978. Altered regulation of mammalian hepatic heme biosynthesis and urinary prophyrin excretion during prolonged exposure to sodium arsenate. *Toxicol. Appl. Pharmacol.* 43:361–371.

Woods, J. S., and Fowler, B. A. 1982. Selective inhibition of δ-aminolevulinic acid dehydratase by indium chloride in rat kidney: Biochemical and ultrastructural studies. *Exp. Mol. Pathol.* 36:306–315.

Woods, J. S., Carver, G. T., and Fowler, B. A. 1979. Altered regulation of hepatic heme metabolism by indium chloride. *Toxicol. Appl. Pharmacol.* 49:455–461.

Woods, J. S., Kardish, R., and Fowler, B. A. 1981. Studies on the action of porphyrinogenic trace metals on the activity of hepatic uroporphyrinogen decarboxylase. *Biochem. Biophys. Res. Commun.* 103:264–271.

Woods, J. S., Fowler, B. A., and Eaton, D. C. 1984. Studies on the mechanisms of thallium-mediated inhibition of hepatic mixed-function oxidase activity: Correlation with inhibition of NADPH-cytochrome *c* (P-450) reductase. *Biochem. Pharmacol.* 33:571–576.

Wu, W.H., Shomin, D., Richards, K. E., and Williams, R. C. 1974. The quaternary structure of δ-aminolevulinic acid dehydratase from bovine liver. *Proc. Natl. Acad. Sci. USA* 71:1767–1770.

Yoshida, T., Okamoto, M., Suzuki, Y., and Hashimoto, Y. 1979. Cadmium-induced alterations in the activities of hepatic δ-aminolevulinic acid synthetase and heme oxygenase in mice. *J. Pharmacobio-Dyn.* 2:84–91, 1979.

Young, P. C. M., Cleary, R. E., and Ragan, W. D. 1977. Effect of metal ions on the binding of 17β-estradiol to human endometrial cytosol. *Fertil. Steril.* 28:459–463.

Chapter 11

Food Additives: A Benefit/Risk Dilemma

C. Jelleff Carr

INTRODUCTION

The use of various substances in the preparation of food for human use has many historic, toxicologic, and economic aspects. Thousands of materials are incorporated into natural foods for preservation, modification, or aesthetic purposes. Only in relatively recent years has the incorporation of such substances as nitrate and nitrite salts, butylated hydroxytoluene, methylparaben, sulfiting agents, urea, caffeine, and tannic acid been considered potentially hazardous and possibly unnecessary. Even such food ingredients as salt, sugar, flavoring agents, and certain plant oils, long considered foods, are now coming under evaluation for possible hazardous effects when added to foodstuffs. This critical reevaluation of human food is a reflection of the growing concern in many quarters about the influence of environmental factors such as diet and lifestyle on health and longevity. The endless controversy surrounding the regulation of cancer-causing substances has resulted in such prestigious reports as the one from the National Academy of Sciences Committee on Diet, Nutrition and Cancer (National Academy of Sciences, 1982). However, clear directives are not to be found, and the numerous reasons for this predictment seem to defy a satisfactory resolution.

PRESENT STATUS OF THE DILEMMA

While the present regulatory climate in the Western World tends to require zero tolerance and tacitly implies absolute safety, the total elimination of "cancer-causing" food ingredients is essentially impossible. It is necessary to balance risks or costs with social benefits, needs, or values in determining the safety of foods and food ingredients. In addition, unnecessary stringent regulation undercuts economy productivity and interferes with social progress to a degree out of proportion with the perceived health hazards.

Today we are developing increasingly sensitive analytical methods for detecting the presence and identity of trace quantities of substances present in foods. Our ability to find and measure levels of chemicals has outrun our ability to assess the significance of these findings. The net result is an agenda for toxicological evaluation and subsequent societal decisions that is mounting beyond any hope of generating the facilities to cope with the demand (Environmental Protection Agency, 1982; Francke and Ng, 1983).

An analysis of this state of affairs reveals a number of significant facts. it is obvious that it is often difficult if not impossible to carry out animal toxicity tests that prove conclusively that a given food substance is safe (hazardous) when administered in the relatively low doses consumed by humans. This is especially true for substances that are not proximate carcinogens. In addition, few animal tests are conducted with the rigor necessary to give proof of safety or hazard that is accepted by all qualified toxicologists. This is clearly illustrated by the studies on sodium nitrite (Carr, 1981; National Academy of Sciences, 1981).

The major element that fuels these debates is the lack of agreement among scientists and professional groups about the often poorly documented experimental or epidemiological evidence. Thus, authorities will differ in their opinions regarding the relative safety of the substance in question. Equally eminent scientists who are expected to pontificate on such issues are often at odds, and the average person is understandably bewildered. The result is that the dispute smolders without clear resolution, and many people dismiss the issue as unimportant or become "desensitized" to the question of food safety. A patchwork of laws and regulations often contested in the courts seems to have been the result. These actions lead to endless discussion, altercation, and dispute. In the interim the food industry loses markets, costs increase, and a general state of confusion prevails. It is obvious that significant regulatory decisions that often have tremendous economic impact must be based on adequate studies that have had peer review before implementation. Tests claimed to be positive in terms of finding a toxic effect, reported in the literature, and then cited in the press as an indictment of a food substance, should not lead to regulatory decisions without proper review. The major effort that is required to mount the costly studies necessary to develop the facts essential for a definitive denouement of such a controversy must be properly financed, planned, and carried out with subsequent peer review. Only in this manner can the regulatory agencies develop the supportable evidence for final regulations acceptable to all parties (Hayes, 1983).

Controversies of this character formed the basis of the work of the Scientific

Committee of the Food Safety Council. The specific goals were to develop acceptable criteria for the safety and wholesomeness of foods and food ingredients. To this end, the report of the Committee, based on nearly 4 years of work, laid out a detailed plan of estimating the risk offered by the ingestion of any component of food (Food Safety Council, 1980).

EVALUATION OF THE GRAS SUBSTANCES

In 1970 the U.S. Food and Drug Administration (FDA), following a presidential directive, initiated a series of implementing actions that led to the formation of a special committee to undertake the novel task of evaluating approximately 400 food ingredients for any potential hazards. In his consumer message of 1967, the President indicated that he did not feel it proper to require exhaustive study of the safety of proposed new food additives, while accepting the safety of food ingredients that had been declared "safe" because they were in common use at the time of the 1958 Food Additives Amendment to the Food, Drug and Cosmetic (FD&C) Act. These food ingredients had been used in foods for preservation, modification, or aesthetic purposes. These substances had become known as GRAS (an acronym for "generally recognized as safe"). In presuming that GRAS substances were safe, based on data available at the time of the 1958 Amendment, the FDA was not required to have a demonstration of safety for the continued use of these substances. On the other hand, FDA would be required to demonstrate these ingredients to be "unsafe" before they could be prohibited in foods.

The Life Sciences Research Office (LSRO), Federation of American Societies for Experimental Biology (FASEB), was selected by FDA to organize the evaluative study and select the committee because of its long experience in conducting independent evaluative studies in the biomedical sciences. A standing committee of qualified scientists was chosen in 1972 representing a number of relevant disciplines. This was the Select Committee on Generally Recognized As Safe (GRAS) Substances that completed their task in 1982. This panel of 11 scientists (SCOGS) undertook the difficult task of evaluating these substances, fully recognizing that in most instances the available information was qualitatively or quantitatively limited.

The general framework for the evaluation process adopted by the Committee proved to be effective. Its central feature was the preparation of consumption surveys, the conduct of special mutagenic and teratogenic tests, the initial collection of toxicological and associated data from the world's literature, the input of information and opinions by interested parties, and the Committee's evaluation itself.

In addition to the expertise of the SCOGS, an efficient and qualified scientific staff of the Life Sciences Research Office, FASEB, supported the studies and provided the necessary report preparation and documentation assistance.

The Select Committee's evaluations were to be made independently of FDA or any other group, governmental or nongovernmental. The FASEB, LSRO, and the Select Committee were to accept the responsibility for each of the several reports. The participating staff, committee members, and outside consultants were to be identified in each report.

A unique feature of this effort involved making the tentative reports prepared on each substance available to the public for review in the office of the Documents Management Branch, FDA, after announcement in the *Federal Register*. An opportunity was provided for any interested person to appear before the SCOGS at a public hearing to make oral presentation of data, information, and views on the substances covered by the reports. The data, information, and views presented at the hearing were considered by the Select Committee in reaching its final conclusions. Final reports were approved by the Director of LSRO, and subsequently by the LSRO Advisory Committee. The Committee's evaluation report on each GRAS substance provided FDA with an analysis of all relevant scientific data expressed as an opinion with regard to the evidence of health effects (Fig. 1).

The Select Committee's deliberations were restricted to a scientific evaluation of potential health hazards posed by each GRAS substance for normal individuals, and, while SCOGS was constantly aware of other factors that FDA was considering in its decision-making process, the Committee did not permit these factors to interfere with the scientific soundness of its conclusions. FDA, in considering revision of regulations with respect to each GRAS substance, regarded the SCOGS reports and conclusions as but one factor in its decision-making process. It is of interest to note that "benefits" were not a part of the SCOGS evaluations (Senti, 1983).

During the 10 years of its work, the Select Committee issued 144 reports presenting its opinions and conclusions and summarized the available information on 468 substances. A listing of these reports is included in the two general overview reports published by the Committee (Select Committee on GRAS Substances, 1977, 1982). The SCOGS overview reports provide detailed information on the framework for evaluation, the problems of interpretation of biological information, and the related background knowledge leading to the final judgments of safety.

The judgment of safety of a food ingredient included assessment of the validity of the toxicologic data; the dynamic nature of food safety criteria; the lack of duplicate studies that insured reproducibility of the reported data; the relevancy of reported findings in subpopulations; bioavailability of the tested substances via absorption from the intestine; and toxicity for human extrapolated from dose ranges as employed in experimental animals.

Based on their many years of experience as a group, the Select Committee made excellent observations on what they termed Extra-Scientific Factors. The members took special pains in making self, as well as group, calibrations from time to time, to reduce the effects of emotion and idiosyncratic biases in making final judgments. They identified the following points: personal leanings on what constitutes safety; differences in the perception of what shall constitute adequate data by the same person for different situations; how much influence "conventional wisdom" has on a decision made; and personal weighting of unconfirmed studies of adverse findings.

It was recognized that these issues influence the decision-making process and vary from person to person, and from time to time in the same person. Therefore, the Select Committee consistently attempted to avoid improper psychological and judgmental overlay and recognized also that subliminal influences inevitably were at work in all meetings of the Committee.

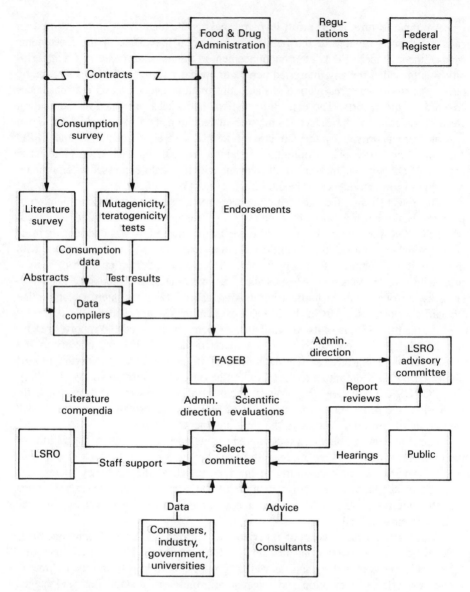

Figure 1 Operational flow in the evaluation of GRAS substances. *(From Select Committee on GRAS Substances, 1977.)*

Two major factors influence the benefit–risk dilemma in assessing the safety of food ingredients. One is the legal requirements that exist for food additives, GRAS, and prior sanctioned substances and laws such as the Delaney Clause regarding carcinogenicity as demonstrated in animals. A description of the technical and legal differences of the terms "food additive," "GRAS," and "Prior Sanctioned Substance" is given in the appendix.

It should be noted that the well-publicized "Delaney Clause" of the 1958 amendment of the FD&C Act does not apply to GRAS substances. For this reason, the
Select Committee's evaluations were not constrained by the serious question about the
safety of a substance found to be carcinogenic even in a single animal study. However, the very existence of this special clause in the law contributed to prolonged
debates on the food safety of numerous substances that had been reported as producing tumors in animals.

Numerous papers are in the literature that point out the problems raised by the
all-or-none absolutism of the Delaney Clause, for example, differences in mechanisms of action of chemical substances, dosage schedules, genetic differences, and
the general significance of extrapolation of animal data to man. These issues led to
critical examination of the often sparse data on many GRAS substances by the Select
Committee. The Committee was successful in arriving at a concluding recommendation in nearly every instance. The final judgments of the Select Committee were
stated in one of the following conclusions:

1 There is no evidence in the available information on ——— that demonstrates or
   suggests reasonable grounds to suspect a hazard to the public when it is used at
   levels that are now current or that might reasonably be expected in the future.
2 There is no evidence in the available information on ——— that demonstrates or
   suggests reasonable grounds to suspect a hazard to the public when it is used at
   levels that are now current and in the manner now practiced. However, it is not
   possible to determine, without additional data, whether a significant increase in
   consumption would constitute a dietary hazard.
3 While no evidence in the available information on ——— demonstrate a hazard
   to the public when it is used at levels that are now current and in the manner now
   practiced, uncertainties exist requiring that additional studies should be conducted.
4 The evidence on ——— is insufficient to determine that the adverse effects reported are not deleterious to the public health when it is used at levels that are
   now current and in the manner now practiced.

In a few instances, no information could be found that was useful in arriving at a
judgment of safety. In these cases the Select Committee noted that there was insufficient data on which to make an evaluation.

It is of interest to learn that only a small fraction of GRAS substances have been
evaluated by an array of tests of safety that are required for the approval of a new
food additive. Gradually, new toxicity information is being developed for those substances the Committee placed in categories three and four.

BENEFITS OF FOOD INGREDIENTS

Benefit–risk issues are well recognized for therapeutic drugs, where possible hazards
of drug therapy are weighed against the often life-saving benefits. In the case of food
additives and GRAS substances, it is extremely difficult to make such risk–benefit

decisions. When millions of people may be the consumers of a food, it is impossible to decide if some or any individual(s) will be unduly exposed to a hazard by a single ingredient. In addition, the perception of what constitutes a benefit will vary from person to person.

A health benefit, such as an essential vitamin or mineral, can be established readily. For such substances, the benefits can be equated against potential hazards. In its work the Select Committee took the position that benefits were not considered in evaluating the health aspects of the GRAS substances, except in the case of certain vitamins and minerals such as vitamins A and D and certain iron compounds. In these special cases the health benefits were considered to outweigh the potential risks, and the substances were considered safe for use in foods with the recognition that over-dosage may prove to be hazardous. Therefore, for GRAS substances no overt attempt was made to arrive at a benefit–risk assessment. The Select Committee assumed that all these substances were originally used as foods or food ingredients for some obvi-ous or easily recognized "benefit" that perhaps had only historical roots. Thus, the difficult task of evaluating benefits was left for the regulatory agency to wrestle with.

Some benefits are readily recognized, and the associated risks can be measured. Such benefit–risk decisions are a part of the legal statutes that address management of risks attendant to the use of chemical substances in society in the United States. Key among these are the Food, Drug and Cosmetic Act, the Federal Meat Inspection Act, the Occupational Safety and Health Act, the Federal Insecticide, Fungicide, and Ro-denticide Act, and the Toxic Substances Control Act (Todhunter, 1983). In most cases the regulatory agencies avoid comparison of economic benefits to risks to human health. Todhunter (1983) has stated,

> The Environmental Protection Agency has attempted to avoid comparison of risk to bene-fit on the basis of weighing economic factors against human health. In the human health area the approach of the agency has been to compare health risks against health benefits to select a suitable risk mitigation goal. Generally, this is some risk level which is for practical purposes nonexistent or of no significance. If it is decided that regulatory action is needed to reach the stated risk goal, then economic risks are balanced against economic benefits and the most cost effective regulatory option is selected.

ARRIVING AT JUDGMENTS

The examples cited in the work of the Select Committee on GRAS substances clearly illustrate the scope of the difficulties encountered by any group attempting a benefit-risk decision for food ingredients. Other committees and numerous individuals have addressed these same issues, and their reports are valuable because in some instances they have reached different conclusions and have developed different views.

A Social and Economic Committee of the Food Safety Council was asked to evaluate and propose techniques for dealing with societal issues and decisions on the level of acceptable risk for substances in foods (Food Safety Council, 1982). After several years of debate, recommendations, and public reviews, their report was not acceptable to the Board of Trustees of the Council. This Board was composed of an equal number of representatives from the public (academia, government, professional societies, consumer, and public–interest organizations) and private (primarily related to the food industry) sectors of society. However, the unique and path-finding dimensions of the Committee's report did establish useful criteria and are worth noting.

Three major categories were identified: *economic, conditions of use in foods,* and *information transfer to the consumer by various techniques.* Two economic approaches were suggested: industrial self-regulation and self-enforcement. Self-regulation places the responsibility for minimizing risks solely on the food industry; self-enforcement requires governmental safety standards for food that the industry is expected to follow without regulatory inspectors overseeing every industry process. The latter is essentially the practice in the United States today. In some cases industry sets its own safety standards, and these are endorsed later by the government. A third economic concept of taxation, to raise the retail price of a good product depending on the level of risk the product entailed for the consumer, was rejected as filled with too many implementation problems.

To control conditions of use of potentially harmful substances, it was proposed to decrease the amount of these substances in foods, restrict the forms of delivery or point of sale, restrict use by age, or disperse the exposure to a single substance by permitting the alternate use of several similar substitute substances. Because all these risk-dispersion ideas would make decisions more complex and demand regulators to make more value judgments, the concept was deemed unsatisfactory. To be useful for managing food risks, risk dispersion as envisaged would require a more thorough biological understanding of how substances interact toxicologically than we now possess.

Information transfer to the consumer provides an opportunity to decide whether to expose oneself to a substance by buying a particular food product or not. In this case the risk–benefit decision is transferred to the ultimate consumer but demands appropriate education. The types of information, the methods of information transfer (e.g., labels, media, and public service announcements), and the difficulties and advantages of this kind of an economic approach to risk management were reviewed in detail by the Committee. The present use of these techniques was pointed out, such as labels for the phenylketonuric that the product contain phenylalanine, and warning signs regarding the suspected hazards of saccharin.

The Social and Economic Committee viewed with favor the concept of consumer education and noted that educational programs are one important way to meet society's needs if we are to move toward a system that allows consumers to assume more personal responsibility for their health. It appears that consumer participation is to become an important subject in risk management in the future. However, as noted, this essentially transfers the matter of the risk–benefit dilemma to the consumer.

To assist in this educational experience, the publication of an authoritative volume, *The Food Additives Book*, by Freydberg and Gortner (1982), is noteworthy. This paperback lists 6212 items of branded packaged foods with an evaluation of the additives and the level of concern for the consumer. The safety ratings this volume provides the consumer give a risk estimate for certain food additives in his diet. Benefits are not considered, but risks can be judged objectively. The book tells the reader why an additive has been used in formulating the food. The authors state:

For the most part, the safety assessments made by the authors have conformed with the judgments arrived at by the Select Committee [GRAS]. . . . In some instances they have not, and, when in disagreement, SCOGS has arrived at a somewhat more severe rating in twice the number of instances as *The Food Additives Book.*

The book is to be used as an information source as a basic shopping list. It also offers the advantage of identifying food ingredients that should be avoided by people who may be hypersensitive to these substances. An additives index makes possible the ready identification of specific additives. It may be that as our awareness of environmental hazards of all kinds increases, "educational volumes" of this character will become necessary guides for proper health decisions. In this respect the committees of the Food Safety Council appear to have supplied a useful dimension to the benefit–risk dilemma.

In a 1979 symposium on "Risks vs. Benefits: Future of Food Safety," most of the issues of the benefit–risk dilemma were reviewed (Massachusetts Institute of Technology, 1979). A philosophical discourse on the nature of benefits noted that "benefits," "wants," and "needs" must be defined and these criteria used in determining the acceptable risks that people are willing to take in relation to their food habits (Darby, 1979). These values change as a result of many influences. When sufficient food is available as in the Western World, we then perceive food benefits as contributing to the fulfillment of nonsurvival requisites. On the other hand, for people who consider food as a requisite for sheer survival, the interpretation of "benefit" is quite different. Thus, the entire benefit–risk equation ceases to be a dilemma for such a population.

In this same symposium, the problems of calculation of risk from animal models were reviewed using carcinogenicity as an example and comparing these issues with risk estimation for effects other than cancer (Wodicka, 1979). The author sarcastically observed that those who fight to the death for a linear conservative model to estimate carcinogenesis are willing to accept tolerances for other toxic effects based on 1% of the no-observed-effect level in animals. The implicit distinction is that cancer never shows a threshold, but other forms of toxicity always do.

Miller (1979) pointed out that animal toxicity tests do not measure endpoints of greatest importance to the consumer. People consuming food are primarily concerned about loss of body function, not necessarily death. Animal toxicity tests rarely measure loss of function—toxicity is related to the eventual endpoint, death. People are concerned about how well they will live, and indeed the fear of carcinogenesis is most often related to the debilitating nature of the disease, not necessarily to the death resulting from it. For these reasons, two different evaluation processes are at work, and thus the benefit–risk dilemma becomes even more difficult to resolve.

It may be noted that the Executive Office of the Assembly of Life Sciences of the National Research Council (NRC) has programs that deal with the questions of risk–benefit in broad terms. A committee on Institutional Means for Assessment of Risks to Public Health is completing a report that encompasses food, pharmaceutical, environmental, occupational, and consumer-product risks regulated by the federal government (National Research Council, 1982). The final report of this committee should be useful in resolving some of the issues of the benefit–risk dilemma.

Risk assessment has been viewed as a useful method to utilize the knowledge available for the evaluation of the hazards to human health resulting from food substances by the Grocery Manufacturers of America. They have petitioned FDA to establish a policy permitting the use of food substances that present an "insignificant" risk to human health, to use risk assessment in determining whether specific substances meet this standard, to consider the totality of a substance for humans, and for the use of independent scientific peer-review committees (Grocery Manufacturers of America, 1982). There has been no recorded action on this petition; however, the regulatory agency has used risk assessment in various ways for a number of years.

One may conclude from the reviews cited that the dilemma of benefit–risk for modern society will likely persist for many years to come. Modern man is acquiring increasing technical knowledge, sophistication, and affluence. His expectations outrun his ability to make satisfactory judgments, and it is equally evident that the technical experts are unable to assist in making these societal decisions.

REFLECTIONS ON THE DILEMMA

Society has adopted a schizoid attitude toward the hazards of modern life. So many extreme risks of everyday life are readily accepted, but for a food even a faint suspicion of some toxicity causes it to become taboo. Perhaps this is because in the public mind the word food is synonomous with "safe to consume," and has been so characterized by the watchdog agency, FDA.

Policy makers are frustrated in their attempts to harmonize uncertain risks with an ill-defined desire to evaluate the benefits of food ingredients. Because the present system does not provide for consistent, predictable, and publicized ways to treat risks and benefits of food additives, a number of thoughtful, interpretative papers, often philosophical, have been published that do make specific recommendations.

One of the earliest studies to address the issues of risk assessment in terms of modern society's search for benefits was the book by Lowrance (1976). He pointed out, contrary to the ideas of many people, that mankind is safer today than ever before in history. Gone are the grim pestilences of the Middle Ages—the dangerous machinery and smoke-clogged alleys of the industrial revolution—we no longer have the cavalier disregard of the early 1900s for arsenical pesticides or canned foods preserved with sulfites, boric acid, and formaldehyde. This picture is bluntly drawn by Bettman (1974) in his volume, *The Good Old Days—They Were Terrible.* Today we have the luxury to worry about subtle hazards that, even if detected in prior years, would have been given only low priority compared beside the much greater hazards of years ago.

An example of how our attitude has changed with respect to foods can be illustrated. Of the millions of cans of food consumed each year, cases of food poisoning, once so common, are now so rare as to make the front pages of newspapers. We seldom consider bacterial food intoxication when we consume canned food. On the other hand, some canned foods now carry a special label, "No salt added"—a titillating decision that has been moved to the consumer as if he really possessed the expertise to make such a health decision. Ignoring the physiological need for salt, most people would cite taste as the benefit of salt in food. The presumed risk is a theoretical concept that high-salt diets predispose to hypertension.

It seems that in the modern world, people's values and expectations have changed and we find ourselves confronted with what appear to be strange new hazards that unfortunately no one seems to know how to evaluate in a satisfactory manner. Without debating the need for measure benefits, Lowrance points out there are "degrees of risk" and "degrees of safety." He concludes that a thing is safe if its risks are judged to be acceptable.

Stumpf (1982) developed the theme of balancing hazards against cultural and human values in food safety assessment. In the case of saccharin, for example, he states that the known facts indicate that there are greater benefits and less overall risks by using than banning saccharin. He calls for the regulatory agencies to take into account various values that the present state of culture has strongly affirmed in their food safety decision—not risk alone. To support his proposition, he stipulates the conditions:

—Values have to be ranked so that survival and the high quality of physical and mental functioning have a priority over economic, aesthetic, and convenience value.

—Assessments of safety must also be ranked according to their degree and probability of risk.

—Benefits are an integral part of the calculus in safety assessments inasmuch as benefits deferred or denied amount to costs and risks.

—Where substitutes are available for suspect substances, there is no justification for using the risk-bearing substance.

—Where all options involve risk, every effort should be made to match the highest benefit with the lowest risk.

—In the real world, where each alternative is a bad one, we should choose the least damaging.

Economists have developed a technique called "benefit–cost analysis" to evaluate programs involving the cost of proposed benefits. For social regulation, cost can be translated to "risk," but unlike material costs, human risk involves potentially toxic effects. The concepts have been explored for consumer and worker safety, product safety (not including foods), and energy and the environment (Miller and Yandel, 1979). These authors conclude from extensive case studies that it is not easy to evaluate the impact of benefit–cost analyses on the regulatory process. However, as the skills of economic analysis are acquired, it appears that they will be employed to a greater degree in the decision-making process of regulatory agencies.

Goldblith (1977, 1980) has reviewed the history of our recent concern about unnecessary and undesirable contaminants in foods, beginning with the 1961 aminotriazole incident in the cranberry bogs that brought disaster to the cranberry industry for several years. He concluded that food processing and food technology can benefit from an analysis of benefits versus risks. However, what is required is the information to adequately evaluate risks and better means of assessing benefits. The former can come from the current research investigations in toxicology; the latter requires some yet-to-be-discovered methodology to place quantitative measures on benefits.

An enormous amount of hard thinking, public discussion by well-informed people, and serious debate by numerous segments of society has been devoted to measuring food additive benefits without agreement. Uniform guidelines for risk assessment determinations are obviously necessary for all regulatory agencies—a factor unfortunately missing in most countries of the world. However, to be acceptable, these uniform rules for decisions must be based on detailed and comprehensive written protocols made publicly available and after peer review. This is the only way the benefit–risk dilemma should be approached and, indeed, appears to be the only mechanism acceptable to society.

APPENDIX

The Federal Food, Drug and Cosmetic Act was amended in 1958 to define a food additive as "any substance the intended use of which results or may reasonably be expected to result, directly or indirectly, in its becoming a component or otherwise affecting the characteristics of any food, including any substance intended for use in producing, preparing, treating, packaging, transporting, or holding food." The amendment required that food additives receive approval of the FDA before they can be added to foods intended for use in interstate commerce, approval being based on scientific data provided by the petitioner to demonstrate the absence of hazard when the substance is used in the amount and manner proposed.

At the time of the 1958 amendment, substances in common use as added food ingredients were exempted from the food additives requirements. These were identified as "Substances Generally Recognized as Safe." This particular category of exempted food ingredients came to be called the GRAS list, and the substances on it, GRAS substances. It totals more than 600 substances, including 100 that are added to cotton fabrics or paper and paperboard used as food-packaging materials.

When the GRAS list was established, it was recognized that explicit approval of substances in food prior to 1958 had been grated for several food ingredients by the FDA or by the U.S. Department of Agriculture. These are the so-called "prior-sanctioned" food ingredients.

REFERENCES

Bettman, O. L. 1974. *The Good Old Days—They Were Terrible*. New York: Random.

Carr, C. J. 1981. The nitrite-cancer controversy. *Regul. Toxicol. Pharmacol.* 1:68–77.

Darby, W. J. 1979. The nature of benefits. Seventeenth Annual Underwood–Prescott Memorial Symposium, September 25, 1979, Cambridge, Mass., p. 37.

Environmental Protection Agency. 1982. Chemical testing industry profile of toxicological testing. National Technical Information Service, Springfield, Va., report 82-140773. Capabilities of U.S. Commercial Toxicological Testing Laboratories.

Food Safety Council. 1980. Proposed system for food safety assessment. Report of the Scientific Committee. The Nutrition Foundation. Washington, D.C.

Food Safety Council. 1982. A proposed food safety evaluation process. Report of the Social and Economic Committee: A new approach: Principles and processes for making food safety decisions, p. 5. The Nutrition Foundation, Washington, D.C.

Francke, D. W., and Ng, S. K. 1983. Characteristics and capabilities of U.S. commercial toxicological testing laboratories. *Regul. Toxicol. Pharmacol.* 3:372–380.

Freydberg, N., and Gortner, W. A. 1982. *The Food Additives Book.* New York: Bantam.

Goldblith, S. A. 1977. The use and abuse of food technology in the quality of our food supply. In *Food and Nutrition in Health and Disease, Ann. New York Acad. Sci.*, 300, eds. N. H. Moss and J. Mayer, pp. 161–166.

Goldblith, S. A. 1980. Risk versus benefits: The future of food safety. *Nutr. Rev.* 38:35–40.

Grocery Manufacturers of America. 1982. Comments by Sherwin Gardner before Public Meeting on Risk Assessment, Assembly of Life Sciences, National Academy of Sciences, February 10, 1982.

Hayes, A. H. 1983. United States Food & Drug Administration approach to risk evaluation and risk management for foods. *Regul. Toxicol. Pharmacol.* 3:152–157.

Lowrance, W. W. 1976. *Of Acceptable Risk—Science and The Determination of Safety.* Los Altos, Calif.: Kaufmann.

Massachusetts Institute of Technology. 1979. Seventeenth Annual Underwood–Prescott Memorial Symposium, September 25, 1979, Cambridge, Mass.

Miller, J. C., and Yandle, B. 1979. Benefit-cost analyses of social regulation. Case studies from the Council on Wage and Price Stability. American Enterprise Institute for Public Policy Research, Washington, D.C.

Miller, S. A. 1979. The new metaphysics. Seventeenth Annual Underwood–Prescott Memorial Symposium, September 25, 1979, Cambridge, Mass., p. 53.

National Academy of Sciences. 1981. The health effects of nitrate, nitrite, and *N*-nitroso compounds. Washington, D.C.: National Academy Press.

National Academy of Sciences. 1982. *Diet, Nutrition and Cancer.* Washington, D.C.: National Academy of Press.

National Research Council. 1982. Annual Report July 1981–June 1982, Assembly of Life Sciences. Washington, D.C.: National Academy Press.

Select Committee on GRAS Substances. 1977. Evaluation of health aspects of GRAS food ingredients: Lessons learned and questions unanswered. *Fed. Proc.* 36:2519–2562.

Select Committee on GRAS Substances. 1982. Insights on food safety evaluation. Life Sciences Research Office, FASEB, Bethesda, Md.

Senti, F. R. 1983. Insights on food safety evaluation: A synopsis. *Regul. Toxicol. Pharmacol.* 3:133–138.

Stumpf, S. E. 1982. Food safety assessment reflecting cultural changes, novel hazards, and human values. *Regul. Toxicol. Pharmacol.* 2:323–330.

Todhunter, J. A. 1983. Risk management strategy under the Toxic Substances Control Act and the Federal Insecticide, Fungicide, and Rodenticide Act. *Regul. Toxicol. Pharmacol.* 3:163–171.

Wodicka, V. O. 1979. Risk and responsibility. Seventeenth Annual Underwood–Prescott Memorial Symposium, September 25, 1979, Cambridge, Mass., p. 45.

Chapter 12

Animal Toxins

R. P. Sharma

M. J. Taylor

INTRODUCTION

Toxins are specific products of living organisms that when introduced into the tissues or body of higher animals, are capable of producing notably toxic effects. Animal venoms are typical of this category, and many of these are typically proteinaceous in character and antigenic in nature. A large number of smaller molecules, which by themselves are not capable of being antigenic, are now considered toxins because of their biologic origin. Chemically the group of toxins may range from complex molecules, many of which are still incompletely characterized, to relatively simple molecules such as formic acid produced by certain arthropods.

It is believed that most animals have developed toxins during evolution to help them survive in the environment. The venoms are used by animals to produce food by either killing or paralyzing the prey or to defend themselves from other predators in the environment. In certain species, the enzymatic secretions may also possess digestive or other metabolic properties. Yet the exact reason for the presence of toxins in some species of animals is not clearly understood. In some cases the toxins found in animals may not be produced by the host itself. For example, the toxins present in certain shellfish organs are produced by protozoan parasites and are merely concentrated in tissues of the host. Animal toxins produce their effects in other animals either by envenomation (bite or sting), by ingestion by people or other predators, or through external contact with the toxin or the venomous animal.

GENERAL CHARACTERISTICS OF ANIMAL TOXINS

A large number of animal toxins are represented by proteinaceous colloidal secretions called *venoms* or venins. Snake venom is a typical example of this class. They are secreted by highly specialized venom glands and can even be toxic to the host if introduced into other tissues. The toxins are confined usually to a smaller part of the animal body. Many of the protein components have enzymatic properties and cause degradation of biological molecules or cellular components. These toxins may be thermolabile and antigenic in nature.

Smaller proteins or peptides present in snake or other animal venoms are often responsible for much of their harm by having very specific biological properties. Their effects are typically produced on the nervous system or other vital systems, e.g., cardiovascular or renal organs. Rapid or even irreversible effects can be produced by these molecules. The proteins and peptides are often susceptible to the proteases present in the digestive tract; the venoms must be introduced parenterally to produce their maximal effect. Ingestion of a venom, however, is not absolutely safe, since the smaller molecules can be absorbed through cuts or ulcerative areas of the mucous membranes in the upper gastrointestinal tract. Often only a very small amount of toxin is needed to produce a toxic response.

A variety of biologically active amines, acids, or other relatively smaller molecules are found as active principles in a variety of animal toxins. Some of these are highly irritant and act as contact toxins. Others may be absorbed by the tissues to produce their degenerative or other specific effects. Yet other types of active components in animal toxins may be alkaloidal or glycosidal in nature. Some of these are extremely toxic and have either generalized or localized effects on vital functions when ingested by people. These toxins are thermostable and not altered by the cooking or other processing of food. In some cases the toxins may be ingested for a long time, since the food may be consumed without the appreciation of toxic hazards associated with it.

There is only a casual relationship between the chemical nature of the toxin and the animal species producing it. The same animal often has venom containing complex mixtures of a variety of toxic products. On the other hand, a single toxin may be present in different species of animals, even ones belonging to different classes. For example, tetrodotoxin, a potent substance associated with the puffer fish, may be found in certain types of amphibian species. Remarkable similarities in toxic components have been noted in snake venoms of animals belonging to different genera, yet a large variation may be found in the venom composition of snakes from the same species.

TOXIC SYNDROMES FROM ANIMAL TOXINS

The toxic effects produced by animal toxins may be as varied as the chemicals associated with them. In venomous poisonings, the toxic effects are generally the result of a bite. Both localized and generalized phenomena are often observed. The local reaction may result either from the destruction of tissue by toxins or as a result of hypersensitivity to the retained material. Tissue destruction leads to necrotizing and subsequent secondary infections. The hypersensitivity reaction may be delayed, taking from a few to several days before maximum damage occurs. An allergic reaction may be immediate if the victim has been sensitized to the venomous components in the past.

Remote or generalized reactions may involve either specific organs or systems or even several systems. The most dangerous toxins affect the central nervous system and may cause damage in one or more areas of the brain. Some of these reactions may be irreversible, even fatal in many instances. The physiologic effects of some toxins are so specific that these toxins have been used as tools in molecular biology to understand normal physiological processes. Some of these illustrations have been indicated later in this chapter. Various types of toxins may possess cardiotoxic, hepatotoxic, or nephrotoxic principles. Generalized allergic reactions leading to the release of vasoactive substances and therefore complex syndromes are observed as a response to toxins in certain individuals.

A variety of toxins may produce simply an irritating effect when they come in contact with the skin or external parts of people or other animals. The effects of such toxins are generally not fatal and are particularly useful to the toxin-producing animals for their survival, since predators often avoid them.

TOXINS IN VENOMOUS SNAKES

Snake venom is a highly complex mixture of proteins, peptides, amines, and a variety of nonproteinaceous substances. The composition of the venom is highly variable, depending on the species, sex, and age of the animal. Nearly 90–95% of the dry venom consists of proteins. Many of these have enzymatic properties and are either directly toxic or facilitate the effects of other toxic components. The small amount of nonprotein material consists of inorganic materials (primarily metals), and organic substances that include nucleotides, carbohydrates, lipids, and biogenic amines. The composition of snake venoms has been reviewed in detail elsewhere (Tu, 1977) and will be only briefly described here. The important toxic factors present in the venom of *Naja naja* are listed in Table 1.

A large number of species and varieties of snakes are found around the world, although a considerable number of species are nonvenomous and therefore harmless. The venomous snakes belong to five major families: Hydrophiidae (sea snakes), Elapidae (cobras and kraits), Viperidae (vipers), Crotalidae (includes pit vipers and rattlesnakes), and Colubridae (the tree snakes).

Enzymes in Snake Venoms

A complex mixture of enzymatic and nonenzymatic proteins are found in snake venoms. Although the nonenzymatic proteins are relatively more toxic, the overall effect of envenomation is a combination of effects produced by both types of proteins. The venom enzymes actively participate in blood coagulation, or may cause anticoagulation, hemorrhage, hemolysis, lysis of cell and mitochondrial membranes, and even

Table 1   Major Toxic Factors Found in *Naja naja* Venom

Factor(s)	Action or effect
L-amino acid oxidase	Conversion of amino acids to keto acids, activation of tissue peptidase
Acetylcholinesterase	May cause muscle paralysis, hydrolyzes acetylcholine
AMPase	Destruction of AMP
L-Arginine esterase	Hydrolysis of arginine
ATPase	Hydrolysis of ATP
DNAase	Destruction of DNA
Exopeptidase	Destroys proteins, causes tissue damage
Hyaluronidase	Hydrolysis of 1–4 linkage of hyaluronic acid, dissolves connective tissue, spreading factor
Invertase	Breakdown of sugars and polysaccharides
Lipase	Hydrolyzes lipids, destroys membranes
NADase	Hydrolyzes NAD
Phosphodiesterase	Hydrolyzes 5'-phosphate on neucleotides, prevents tissue repair, hypotension
Alkaline phosphatase and acid phosphatase	Destroy various phosphates, including nucleotides
Phospholipase A, B, C.	Hydrolyze phosphatidylcholine and cause damage to cellular membranes
Protease	Proteolytic, tissue damage
Antifibrinolysin, antiprothrombic factor, antithromboplastic factor, and fibrinolysin	Interfere with the clotting mechanism, induce hemorrhage
Cardiotoxin	Cardiovascular damage
Hemorrhagin	Induce hemorrhage
Neurotoxin	Peptides, polypeptides, and amines, cause neurotoxic effects
Complement (C-3) inhibitor	Prevents complement activity, interferes with the immune mechanisms

affect axonal conduction. Some of the enzymes found in venoms are briefly described here.

Phospholipase A_2 (also known as lecithinase) is the most common enzyme found in various snake venoms. The enzyme has been isolated from Elapidae, Viperidae, and Crotalidae species. This enzyme is extremely stable and resistant to heat denaturation. The molecular weight of the enzyme is in the order of 9,000–15,000, except in certain species it is present as a dimer (20,000–30,000 daltons). The amino acid sequences of several types of phospholipase A_2 have been described. The enzyme has a high specificity for hydrolyzing phosphatidylcholine at the β (C_2) position. Some venoms contain more than one type of phospholipase A_2. The effect of this enzyme is highly apparent on membrane structures. It causes disintegration of mitochondria and subsequent disruption of electron transport. The release of vesicle-bound acetylcholine at nerve endings has been observed, including those in the central nervous system, even though the enzyme has a limited ability to cross the blood–brain barrier. Increase in cell-membrane permeability has been reported, along with a high hemo-lytic property. The LD50 of the purified enzyme is considered to be about 8 mg/kg in mice, given parenterally.

• The *phosphodiesterases* present in the snake venoms include exonucleases, en-donucleases, and enzymes that hydrolyze adenosine triphosphate (ATP) into adeno-sine monophosphate (AMP) and pyrophosphate. Most of these enzymes have not been purified. The snake-venom exonucleases hydrolyze nucleotides of any chain length. Both RNA and DNA may be employed as a substrate. The enzymes also hydrolyze nicotinamide dinucleatide (NAD) into nicotinamide mononucleotide and AMP. Little is known about the chemical structures of these enzymes. Small amounts of endonucleotidases (RNAase and DNAase) have been reported in snake venoms. It is suggested that even the exonuclease in snake venom may have a limited activity as an endonuclease. All five families of venomous snakes have been known to possess these enzymes.

Several specific and nonspecific *phosphomonoesterases* (phosphatases) have been described in various venoms. Certain venoms contain both acid and alkaline phospha-tases, whereas others may have only one or the other type. The specific phosphatases may include 5′-nucleotidase, which has high specificity to 5′-AMP and also hydro-lyzes 5′-CMP and 5′-UMP.

L-Amino acid oxidase, a nonhydrolytic enzyme, has been described in snake venoms. The property of this enzyme is to convert free amino acids into α-ketoacids. The molecular weight of this enzyme ranges from 85,000 to 153,000, with enzymes of 130,000 daltons most consistently reported. Isozymes with similar specific activi-ties have been suggested. The LD50 of the purified enzyme is reported to be 9 mg/kg in mice.

A variety of *proteolytic enzymes* have been recognized in snake venoms. Crotali-dae venoms possess strong proteolytic activity, whereas other venoms may have ei-ther weak or no proteolytic action. The proteases are not highly lethal but may have strong local effects. Both endo- and exopeptidases are found, although the exopepti-dase activity is limited to di- and tripeptides. Other proteases include collagenase and elastase. Several other esterases, such as arginine ester hydrolase, have been de-scribed in Elapidae and Hydrophiidae venoms. These are obviously distinct from the proteolytic enzymes.

A heat-sensitive *acetylcholinesterase* has been isolated from the venoms of Ela-pid and Hydrophiid snakes. The enzyme has a molecular weight of 103,000 daltons. This enzyme has similar specificity but is much smaller than the similar one isolated from other sources like electric eel. Other analogs of choline esters are hydrolyzed by this enzyme. The biological significance of this enzyme in venom is not clear.

Hyaluronidase, an enzyme effective in hydrolyzing hyaluronic acid (a mucopoly-saccharide found in connective tissue), is present in many venoms, including those from snakes. This is often referred to as a "spreading factor" because of its ability to facilitate diffusion of toxins or other materials in tissues. Nearly all venomous snakes, with the possible exception of Hydrophiidae, possess this factor.

Other less-frequent enzymes found in snake venoms include amylases, NAD nucelosidase, glutamic–pyruvic transaminase, and lactate dehydrogenase. In addition, there are several enzyme inhibitors present in snake venoms. These include phospholipase A_2 inhibitor, acetylcholinesterase inhibitor, angiotensinase inhibitor, and the proteinase inhibitor.

Neurotoxic Proteins in Snake Venoms

At least two distinct types of neurotoxic proteins, with different pharmacological properties, have been found in snake venoms. The first are the postsynaptic neurotoxins that combine with the postsynaptic acetylcholine receptors and resemble *d*-tubocurarine in their action. Although these proteins from different species of snakes may be slightly different in their chemical structures, there are remarkable similarities noted in their specific amino acid sequences. More than 50 such proteins have been sequenced for their amino acid residues, and these illustrate the presence of a number of "invariant" amino acids. The proteins generally fall into two major categories, the "short" ones with 60–62 amino acids and the "long" ones with 71–74 amino acid residues. The short neurotoxic proteins are structurally similar to "cardiotoxins" present in elapid venoms (see later).

The amino acid sequences of a number of postsynaptic neurotoxins have been reviewed (Tu, 1977; Yang, 1978). A number of homologous toxins, including those with cardiotoxic properties, have three identical residues: Tyr 25, Gly 44, and Pro 50. In addition there are eight half-cystine residues (3, 17, 24, 45, 49, 60, 61, 66) present that are responsible for the folding of the protein molecule. Additional invariant residues include Try 29, Asp 31, Arg 37, and Gly 38 in these neurotoxic compounds.

Pharmacological and toxic properties of these neurotoxins have been studied in detail and reviewed (Tamiya et al., 1978; Tu, 1977; Yang, 1978). The LD50 of cobra neurotoxin given intravenously in mice is estimated to be 50–150 μg/kg. On a molar basis this is considerably more potent than *d*-tubocurarine. The toxin causes respiratory paralysis and asphyxiation, often accompanied by violent spasms. The neuromuscular blockage induced by the long neurotoxins is virtually nonreversible. Because of this latter property, some of the purified neurotoxins have been usefully employed in characterizing the acetylcholine receptor.

The second type are presynaptic neurotoxins, which have been relatively less studied. These proteins are partly similar in structure to phospholipase A. Some of the presynaptic proteins isolated from venoms include crotoxin (from South American rattlesnake), β-bungarotoxin (Taiwan krait), notexin (Australian tiger snake), and taipoxin (Australian taipan). Toxins II-B-2 and III-A and B from Indian krait are also presynaptic in nature. All these are sightly larger in molecular weight than the postsynaptic neurotoxins.

The presynaptic neurotoxins are much more potent than the postsynaptic ones in inducing paralysis. Although their effect somewhat resembles the botulinum toxin, the two are different in their mechanism and indeed are antagonistic in their function.

Cardiotoxins and Cytotoxins

A number of basic proteins, other than neurotoxins, have been found in snake venoms, particularly from Elapid snakes. The structures of these proteins have a remarkable resemblance to the neurotoxic components of venoms (Tu, 1977). The cardiotoxins are similar to the short neurotoxins and have an LD50 of 1.5 mg/kg in mice. These proteins cause systolic arrest of amphibian or mammalian heart. They also cause irreversible polarization of muscle-cell membrane. The contraction of guinea pig ilium produced by these proteins can be antagonized by atropine. Several larger cardiotoxins have also been described.

The cardiotoxic proteins also possess cytotoxic properties in various cell cultures. In addition, venoms from Crotalids and Viperids contain additional cytotoxic components that can cause cell lysis in culture. The amino acid sequence of some of these cytotoxic proteins is identical to those described for cardiotoxic substances.

Effects of Envenomation

The overall hazard of a snake bite is a combination of the relative potency of its venom and the amount that a particular snake may release during the bite. Some species can yield as much as 720 mg dry venom from their glands and can be far more toxic than another species with a low yield, even though the toxicity of venom may be higher in case of the latter. The relative potencies of several venoms from selected species are listed in Table 2.

Various factors influence the severity of a snake bite. Apart from the toxicity of venom, the size of snake is also important, since large snakes are likely to have larger venom glands. In most cases the venom gland is nearly emptied when a snake bites its victim. Therefore, the period elapsed between the last prey and the bite may be important if the supply of the venom is not fully replenished in the gland. Juveniles and yearlings have more toxic venoms than the adult snakes. Toxicity of rattlesnake and copperhead venoms reaches a peak at the age of 6–9 months, after which a slight decrease may be noticed. There are no definite differences based on the sex of the snakes. Toxicity of a snake bite, of course, is largely dependent on the species of snake, the size of the victim, and whether all the venom was released during the bite.

Venoms from snakes of the Hydrophiidae family contain potent neurotoxins that are among the most toxic substances in the world; they are more toxic than terrestrial snakes, including copperheads, rattlesnakes, kraits, and cobras (Tu, 1974). Sea-snake bites are common among fishermen in coastal areas. Sea snakes are found in the coastal waters of Baja California, Mexico, Central and South America, Southeast Asia, the Far East, Australia, Indonesia, Burma, India, Iran, the Arabian peninsula, and eastern Africa. The amount of crude venom from sea snakes is very small, ranging from 0.2 to 19 mg/snake depending on the size of the animal. Sea-snake bites are characterized by generalized myalgia, starting 30 min to 1 h after the bite. Aches, pain, and stiffness occur when arm, thigh, neck, or trunk muscles are moved. Myoglobinurea becomes evident 3–6 h after the bite.

Table 2   Poisonous Snakes, Their Origin, and Relative Toxicity of Venom[a]

Species	Common name	Origin	LD50, iv, mice (mg/kg)
Family: *Hydrophiidae* (sea snakes)			
Enhydrina schistosa	Sea snake	Worldwide	2.3
Hydrophis cyanocinctus	Sea snake	Africa, Asia	4.8
Hydrophis spiralis	Sea snake	Africa, Asia	5.0
Hydrophis melanosoma	Sea snake	East Indies	8.0
Kerilia jerdoni	Sea snake	Asia	10.6
Family: *Elapidae* (cobras)			
Micrurus fulvius fulvius	Eastern coral snake	Southeastern and southwestern United States	0.006
Dendroaspis jamesoni	Jameson's mamba	Africa	0.008
Dendroaspis polylepis	Black mamba	Africa	0.011
Naja haje	Egyptian corbra	Africa	0.02
Hemachatus haemachates	Ringhal's cobra	Africa	0.03
Bungarus caeruleus	Indian krait, blue krait	India, Ceylon	0.05
Bungarus ceylonicus	Sinhalese krait	Ceylon	0.06
Naja nivea	Cape cobra	South Africa	0.06
Dendroaspis angusticeps	Green mamba	Africa	0.06
Bungarus fasciatus	Banded krait	Southeast Asia	0.07
Bungarus multicinctus	Many-banded krait	China	0.07
Naja melanoleuca	Black forest cobra	Africa	0.5
Naja naja	Common cobra	Asia	0.5
Naja nigricollis	Spitting cobra	Africa	1.0
Ophiophagus hannah	King cobra	Asia	1.5
Family: *Viperidae* (vipers)			
Vipera russelli	Russell's viper	Middle East, Asia	0.1
Causus rhombeatus	Night adder	Africa	0.18
Bitis nasicornis	Rhinoceros viper	Africa	1.0
Echis carinatus	Saw-scale viper	Middle East	1.0
Bitis caudalis	Sand viper	South Africa	1.2
Bitis arietans	Puff adder	Africa	2.0
Bitis gabonica	Gaboon viper	Africa	2.0
Family: *Crotalidae* (pit vipers)			
Ancistrodon acutus	Sharp-nosed viper	China	0.04
Crotalus aculatus	Mojave rattlesnake	Western United States	0.2

(See footnote on p. 447.)

Table 2   Poisonous Snakes, Their Origin, and Relative Toxicity of Venom[a]
(*Continued*)

Species	Common name	Origin	LD50, iv, mice (mg/kg)
Sistrurus catenatus catenatus	Massasauga	Central United States	0.6
Ancistrodon bilineatus	Mexican moccasin	Central America	1.0
Trimeresurus popeorum	Bamboo viper	Southeast Asia	1.0
Ancistrodon halys	Pallas' viper	China	1.2
Crotalus durissus terrificus	Tropical rattlesnake	Central and southern United States	1.2
Bothrops atrox	Barba amarilla	Central America	1.4
Trimeresurus albolabris	White-lipped viper	Southeast Asia	1.5
Trimeresurus purpureomaculatus	Mangrove viper	Southeast Asia	1.5
Crotalus viridis viridis	Prairie rattlesnake	Western United States	1.5
Lachesis muta	Bushmaster	Central America	1.5
Bothreps schlegelii	Schlegil's viper	Central America	1.6
Crotalus adamanteus	Eastern diamond-back rattlesnake	Southeast United States	2.0
Bothrops nummifer	Jumping viper	Central America	2.4
Crotalus cerastes cerastes	Sidewinder	Western United States	2.6
Trimeresurus wagleri	Wagler's pit viper	Southeast Asia	3.0
Calloselasma rhodostoma	Malayan pit viper	Southeast Asia	3.6
Ancistrodon piscivorus piscivorus	Cottonmouth water moccasin	Southeast and southwest United States	4.0
Crotalus atrox	Western diamond-back rattlesnake	Western United States	4.0
Crotalus ruber	Red-diamond rattlesnake	Western United States	4.0
Trimeresurus flavoviridis	Habu	Southeast Asia	4.3
Bothrops nasuta	Hognosed viper	Central America	4.6
Ancistrodon contortrix controtrix	Southern copper-head, northern copperhead	Southeast and northeast United States	8.0
Sistrurus miliarius barbouri	Ground rattler	Southeast United States	10.0
Family: *Calubridae* (tree snakes)			
Dispholidus typus	Boomslang	Central and South Africa	0.0012
Thelotornis kirtlandi	Vine snake	Central and South Africa	0.021

[a]Compiled from Tu (1977), Barne (1968), and Christensen (1968).

The family Elapidae comprises a large group of different species of snakes, including cobras, coral snakes, kraits, and death adders. Neurotoxins from Elapid snakes cause death in untreated subjects within 24–48 h. The venoms are complex, as is the symptomology of elapid bites. The major symptoms are characteristic of a competitive block of cholinoceptive receptors. Drowsiness, thirst, nausea, muscle weakness, and flaccid paralysis of facial muscles, which extends to the limbs, are observed as the degree of poisoning progresses. Finally, respiratory distress and death occur (Watt et al., 1974).

Viperidae venoms are less toxic than Elapidae and Hydrophiidae venoms but more potent than Crotalidae venoms. Venoms from viperids produce a paralytic effect in the central nervous system, circulatory failure, intravascular clots, hemorrhage, and direct paralytic action.

The snakes of the Crotalidae family contain venoms with a greater array of biologically active components than either Elapidae or Hydrophiidae venoms, and have a more complex spectrum of pharmacologic actions. The toxin produced by these animals (termed *crotoxin*) has neurotoxic activity, and in addition has blood clotting, hemolysis effects, causes an immediate and transitory fall in blood pressure, and finally respiratory disturbance.

The family Colubridae is the largest family of snakes, including about 250 genera and over 1000 species. Because of the anatomical location of their fangs (posterior maxillary), there are few clinically significant envenomations by these animals. However, deaths have been occasionally reported. The venoms are not fully characterized and have various enzymatic and neurotoxic properties. The venom components have immunologic cross-reactivity with sera against venoms of other families and are believed to be qualitatively similar (Boquet and Saint-Girons, 1972).

The management of snake bite requires immediate attention to make the effort successful. The first priority should be to prevent the absorption of venom at the site of envenomation. Suction and washing of the wound are helpful (suction by mouth should be avoided). Cold packs and tourniquet have been suggested to decrease the blood flow. The use of antivenin is the most beneficial measure in therapy; if possible, specific antivenin should be employed. Often an allergic reaction may be observed following injection of antisera. Other symptomatic treatments, including those for pain, blood loss, allergy, and/or local tissue damage, are helpful.

TOXIC LIZARDS

The two species of heloderma, *Heloderma suspectum* (Gila monster) and *H. horridum* (Mexican beaded lizard), are known to be toxic by the production of venoms. The upper teeth in these animals are grooved, and there are four venom glands on each side that bathe the teeth from the top. In case of a bite, all the upper teeth are dangerous. When these lizards bite, they hold on in a chewing fashion, and this process helps the delivery of venom more efficiently than a simple bite. The toxic effects in the victim include pain and swelling at the site of envenomation, which progresses upward in the body. Cardiovascular shock and depression of central nervous system may follow, although fatalities are rare. Cases of such lizards biting humans are infrequent.

AMPHIBIAN POISONS

The common poisonous amphibia include frogs, toads, and salamanders. The poisonous material is usually contained in skin glands, which are often distributed throughout the body surfaces. The glands in some cases may be localized, such as the parotid glands. Various amphibian species are not truely venomous since they are unable to inject toxic substance into their prey. These animals indeed have toxic secretions that act as a defense mechanism toward predators. In most cases the toxic secretions are offensive in odor or highly irritant, so that a predator easily learns to avoid them. However, some extremely toxic substances have been isolated from these animals. The chemicals are highly variable in composition and toxicity potential. However, unrelated animal species may sometimes exhibit remarkable similarity in the types of toxic materials present in their tissues.

The various types of toxic materials that have been characterized include biogenic amines and their derivatives, peptides, proteins, and a variety of alkaloids (Daly and Witkop, 1971). Of these, only some of the alkaloids are extremely toxic. Some nontoxic alkaloids and substituted amines are responsible for the irritant nature of skin secretions and may possess important physiological function in the host itself (e.g., skin coloration). Some of the major toxic constituents of these toxins are described as follows.

Biogenic Amines

A variety of amines—namely, norepinephrine, serotonin, histamine, and their derivatives—have been reported in skin secretions of frogs and toads. Amines in amounts of more than 1 mg/g skin have been found in various anurans. The most common of these are serotonin and its methyl derivatives (Table 3). Derivatives of

Table 3   Various Biogenic Amines Found in Frogs and Toads

Class of amine	Chemical	Families of animals
Indoleamine derivatives	Tryptamine, serotonin, N-methyl serotonin, bufotenine, bufotenin sulfate ester, bufotenidine, dehydrobufotenine, bufothionine	*Leptodectylus,* Hylidae, Ranidae, Discoglossidae, Bufonidae
Phenolic quaternary amines	Tyramine, leptodectyline, p-OH-leptodectyline	Anurans
Catecholamines	Epinephrine, norepinephrine, dopamine, epinine	Bufonidae
Histamine	Histamine, N-methyl histamine, N-acetyl histamine, N,N-dimethyl histamine, spinaceamine, 6-methylspinaceamine	*Leptodectylus,* Hylidae

various indolamines are present in secretions of *Hyla, Rana,* and *Bufo* species. One of the common indolamine derivatives found in the largest amount is N,N'-dimethylserotonin or bufotenine. The structures of selected amine derivatives are indicated in Fig. 1.

A phenolic quarternary amine, leptodectyline, has been reported in anurans. Smaller amounts of *p*-hydroxyleptodectyline and tryptamine are also found in their skins. Catecholamines have been reported in the glands of toads of the genus *Bufo*, the major amine of this class being epinephrine. Histamine and its derivatives have been reported in anurans from the genera *Leptodectylus* and *Hyla*. Most of these biogenic amines are irritant to mucous membranes and hence are strong deterrents to predators.

Peptides and Proteins

A variety of peptides, some of which have hypotensive potential and are hence extremely toxic, have been isolated from certain frogs (Table 4). All toxic peptides (bradykinin, caerulein, and physalaemin) produce strong vasodilation and cause stimulation of smooth muscles. In addition, these peptides also possess irritant properties.

Toxic hemolytic proteins of high molecular weight have been described in the skins of anurans. Most of these are not well characterized but are known to be very toxic (Mar and Michl, 1976).

Alkaloids from Amphibian Skins

A number of toxic alkaloids have been found in a variety of poisonous toads and frogs (Table 5). One of the most toxic of these, batrachotoxin, is a steroidal alkaloid found

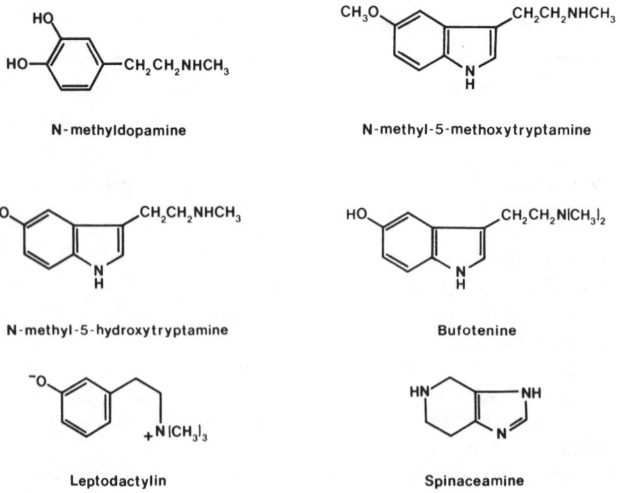

Figure 1 Some biogenic amine derivatives found in amphibian venoms.

Table 4 Representative Toxic Peptides from Amphibians

Peptide	Structure	Species associated
Bradykinin	Arg-Pro-Pro-Gly-Phe-Ser- Pro-Phe-Arg	*Rana temporaria,* *Phyllomedusa rohdei,* *Acaphus truei*
Physalaemin	Pyroglu-Ala-Asp-Pro- Asp(NH$_2$)-Lys-Phe-Tyr- Gly-Leu-Met(NH$_2$)	*Physalaemus fuscumaculatus,* *Phyllomedusa rohdei*
Caerulein	Pyroglu-Glu-Asp-Tyr(SO$_3$H)- Tyr-Gly-Trp-Met-Asp-PheNH$_2$	*Hyla caerulea,* *Leptodectylus* sp.

in dentrobates. Over 1000 biologically active alkaloids have been described in these animals (Daly, 1982). Over a dozen derivatives of batrachotoxin are naturally found in amphibia.

Batrachotoxin The Colombian arrow poison frog (*Phyllobates aurotaenia*) contains a mixture of deadly alkaloids of this family. The structure of batrachotoxin is indicated in Fig. 2. One adult frog may contain 50 μg labile active toxin and equal amounts of other less toxic substances. The lethal dose of batrachotoxin in mammals has been suggested to be nearly 2 μg/kg. This makes it one of the most toxic chemicals known (other than some toxins of bacterial origin). Homobatrachotoxin (2-ethyl, 4-methyl-pyrrol-3-carboxylate analog) is the other major congener and has a similar toxic potential.

Table 5 Miscellaneous Toxins Isolated from Frog and Toad Tissues

Toxin	Nature	Toxic dose (mg/kg)[a]
Batrachotoxin	Alkaloid (several congeners isolated)	0.002
Pumiliotoxin C	Alkaloid	>20
Histrionicotoxins	Alkaloid	>5
Pumiliotoxin A and B	Alkaloid	2.5(A), 1.5(B)
Gephyrotoxin	Alkaloid	>10
Chiriquitoxin	Alkaloid	—
Zetekitoxin	Alkaloid	0.08 (ip)
Tetrodotoxin	Alkaloid	0.008
Bufogenins	Steroidal	—
Bufotoxins	Steroidal alkaloid	—

[a]LD50 in mice (subcutaneous, except as noted). Most chemicals found in skin extracts, except chiriquitoxin also found in eggs and tetrodotoxin in eggs only. Based on Daly (1982) and Brown et al. (1977).

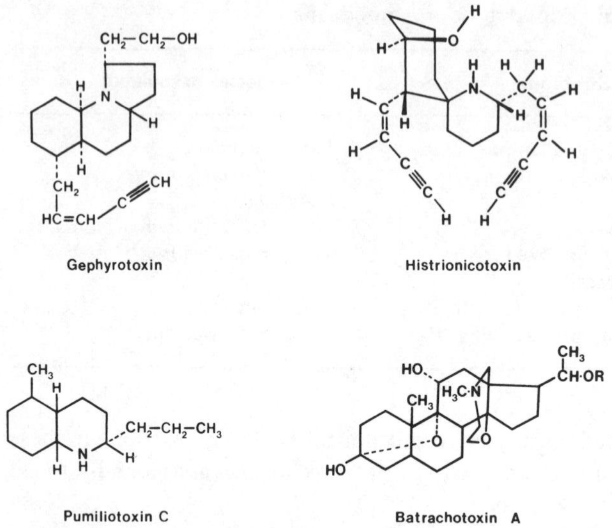

Gephyrotoxin

Histrionicotoxin

Pumiliotoxin C

Batrachotoxin A

Figure 2 Structures of selected toxins from amphibian venoms. In batrachotoxin A, R=H, whereas in batrachotoxin, which is one of the most toxic compounds of this class,

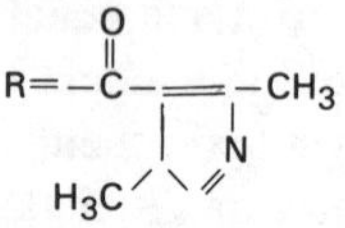

Because of its extreme toxicity and unique pharmacologic activity, batrachotoxin has been investigated in detail (Albuquerque et al., 1971). The alkaloid and its congeners depolarize neurons and muscle cells by a specific interaction with sodium channels. The voltage-dependent sodium channel binds the toxin and prevents the physiological inactivation of the channel. This leads to a massive sodium influx and persistent membrane depolarization. This effect of batrachotoxin is similar to certain other alkaloids such as veratridine and aconitine, but the latter two are relatively less potent and may indeed act as antagonists when simultaneously present with batrachotoxin. Tetrodotoxin and saxitoxin may reverse the depolarization produced by batrachotoxin. The blockade by tetrodotoxin appears to be mediated by sites different from those binding batrachotoxin. Local anesthetics act as competitive antagonists to the batrachotoxin-induced depolarization.

Batrachotoxin produces structural damage to nerves and muscles. This damage is believed to be secondary to depolarization and subsequent massive acetylcholine release. For this reason, the alkaloid is a potent cardiotoxic agent, leading to arrythmia and cardiac arrest. These cardiac effects are not related to cardiac glycosides, since no inhibition of Na^+, K^+-ATPase is produced by batrachotoxin at toxic doses. The cardiac effects are antagonized by tetrodotoxin. Batrachotoxin has no apparent effect on calcium channels, although axonal conduction is effectively inhibited by this alkaloid.

Steroids in Toad Skins

Skins of toads of *Bufo* species contain a mixture of digitalis-like steroidal compounds that have been called *bufogenins* (Meyer and Linde, 1971). The compounds are C_{24} steroids (Fig. 3) and have potent cardiotoxic properties. The yield of such steroids from a single animal is highly variable: up to 1200 mg has been isolated from one animal skin. Some of the bufogenins with a known structure include arenobufogenin, argentinogenin, bufalin, 3-epibufalin, bufalon, bufarenogin, bufotalidin, bufatalinin, bufatalon, cinobufagin, cinobufaginol, cinobufatalin, desacetylbufotalin, desacetylcinobufagenin, desacetylcinobufotalin, gamabufotalin, hellebrigenol, resibufagenin, artebufogenin, and telocinobufagin (Meyer and Linde, 1971).

Bufotoxin

In addition to bufogenins, toad skin contains different types of steroidal compounds called bufotoxins (Meyer and Linde, 1971). These toxins are conjugates of bufogenins and suberylarginine. These nitrogenous chemicals are still not adequately characterized. One of these compounds, *bufotoxin*, consists of an anhydrous compound of steroid bufotalin as the steroidal residue. Others include cinobufotoxin, gamabufotoxin, and marinobufotoxin.

There are additional nitrogen-containing steroids found in the skins of various toads. Many of these have not been investigated and have potent cardiac properties. Their diuretic properties were recognized in China and Japan well before the use of digitalis for this purpose.

Zetekitoxins

A mixture of low-molecular-weight toxins was isolated from the skin of *Atelopus zeteki* (found only in Panama) and was named *zetekitoxin* by Brown and co-workers

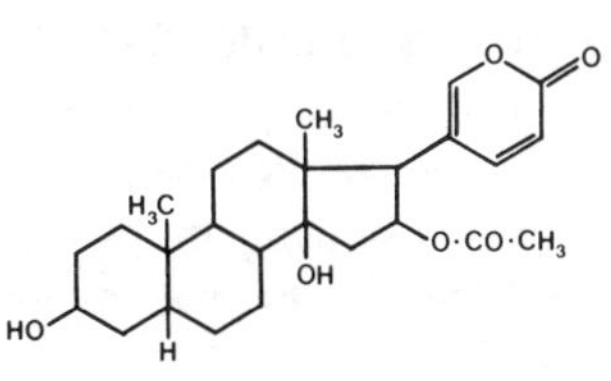

Bufotalin

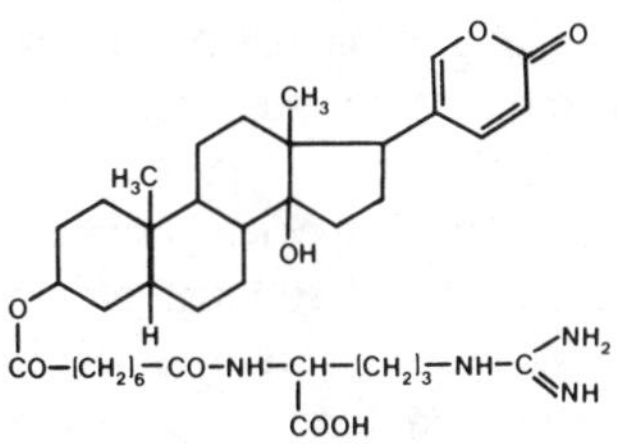

Bufotoxin

Figure 3 Steroids isolated from toad venoms.

(1977). One major fraction of this toxic mixture was separated by electrophoresis and called zetekitoxin AB. This fraction had an LD50 of approximately 11 μg/kg intraperitoneally in mice. The second, less toxic, fraction, *zetekitoxin C,* was found to have an intraperitoneal LD50 of 80 μg/kg in mice. These water-soluble toxins were reported to be neither polypeptide nor steroid or carbohydrate in nature. In higher animals, like dogs and cats, these toxins produce prolonged hypotension. During the hypotension phase, the pressure response to epinephrine or norepinephrine was not altered. The toxin blocked arterial vasoconstriction caused by an electrical stimulation in a rabbit ear; the effect was antagonized by *d*-amphetamine. The toxin did not block α-adrenergic receptors but in high concentrations (10 μg/l) partially blocked β-adrenergic receptors. The animals that produce zetekitoxin are not affected by the toxin.

Chiriquitoxin

The eggs of Costa Rican frog, *Atelopus chiriquiensis,* contain tetrodotoxin and a tetrodotoxin-like compound called chiriquitoxin (Pavelka et al., 1977). Chiriquitoxin is a congener of tetrodotoxin and also a potent neurotoxin similar to the latter compound. Chiriquitoxin has a large group of 104 mass units substituting the —CH₂OH group at C_6 of tetrodotoxin. In addition to its effect, similar to tetrodotoxin on sodium channels of nerve and muscle fibers, chiriquitoxin also has an effect on potassium channels (Kao, 1981). The two toxic alkaloids bind to the same receptor site on the membrane, and tetrodotoxin antagonizes the effect of chiriquitoxin on K^+ channels.

Table 6 presents the occurrence of various toxins in different amphibian species. The variety of toxic components present in several types of animals is apparent.

Venoms from Salamanders

The fire salamander (*Salamandra maculosa*) has been historically considered poisonous. The venom is produced in skin glands and contains a mixture of toxic alkaloids. The relative toxicity of individual alkaloids is still not well known. The toxic effects of crude poison include restlessness, epileptic convulsions, dilated pupils, weak respiration, and cardiac arrythmia, followed by intermittant convulsions, paralysis of hindlimbs, and death. The poisoned animals show hemorrhages in internal organs (Habermehl, 1971).

Several major alkaloids have now been isolated. These are somewhat similar to steroids but not truely steroidal in structure. The main alkaloid is samandarin, along with other minor compounds, including samandenon, *O*-acetyl samandarin, samandaridin, and cycloneosamandaridin (Fig. 4). In addition, other minor steroidal alkaloids and certain nonsteroidal alkaloids are also present.

A different type of toxin has been isolated from *Pseudotriton* species (*P. ruber* and *P. montanus*), the plethontid salamanders. The toxin, named pseudotritontoxin (Brandon and Huheey, 1981), is an incompletely characterized large molecule (greater than 200,000 daltons) and has properties similar to tetrodotoxin. It produces hyperextension of hindlimbs and lower back, extreme irritability, hypothermia, pro-

Table 6 Occurrence of Various Toxins in Different Species of Amphibians

Species	Chemical												
	Epine-phrine	Serotonin	Bufotenin	His-tamine	Lepto-dactylin	Active peptides	Hemolytic proteins	Bufo-toxin	Batracho-toxin	Piperidine alkaloids	Zeteki-toxin	Tetrodo-toxin	Saman-darine
Bufo	X	X	X					X					
Leptodactylus		X	X	X	X								
Hyla		X	X	X		X	X						
Rana		X	X			X	X						
Bombina		X				X	X						
Phyllobates									X				
Dendrobates										X			
Atelopus											X	X	
Salamandra													X
Taricha												X	

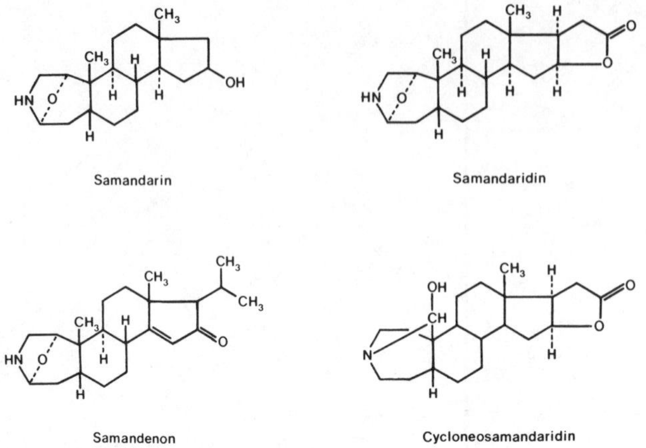

Figure 4 Representative toxins found in venoms from salamanders.

longed debility, and coma followed by death within 12–48 h. The LD50 values of crude skin extracts were reported to be between 100 and 500 mg/kg, depending on the origin of the toxin.

TOXIC PRINCIPLES ASSOCIATED WITH FISHES

Marine organisms produce many toxic substances. However, only a relatively small number of these are involved in human and food poisoning. In some areas of the world, Japan for example, poisoning from sea foods has accounted for two-thirds of all food-poisoning cases. Many of the marine toxicants involved in cases of food poisoning are produced by microorganisms such as various forms of marine algae accumulated in edible marine animals consumed by humans. Most of the toxicants from marine animals are quite stable to heat processing or cooking, and are refractory to the action of the digestive enzyme of humans. Some of the marine toxins are produced intrinsically (e.g., tetrodotoxin).

Puffer-Fish Toxicity

Poisonous puffer fishes (family Tetrodontidae) are the best known source of tetrodotoxin. About 80 fishes of the family Tetrodontidae are known to contain tetrodotoxin. Invariably, the ovaries of puffer fish contain the highest concentration of toxin, followed by the liver and the intestines; muscles contain the lowest amount of toxin. Puffer fishes are considered to be delicious in winter, the time when the concentration of tetrodotoxin in the ovaries and liver is highest; in summer they are relatively nontoxic. Human poisoning most frequently occurs from contamination of the edible parts of the fish by toxic ovaries or liver; ingestion of internal organs by uniformed people also causes toxicity.

The molecular formula of tetrodotoxin has been reported as $C_{11}H_{17}N_3O_8$, with a molecular weight of 300, and pK$_a$ of 8.7 (see Fig. 5). Even relatively small alterations in the chemical structure abolish its pharmacological activity. Crystalline tetrodotoxin is practically insoluble in water and organic solvents. The pure toxin can be dissolved in weak acid. Stability of tetrodotoxin to heating in aqueous solution is markedly dependent on the pH of the solution. At about pH 7.0, little or no inactivation occurs during boiling in water for 30–60 min or autoclaving for 1 h at 120 °C. The toxin can be partially or completely inactivated by heating in acid solutions at pH 4.0 or below or in alkaline solutions at pH 9.0 or above. Tetrodotoxin can be more readily inactivated in alkaline medium rather than in acid medium. Ordinary cooking will not inactivate the toxin.

Toxic signs and symptoms generally appear in 30–60 min after intoxication by tetrodotoxin and include numbness of the lips, tongue, and fingers, and anxiety, nausea, and vomiting. Numbness becomes more marked; muscular paralysis of extremeties without loss of tendon reflexes occurs; severe hypertension, ataxia, and motor incoordination become more severe; paralysis develops; consciousness is maintained but speaking is difficult because of paralysis; and death occurs due to respiratory failure.

Tetrodotoxin blocks neural conduction by a highly specific effect on the movement of sodium ions and not of potassium ions across cell membranes of common excitable cells (Kao, 1972). The lethal dose of tetrodotoxin is approximately 1–2 mg for adults, when taken orally. The minimal lethal dose of tetrodotoxin for the mouse is approximately 8 μg/kg. In experimental animals, intravenous administration of doses of 1–5 μg/kg crystalline tetrodotoxin produced a rapid weakening of muscular contraction and paralysis, depression in respiration, and profound severe hypertension. Tetrodotoxin has a direct paralyzing action on sketetal (striated) muscles and on nerve fibers.

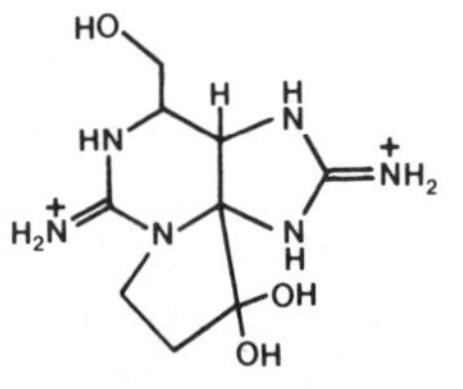

Saxitoxin

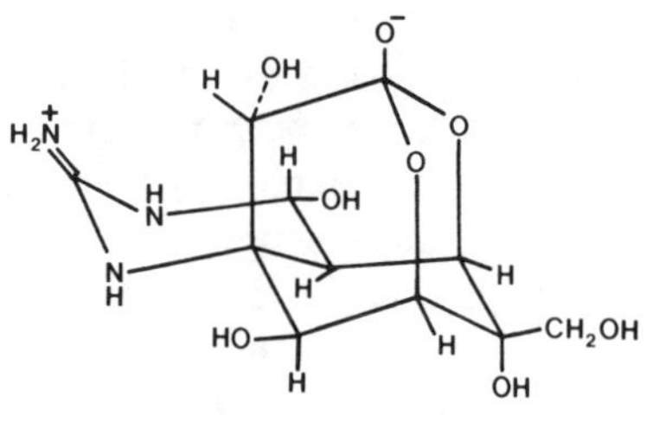

Tetrodotoxin

Figure 5 Structures of tetrodotoxin and saxitoxin.

Ciguatoxin

Poison-causing ciguatera originates in some of the marine algae and gets into fish through the food chain. Ciguatera poisoning is common throughout the Caribbean area and much of the Pacific area particularly in the torrid zones. The alga that produces ciguatoxin is *Schizothrix calcicola*. Both water and lipid extracts of this alga contained the toxins and produced symptoms in mice and mongoose.

Ciguatoxin is a viscous, ultra violet- (UV-) transparent oil, quite stable to heat used in ordinary cooking, and can be dried without loss of potency. Ciguatoxin is easily soluble in lipid solvents, but less soluble in water. Clinical ciguatoxin symptoms are neurological and gastrointestinal disturbances including tingling of the lips, mouth and fingertips, itching of the skin, reversal of temperature sensation, loss of motor ability, vomiting, and diarrhea. Ciguatoxin poisoning is rarely fatal but often prolonged.

Other Toxins and Venoms from Fishes

Toxins from the eggs of two marine fish, the northern blenny of Japan and the cabezon of western North America, are lipoproteins that produce toxic effects several hours after their ingestion. A severe illness that includes headache, diarrhea, vomiting, chest pain, and sometimes coma or death is produced by the lipoprotein toxins. Death usually occurs due to respiratory failure.

COELENTERATES

Several members of the phylum Coelenterata are among the most dangerous creatures inhabiting the oceans. The coelenterates are divided into three classes: Hydrazoa, Scyphozoa, and Anthozoa. The Scyphozoans are known as the true jellyfish. *Physalia physalis* (the Portuguese man-of-war) is a hydrazoan, not to be confused with the true jellys. Ironically, it is the most widely known Coelenterate. The class Anthozoa is comprised of the sea anemones.

A comparison of nematocysts and their respective toxins has been presented by Burnett and Calton (1977). A detailed discussion on the nature of coelenterate nematocysts was presented by Halstead and Courvillue (1965). The nematocyst is the toxin-discharging organ of the coelenterate, located numerously on the tentacles, each acting independently of its neighbors. The total toxin dose to a victim is dependent on the number of effective nematocyst discharges. Jellyfish toxins are primarily proteins of varying molecular weights. Severe cutaneous pain is a common factor of jellyfish envenomations. Many of the jellyfish toxins are cardiotoxic. *Chironex fleckeri* is reputed to be the most dangerous inhabitant of the seas. Its envenomation is most often fatal, with death occurring within minutes after the victim is stung.

Coelenterate venoms are primarily proteinaceous compounds. Six enzymatic activities have been associated with nematocysts isolated from *Physalis physalis*: ATPase, nonspecific aminopeptidases, RNAase, DNAase, AMPase, and fibrinolysin (Burnett and Calton, 1974). The isolated peptides contain high levels of glutamic acid and low levels of aromatic acids. Collagenase (Lal et al., 1981) and endonuclease (Neeman et al., 1981) have been reported for venoms isolated from *Physalia physalis* nematocysts, having molecular weights of 25,000 and 75,000 daltons, respectively. Several enzymatic activities have also been observed for extracts from *Stomolophus melagris* nematocysts, including 5-nucleotidase, hyaluronidase, acid and alkaline phosphatases, phosphodiesterase, leucine aminopeptidase, and protease (Toom and Chan, 1972). Nematocysts prepared from *Chrysaora* spp. have been shown to have the following activities: ATPase, RNAase, DNAase, hyaluronidase, acid protease, alkaline protease, and nonspecific amino peptidase (Burnett and Calton, 1977). The anemone *Actina cari* is known to produce hemolytic proteins, caritoxin I, II, and III, all of which are basic proteins with molecular weights ranging from 20,000 to 25,000 daltons (Macek et al., 1982). The LD50 of caritoxin I in mice (iv) is 22 μg/kg. The toxic peptides isolated from *Anemonia sulcata* have molecular weights ranging from 2600 to 4700 daltons (Alsen, 1983). Bernheimer and Avigad (1981) have isolated cytolysins from seven sea anemones with molecular weights ranging from 10,000 to 100,000 daltons.

Pharmacological activities have been discovered for coelenterate venoms. A peptide fraction ($>300,000$ daltons) isolated from *Stomolophus melagris* was shown to produce cardiac arrhythmias in mice and was also associated with hyperkalemia and hyponatremia (Larsen and Price, 1978). ATX II, isolated from *Anemonia sulcata*, has been associated with pronounced inotropic effects (Alsen, 1983). Powerful positive inotropic effects without any chronotropic effects have been demonstrated for venoms obtained from *Anthopleura xanthogranmica* (Norton, 1981). Pressor activity was demonstrated for fractions with molecular weights $<100,000$ daltons. The toxic action of venom from the sea nettle (*Chrysaora* spp.) on frog heart and sartorius muscle resulted from the toxin's ability to increase Na^+ permeability (Shryock and Bianchi, 1983). The depolarizing effects of the toxin were not altered by tetrodotoxin, d-tubocurarine, or by changing the external Ca^{2+} level (Warnick et al., 1981). Altered membrane permeability to Na^+, caused by toxic isolates from *Stomolophus melagris*, is due in part to its effect on ATPase (Toom and Phillips, 1978).

Antigenic properties were observed for venomous extracts obtained from *Chironex fleckeri* (Baxter et al., 1968) and *Actinia equina* (Ferlan and Lebez, 1974). An effective antivenom antibody capable of neutralizing the lethal activity of an iv challenge of crude *Physalia physalis* venom has been produced (Gaur et al., 1982).

Nuclear alterations and dissolution of intracellular collagen was observed in CHO (Chinese hamster ovary) K-1 cells that had been exposed to venom from either *Chrysaora* spp. or *Physalia* spp. (Neeman et al., 1980). It was hypothesized by the authors that the observed changes resulted from collagenase, protease, and lectin-like activities of the venoms. *Chrysaora* spp. venom significantly decreased the oxygen uptake by mitochondria, actively oxidizing exogenous NADH (Watrous and Blasett, 1978).

Acute renal failure was reported for a 4-year-old girl stung by a Portuguese man-of-war (*Physalia physalis*) (Guess et al., 1982). Burnett et al. (1983) have reported on practical methods of first aid for treating stings from *Physalia* spp. and *Chrysaora* spp. Inflamed areas of skin can be rinsed with vinegar or a solution of baking soda for stings from *Physalia* and *Chrysaora,* respectively. Verapamil, a calcium antagonist, has been shown to be an effective agent in delaying time to death in mice after receiving an iv injection of *Chironex* spp. venom (Burnett and Calton, 1983).

DINOFLAGELLATES

Both paralytic and neurotoxic shellfish poisoning have been associated with the blooming phenomena of toxic dinoflagellates. The blooms are frequently referred to as red-tide, red-water, or brown water. The red color results primarily from the xanthophyll pigment peridinin (Strain et al., 1944). The etiology of paralytic and neurotoxic shellfish poisonings begins with the ingestion of contaminated molluscus, clams, and mussels, which have accumulated dinoflagellate toxins within their body tissues (Hughes, 1979). Inhalation of sea-spray-associated toxic dinoflagellate fragments has been reported and linked to respiratory irritation in humans (Baden et al., 1982).

Several toxic fractions have been isolated in conjunction with shellfish poisoning. Table 7 identifies the sources and names of several known toxic isolates. Paralytic shellfish poisoning most likely results from a combination of the toxic fractions. Baden et al. (1982) believe that T34 and GB-2 isolated by Shimizu (1978) may in fact be the same compound. It is possible that the array of toxic constituents observed may arise from metabolic rearrangement within contaminated molluscs (Boyer et al., 1979). Bates et al. (1978) have reported on the occurrence of saxitoxin and other dinoflagellate toxins. Ciguatoxin has recently been shown to be produced by the benthic dinoflagellate *Gambierdiscus toxicus* (Bagnis et al., 1980).

Structural characterizations of dinoflagellate toxins are limited to the following: saxitoxin (Schantz et al., 1975), brevetoxin B (Lin et al., 1981), ciguatoxin, and gonyautoxin II. Saxitoxin (Fig. 5), associated with paralytic shellfish, is water-soluble and is produced primarily by *Gonyaulax* spp. The toxins associated with neurotoxic shellfish are lipoidal in nature (Alam et al., 1982).

Known LD50 values for dinoflagellate toxins are indicated in Table 8. The minimum lethal dose for saxitoxin in humans is 0.5 mg. Interspecies toxicity of saxitoxin,

Table 7 Species Source and Toxic Isolate of Several Dinoflagellate Toxins

Source	Compound[a]	Reference
Ptychodiscus brevis	T17, T34	Baden et al. (1979)
Ptychodiscus brevis	T_2, T_4	Risk et al. (1979)
Ptychodiscus brevis	$GBTX_\alpha$, $GBTX\beta$	Padilla et al. (1979)
Gonyaulax tamarensis	Saxitoxin, neosaxitoxin	Boyer et al. (1979)
Gonyaulax excavata	Gonyautoxins I, II, III, IV, neosaxitoxin	Oshima and Yasumoto (1979)

[a]The letters symbolize the toxic fractions isolated by various investigators as indicated.

Table 8   LD50 Values for Several Dinoflagellate Toxins

Compound	LD50 (mg/kg)	Animal	Route	Reference
T17	0.15	Mouse	ip	Baden et al. (1979)
	0.52	Mouse	po	Baden and Mende (1982)
	0.094	Mouse	iv	Baden and Mende (1982)
T34	0.20	Mouse	ip	Baden and Mende (1982)
	6.60	Mouse	po	Baden and Mende (1982)
	0.20	Mouse	iv	Baden and Mende (1982)
	0.011[a]	Fish		Baden et al. (1981)
T_{46}	5[b]	Fish		Risk et al. (1979)
T_{47}	30[c]	Fish		Risk et al. (1979)
GBTX	0.5	Mice	ip	Ellis et al. (1979)
Saxitoxin	10.0	Mice	ip	Halstead (1981)
	263	Mice	po	Halstead (1981)
	2.4	Mice	iv	Halstead (1981)

[a]LC50, mg/l.
[b]LC50, ng/ml.
[c]LC50, ng/ml.

administered orally, varies between 91 μg/kg for pigeons to greater than 360 μg/kg for mouse and monkey (Shimizu, 1978).

Table 9 describes known pharmacologic and toxicologic properties of dinoflagellate toxins. Systemic symptomatology of paralytic shellfish poisoning in humans includes facial paresthesia, nausea, vomiting, diarrhea, dysphonia, dysphagia, and ataxia (Pasquini and Andreucci, 1979). Symptoms may appear within minutes after ingestion. Deaths have been reported from respiratory paralysis with 2–24 h, depend-

Table 9   Pharmacological and Toxicological Effects of Dinoflagellate Toxins

Compound	Biological effect	Reference
T_{46}	Stimulated differential release of amino acid neurotransmitters from mammalian cortical synaptasomes, loss of K^+, stimulated respiration, acetylcholine release from guinea pig ileum	Risk et al. (1982)
T17	Caused bronchoconstriction in guinea pig	Baden et al. (1982)
GBTX	Respiratory failure, cardiac arrhythmia, toxin appears to activate the Bezold–Jarisch reflex and produce catecholamine release	Ellis et al. (1979)

ing on dose. The symptoms elicited by T17, an isolate from *Ptychodiscus brevis* (*Gymnodium breve* syn.) in mice, include tremors, marked muscular contractions or fasciculations, straub tail phenomenon, labored breathing, salivation, lacrimation, urination, defecation, compulsive chewing motions, and rhinorrhea (Baden and Mende, 1982).

Saxitoxin is a neurotoxin that effectively blocks Na^+ transport channels in the membranes of excitable cells (Kao, 1974). All skeletal muscles, including respiratory muscles, are affected by saxitoxin. Kao (1981) suggested receptor-site competition between saxitoxin and tetrodotoxin.

The effect of T34 (Baden et al., 1981) and ciguatoxin (Hokama et al., 1980) on components of the murine immune system has been investigated. T34, administered ip up to a dose of 0.1 mg/kg 1 day prior to or 1 day following antigenic sensitization (sheep red blood cells), had no effect on anti-sheep red blood cell antibody production. Ciguatoxin had a suppressive effect on the ability of mouse lymphoid cells to respond to mitogen stimulation.

VENOMOUS MAMMALS

Very few species of mammals possess a venom-producing and -releasing apparatus. In the platypus (*Ornithorphynchos anatinus*), a venom apparatus is found only in the male animals. It consists of a movable horny spur on the inner side of each hind limb near the heel. This is connected to a poison gland. The venom is not highly toxic, and there have been only a few instances where humans have been attacked. The symptoms may include swelling at the site, intense pain that develops shortly after the attack, and hypotension.

The spiny anteater (*Tahyglossus* spp. and *Zaglossus* spp.) has anatomical apparatus similar to that in platypus. Poisoning is again rare. A few other mammalian species have been suggested to be toxic. These include *Solenodon pardoxus* and *Sorex* spp. (shrews). The submaxilary secretions of these animals are toxic, and envenomation may occur during a bite.

TOXIC INSECTS AND ARACHNIDS

Toxic insects are venomous arthropods. Their toxicity has been documented throughout the history of the world. The venomous arthropods possess one or more venom glands and a mechanism or apparatus to inflict a wound or inject the venomous material into the victim. The venomous arthropods include spiders, scorpions, bees, wasps, hornets, ants, beetles, and caterpillars. A list of various arthropods, the nature of their venoms, and a brief summary of their biological effects is provided in Table 10.

Venom and its extruding mechanisms are perhaps evolved in these insects for two main reasons, defense and nutrition. For nutritional purposes, the insects usually have a biting apparatus by which they can feed themselves. In other cases the stinging mechanism is only to release the venom from an exocrine gland. In case of caterpillars and beetles, direct bodily contact, either internally or externally, is required to get the venom into victim's tissues.

Table 10 Venomous Insects and Arachnids[a]

Type or species	Venom type and constituents	Effects of venom
Bees		
Apis dorsata (India) *Xilociepa brasi-lianorum* (Brazil)	Formic acid	Nausea, vomiting, sphincter relaxation, dyspnea, convulsion
Apis mellifera (honey bee)	Formic acid Mellitin (contains amino acids, lipids, sugars and proteins)	Local edema, irriation, hemolysis, cardiac arrest, histamine liberation in sensitized individuals; LD50 mice, 3–4 mg/kg
Wasps and hornets	Formic acid, serotonin, acetyl-choline, histamine, kinins	Pain, proteolysis, vasocactive effects, hemolysis
Ants	Formic acid, kinins, histamine-releasing factors, hyaluronidase, cell-lysing factors	Weal, erythema, edema, chills, tachycardia
Spanish fly (beetles)	Cantheridin	Blistering, necrosis
Scorpions	Somewhat similar to snake venom, contains neurotoxic and hemolytic factors	Pain, locomotor disturbance, excitation, convulsions, tachycardia
Spiders	Neurotoxic venom	Elevation of blood pressure, internal hemorrhage
Ticks	Neurotoxic factors	Itching, dermatitis, acute ascending flaccid paralysis
Caterpillars	Hemolytic, proteolytic, hyaluronidase	Urticaria, blood-pressure rise followed by fall
Centipedes and milli-pedes	Phenols, quinones, cyanogenic factors	Local inflammation, erythema, edema, purpura

[a]Summarized from Diniz and Corrado (1971).

463

Wasps, Bees, Hornets, and Ants

A large number of deaths are caused by bites of wasps, bees, ants, and hornets, and most of these result from hypersensitivity. Nearly 20% of the U.S. population is allergic to such venoms. During a 10-year period ending in 1959, 460 deaths were reported in the United States due to venomous animals; 50% of these were caused due to stings by hymenopterans. In these insects the stinger is smooth, resembles a hypodermic needle, and is usually withdrawn after stinging. The honeybee has a barbed tip that remains at the site of injection.

The venoms produced by wasps, bees, and hornets have been reviewed in detail elsewhere (Tu, 1977; O'Connor and Peck, 1978; Rathmayer, 1978; Edery et al., 1978; Beard, 1978; and Habermehl, 1981). The present discussion summarizes some of the information presented by the above authors.

The venoms of the wasp, bee, and hornet contain biogenic amines, polypeptides, kinins, and, to a lesser extent, enzymes. The biogenic amines include histamine, serotonin, acetylcholine, dopamine, and noradrenaline. Acetylcholine content of hornet venom is approximately 5% on a dry-weight basis. Several large peptides have been identified, including apamin, mellitin (a family of proteins), and a mast-cell degranulating peptide. Enzymes that have been identified are hyaluronidase, phospholipase A_2, esterases, acid and alkaline phosphatases, and hexosaminidase. Mellitin and phospholipase A_2 exhibit synergism toward the lysis of erythrocytes.

Known pharmacological and toxicological properties of the honeybee (*Apis meliffera*) venom and its components are acetylcholinesterase inhibition, anaphylactogenity, antigenicity, blood-pressure depression, cardiac antiarrhythmic effects, and CNS excitation and inhibition. [^{125}I]Apamin (honeybee toxin) was observed to be distributed over brain regions in a nonspecific manner (Habermann and Horvath, 1980). The 24-h LD50 values in mice for the venoms of 26 hymenopteran species have been reported (Schmidt et al., 1980). The authors also tabulated quantities of venoms obtained per insect. Toxicities ranged from 0.25 to 117.5 mg/kg body weight following ip injection.

The fire ants, *Solenopis* spp., are the most notorious ants in the United States and are imposing an ever-increasing threat to humans living in the Gulf Coast states and Hawaii. An estimated 10,000 stings occur yearly. Their stings cause pain, a burning sensation, edema, redness, itch, pustules, necrosis, and scarring. The ant venoms contain, in addition to the substances identified above, piperidine alkaloids.

No specific antivenin is available, and the management of such bites usually requires a symptomatic therapy involving antihistamines to prevent or counteract allergic reactions and systemic or local pain-relieving substances.

Beetles

These belong to the order Coleoptera and possess a potent contact poison, cantharidin. Cantharidin produces a large vesicle in the skin or the mucous membrane, and deep necrosis may develop later. Cantharidin has been suggested as an aphrodisiac, and deaths have resulted from swallowing this highly irritant chemical. In case of internal administration, serious lesions of mucous membranes develop, leading to vomiting and bloody diarrhea. Swallowing may be interfered with because of esophageal spasms and is associated with intense thirst. The poison may be absorbed and causes renal damage, producing hemorrhagic nephritis, albuminurea, and hematurea. Fatal uremia may result following anurea. Treatment is symptomatic.

Scorpions

Approximately 650 species have been described, belonging to six or seven recognized families. In the United States, scorpions of medical importance are members of the genus *Centruroides* of the family Buthidae. The families Chactidae and Buthidae account for the greatest number of species and hence have received the greatest attention. Scorpion venoms have been reviewed in detail (Tu, 1977; Stahnke, 1978; Shulov and Levy, 1978; Bucherl, 1978; Diniz, 1978; Goyffon and Kovoor, 1978; and Habermehl, 1981).

Scorpions generally occur in arid regions of various continents and produce a venom similar to snake venom. On a weight basis the scorpion venom may be more toxic than snake venom, but human fatalities are less frequent because of the small size of the venom gland and amount of venom released. Deaths are usually in small children and old people. The venom is injected into the victim via a stinger located on the tip of the tail. The gland is situated in the terminal segment of their body.

Scorpion venoms are comprised primarily of proteinaceous compounds, both enzymatic and nonenzymatic. Characterized peptides contain 57–78 amino acid residues; most are 62–66 residues in length. The peptides do not contain methionine. All contain four disulfide bridges. Twenty-two toxic proteins were isolated from 5 scorpions of the family Buthidae, of which 20 were active in mammals. Enzymatic compounds include phospholipase A_2, acetylcholinesterase, hyaluronidase, phosphomonoesterase, 5′-nucleotidase, gelatinase, and protease activities. Nonenzymatic constituents include numerous free amino acids, 5-hydroxytryptamine, glycosaminoglycans, hyaluronic acid, and hexosamine. LD50 values of scorpion venom in mice ranged from a low of 9 to a maximum of 810 μg toxin/kg body weight.

Numerous human encounters with scorpions have provided much information regarding the symptomology of scorpion envenomation. Pain, local edema, antigenicity, and fever are pronounced 1–20 h after the sting. Discoloration, sweating, pallor, restlessness, anxiety and confusion, salivation, nausea, abdominal cramps, chest pains, and headaches have also been recorded. Symptoms may also include respiratory difficulties, temporary blindness, defecation, penile erection, respiratory arrest, hypertension, and cardiac failure. Increased urinary excretion of catecholamines and their metabolites has been detected. Serum potassium increases and sodium decreases. Congestion and hemorrhage in various organs, pulmonary edema, infiltration of monocytes and lymphocytes, and deposition of fat droplets have been observed as well.

Pharmacological activities produced by scorpion venoms are numerous. Scorpion venoms are known to block nerve-impulse transmission at presynaptic sites of both cholinergic and adrenergic nerves. The venoms affect contractility and relaxation of smooth muscle and cause positive ionotropisms; tachycardia, hypertension, arryth- mias, bradycardia, and hypotension have all been observed. In vitro inhibition of the angiotension-converting enzyme has been reported (Longnecker et al., 1980). Scor- pion venoms have also been investigated for their ability to cause the aggregation of platelets (Longnecker and Longnecker, 1981).

Centruroides sculpturatus is the only scorpion in the United States that has a potentially lethal venom. In Arizona it is responsible for more deaths than any other venomous animal. Although antivenins are available in regions where scorpions are a problem, most of the treatment involves symptomatic management.

Centipedes and Millipedes

These arthropods cause more nuisance because of their appendages causing irritation upon contact to the skin and also due to their appearance. Some of these are also capable of injecting toxic substances composed of phenols, quinones, or cyanogens via a pair of hollow jaws that serve as fangs. The species that secrete cyanogenetic factors also secrete a catalyst to release free cyanide. The common symptoms involve erythema, edema, inflammation, purpura at the site of bite, and rarely generalized systemic effects. Usually the episodes are short-lasting.

Spiders and Ticks

Poisonous spiders usually occur in warm climates. The most dangerous are the black widow (*Lactrodectus mactens*) and the brown recluse spider (*Loxoscales reclusa*). The bite of a black widow is similar to a needle puncture and causes pain that may last for hours.

Several enzymes have been isolated from spider venoms: hyaluronidase, prote- ases, esterases, alkaline phosphatase, and phosphodiesterase. The presence or ab- sence of any one of the above enzymes depends on the species of spider (Tu, 1977). Spider venoms also contain nonprotein compounds: 5-hydroxytryptamine, α- aminobutyric acid, gluatmic and aspartic acids, histamine, and serotonin have been detected.

LD50 values for the venom of the black widow spider in several animal species have been reported by Habermehl (1981). The rat LD50 value is 0.21 mg/kg body weight. The frog is exceptionally resistant to the toxin: the LD50 is equal to 145 mg/ kg body weight. A neurotoxin with a molecular weight of 130,000 daltons has been isolated form the venom of the black widow (Grasso, 1976). The neurotoxic venom acts on the myoneural junctions, causing an ascending motor paralysis. Feeble pulse, cold skin, labored breathing and speech, light stupor, and delirium may follow. The symptoms are somewhat similar to and may be confused with acute abdominal dis- eases. The syndrome elicited by envenomation from black widow spiders is referred to as latrodectism; intense feelings of anxiety or mortal fear have been reported.

Moderate tachycardia is observed initially, followed by a marked bradycardia. Britos et al. (1978) reported a significant reduction of both brain and heart levels of noradrenaline. They observed no change in the levels of heart or brain 5-hydroxytryptamine (5-HT); heart levels of acetylcholine were seen to increase. Death may occur from the venom, depending on the victim's physical condition, age, and the location of the bite. The brown recluse spider bite induces pain that becomes progressively severe. In about 8 hr or so, a bleb surrounded by erythema may develop. The bleb then sloughs off, revealing a zone of intense ischemia with ecchymosis and edema. In 24–48 h the erythema may be intense and the central zone darkens and appear like a black eschar. The resulting necosis may be slow to heal and leaves a residual scar. Hemolytic crisis ultimately resulting in death has been reported. No specific antivenin is available for the brown recluse spider venom.

The tick may cause an ascending flaccid paralysis caused by the release of toxins during the bite. The problem rarely occurs in people but is commonly encountered in infested animals. The toxin is not well-characterized but is believed to interfere with acetylcholine release at the neuromuscular junction in the vicinity of the biting site.

REFERENCES

Alam, M., Sandvja, R., Hassain, M. B., and Van Der Helm, D. 1982. *Gymnodinium breve* toxins. *J. Am. Chem. Soc.* 104:5232–5234.

Albuquerque, E. X., Daly, J. W., and Witkop, B. 1971. Batrachotoxins: Chemistry and pharmacology. *Science* 172:995–1002.

Alsen, C. 1983. Biological significance of peptides from *Anemonia sulcata. Fed. Proc.* 42:101–108.

Baden, D. G. and Mende, T. J. 1982. Toxicity of two toxins from the Florida red tide marine dinoflagellate, *Ptcyhodiscus brevis. Toxicon* 20:457–461.

Baden, D. G., Mende, T. J., and Block, R. E. 1979. Two similar toxins isolated from *Gymnodinium breve.* In *Toxic Dinoflagellate Blooms,* eds. D. L. Taylor and H. H. Seliger, pp. 327–334. New York: Elsevier/North Holland.

Baden, D. G., Mende, T. J., Lichter, W., and Willham, L. 1981. Crystallization and toxicology of T34: A major toxin from Florida's red tide organism (*Ptychodiscus brevis*). *Toxicon* 19:455–462.

Baden, D. G., Mende, T. J., Bikhazi, G., and Leung, I. 1982. Bronchoconstriction caused by Florida red tide toxins. *Toxicon* 20:929–932.

Bagnis, R., Chanteau, S., Chungue, F., Hurtel, J. M., Yasumoto, T., and Inoue, A. 1980. Origins of ciguatera fish poisoning: A new dinoflagellate, *Gambierdiscus toxicus* atachi and Iukyuyo, definitively involved as a causal agent. *Toxicon* 18:199–208.

Barne, M. 1968. Venomous sea snakes (Hydrophiidae). In *Venomous Animals and Their Venoms,* eds. W. Buchrel, E. E. Buckley, and V. Denlofeu, vol. 1, pp. 285–308. New York: Academic.

Bates, H. A., Kostriken, R., and Rapoport, H. 1978. The occurrence of saxitoxin and other toxins in dinoflagellates. *Toxicon* 16:595–601.

Baxter, E. H., Marr, A. G., and Lane, W. R. 1968. Immunity to the venom of the sea wasp *Chironex fleckeri. Toxicon* 6:45–50.

Beard, R. L. 1978. Venoms of Braconidae. In *Arthropod Venoms,* ed. S. Bettini, pp. 773–800. New York: Springer-Verlag.

Bernheimer, A. W., and Avigad, L. S. 1981. New cytolysins in sea anemones from the west coast of the United States. *Toxicon* 19:529–534.

Boquet, P., and Saint-Girons, H. 1972. Etude immunologique des glandes salivaires du vestibule buccal de guelques colubridae opistoglyphes. *Toxicon* 10:635–644.

Boyer, G. L., Wichmann, C. F., Mosser, J., Schantz, E. J., and Heinrich, K. S. 1979. Toxins isolated from Bay of Fundy scallops. In *Toxic Dinoflagellate Blooms,* eds. D. L. Taylor and H. H. Seliger, pp. 373–376. New York: Elsevier/North Holland.

Brandon, R. A., and Huheey, J. E. 1981. Toxicity in the plethodontid salamanders *Pseudotriton ruber* and *Pseudotriton montanus* (Amphibia, Caudata). *Toxicon* 19:25–31.

Britos, S. A., Orsinger, O. A., and Fulginita, S. 1978. Effects of venom gland extract of the black widow spider on rat brain and heart levels of noradrenaline, 5-hydroxytryptamine and acetylcholine. *Toxicon* 16:393–395.

Brown, G. B., Kim, Y. H., Kuntzel, H., and Mosher H. S. 1977. Chemistry and pharmacology of skin toxins from the frog *Atelopus zeteki* (Atelopidtoxin: Zetekitoxin). *Toxicon* 15:115–128.

Bücherl, W. 1978. Venoms of Tityinae. In *Arthropod Venoms,* ed. S. Bettini, pp. 371–378. New York: Springer-Verlag.

Burnett, J. W., and Calton, G. J. 1974. The enzymatic content of the venoms of the sea nettle and Portuguese man-o'war. *Comp. Biochem. Physiol.* 47B:815–820.

Burnett, J. W., and Calton, G. J. 1977. Review article. The chemistry and toxicology of some venomous pelagic coelenterates. *Toxicon* 15:177–196.

Burnett, J. W., and Calton, G. J. 1983. Response of the box-jellyfish (*Chironex fleckeri*) cardiotoxin to intravenous administration of verapamil. *Med. J. Aust.* 2:192–194.

Burnett, J. W., Rubinstein, H., and Calton, G. J. 1983. First aid for jellyfish envenomation. *South Med. J.* 76:870–872.

Christensen, P. A. 1968. The venoms of Central and South African snakes. In *Venomous Animals and Their Venoms,* eds. W. Buchrel, E. E. Ruckley, and V. Deulofeu, vol. 1, pp. 437–461. New York: Academic.

Daly, J. W. 1982. Biologically active alkaloids from poison frogs (Dendrobatidae). *J. Toxicol. Toxin. Rev.* 1:33–86.

Daly, J. W., and Witkop, B. 1971. Chemistry and pharmacology of frog venoms. In *Venomous Animals and Their Venoms,* eds. W. Bucherl and E. E. Buckley, vol. II, pp. 497–519. New York: Academic.

Diniz, C. R. 1978. Chemical and pharmacologic aspects of Tityinae venoms. In *Arthropod Venoms,* ed. S. Bettini, pp. 379–394. New York: Springer-Verlag.

Diniz, C. R., and Corrodo, A. D. 1971. Venoms of insects and arachnids. In *Pharmacology and Toxicology of Naturally Occurring Toxins,* ed. H. Raskova, vol. II, pp. 117–140. Oxford: Pergamon.

Edery, H., Ishay, J., Gitter, S., and Joshua, H. 1978. Venoms of Vespidae. In *Arthropod Venoms,* ed. S. Bettini, pp. 691–772. New York: Springer-Verlag.

Ellis, S., Spikes, J. J., and Johnson, G. L. 1979. Respiratory and cardiovascular effects of *G. breve* toxin in dogs. In *Toxic Dinoflagellate Blooms,* eds. D. L. Taylor and H. H. Seliger, pp. 431–434. New York: Elsevier/North Holland.

Ferlan, I., and Lebez, D. 1974. Equinatoxin, a lethal protein from *Actina equina*—I. Purification and characterization. *Toxicon* 12:57–61.

Gaur, P. K., Anthony, R. L., Calton, G. J., and Burnett, J. W. 1982. Isolation of hybridomas secreting monoclonal antibodies against *Physalia physalis* (Portuguese man-o'war) nematocysts venom. *Toxicon* 20:419–425.

Goyffon, M., and Kovoor, J. 1978. Chactoid venoms. In *Arthropod Venoms,* ed. S. Bettini, pp. 395–418. New York: Springer-Verlag.

Grasso, A. 1976. Preparation and properties of a neurotoxin purified from the venom of black widow spider (*latrodectus mactans tdecimguttatus*). Biochim. Biophys. Acta 439:406–412.

Guess, H. A., Saviteer, P. L., and Morris, D. R. 1982. Hemolysis and acute renal failure following a Portuguese man-of-war sting. *Pediatrics* 70:979–981.

Habermann, E., and Horvath, E. 1980. Localization of apamin after application to the central nervous system. *Toxicon* 18:549–560.

Habermehl, G. 1971. Toxicology, pharmacology, chemistry, and biochemistry of salamander venom. In *Venomous Animals and Their Venomas,* eds. W. Bucherl and E. E. Buckley, vol. II, pp. 569–584. New York: Academic.

Habermehl, G. G. 1981. *Venomous Animals and Their Toxins.* New York: Springer-Verlag.

Halstead, B. W. 1981. Current status of marine biotoxicology—An overview. *Clin. Toxicol.* 18:1–24.

Halstead, B. W., and Courvillue, D. A. 1965. *Poisonous and Venomous Marine Animals of the World,* vol. 1. Washington, D.C.: U.S. Government Printing Office.

Hokama, Y., Okubo, C. M., Cripps, C., Matsukawa, L. A., and Kimura, L. H. 1980. The effect of purified ciguatoxin on mitogen responses of mouse spleen lymphoid cells. *Res. Commun. Chem. Pathol. Pharmacol.* 29:397–400.

Hughes, J. 1979. Epidemiology of shellfish poisoning in the United States. In *Toxic Dinoflagellate Blooms,* ed. D. L. Taylor and H. H. Seliger, pp. 23–28. New York: Elsevier/North Holland.

Kao, C. Y. 1972. Pharmacology of tetrodotoxin and saxitoxin. *Fed. Proc.* 31:1117–1123.

Kao, C. Y. 1974. Differences between the actions of tetrodotoxin and saxitoxin. In *Bioactive Compounds from the Sea,* eds. H. J. Humm and C. E. Lane, pp. 115–121. New York: Dekker.

Kao, C. Y. 1981. Tetrodotoxin, saxitoxin, chiriquitoxin: New perspectives on ionic channels. *Fed. Proc. Fed. Am. Soc. Exp. Biol.* 40:30–35.

Lal, D. M., Calton, G. J., Neeman, I., and Burnett, J. W. 1981. Characterization of *Physalia physalis* (Portuguese man-o'war) nematocyst venom collagenase. *Comp. Biochem. Physiol.* 70B:635–638.

Larsen, J. B., and Price, W. J., Jr. 1978. Some physiological effects of fractionated jellyfish toxins. *Toxicon (Suppl.)* 1:517–526.

Lin, Y. Y., Risk, M., Ray, S. M., Van Enger, D., Clardy, J., Golik, J., James, J. C., and Nakanishi, K. 1981. Isolation and structure of brevetoxin B from the "red tide" dinoflagellate *Ptcyodiscus brevis* (= *Gymnodinium breve*). *J. Am. Chem. Soc.* 103:6773–6775.

Longnecker, G. L., and Longnecker, H. E. 1981. *C. Sculpturatus* venom and platelet reactivity: Possible role in scorpion venom induced defibrination syndrome. *Toxicon* 19:153–157.

Longnecker, G. L., Longnecker, H. E., and Watt, E. 1980. Inhibition of angiotension converting enzyme by venom of the scorpion. *Toxicon* 18:667–670.

Macek, P., Sencic, L., and Lebez, D. 1982. Isolation and partial characterization of three lethal and hemolytic toxins from the sea anemone *Actinia cari. Toxicon* 20:181–185.

Mar, A., and Michl, H. 1976. A study of the high molecular weight hemolysin from the skin secretion of the amphibian *Bombina variegata. Toxicon* 14:191–195.

Meyer, K., and Linde, H. 1971. Collection of toad venoms and chemistry of the venom steroids. In *Venomous Animals and Their Venoms,* eds. W. Bucherl and E. E. Buckley, vol. II, pp. 521–556. New York: Academic.

Neeman, I., Calton, G. J., and Burnett, J. W. 1980. An ultrastructural study of the venoms from the sea nettle (*Chrysaora quinquecirrha*) and Portuguese man-of-war (*Physalia physalis*) on cultured Chinese hamster ovary K-1 cells. *Toxicon* 18:495–501.

Neeman, I., Calton, G. J., and Burnett, J. W. 1981. Purification of an endonuclease present in *Chrysaora quinquecirrha* venom. *Proc. Soc. Exp. Biol. Med.* 166:374–382.

Norton, T. R. 1981. Cardiotonic polypeptides from *Anthoplevra xanthogrammica* (Brandt) and *A. elegantissima* (Brandt). *Fed. Proc.* 40:21–25.

O'Connor, R., and Peck, M. L. 1978. Venoms of Apidae. In *Arthropod Venoms,* ed. S. Bettini, pp. 613–660. New York: Springer-Verlag.

Oshima, Y., and Yasumoto, T. 1979. Analysis of toxins in cultured *Gonyaulax excavata* cells originating in Ofunato Buy, Japan. In *Toxic Dinoflagellate Blooms,* eds. D. L. Taylor and H. H. Seliger, pp. 377–380. New York: Elsevier/North Holland.

Padilla, G. M., Kim, Y. S., Raukman, E. J., and Rosen, G. M. 1979. Physiological activities of toxins from *Gymnodinium breve* isolated by high performance liquid chromatography. In *Toxic Dinoflagellate Blooms,* eds. D. L. Taylor and H. H. Seliger, pp. 351–354. New York: Elsevier/North Holland.

Pasquini, V. M., and Andreucci, G. 1979. Saxitoxin and tetrodotoxin intoxication: Report of 16 cases. *Vet. Hum. Toxicol.* 21:107–110.

Pavelka, L. A., Kim, Y. H., and Mosher, H. S. 1977. Tetrodotoxin and tetrodotoxin-like compound from the eggs of the Costa Rican frog *Atelopus chiriquiensis. Toxicon* 15:135–139.

Rathmayer, W. 1978. Venoms of Sphecidae, Pompilidae, Mutillidae, and Bethylidae. In *Arthropod Venoms,* ed. S. Bettini, pp. 661–690. New York: Springer-Verlag.

Risk, M., Lin, Y. Y., MacFarlan, R. D., Sadagopa, R., Smith, L. L., and Trieff, N. M. 1979. Purification and chemical studies on a major toxin from *Gymnodium breve.* In *Toxic Dinoflagellate Bloosm,* eds. D. L. Taylor and H. H. Seliger, pp. 335–344. New York: Elsevier/North Holland.

Risk, M., Norris, P. J., Coutinho-Netto, J., and Bradford, H. F. 1982. Actions of *Ptychodiscus brevis* red tide toxin on metabolic and transmitter-releasing properties of synatosomes. *J. Neurochem.* 39:1485–1488.

Schantz, E. J., Modl, J. D., Stanger, D. W., Shavel, J., Riel, F. J., Bowden, J. P., Lynch, J. M., Wyler, R. S., Riegel, B., and Sommer, H. 1975. Paralytic shellfish poisoning, IV. *J. Am. Chem. Soc.* 79:5230–5235.

Schmidt, J. O., Blum, M. S., and Overal, W. L. 1980. Comparative lethality of venoms from stinging hymenoptera. *Toxicon* 18:469–474.

Shimizu, Y. 1978. Dinoflagellate toxins. In *Marine Natural Products Chemical and Biological Perspectives,* ed. P. J. Scheuer, vol. 1, pp. 1–32. New York: Academic.

Shryock, J. C., and Bianchi, C. P. 1983. Sea nettle (*Chrysaora quinquecirrha*) nematocyst venom: Mechanism of action on muscle. *Toxicon* 21:81–95.

Shulov, A., and Levy, G. 1978. Venoms of Buthinae. In *Arthropod Venoms,* ed. S. Bettini, pp. 309–370. New York: Springer-Verlag.

Stahnke, H. L. 1978. The genus *Centruroides* (Buthidae) and its venoms. In *Arthropod Venoms,* ed. S. Bettini, pp. 279–308. New York: Springer-Verlag.

Strain, H. H., Manning, W. M., and Hardin, G. H. 1944. Xanthophylls and carotenes of Diatoms, Brown Algae, Dinoflagellates, and Sea-Anemones. *Biol. Bull.* 86:169–191.

Tamiya, N., Ishikawa, Y., Menez, A., Hori, H., and Yoshida, A. 1978. The structure of snake neurotoxins and their affinity for the acetylcholine receptor. In *Toxin, Animal, Plant and Microbial,* eds. P. Rosenberg, pp. 243–253. Fairlawn, NJ: Oxford University Press.

Toom, P. M., and Chan, D. S. 1972. Enzymatic activities of venom from the jellyfish *Stomolophus meleagris. Comp. Biochem. Physiol.* 43B:435–441.

Toom, P. M., and Phillips, T. D. 1978. Some effects of purified components of jellyfish toxin on adenosine triphosphate activities. *Toxicon (Suppl.)* 1:527–538.

Tu, A. T. 1974. Sea snake venoms and neurotoxins. *J. Agric. Food Chem.* 22:36–43.

Tu, A. T. 1977. *Venoms: Chemistry and Molecular Biology.* New York: Wiley.

Warnick, J. E., Weinreich, D., and Burnett, J. W. 1981. Sea nettle (*Chrysaora quinquecirrha*) toxin on electrogenic and chemosensitive properties of nerve and muscle. *Toxicon* 19:361–371.

Watrous, J. J., and Blasett, J. W. 1978. A reinvestigation of the action of *Chrysaora quinquecirrha* (sea nettle) toxin on rat liver mitochondria. *Toxicon* 16:300–302.

Watt, D. D., Babin, D. R., and Meejnek, R. V. 1974. The protein neurotoxins in scorpion and elapid snake venoms. *J. Agric. Food Chem.* 22:43–51.

Yang, C. C. 1978. Chemistry and biochemistry of snake venom neurotoxins. In *Toxin, Animal, Plant and Microbial,* ed. P. Rosenberg, pp. 261–292. Fairlawn, NJ: Oxford University Press.

Chapter 13

Asphyxiant Gases

Allen Brands

INTRODUCTION

Asphyxiant gases are used by industry in manufacturing, are byproducts of manufacturing processes, or are the products of a chemical reaction or a chemical process such as combustion or degradation of organic materials that is toxic to the human body. Some are produced by slow vaporization of products used in materials for construction.

A particular gas may be an irritant, it may affect cellular metabolism, or it may produce antibodies. The toxicity generally results from inhalation of the gas. However, some gases may be local irritants to the eyes and skin also. Asthmatics generally have more severe reactions to the irritant gases than nonasthmatics. Some gases are noxious, some odorless, and many are irritating.

Some of the gases are extremely poisonous and require strict monitoring to prevent severe adverse effects. Some produce toxicity through repeated or continuous exposure. As a protection to the public, the National Institute of Occupational Safety and Health (NIOSH) has established upper limits on most gases that may be present in the environment.

472

Prevention is the best protection from the toxic effects of the gases, by avoidance, adequate ventilation, and continuous monitoring.

AMMONIA

Ammonia is a colorless gas with a very pungent odor, mp $-77.7\,°C$, bp $-33.35\,°C$. Inhalation of concentrated vapors of ammonia causes edema of the respiratory tract, spasms of the glottis, and asphyxia. Treatment must be prompt to prevent death (Merck, 1976).

Close et al. (1980) reported on the acute and chronic effects of ammonia burns of the respiratory tract caused by a tank truck carrying anhydrous ammonia that exploded on a highway, releasing a massive cloud of ammonia fumes. Two patients that were directly exposed to high concentrations of the gas showed epithelial defects of the cornea, full-thickness burns of the face, and second- and third-degree burns of the nasal passages, soft palate, pharynx, and larynx. Both required an emergency airway and were treated with steroids, antibiotics, and mechanical ventilation. Even though both patients had significant burns of the larynx, later examinations showed only slight scarring of the vocal cords. Both recovered with no meaningful pulmonary sequelae. Another patient exposed for a longer period of time sustained burns of the entire airway in addition to the burns sustained by the above two patients, and died 18 days after the accident. Autopsy revealed full-thickness burns of the entire respiratory tract, acute necrotizing tracheobronchitis, and bilateral pneumonia. One patient several hundred feet from the accident sustained mild erythema of the face and conjunctival irritation with no epithelial corneal defect, and first- and second-degree burns of the oral cavity, oropharynx, and larynx. A chest X-ray revealed bilateral parenchymal infiltrate. The patient's condition became stable for a period of time, then deteriorated, with dyspnea, increased secretions, and bilateral pneumonia. Prednisone and cephalosporin were administered. A year later, lung scans showed extensive bilateral ventilation and perfusion, abnormalities that were relatively unchanged from 8 months earlier. The patient had been relatively stable clinically, but ventilatory assistance through a tracheostomy was necessary. Another patient who drove into the ammonia cloud several minutes after the accident was exposed for about half an hour. The patient sustained mild erythema of the face with mild conjunctival irritation, but no corneal epithelial defect was noted. The nose and throat were not examined. Later, after improvement, lower-lobe pneumonia developed and was treated with gentamicin sulfate. Severe progressive hoarseness developed, and an examination showed fibrinous patches over the soft-palate mucosa and edema and exudate throughout the larynx. Pulmonary-function studies showed a combined obstructive and restrictive lung disorder. Since discharge the patient has required intermittent positive-pressure breathing treatment, antibiotics, acetylcysteine, and oxygen infrequently for bronchiectasis. The patient has a normal voice and a normal larynx. Four patients that died in the accident prior to medical treatment had at autopsy full-thickness burns of the entire tracheobronchial tree and pulmonary edema. The authors stated that early intubation or tracheotomy is lifesaving, and removal of sloughed mucosa from major airways is essential. Lower concentrations of anhydrous ammonia vapor inhaled over a long period of time can result in extensive burns of the entire tracheobronchial tree, but may not result in acute upper-airway obstruction, with small-airway injury and pulmonary edema occurring. Aggressive treatment of pulmonary injury is essential for patients exposed to moderate amounts of anhydrous ammonia gas over long periods of time, even though they show few if any clinical or laboratory findings. Serial pulmonary-function studies, and perfusion and ventilation lung scans are the most accurate laboratory studies to determine chronic pulmonary sequelae.

Hoeffler et al. (1982) reported the death of a patient 3 years after exposure to anhydrous ammonia gas. Two years after the exposure, the patient's chest roentgenograms suggested cystic bronchiectasis due to the presence of lower-lobe saclike structures. Autopsy findings included bilateral cylindrical and saccular bronchiectasis involving the right middle lobe, lingula, and lower lobes of the lungs. There was no evidence of obliterative bronchiolitis. The authors stated that "speculation remains as to whether the bronchiectasis resulted from the chemical burn or subsequent bacterial bronchitis."

The follow-up of six patients that were involved in industrial-plant accidents with ammonia were reported by Walton (1973). Airway obstruction was severe at the time of the accidents. Recovery was rapid at first, then was more gradual. The forced vital capacity, which was low at first, improved in each patient except the one with the least severe exposure. The report stated that the forced expiratory volume test is the best single test for following airway disturbances in such patients. There were airway damage and reduced gas transfer in these patients for up to 3 years. A patient arrived at a hospital intensive care unit after being exposed to anhydrous liquid ammonia from a refrigeration unit (White, 1971). The patient was unconscious and cyanotic, with pinkish foaming at the mouth and nose. All extremities were spastic. The patient was transferred to a university hospital to do blood-gas studies. With 60% oxygen, blood gases were near normal. Treatment was blood plasma with intravenous fluids. Local steroids and antibiotics were used for the eyes. Kaomycin was prescribed for aerobacteria shown by sputum culture. Arterial blood gases showed mild hypoxia at discharge. After 6 months the patient was working, had normal vision, and, except for a mild cough, no pulmonary symptoms. Fourteen persons were accidently exposed to ammonia gas on board a fishing vessel (Montague and Macneil, 1980). The patients' physical findings varied and included inflammation of the pharynx and conjunctiva, with corneal burns in two patients. Five patients had normal chest examination and were discharged on the second hospital day. Nine patients had a mean duration of 6.3 days hospitalization. All patients received a single dose of hydrocortisone sodium succinate intravenously, and nebulized dexamethasone and oxygen in the examining room. Five patients were treated with intravenous aminophyllin and nebulized salbutamol for signs of airway obstruction. Two patients with fever and productive cough received oral penicillin. Long-term follow-up was not possible on any patient.

Accidental inhalation of anhydrous ammonia gas used as a soil fertilizer was reported by Dalton and Bricker (1978). They had treated 6 patients over a period of 7 years. Three patients required a tracheostomy and use of a mechanical ventilator. One patient died, and autopsy findings included chronic interstitial pneumonitis and pulmonary hyaline membrane formation. For treatment, the authors recommended a tracheostomy immediately if there are facial or pharyngeal burns, because of laryngeal edema possibly developing during the first 24 h. A subclavian venous catheter is helpful to monitor central venous pressure and management of intravenous fluids and medications. Steroids, antibiotics, bronchodilators, and diuretics have been used for treatment of shock, burns, and associated injuries and were recommended. The authors recommended, "Close monitoring of (1) electrocardiogram, (2) arterial pressure, (3) arterial blood gases, (4) central venous pressure, and (5) hourly urine output is carried out for the first three to four days. Immediate chest x-ray and serial x-rays at 12-hour and then 24-hour intervals is recommended." Laryngeal edema increases during the first 48 h after exposure to ammonia gas.

Sobonya (1977) reported on the pathological findings of a fatal anhydrous ammonia inhalation. The findings included purulent cavity pneumonia; some bronchioles and the smallest bronchi had mucous plugging and mural thickening; gram-negative bacilli were present; there was denudation of the epithelium of the main and lobar bronchi; bronchial glands were enlarged; and some small airways were filled with collagenous tissue. The parenchyma had no emphysematous lesions. The alveolar parenchyma was normal or showed hyperemia, alveolar edema, and recent hemorrhage microscopically.

Hatton et al. (1979) tested the urine samples of four patients exposed to ammonia gas and reported that there was a significantly higher excretion of total hydroxylysine metabolites in the urine that could be documented either immediately or 1 day after exposure. The metabolites that increased were glucosylgalactosylhydroxylysine and galactosylhydroxylysine, as measured 1–3 days after exposure. The authors felt that the ammonia in the lower airways and alveoli caused degradation of the structural proteins, including collagen.

Ferguson et al. (1977) reported that humans can adapt to continuous exposure to 100 ppm of ammonia gas after acclimation with no observed effect on the general health. Occasional exposure to 200 ppm was easily tolerated. An allergic reaction to an aromatic ammonia inhalant ampule by an athlete was reported by Herrick and Herrick (1983). The allergic symptoms included rhinitis, rhinorrhea, conjunctivitis, dizziness, severe headache, wheezes, shortness of breath, and periorbital swelling so the patient could not see. Treatment was with epinephrine subcutaneously and with intravenous diphenhydramine hydrochloride, with resolution of the symptoms. It was reported that the use of ammonia inhalants is common among athletes engaging in weight lifting, discus throwing, hammer throwing, and shot putting. The use of aromatic ammonia inhalation to suppress self-injurious behavior in two retarded children was reported by Baumeister and Baumeister (1978). The authors point out that such treatment should be a last treatment measure.

Kapeghian et al. (1982) studied the toxicity of ammonia gas in mice and found that there was a progressive decrease in body weight so the animals appeared to be in a state of starvation. Acute ammonia gas exposure caused congestion and hemorrhage of lung tissue, and alveolar disruption, with late sequelae causing degenerative changes in the liver apparently related to the decline in the nutritional state. Appleman et al. (1982) found hemorrhagic lungs in rats exposed to ammonia gas.

CARBON MONOXIDE

Carbon monoxide (synonym monoxide) is an odorless, colorless, tasteless, flammable gas. mp —199 °C, bp —191.5 °C (Merck, 1976; National Institute for Occupational Safety and Health, 1978a).

Carbon monoxide (CO) is an asphyxiant gas that can combine with myoglobin and hemoglobin in competition with oxygen. Carbon monoxide has an affinity for hemoglobin about 200 times greater than oxygen. It blocks electron transport in the mitochondria by inhibiting the ferrous form of the carrier cytochromes aa_3. This blocks the electron flow between the cytochrome oxidase complex and oxygen (Stryer, 1981; Lehninger, 1982b). Carbon monoxide causes damage by hypoxia, which primarily affects the brain and myocardium (Winter and Miller, 1976).

Symptoms of carbon monoxide poisoning, depending on the individual and the severity of the poisoning, may include agitation, confusion, headache, dizziness, ataxia, syncope, nausea, cyanosis, fever, a cherry-red color to the skin, mucous membranes, and fingernails, and blistering of the skin. However, the cherry-red color of the skin is not always present. Unconsciousness and death may result. Carbon monoxide poisoning may also cause memory and concentration deficit, tachycardia, tachypnea, rapid eye movement, brisk deep-tendon reflexes, pulmonary edema, hyperkalemia, hypocalcemia, seizures, and impaired renal function (Strohl et al., 1980; Arena, 1979a; Larkin et al., 1976; Abbott, 1972; Zimmerman and Truxal, 1981; National Institute for Occupational Safety and Health, 1978a). Headache, nausea, and dizziness are the first symptoms.

The National Institute for Occupational Safety and Health (1978a) reported that exposure to concentrations of 4000 ppm and above can cause coma with a premonitory warning of dizziness and transient weakness. Exposure to 500–1000 ppm causes headache, tachypnea, nausea, weakness, dizziness, mental confusion, and hallucinations in some instances, and may result in brain damage. Concentrations of 50 ppm greatly increases the risk of angina pectoris and coronary infarctions due to decreased oxygen in the blood and in myoglobin of heart muscle. Reaction to a given blood level of carbon monoxide is variable. Some persons may remain normal at carboxyhemoglobin levels of 55%, while others with a level of 38% may be comatose. Carbon monoxide combines with hemoglobin to form carboxyhemoglobin, and this results in a shift of the oxygen saturation curve to the left (Longo, 1970) and increases the affinity of hemoglobin for oxygen so that oxygen is not readily released to the tissues.

Carbon monoxide poisoning and metabolic acidosis are often the major problems of fire victims with smoke inhalation (Strohl et al., 1980). In a study by Treitman et al. (1980), carbon monoxide was found to exceed the short-term exposure limit of 400 ppm in virtually all fire environments studied. Judgment, visual accuity, and decision-making may be impaired in fire fighters by low concentrations of carbon monoxide. Birky and Clarke (1981) stated that a 50% carboxyhemoglobin level was considered lethal and that 60% of the victims fall into this category. Cardiovascular disease may contribute to fatalities at less than 50% carboxyhemoglobin, as such individuals may already have reduced oxygen supply to the heart. However, most of the victims with significant heart disease studied had carboxyhemoglobin levels greater than 50%, suggesting that the heart disease may have contributed to the inability to escape the fire and smoke.

Abbot (1972) described the slow recovery from carbon monoxide poisoning. The patient appeared to develop decerebrate rigidity as a result of the poisoning. He developed a urinary-tract infection and bronchopneumonia. The electroencephalo-gram (EEG) showed dominant generalized delta-wave activity down to 1 cycle/sec on day 7, which was symmetrical and more marked in the anterior than posterior re-gions. The patient was mute and showed no comprehension of speech. There were occasional spasms. There was a continued loss of muscle power in all 4 limbs after 48 days. A grand mal seizure occurred on day 62. The patient was discharged after 71 days, and he felt he was entirely normal at 84 days after admission.

A carbon monoxide poisoning of a 13-year-old boy was reported by Zimmerman and Truxal (1981). Physical examination revealed no response to painful stimuli be-low T-4. There were frequent episodes of tonic contraction of the extremities, with flexion of the neck. There was no response to plantar stimulation, and lower-extremity deep-tendon reflexes were absent. The patient initially was unresponsive to commands, had bizarre facial grimacing, and had tetanic-like contractions of the upper extremities. Medium- to high-voltage 2–4 cps bilateral activity was revealed by an EEG, interpreted as encephalopathy. There was acute renal failure due to myone-crosis, and dialysis was required for 3 weeks.

A fatal case of acute renal failure due to muscle necrosis in carbon monoxide poisoning was reported by Loughridge et al. (1958). The histological findings were those of acute tubular necrosis. The brain was edematous. There was acute conges-tion of the liver, and the kidneys were pale and swollen. The muscle necrosis was in one lower limb and was probably due to pressure stopping the flow of blood for the period of time the patient was immobilized. The authors pointed out the importance of frequent clinical and laboratory assessment and that such victims should have twice-daily estimations of serum electrolytes.

Sone et al. (1974) reported on the effect of carbon monoxide poisoning revealed by chest roentgenograms. A ground-glass appearance indicating lung edema was the most common roentgen finding. The abnormal roentgen findings cleared in 3–5 days.

Shafer et al. (1965) reported on myocardial disease resulting from acute carbon monoxide poisoning. Ten months after exposure the patient was admitted to the hospi-tal because of chest pains that occurred chiefly in the precordial region and radiated to the axilla and left shoulder. A diastolic gallop was heard at the initial examination. The electrocardiogram (ECG) indicated evidence of myocardial damage. Myocardial toxicity following carbon monoxide poisoning was also reported by Anderson et al. (1967). One patient on day 5 after exposure developed ventricular fibrillation and died. At postmortem, a mural thrombus was found near the apex of the left ventricle. A thromboembolus occluded a terminal branch of the left anterior descending coro-nary artery. Individual muscle fibers were swollen and necrotic. In other patients that recovered, the results of electrocardiograms included ST segment depression, QT interval prolongation, and inverted T waves in precordial leads. The electrocardiograms were normal after 1–2½ months. The neurological and psychiatric damage to four patients exposed to a high concentration of carbon monoxide was described by Garland and Pearce (1967). The findings included blindness, object agnosia, temporospatial disorientation, dysphasia, transient deafness, parkinsonism, epilepsy, depression, and psychosis.

Garvey and Longo (1978) investigated the effect of low-level maternal carbon monoxide exposure on the rat fetus and found a reduction in the number of successful pregnancies, and altered growth and development of various fetal organ systems. In the monkey, Ginsberg and Myers (1974) found that a single acute maternal exposure to carbon monoxide led to alterations in fetal homeostasis and severe brain injury or death of the fetus. Fetal bradycardia, metabolic acidosis, and hypotension in the fetus were results of severe hypoxia.

Smith (1965) at autopsy found severe arteriolitis of the midbrain and eschemia of the globus pallidus.

Smith (1965) also found decerebrate rigidity, plantar responses that were extensor, extrapyramidal damage with tremor and rigidity, and expressionless features.

The first treatment for carbon monoxide poisoning is to provide adequate oxygen. The more oxygen, within limits of toxicity, the more effective the treatment. The use of 100% oxygen at atmospheric pressure or in a hyperbaric chamber up to 2.5 atm is recommended (Klaassen, 1980a; Winter and Miller, 1976). Since oxygen is carried in plasma in the dissolved state, administration of 100% oxygen can supply one-third of the oxygen requirements in dissolved form (Strohl et al., 1980; Garland and Pearce, 1967). Screening for the detection of immediate or delayed myocardial toxicity for several days is indicated with serial ECGs and lactate dehydrogenase (LDH), serum glutamic–oxaloacetic transaminase (SGOT), and creatine phosphokinase (CPK) determinations, as myocardial toxicity does not correlate with the carboxyhemoglobin level (Arena, 1979a).

ETHYLENE OXIDE

Ethylene oxide (synonyms: oxirane, ethene oxide, 1,2-epoxyethane) is a colorless, highly flammable gas, mp −111 °C, bp 10.7 °C.

Ethylene oxide is irritating to the eyes, nose, and throat, and may cause coughing and vomiting. In high concentrations it can cause pulmonary edema (Merck, 1976). Symptoms include headache, nausea, dyspnea, drowsiness, and weakness. Ficarra (1980) categorizes ethylene oxide as a possible carcinogenic substance. It is considered a mutagenic alkylating agent.

Garry et al. (1979) studied the effects of occupational exposure of hospital personnel in a sterilizing room during ethylene oxide gas sterilization of materials for use by the hospital. The maximum concentration of the gas was 36 ppm. Symptoms reported by the exposed personnel were sore throat and dry mouth, diarrhea, conjunctival irritation, headache, nausea, speech difficulty, recent memory loss, weakness, dizziness, and incoordination. There was an increase in the frequency of sister-chromatid exchange in lymphocytes as compared to controls.

Three adult males exposed to ethylene oxide at concentrations up to 400 ppm developed sensorimotor peripheral neuropathy. Weakness, paresthesia, headache, and nausea were presenting symptoms. Neurological examination revealed decreased deep-tendon reflexes, decreased lower-extremity sensation, and weakness. Two months after onset of symptoms, decreased nerve-action potentials and muscle-action potentials, as measured by nerve conduction studies, were present (Gross et al., 1978).

Male rats exposed to 1000 ppm ethylene oxide for 4 h showed some signs of toxicity that included central depression, diarrhea, and ocular and respiratory irritation. No deaths occurred, and the rats appeared normal within 24 h following exposure (Embree et al., 1977). When the rats were mated, there was a significant increase in postimplantal fetal deaths, which occurred only during the first 5 weeks of a 10-week experiment following the exposure to ethylene oxide gas. There was also a decrease in the number of rats that became pregnant per number mated.

Snelling et al. (1982) exposed pregnant rats to either 10, 33, or 100 ppm ethylene oxide gas for 6 h/day on days 6–15 of the gestation period. From the results it was concluded that ethylene oxide gas by inhalation at these concentrations was not teratogenic.

In a study of the effects of ethylene oxide gas inhalation on sister-chromatid exchanges in rabbit lymphyocytes, it was found that there was an increase in the sister-chromatid exchanges after exposure to 50 ppm and 250 ppm of gas, but no detectable increase at 10 ppm (Yager and Benz, 1982). It was concluded that ethylene oxide results in a dose-related sister-chromatid exchange effect and that sister-chromatid exchange is a sensitive indicator to ethylene oxide exposure.

The exposure of male mice to ethylene oxide gas by Sega et al. (1981) resulted in alkylation in sperm cells in the mid to late spermatid stages. The protamine from caudal sperm was alkylated about seven times more than was found in the early spermatid and late spermatocyte stages.

Ehrenberg et al. (1974) studied the degree of alkylation of proteins in various organs of mice by ethylene oxide gas inhalation. Protein alkylation in the liver was about twice that in the spleen, brain, and testes at high doses of ethylene oxide gas, but not at lower levels of the gas.

FLUOROCARBONS

Characteristics of some important fluorocarbons are as follows.

Carbon tetrafluoride (synonyms: tetrafluoromethane, Freon-14) is a colorless, odorless gas, thermally stable, with mp $-183.6\,°C$, bp $-127.8\,°C$.

Cryofluorane (1,2-dichloro-1,1,2,2-tetrafluoroethane, synonyms: Freon 114, Frigen 114, Arcton 33) is a colorless, practically odorless, nonflammable gas, with mp $-94\,°C$, bp $4.1\,°C$.

Dichlorodifluoromethane (synonyms: Freon 12, Frigen 12; Arcton 6, Genetron 12, Halon, Isotron 2) is a colorless, practically odorless, nonflammable gas, with mp $-158\,°C$, bp $-29.8\,°C$.

Trichlorofluoromethane (trichloromonofluoromethane, fluorotrichloromethane, synonyms: Freon 11, Frigen 11, Arcton 9) has a faint ethereal odor and is nonflammable. It is a liquid at temperatures below 23.8 °C, with mp −111 °C, bp 23.7 °C (Merck, 1976).

Freon is the trademark name of E. I. DuPont de Nemours & Co. The Freons are a class of compounds that are used in refrigeration and have been used as propellants in aerosol sprays. The Freons are identified by a number after the name—Freon 11, 12, etc. The first digit on the right indicates the number of fluorine atoms, the second digit from the right is one more than the number of hydrogen atoms, and the third digit from the right is one less than the number of carbon atoms but is omitted if zero. The number of chlorine atoms equals the number of carbon bonds not occupied by fluorine or hydrogen atoms.

Many deaths have been reported from sniffing volatile hydrocarbons, among which are the propellants used in aerosol spray cans and atomizers. The deaths have occurred from collecting household-use aerosol sprays in a plastic bag and inhaling the contents of the bag. The aerosol propellant was toxic to the cardiovascular and respiratory systems (Bass, 1970; Aviado, 1975). The deaths were sudden and followed physical exertion after inhalation of the aerosol propellant gas. No anatomical cause of death was found at autopsy.

Aviado (1978) reported that these gases induced cardiac arrhythmias by sensitization of the heart to epinephrine, depression of myocardial contractility, reduction in cardiac output, and reflex increase in sympathetic and vagal impulses to the heart by irritation of the mucosa in the upper and lower respiratory tract.

In a report by Bass (1970) on three sudden deaths in which the victims inhaled the aerosol propellant from a bag, each victim very shortly after inhaling the gas engaged in a physical activity (e.g., running) and collapsed and died. In each case there was no anatomical cause of death at autopsy. The author described the events as sudden death that occurred after sniffing followed by some exercise or stressful situation.

In a study using dogs, it was found that fluorocarbons used as propellants sensitize the cardiac muscle to epinephrine. The authors suggested that the heart is more sensitive to epinephrine because of hypoxia and exposure to the compound (Reinhardt et al., 1971). It seems that there may be a disturbance in the normal conduction of the electrical impulse through the heart, probably due to a local disturbance in the electrical potential across the cell membrane. However, a precise explanation could not be given for the sensitization of the heart.

Sakata et al. (1981) studied the toxic effects of Freon 12 in rabbits and mice. The toxic symptoms in rabbits were reeling, foreleg weakness, falling down, flow of mucus from the mouth and nose, mydriasis, lacrimation, violent movement of the body and extremities, cyanosis, and death. The autopsy findings were bulging of lungs, subplural hemorrhage, and a colorless mucus fluid in the trachea and bronchus. Pulmonary emphysema, congestion, hemorrhage in lungs, and interalveolar septum thickening were histological findings.

In examining the metabolic effects of fluorocarbon (FC) 11 and FC 12 in rats, rabbits and dogs, Paulet et al. (1975a) reported that FC 12 had no effect, but FC 11 at 5% caused a decrease in oxygen uptake, an increase in glycemia and lactacidemia, a reduction in hepatic glycogen secretion, a decrease in blood urea, a small increase in free fatty acids, and an increase in the respiratory quotient. It was felt that the effects were the result of a slower cellular oxidation. The metabolic changes were reversed when inhalation ceased.

FC 11 and FC 12 were found in the blood, cerebrospinal fluid (CSF), urine, and bile 1 min after inhalation in the dog and rabbit by Paulet et al. (1975b). Elimination of 98% of the gases was through the pulmonary system.

Similar results were obtained by Blake and Mergner (1974), who reported that essentially all of the inhaled FC 11 and FC 12 was exhaled intact within 1 h. Only traces were found in exhaled CO_2 and urine. They concluded that little biotransformation of these gases takes place.

Taylor et al. (1971) found that inhalation of an FC 12 and FC 114 mixture in 61% oxygen produced ventricular premature beats and ventricular tachycardia in monkeys, which began at an average of 39 sec. The authors stated that the arrythmias were mediated through beta-adrenergic receptors, or from a direct toxic effect on the heart that was nonadrenergic.

In a study of the cardiopulmonary effects of FC 11, FC 12, and FC 21 on dogs by Belej and Aviado (1975), it was found that the low-pressure compounds, FC 11 and FC 21, were more toxic than the high-pressure compound, FC 12. While FC 12 and FC 21 produced bronchoconstriction, FC 11 produced bronchodilation. It was felt that the bronchodilation caused by FC 11 was due to the stimulation of the beta-adrenergic receptors of bronchial smooth muscles, as propanolol administration prevented the bronchodilation. FC 11, FC 12, and FC 21 produced hypotension and tachycardia. These compounds sensitized the cardiac muscle to epinephrine.

A technique using partial asphyxia was utilized by Taylor and Harris (1970) and Harris (1973). After breathing FC 11, FC 12, and FC 114, mice were asphyxiated for 4 min, then allowed to breath room air. It was found that the inhalants sensitized the hearts of the mice to asphyxia-induced sinus bradycardia, atrioventricular (AV) block, and ventricular T-wave depression. The authors suggested that the gases produce cardiac toxicity and may have been the cause of sudden asthma deaths. Four minutes of asphyxiation in mice that did not receive the gases did not produce the toxic results.

Arena (1979b) reported that in experiments on dogs, sinus-node suppression occurred and frequently included sinus bradycardia, AV dissociation, and electric asystole or ventricular fibrillation. The result is immediate and tragic. Epinephrine or isoproterenol is contraindicated. The treatment recommended was resuscitation with cardiac massage, defibrillation, and pacing.

FORMALDEHYDE

Formaldehyde (synonyms: methanal, oxomethane, oxymethylene, methylene oxide, formic aldehyde, methyl aldehyde) is a flammable, colorless gas at ordinary temperatures, with pungent, suffocating odor, mp $-92\,°C$, bp $-19.5\,°C$ (Merck, 1976).

Formaldehyde is used in the manufacture of some building materials and foam insulation, thus exposing employees in the manufacture of such products and the general public where these products were used as building materials to formaldehyde vapors. Common symptoms resulting from exposure to low concentrations of formaldehyde vapors are eye irritation, respiratory-tract irritation, headache, and tiredness (Arena, 1979c; Olsen and Dossing, 1982; National Research Council, 1981). When persons were exposed to formaldehyde vapors in their work environment but were not exposed in their nonworking environment, such as weekends, relief from the symptoms occurred (Olsen and Dossing, 1982; Alexanderson et al., 1982; Arena, 1979c).

A study was done by questionnaire to employees at mobile day-care centers that had urea–formaldehyde-glued particle board for indoor paneling and to employees at institutions where no particle boards had been used in the buildings for controls. The staff in the mobile day-care centers had "a significantly higher frequency of irritation of the eyes and upper respiratory tract, unnatural drowsiness, headache, menstrual irregularities, and use of analgesics." The median formaldehyde concentration in the mobile day-care centers was 0.43 mg/m^3, with ventilation less than 0.5 changes/h. There was relief from the symptoms after the end of the working day, and on weekends and holidays (Olsen and Dossing, 1982). Alexandersson et al. (1982) conducted a study on the effects of formaldehyde vapors on pulmonary function. They found that there was a reduction in forced expiratory volume, in percent forced expiratory volume, and in maximum mid-expiratory flow, and an increase in closing volume in percentage of vital capacity at the end of the working day. The study was conducted at carpentry works. The subjects had been employed for more than 1 year and had been regularly exposed to formaldehyde vapors. The average concentration of formaldehyde in the air was 0.45 mg/m^3. Some subjects also experienced symptoms involving the eyes, nose, and throat, dyspnea, and chest oppression. On Monday morning, after 2 days of nonexposure to formaldehyde, lung function was normal. The authors stated that the changes in lung function were moderate, would not decrease the subjects' physical capability, and were reversible, and no chronic effects were established.

Cockcroft et al. (1982) reported that two carpenters had developed asthma from working with cedar urea–formaldehyde particle board. Both developed nasal and chest symptoms after cedar urea–formaldehyde sawdust exposure. One also developed an equivocal early asthma response and the other a dual asthmatic response. Symptoms in neither appeared after exposure to spruce or cedar sawdust. One patient, after 2 h of exposure to cedar urea–formaldehyde sawdust, developed a burning sensation in the chest, sore throat, headache, cough, and sputum. Confusion, nausea, and vomiting occurred 12 h later. Boggs (1983) pointed out in a letter on the above report that the asthma may have been caused by industrial-secret chemicals in the cedar urea–formaldehyde particle board rather than by the formaldehyde. Cockcroft et al. (1983) concurred by restating that it was a component of the urea–formaldehyde resin system that was responsible. In another study by Nethercott et al. (1982), formaldehyde was presumed to be the cause of erythema multiforme in four workers employed in the manufacture of printed circuit boards. The patients had been employed at the plant for 6–8 weeks before the development of erythema multiforme. The patients developed pyrexia, coughing, widespread erythmeatous plaques, target lesions, and vesicles, with vesicles on the oral mucosa and genitals. One patient had hepatic inflammation that was confirmed by liver biopsy, which revealed fine fat deposits in the hepatocytes. Two patients had a positive reaction to a formalin skin test. None was positive to a skin test for the other chemicals used. The authors felt that formaldehyde was the most likely chemical agent responsible. Triamcinalone cream, oral prednisone, and betamethasone-17-valerate cream were used in treatment.

A man who had worked as a textile engineer with 25 years of occupational exposure to low concentrations of formaldehyde developed squamous-cell carcinoma of the nasal cavity (Halperin et al., 1983). His first symptoms appeared 21 years after the initial exposure and included infrequent right-sided midfacial and right-sided nasal discomfort. Later the frequency of facial pain increased, and nasal obstruction developed. Examination revealed bilateral nasal polyps in the middle meatus and a nasal tumor on the right side that extended to the nasopharynx. Surgery was performed followed by radiation therapy. After 3 years there was no clinical evidence of a recurrence. The authors point out that this one case "does not at all establish that formaldehyde causes cancer of the nasal cavity in man." They do mention that formaldehyde is a biologically plausable carcinogen as it is a reactive alkylating agent. Kreiger (1983) wrote that the risk of nasal cancer due to formaldehyde is small. Marsh (1982) conducted a mortality analysis of chemical-plant workers exposed to formaldehyde on deaths that occurred between 1950 and 1976. He found no statistically significant differences in mortality of the formaldehyde-exposed group as compared to United States men and men from the local county area. There was no mention of sinonasal cancer as a cause or contributory cause of death. The mortality experience of embalmers was investigated by Walrath and Fraumeni (1983). They reported significantly elevated mortality from cancers of the skin, kidney, and brain for those licensed only as embalmers as compared to those licensed also as funeral directors. Skin-cancer mortality (including melanoma) was significantly elevated, especially among those licensed for more than 35 years. Mortality from kidney and brain cancers was significantly greater. However, there was no excess mortality from cancers of the nasal passages or respiratory tract.

Kreiger and Garry (1983) measured some toxic effects of formaldehyde on human lymphocyte cultures. The results showed significant cytotoxic responses. Formaldehyde appeared to be a weak inducer of sister-chromatid exchanges, showing a possible induction threshold effect. Mitotic inhibition doses of formaldehyde seemed to be affected by blood-donor factors or initial viable cell number.

The effects of inhalation of formaldehyde in rats and mice were studied by Jaeger and Gearhart (1982). They found that mice were more sensitive than rats to the irritant effects of formaldehyde. Mice had a similar reduction in tidal volume but a larger decrease in respiratory rate and, as a consequence, in minute volume. Mice had a greater decrease in carbon dioxide production and a greater decrease in body temperature. The authors hypothesized that a method for animals to avoid the irritant effect of gases was to decrease ventilation. Albert et al. (1982) reported that inhalation of formaldehyde or formaldehyde in combination with hydrogen chloride by rats resulted in nasal cancer. The toxic and mutagenic effects of formaldehyde on *Salmonella typhimurium* were studied by Temcharoen and Thilly (1983). They found that formaldehyde was toxic and mutagenic to the bacteria. The toxic and mutagenic effects were concentration- and time-dependent.

HYDROGEN CYANIDE

Hydrogen cyanide (synonyms: hydrocyanic acid, prussic acid, formonitrile) is a colorless or pale-blue liquid or gas with a bitter almond odor, intensely poisonous, with mp -14.4 to $-16.8\,°C$, bp $26\,°C$ (National Institute for Occupational Safety and Health, 1978b). The oral injestion of cyanide salts is mentioned in this section as the action is similar to inhalation of the gas.

Hydrogen cyanide is extremely poisonous and acts very rapidly, with death occurring within a few minutes from respiratory failure. Cyanide reacts with the trivalent iron of cytrochrome oxidase (aa_3) in mitrochrondia, thereby blocking the reduction of oxygen required for cellular respiration, resulting in cytotoxic hypoxia. The transfer of electrons from cytochrome oxidase to oxygen is blocked (National Institute for Occupational Safety and Health, 1978b; Klaassen, 1980b; Finelli, 1981; Lehninger, 1982b).

Early symptoms of toxic reactions to lower levels of exposure to HCN may include weakness, headache, confusion, and occasionally nausea and vomiting; the rate and depth of respiration increases and later becomes slow and gasping. High concentrations of HCN may cause almost instantaneous collapse, cessation of respiration, and death. At 270 ppm HCN is immediately fatal to humans; 180 ppm is fatal after 10 min, 135 ppm after 30 min, and 110 ppm in 1 h. Some symptoms may occur in humans after several hours of exposure to 18–36 ppm HCN. Humans can tolerate exposure to 45–54 ppm HCN for $1/2$–1 h without immediate or delayed effects (National Institute for Occupational Safety and Health, 1978b). Respiration is at first stimulated in cyanide poisoning, due to the chemoreceptive cells of the carotid and aortic bodies responding to decreased oxygen. Then hypoxic convulsions occur, with respiratory arrest resulting in death (Klaassen, 1980b; Smith, 1980). The venous blood may be bright red because of the high concentration of oxyhemoglobin, resembling arterial blood (Arena, 1979d; Klaassen, 1980b).

Lactic acid acidosis and pulmonary edema were reported to result from cyanide poisoning (Graham et al., 1977; Shragg et al., 1982). The blocking of the cytochrome oxidase increases the generation of lactic acid, with a resultant fall in plasma bicarbonate to buffer the acid.

Finelli (1981) reported on a cyanide poisoning in which a computed tomography showed symmetrical globus pallidus infarctions with an infarction of the left cerebellar hemisphere.

Treatment must be immediate to be life-saving. If breathing has ceased or is labored, artificial respiration is begun immediately. First, amyl nitrate inhalant and intravenous sodium nitrite are administered. The nitrites form methemoglobin, which binds to cyanide ions in the blood. The ferric iron in methemoglobin competes with cytochrome oxidase for cyanide and forms cyanmethemoglobin. Methemoglobin has a greater affinity for cyanide than cytochrome oxidase. This leads to a resumption of cellular oxidative metabolism by dissociation of the cyanide–cytochrome complex.

Secon, a 25% solution of sodium thiosulfate, is injected intravenously. The thiosulfate converts cyanide to thiocyanate, which is relatively nontoxic. When a cyanide has been injested orally, a gastric lavage should be performed to remove any of the cyanide remaining in the stomach (Arena, 1979d; Smith, 1980; Klaassen, 1980b).

HYDROGEN SULFIDE

Hydrogen sulfide (synonyms: sulfurated hydrogen, hydrosulfuric acid, hepatic gas, sulfur hydride, rotten egg gas, and stink damp) is a colorless, heavier-than-air gas with an offensive odor of rotten eggs and a sweetish taste. It is flammable and highly poisonous, with mp −85.49°C, bp −60.33°C (Merck, 1976).

Hydrogen sulfide occurs in coal pits, gas wells, sulfur springs, and from decaying organic matter containing sulfur. It also occurs as a by-product of some industrial plants. There have been accidental poisonings in tanneries, glue factories, fur-dressing and felt-making plants, and in beet-sugar factories (Hamilton and Hardy, 1974). It may occur in relatively unlikely places. Peters (1981) reported on the poisoning of a person in a hospital while cleaning the plaster of paris sludge in a cast-room drain with a strong acid industrial cleaner. It was reported that there was a calcium sulfide sludge in the drain that was the product of anaerobic degradation of the plaster of paris. The acid in the cleaner released the hydrogen sulfide gas by its action on the calcium sulfide sludge in the drain. This result was proven by laboratory tests in which concentrated sulfuric acid released hydrogen sulfide gas from black plaster of paris sludge.

Poisoning among fisherman has been reported with hydrogen sulfide gas being produced by the anaerobic decay of insufficiently refrigerated fish stored in an unventilated hold of a fishing vessel (Glass et al., 1980). Manure is a potent source of hydrogen sulfide, and deaths have been reported in which farm workers were exposed to the gas evolving from manure storage tanks and from gutters for carrying manure from the barn (Morse et al., 1981; Osbern and Crapo, 1981). One report used the term "dung lung" in a report of toxic exposure to liquid manure. Sewers may be a source of hydrogen sulfide gas due to waste products being discharged by some industrial plants.

The offensive odor is the first indication of the presence of hydrogen sulfide gas. However, the odor should not be used as a warning signal, as at concentrations of approximately 150 ppm or greater, rapid paralysis of the olfactory nerve occurs (Stine et al., 1976). Hydrogen sulfide is toxic and irritating when inhaled, if it comes in contact with the eyes, nose, throat, or skin, or if it is swallowed. When inhaled in concentrations of 1000–2000 ppm, 1 or 2 breaths of this contaminated air can cause almost immediate loss of consciousness and almost immediate death, as noted by Adelson and Sunshine (1966). They described the anatomic and laboratory findings in three persons who died in a sewer from hydrogen sulfide asphyxia. The three had similar findings at autopsy. Externally they had a grayish-green cyanosis. Internally there was hemorrhagic pulmonary edema. The blood and viscera had a peculiar greenish cast. The cerebral and nuclear masses were greenish purple.

The toxicity of hydrogen sulfide is comparable to the toxicity of hydrogen cyanide. They both interrupt the respiratory electron transport chain by reversibly binding cytochrome oxidase (Stine et al., 1976; Ravizzo et al., 1982). The National Institute for Occupational Safety and Health (1978c) reported that hydrogen sulfide is a leading cause of death in the workplace.

Ravizzo et al. (1982) described their findings in a person who was overcome by hydrogen sulfide gas and recovered with treatment. The patient arrived at the hospital 35 min after losing consciousness. He was found to have distonic reaction to painful stimuli, tonic contraction of the neck and upper arm muscles, and bilateral mydriasis response to light. There were cyanosis, tachypnea, 120/80 blood pressure, and a heart rate of 140 beats per minute. Pulmonary edema and hypoxia were present. Arterial blood gases had a PaO_2 of 48 mm Hg, and there was metabolic acidosis with a pH 7.21, BE —8. Stine et al. (1976) reported an arterial blood pH of 6.97 for a patient that recovered.

Brief exposure to hydrogen sulfide at high concentrations has caused conjunctivitis and keratitis. Exposure at very high concentrations has caused unconsciousness, respiratory paralysis, and death. There is evidence that hydrogen sulfide at low concentrations has caused disorders of the nervous system and of the cardiovascular and digestive systems, and affects the eyes (National Institute for Occupational Safety and Health, 1978c).

Hydrogen sulfide causes respiratory paralysis with asphyxia at high concentrations. A single breath of hydrogen sulfide at concentrations of 1000–2000 ppm may cause coma with fatal results. Excessive exposure to 50 ppm can cause rhinitis, pharyngitis, bronchitis, and pneumonitis, as well as conjunctivitis with pain and photophobia, which may progress to keratoconjunctivitis and vesiculation of the corneal epithelium. Olfactory fatigue occurs rapidly at high concentrations. Repeated exposure results in increased susceptibility, so that concentrations previously tolerated may cause adverse effects (National Institute for Occupational Safety and Health, 1978c).

The first and foremost action for a person exposed to hydrogen sulfide is to move the affected person to fresh air at once. If the gas gets into the eyes, immediately wash with copious amounts of water. Contact lenses should not be worn when working with this chemical. If the gas gets on the skin, or if it gets on clothing and penetrates to the skin, remove the clothing and thoroughly wash the skin with water (National Institute for Occupational Safety and Health, 1978c). Treatment of acute hydrogen sulfide poisoning has varied. In one poisoning (Ravizzo et al., 1982), the patient was treated with intermittent positive-pressure ventilation with positive-end respiratory pressure and with thiopental at 30 mg/kg for cerebral protection. Stine et al. (1976) used 40% oxygen with a face mask, amyl nitrite inhalations, intravenous sodium nitrite, and intravenous sodium thiosulfate. No sodium bicarbonate was administered. In another successful treatment reported by Peters (1981), the patient was placed on 40% oxygen with a face mask after an ampule of sodium bicarbonate. Then about half an hour later amyl nitrite inhalation and sodium nitrite and sodium thiosulfate by intravenous push were given.

The literature has reported (Smith and Gosselin, 1964, 1966; Smith et al., 1976) that methemoglobin binds with the sulfide to form sulfmethemoglobin, a tightly bound complex. Nitrites oxidize hemoglobin to form methoglobin. Two reports (Smith and Gosselin, 1966; Smith et al., 1976) felt that the thiosulfate injection should be omitted, and one (Smith et al., 1976) felt that it had not been demonstrated that oxygen had a protective or antidotal effect, even though it was widely recommended as the antidote of choice.

Because of reports of pulmonary infections following exposure to hydrogen sulfide, Rogers and Ferin (1981) conducted an experiment on rat lung to determine the effect of hydrogen sulfide on bacterial inactivation. It was reported that the alveolar macrophage was impaired and there was decreased mucociliary activity.

ISOCYANATES

Toluene 2,4-Diisocyanate (synonyms: 2,2-diisocyanatotoluene, 2,4-tolylene diisocyanate, TDI, nacconat 100) is a liquid at room temperature with a sharp pungent odor and mp 19.5–21.5 °C, bp 251 °C (Merck, 1976).

Several isocyanates are used in the manufacture of products for insulation, coatings, paints, cushions, clothing, automobiles, and aircraft. These include toluene 2,4-diisocyanate (TDI), diphenyl methane diisocyanate (MDI), and hexamethylene diisocyanate (HDI) (Sangha and Alarie, 1979). TDI is sufficiently volatile at room temperature for measurable concentrations to be found in the room air (O'Brien et al., 1979).

The isocyanates can induce hypersensitivity and asthmatic reactions in humans exposed to the vapors, with symptoms of shortness of breath, wheezing, cyanosis, and dermal reactions (Karol et al., 1979; O'Brien et al., 1979; Danks et al., 1981).

A patient employed as a foundary worker who was exposed to diphenyl methane diisocyanate at work developed dyspnea and restrictive breathing (Malo and Zeiss, 1982). Symptoms documented for the patient were general malaise, fever, increased leukocyte count, and lung-function impairment. There were elevated concentrations of specific immunoglobin G (IgG) antibodies. The bronchial reactions appeared to be primarily the result of isocyanate exposure.

Isocyanates are irritant chemicals that primarily affect the respiratory system. Charles et al. (1976) reported that one patient exposed to isocyanate vapor had a lung biopsy performed. Microscopic examination revealed that acute inflammation to end-stage fibrosis was present. It was suggested by the authors that the cause was a hypersensitivity response to an inhaled allergen. The authors felt that instead of an asthmatic syndrome, patients develop a hypersensitivity pneumonitis.

O'Brien et al. (1979) found that in a plant handling diisocyanates, 16 of 24 workers who had respiratory diseases also had an asthmatic reaction to toluene disso-cyanate. Some of the 16 workers had an asthmatic reaction to diphenyl methane diisocyanate and/or hexamethylene diisocyanate as well.

A group of 35 firemen were exposed to chemical fumes that included toluene diisocyanate while fighting a fire in a factory (Axford et al., 1976). Four years later, 43% of the firemen had evidence of long-term damage to the respiratory system. The authors stated that while the evidence that the lung damage was caused by toluene diisocyanate exposure is inconclusive, it could have been the responsible chemical.

Baur and Fruhmann (1981) reported that a subgroup of patients with toluene diisocyanate asthma suffer from an IgE-mediated hypersensitivity to isocyanates. The authors suggested that there is a cross-reactivity to *p*-tolyl (mono)isocyanate, diphenyl methane diisocyanate, diphenyl methane 4-(mono)isocyanate, and hexamethylene diisocyanate. However, Danks et al. (1981) reported that they were unable to detect IgE antibodies against *p*-tolyl (mono)isocyanate human serum conjugate in patients with respiratory disease induced by toluene diisocyanate. It was felt by Davies et al. (1977) that toluene diisocyanate has beta-adrenoceptor blocking activity, which could contribute to asthma.

The immunological response in guinea pigs that inhaled various concentrations of toluene diisocyanate was investigated by Karol (1983). The antibody response was concentration-dependent. Antibodies were not detected in animals exposed to 0.12 ppm toluene diisocyanate. Pulmonary sensitivity was not found in animals exposed to 0.12 ppm but did occur at concentrations of 0.36 ppm or greater. Exposure concentrations of 2 ppm and higher were pneumotoxic.

Guinea pigs were sensitized with toluene diisocyanate/hexamethylene diisocyanate human serum conjugates and then challenged with toluene diisocyanate/hexamethylene diisocyanate coupled to transferrin, a different protein carrier (Chen and Bernstein, 1982). Positive responses were obtained. The authors felt that the use of guinea pigs with their procedure was a reliable animal model of studying allergic responses to diisocyanates.

Using peripheral leukocytes of human blood, VanErt and Battigelli (1975), examined the effect of toluene diisocyanate in blocking beta-adrenergic receptors stimulated by isoproterenol, norepinephrine, epinephrine, and glucagon. The toluene diisocyanate reduced the catecholamine effect ón cyclic adenosine monophosphate and also inhibited the antigenic release of histamine.

McKay and Brooks (1983) investigated the effects of toluene diisocyanate on the beta-adrenergic receptor function using frog erythrocyte membranes and guinea pig trachial smooth-muscle responsiveness. It was found that toluene diisocyanate inhibited isoproterenol-stimulated erythrocyte adenylate cyclase activity in a dose-dependent manner. However, toluene diisocyanate had no effect on isoproterenol-induced trachial smooth-muscle relaxation. The authors suggested that toluene diisocyanate-induced asthma may be caused by mechanisms other than direct beta-adrenergic blockade. In this and a previous study (McKay et al., 1981), it was concluded that toluene diisocyanate exerts a nonspecific effect on the beta-adrenergic/adenylate cyclase system of frog erythrocyte membrane preparations.

A study to investigate the effect of different concentrations of toluene diisocyanate on the levels of cyclic adenosine monophosphate produced by isoproterenol, prostaglandin E, and histamine on human eryuthrocytes was conducted by Davies et al. (1977). It was found that toluene diisocyanate reduced the levels of cyclic adenosine monophosphate produced by isoproterenol and prostaglandin E, but not that produced by histamine. The authors suggested that obstructive airway disease may be caused by toluene diisocyanate through pharmacological mechanisms, and it may be a partial agonist.

Brown et al. (1982) reported that hexamethyl isocyanate, hexyl isocyanate, and

2,6-toluene diisocyanate completely inhibited purified human serum cholinesterase at molar concentrations of 4:1 to 8:1 (isocyanate:enzyme), while a molar concentration of 50:1 was required for 50% inhibition by 2,4-toluene diisocyanate. It was felt that the cholinesterase inhibition may be responsible for respiratory symptoms caused by exposure to the isocyanates.

Using mice, Sangha and Alarie (1979) investigated sensory irritation produced by single and repeated exposures to toluene diisocyanate. It was reported that the level of response as measured by a decrease in respiratory rate was dependent not only on concentration but also on the duration of the exposure. A similar study using mice investigated the effects of phenyl isocyanate, o-toluene isocyanate, p-toluene isocyanate, 1,6-hexamethylene diisocyanate, and hexylisocyanate. The results were similar to those obtained with toluene diisocyanate (Sangha et al., 1981).

NITROGEN DIOXIDE

Nitrogen dioxide (synonyms: nitrogen tetroxide, NTO, dinitrogen tetroxide, nitrogen peroxide; Formula NO_2 and N_2O_4) is a dark-brown fuming liquid or gas with a pungent, acrid odor, mp $-9.3\,°C$, bp $21.15\,°C$ (Merck, 1976).

Nitrogen dioxide is highly toxic and can adversely affect the body if inhaled or if it comes in contact with the eyes or skin. According to the National Institute for Occupational Safety and Health, (1978d):

> Exposure may cause severe breathing difficulties which are usually delayed in onset and which may cause death. Recovery may be slow (2 to 3 weeks) with possible relapse and possible permanent lung damage. Pneumonia may occur. Irritation of the eyes, nose, throat, and skin may occur with acute exposures.

The acute phase resulting from inhalation of nitrogen dioxide may include chest pain, profuse sweating, marked breathlessness, coarse crepitations throughout both lungs, sinus tachycardia, cough with production of yellow sputum or a dry irritating cough, hypoxemia, alveolar hyperventilation, cyanosis, cold clammy extremities, and pulmonary edema (Jones et al., 1973; Fleming et al., 1979; Scott and Hunt, 1973; Hatton et al., 1977; McCabe, 1977).

Silo-fillers' disease is caused by nitrogen dioxide being produced for a few days after silo filling and persons entering the silo too soon (McCabe, 1977; Scott and Hunt, 1973). Scott and Hunt state that a history is of major importance in the diagnosis of silo-fillers' disease.

A second phase as a result of nitrogen dioxide poisoning may occur days or weeks after an acute exposure, with headache, tiredness, sweating, aching pains, dyspnea, cough and sometimes emphysema (Jones et al., 1973; Fleming et al., 1979; National Institute for Occupational Safety and Health, 1978d). Extensive mucosal edema and inflammatory-cell exudation are found in the lungs on pathologic examination of the acute lesion. The delayed lesion shows the histologic appearance of bronchiolitis obliterans. Both stages show a reduction in lung volume and diffusion capacity. Jones et al. (1973) reported bronchiolitis obliterans as being present in one patient and the clinical features present in a second. Hatton et al. (1977) reported that there was an increase in urinary excretion of hydroxylysine metabolites by 3 astronauts accidently exposed to nitrogen dioxide gas for 4 min and 40 seconds. The authors felt that the increase in the urinary metabolites was due to the gas causing acute pulmonary lesions with lung collagen degradation. Other symptoms were tightness of the chest, retrosternal burning sensation, inability to inhale deeply, and a nonproductive cough. Blood-gases analysis indicated mild respiratory alkalosis and hypoxia with hyperventilation. Similar results were obtained by blood-gas measurements by Scott and Hunt (1973), Jones et al. (1973), and Fleming et al. (1979). Orehek et al. (1976) exposed asthmatic patients to 0.1 ppm nitrogen dioxide for 1 h and found that the gas increased the bronchial sensitivity of these asthmatic patients to the bronchoconstrictor agent, carbachol. According to the National Institute for Occupational Safety and Health (1978d):

> The effects expected in humans from exposure to nitrogen dioxide for 60 minutes are: 100 ppm, pulmonary edema and death; 50 ppm, pulmonary edema with possible subacute or chronic lesions in the lungs; 25 ppm, respiratory irritation and chest pain.

Rabbits exposed to concentrations of 7, 14, and 28 ppm nitrogen dioxide gas, continuously or intermittently, resulted in an increase of polymorphonuclear leukocytes in the lungs (Gardner et al., 1977). An increase in pulmonary infection with streptococci occurred in mice with increases in nitrogen dioxide concentration. Sherwin and Richters (1982) found that mice exposed to ambient levels of the gas, 0.34 ppm, 6 h/day for 6 weeks, had an increase in the number and size of type II cells in the lung. It was believed that the increase was due to damage and loss of type I cells. Similar findings were reported in beagle dogs by Johnson et al. (1982) and in rats by Wright et al., (1982).

A study of the effect of nitrogen dioxide on the lungs of beagle dogs was done by Guidotti (1980). In the study, the upper airway was bypassed with a bronchial cannulation system so that one lung received 37 ppm of the gas and the other lung received room air. Oxygen uptake in the exposed lung dropped abruptly, 65% in 30 min, but was reversible. Pathologically, the exposed lung had a disorganization and loosening of interstitial structure, an increase in the number of vesicles, and an increase in the dimension of capillar endothelium. Johnson et al. (1982) exposed beagle dogs to a concentration of 70 ppm nitrogen dioxide for 6 h to simulate an accidental exposure. They reported a productive cough, an increase in respiratory frequency, ausculatory rales, interstitial lung density radiographically, FRC, alveolar dead space, and lung weight. There was a decrease in tidal volume and in percentage alveolar ventilation. White foam was present in the airways, with excessive pulmonary air trapping. The loss of airway cilia at 0.1 day postexposure (DPE) returned to normal at 14 DPE. At 2 DPE the coughing stopped, and the breathing-pattern changes were characteristic of restrictive and not obstructive pulmonary dysfunction. It was felt that irritant-receptor stimulation resulted in the cough and the bronchial restriction. Hamsters were exposed to various concentrations of nitrogen dioxide by DeNicola et al. (1981). The deep-lung damage was measured biochemically and cytologically by examining pulmonary fluid. There was a 10-fold increase in neutrophils at the lowest level of the gas exposure. The authors considered this test a sensitive indication of pulmonary injury histologically. Biochemically, there was an increase in soluble protein and sialic acid in the lavage fluid.

Oxygen and carbon dioxide exchange was lowered in mice after exposure to 20 ppm nitrogen dioxide for 24 h. The mice recovered in 3 days (Suzuki et al., 1982). Rats continuously exposed to 15 ppm nitrogen dioxide for up to 17 months had increases in lung volume and lesions of small airways and adjacent alveoli (Juhos et al., 1980). Rats exposed for 17 months had the lung volume tripled, while the caliber of terminal bronchioles decreased to 45.6% less than the controls.

Kleinerman (1979) exposed hamsters to 30 ppm nitrogen dioxide for 22 h/day for 3 weeks. there was a general loss of body weight and an increase in lung weight. A decrease in total lung collagen occurred within 4 days and in elastin within 10 days. Total lung collagen returned to preexposure levels by day 14 of exposure. Total lung elastin did not return to normal until the exposure was terminated. The authors suggested that the alveolar macrophages secreted enzymes that may cause the loss of elastin and collagen. A study by Drozdz et al. (1977) of guinea pigs after exposure to nitrogen dioxide gas at 2 mg/m^3 revealed a decrease in total collagen content of the lungs, an increase in skin collagen, and an increase in collagen catabolite levels in blood serum and urine. In the skin there was an increase of soluble fractions and a decrease of insoluble fractions of collagen. Nitrogen dioxide may cause a metabolic defect by activating the catabolic processes to decrease the total collagen content of lung tissue.

Multiple exposures of hamsters to 10 ppm nitrogen dioxide by Creasia et al. (1977) caused multiple waves of DNA synthesis. However, the synthetic activity stimulation diminished with repeated exposure. The shorter the exposure-free interval, the quicker the decline in DNA synthesis by subsequent exposure. The response was measured by [^{3}H]thymidine labeling. Gooch et al. (1977) reported that inhalation of nitrogen dioxide by mice caused no increase in either chromatid or chromosome-type aberrations on leucocyte or spermatocyte chromosomes.

Graham et al. (1982) studied the effect of ambient concentrations of nitrogen dioxide on selected hepatic enzymes of mice and found no change in activity. Exposure of rats by Kaya and Miura (1982) to nitrogen dioxide increased the ratio of arachidonic acid (20:4) to total fatty acid content and decreased palmitic acid (16:0) and/or stearic acid (18:0) in red-cell membranes, so that at 4 ppm and 10 ppm, the ratio of unsaturated fatty acid was raised 1.25- and 1.33-fold, respectively. Arachidonic acid in serum also increased with a slight decrease in oleic (18:1) and linoleic (18:2) acids. The fatty acid composition of serum phosphatidylcholine paralleled serum fatty acid composition. The authors felt that nitrogen dioxide inhalation stimulated fatty acid metabolism by the liver.

Mice exposed to 0.3 ppm of nitrogen dioxide for 8 h/day, 5 days a week for 6 weeks had an increase in the weight of the spleen, an increase in the size of spleen lymphoid nodules, a smaller increase in spleen cell number, and a greater preponderance of red cells in the red pulp (Kuraitis et al., 1981). Acute exposure of mice to nitrogen dioxide by Hidekazu et al. (1981) resulted in the suppression of antibody responses, which was more apparent in males than in females. A decrease in the total cell number in the spleen and thymus was also found after acute exposure to 20 ppm and 40 ppm for 12 h. Exposure to 5 ppm did not affect the antibody response. The authors suggested "that the processes of differentiation and proliferation of T and B cells are more susceptible to nitrogen dioxide exposure than any other processes of primary antibody responses." Joel et al. (1982) exposed sheep to 5 ppm nitrogen dioxide, 1½ h/day for 10–11 days, and found reduced pulmonary immune response 2 days after termination of the exposure, but had no affect 4 days after exposure. The results suggested that intermittent, short-term exposure to 5 ppm nitrogen dioxide may temporarily alter pulmonary immune response.

The initial medical examination of a patient exposed to nitrogen dioxide gas should include a complete history and physical examination, chest roentgengram for lung damage, and FVC and forced expiratory volume (FEV) (1 sec) for impaired pulmonary function. Depending on the severity, annual or more frequent medical examinations should be performed (National Institute for Occupational Safety and Health, 1978d). Treatment included corticosteroids, with oxygen being used by some (McCabe, 1977; Scott and Hunt, 1973; Jones et al., 1973; Fleming et al., 1979; Hatton et al., 1977).

NITROUS OXIDE

Nitrous oxide (synonyms: dinitrogen monoxide, laughing gas, hyponitrous acid anhydride, factitious air) is an asphyxiant, colorless gas, with slightly sweetish odor and taste; it is very stable and rather inert at room temperature. It supports combustion like oxygen when it is in the proper concentration with a flammable anesthetic, such as ether.

Nitrous oxide is a simple asphyxiant gas. It is used for inhalation anesthesia and analgesia, and also as a propellant in cartridges for whipped-cream dispensers (Merck, 1976). Nitrous oxide exchanges with nitrogen in the body. The blood-gas partition coefficient is 34 times that of nitrogen. As a result, pockets of trapped nitrous oxide gas expand as nitrogen leaves and is replaced by larger amounts of nitrous oxide. This may result in increased pressure (Marshall and Wollman, 1980).

While nitrous oxide has been considered chemically inert in the body, Hong et al. (1980), demonstrated by in vitro studies that nitrous oxide was reduced by intestinal bacteria to nitrogen at 5% oxygen tension, which was comparable to the normal oxygen tension found in the intestine. The reduction was significantly inhibited by antibiotics. The authors suggested that the reduction may take place with the formation of free radicals through a single electron transfer. It was estimated that 1.3 mg nitrogen would be generated during a 3-h period of anesthesia with 75% nitrous oxide. Nunn and Chanarin (1978) stated that most anesthesiologists had been believing that nitrous oxide was eliminated unchanged.

Severe bone-marrow depression that occurred after the treatment of tetanus in a patient by prolonged nitrous oxide anesthesia was reported by Lassen et al. (1956). The general anesthesia was 50% nitrous oxide and 50% oxygen. There was a large decrease in granulocytes by day 4, and the nitrous oxide was discontinued. The white-cell count returned to normal after a few days. Wilson et al. (1956) and Sando and Lawrence (1958) reported similar findings of bone-marrow depression with granulocytopenia in patients treated with nitrous oxide as one of the drugs for tetanus. Rats exposed to nitrous oxide showed evidence of bone-marrow injury by day 3, with recovery occurring within 3 days after resumption of breathing air (Kripke et al., 1977).

Nitrous oxide produces a reversible megaloblastosis in bone marrow with a few hours exposure (Kondo et al., 1979; Goodman et al., 1979).

The activity of the enzyme methionine synthetase is decreased by nitrous oxide with the displacement of cobalamin from the enzyme. The enzyme activity slowly recovered when nitrous oxide was discontinued (Kondo et al., 1981). The activity of methionine synthetase in the liver of mice progressively decreased as the exposure times to nitrous oxide increased.

Amess et al. (1978) found that some patients undergoing cardiac bypass surgery that received nitrous oxide ventilation for periods up to 24 h had bone-marrow depression. Eight patients that received 50% nitrous oxide with 50% oxygen had megaloplastic bone-marrow aspirates and abnormal deoxyuridine-suppression tests at the end of the ventilation. The deoxyuridine-suppression test is used to assess abnormalities in DNA synthesis (Amos et al., 1982). Skacel et al. (1983) reported a rise in serum folate and a fall in serum methionine levels in patients receiving nitrous oxide. Cullen et al. (1979) reported that a 24-h exposure to nitrous oxide results in an increase in the proportion of early S-phase cells and a decrease in late S, G_2, and mitotic cells, resembling changes seen following the use of S-phase-specific cytotoxic drugs.

Polyneuropathy from chronic inhalation of nitrous oxide has been reported (Layzer, 1978; Layzer et al., 1978; Sahenk et al., 1978). Sahenk et al. (1978) reported on the symptoms developed by a patient that inhaled nitrous oxide cartridges through a whipped-cream dispenser. The symptoms included numbness of the hands and feet with loss of perception for pinprick and light touch on the toes and fingers, decreased vibratory sense on the feet, loss of fine coordinated movements, and unsteady wide-based gait. Neuropathy in dental personnel due to nitrous oxide exposure was reported by Brodsky et al. (1980). The neuropathy resembled the neuropathy of pernicious anemia. Such exposure could be an occupational hazard. However, Dyck et al. (1980) examined dental personnel with recurring myeloradiculoneuropathic syndromes that could not be attributed to nitrous oxide exposure. In a study of rats exposed to high levels of nitrous oxide for 6 months, no clinical neuromuscular or neurologic abnormalities were found (Dyck et al., 1980). The authors felt that their study found that the prudent use of nitrous oxide in the clinical situation was not associated with findings or symptoms of neurotoxicity. Korttila et al. (1981) stated that the administration of nitrous oxide impairs mental and psychomotor function during and after administration. Hand–eye coordination was impaired, and the authors stated that outpatients receiving nitrous oxide need supervision for 20–30 min after administration. Van Der Westhuyzen et al. (1982) stated that fruit bats are an animal model for the neurological damage that occurs in humans with vitamin B_{12} deficiency, and they found vitamin B_{12} analogs absent in the plasma of fruit bats exposed to nitrous oxide.

Nitrous oxide at 70–75% caused fetal resorption, skeletal anomalies, and other teratogenic effects in pregnant rats when exposure to nitrous oxide was on day 9 of gestation (Lane et al., 1980). Vierra et al. (1983) reported that pregnant rats exposed to 0.5% nitrous oxide in air had a significant reduction in litter size, with no evidence of fetal resorption or skeletal malformation. A reduction in mature spermatozoa in rats exposed to 20% nitrous oxide for 35 days was found by Kripke et al. (1976). The antispermatogenic effect appeared to be reversible.

Koblin et al. (1981) examined the inactivation of methionine synthetase by nitrous oxide in mice by measuring enzyme inactivation as a function of nitrous oxide concentration and exposure time. It was found that the methionine synthetase activity in the liver progressively decreased as exposure times increased. Methionine synthetase activity decreased to 5% of the control value after 4 h of exposure to 0.8 atm nitrous oxide. Brain methionine synthase activity was reduced also. The methionine synthetase activity returned to nearly normal 2–4 days after exposure.

SULFUR DIOXIDE

Sulfur dioxide (synonyms: sulfurous anhydride, sulfurous oxide) is a colorless, nonflammable gas, with a strong, suffocating odor, mp −72 °C, bp −10 °C (Merck, 1976).

The federal standard for limits to exposure of sulfur dioxide in air is 5 ppm (13 mg/m³). However, experimental and epidemiologic studies have prompted the National Institute for Occupational Safety and Health (NIOSH) to conclude that this standard of 5 ppm can increase airway resistance, thereby causing adverse respiratory effects. Some persons are more sensitive to sulfur dioxide than are others to these effects (Sittig, 1981). Sulfur dioxide is irritating to the upper-respiratory-tract mucus membranes, with rhinitis, cough, and dryness of the throat resulting from chronic effects. Chronic exposure may cause increased mucus secretion, dyspnea, fatigue, and cough. Acute exposure can cause death from asphyxia.

Woodford et al. (1979) reported an incident in which a patient developed obstructive lung disease from an acute sulfur dioxide exposure as a result of a canister of sulfur dioxide rupturing. The patient was in a high concentration of the gas for 15–20 min and had burning of the eyes, rhinorrhea, cough, and almost passed out. He was given first aid with oxygen and admitted to the hospital. His chest roentgenogram was almost clear at the time of discharge, 7 days after admission. However, after 7 days he was again hospitalized with a severe constant cough and wheezing. He was dyspneic at rest. The chest film showed hyperinflation, which was not present previously. After 10 days he developed pulmonary edema and was transferred to a major medical center where he required a respirator. He was treated with digoxin, aminophyllin, chloramphenicol, and corticosteroids, and discharged on digoxin, aminophyllin, and prednisone. After 20 months he still had moderately severe obstructive impairment. A report by Charan et al. (1979) on five persons who were acutely exposed to very high concentrations of sulfur dioxide in an industrial accident stressed the need to follow parameters of pulmonary function in nonfatal cases. Two of the persons with the highest exposure died immediately, and histologic examination showed extensive sloughing of the large- and small-airway mucosa with hemorrhagic alveolar edema. The mucosa of the large airways was completely denuded in several places. Three survivors had severe conjunctivitis and superficial corneal burns, irritation and soreness of the nose and throat, tightness in the chest, and intense dyspnea.

A fatality resulting from sulfur dioxide inhalation in which the patient was hospitalized, discharged, readmitted to the hospital after 10 days, and died 17 days after the date of the accident was reported by Galea (1964). During the second hospitalization, the patient received antibiotics, oxygen, corticoids, ouabain, and aminophyllin. The autopsy findings were unremarkable except for those of the respiratory organs. No pleural adhesions or effusions were present. The lungs had a marble appearance and were voluminous, feathery, and pillowy in consistency. There was no elastic rebound on compression. The lungs resembled acute emphysema of a diffuse type. The tracheal surface mucosa was ulcerated. The immediate cause of death was presumably due to acute emphysematous changes due to extensive peribronchiolar fibrosis and bronchiolitis obliterans.

Sheppard et al. (1980) compared the bronchomotor responsiveness of persons with mild asthma with normal persons and normal persons with atopic rhinitis. Asthmatic subjects had significant increases in specific airway resistance (SR_{aw}) during exposure to 1, 3, and 5 ppm sulfur dioxide. The normal and atopic subjects had a significant increase in SR_{aw} only at 5 ppm and this was significantly smaller than in asthmatics. It was also found that atropine blocked the response to sulfur dioxide in asthmatic and nonasthmatic subjects. The results indicate that bronchoconstriction caused by sulfur dioxide is mediated by parasympathetic pathways. In another study it was found that exercise increased bronchoconstriction due to sulfur dioxide in asthmatic patients (Sheppard et al., 1981a). This increase due to exercise was probably due to an increase in air being inhaled through the mouth. The inhibitory effect of atropine and sodium cromoglycate on bronchoconstriction in normal and asthmatic subjects was reported by Snashall and Baldwin (1982). Sulfur dioxide was used to obtain a bronchial response. Atropine decreased the bronchial response to sulfur dioxide in normal subjects but not in asthmatic subjects. Sodium cromoglycate decreased the response in both normal and asthmatic subjects. Sheppard et al. (1981b) also reported that sodium cromoglycate decreased sulfur dioxide-induced bronchoconstriction in asthmatics. The response of adolescent asthmatic patients to a mixture of 1 ppm sulfur dioxide and 1 mg/m^3 of sodium chloride droplet aerosol was tested by Koenig et al. (1980). There were significant decreases in $\dot{V}_{max50}$ and $\dot{V}_{max75}$ when the group was exposed to sulfur dioxide and sodium chloride droplet aerosol, but no significant changes were noted on exposure to filtered air or sodium chloride droplet aerosol alone. Koenig et al. felt that the site of the effect was in the small airways. Koenig et al. (1980) reported a dose–response relationship to sulfur dioxide in adolescent asthmatics.

Speizer and Frank (1966) studied the absorption and desorption of sulfur dioxide by the human nose. During exposures of 30 min, most of the sulfur dioxide was removed by the nose. The concentration of sulfur dioxide in the mask was about 16 ppm; 1–2 cm within the nose it was 13.8 ppm; and in the pharynx it was 0.3 ppm. Expired gas in the pharynx was 0.4 ppm, and at the nose 2 ppm. The capacity for the nose to absorb the sulfur dioxide is due to the high solubility of the gas in tissue fluids. Other factors may be the gas combining capacity with nasal mucosa and blood, along with the rate at which the circulation removes the gas from the mucosa. The nasal mucus flow rate in humans was studied by Andersen et al. (1974) during 6-h exposures to 1, 5, and 25 ppm sulfur dioxide. The mucus flow rate decreased as the concentration of the gas increased. Subjects with initially slow mucus flow rates had more discomfort. The pharyngeal air samples contained less than 1% of the inhaled sulfur dioxide, which agreed with Speizer and Frank's (1966) results. It was reported that mucociliary transport is a defense mechanism against airborne pollutants, and mucostasis could probably result in an increase in the subjects' susceptibility. In the week following exposure to sulfur dioxide, there was a high rate of upper-respiratory infection.

Mannix et al. (1982) studied the effect of a model sulfur pollutant atmosphere on the clearance of particles from the lungs of rats and found no significant alteration in early or late clearing rates. The model pollutant was 5 ppm sulfur dioxide and 1.5 mg/m^3 of sulfate aerosol at 80–85% relative humidity.

Haider et al. (1981) found a significant depletion of total lipids and free fatty acids in all brain regions in guinea pigs after exposure to 10 ppm sulfur dioxide for 1 h daily for 21 days. The guinea pigs exhibited nasopharyngitis, somnolence, staggering, itching, pruning, and shin and eye irritation. Phospholipids and cholesterol increased in the cerebral hemisphere and decreased in the cerebellum. Cholesterol decreased in the brainstem. Free fatty acids decreased in the cerebral hemisphere, cerebellum, and brainstem. Esterified fatty acids decreased in the cerebral hemisphere and brainstem and increased in the cerebellum. It was concluded that an increase in lipase activity by sulfur dioxide contributed to the reduction of total lipids in the brain region. A study on rats by Haider et al. (1982) with exposure to 10 ppm sulfur dioxide for 1 h/day for 30 days resulted in a reduction of total lipids in all brain areas. Malonaldialdehyde formed by sulfur dioxide exposure increased in different regions of the brain. Peroxidation of lipids was enhanced, and lipase activity was elevated in the cerebral hemisphere.

REFERENCES

Abbott, D. F. 1972. Slow recovery from carbon monoxide poisoning. *Postgrad. Med. J.* 48:639–642.

Adelson, L., and Sunshine, I. 1966. Fatal hydrogen sulfide intoxication. *Arch. Pathol.* 81:375–380.

Albert, R. E., et al. 1982. Gaseous formaldehyde and hydrogen chloride induction of nasal cancer in the rat. *JNCI* 68:597–603.

Alexandersson, R., et al. 1982. Exposure to formaldehyde: Effects on pulmonary function. *Arch. Environ. Health* 37:279–283.

Amess, J. A. L., et al. 1978. Megaloblastic haemopoiesis in patients receiving nitrous oxide. *Lancet* 2:339.

Amos, R. J., et al. 1982. Incidence and pathogenesis of acute megaloblastic bone-marrow change in patients receiving intensive care. *Lancet* 2:835–838.

Andersen, I., et al. 1974. Human response to controlled levels of sulfur dioxide. *Arch. Environ. Health* 28:31–39.

Anderson, R. F., et al. 1967. Myocardial toxicity from carbon monoxide poisoning. *Ann. Int. Med.* 67:1172–1182.

Appelman, L. M., et al. 1982. Acute inhalation toxicity study of ammonia in rats with variable exposure periods. *Am. Ind. Hyg. Assoc.* 43:662–665.

Arena, J. M. 1979a. *Poisoning,* 4th ed., p. 242. Springfield, Ill.: Thomas.

Arena, J. M. 1979b. *Poisoning,* 4th ed., p. 625. Springfield, Ill.: Thomas.

Arena, J. M. 1979c. *Poisoning,* 4th ed., p. 244. Springfield, Ill.: Thomas.

Arena, J. M. 1979d. *Poisoning,* 4th ed., pp. 153–155. Springfield, Ill.: Thomas.

Aviado, D. M. 1975. Toxicology of aerosols. *J. Clin. Pharmacol.* 15:86–104.

Aviado, D. M. 1978. Physiological and biochemical responses to specific groups of inhalants. *Fed. Proc.* 37:2508.

Axford, A. T., et al. 1976. Accidental exposure to isocyanate fumes in a group of firemen. *Br. J. Ind. Med.* 33:65–71.

Bass, M. 1970. Sudden sniffing death. *JAMA* 212:2075–2079.

Baumeister, A. A., and Baumeister, A. A. 1978. Suppression of repetitive self-injurious behavior by contingent inhalation of aromatic ammonia. *J. Autism Child. Schizophr.* 8:71–77.

Baur, X., and Fruhmann, G. 1981. Specific IgE antibodies in patients with isocyanate asthma. *Chest* 80:1 (suppl.):73s–76s.

Belej, M. A., and Aviado, D. M. 1975. Cardiopulmonary toxicity of propellants for aerosols. *J. Clin. Pharmacol.* 15:105–115.

Birky, M. M., and Clarke, F. B. 1981. Inhalation of toxic products from fires. *Bull. NY Acad. Med.* 57:997–1013.

Blake, D. A., and Mergner, G. W. 1974. Inhalation studies on the biotransformation and elimination of trichlorofluoromethane and dichlorofluoromethane in beagles. *Toxicol. Appl. Pharmacol.* 30:396–407.

Boggs, P. B. 1983. To the editor. *Chest* 83:584.

Brodsky, J. B., et al. 1980. Occupational exposure to N_2O and neurological disease. *Anesthesiology* 53:S367.

Brown, W. E., et al. 1982. Inhibition of cholinesterase activity by isocyanates. *Toxicol. Appl. Pharmacol.* 63:45–52.

Charan, N. B., et al. 1979. Pulmonary injuries associated with acute sulfur dioxide inhalation. *Am. Rev. Respir. Dis.* 119:555–560.

Charles, J., et al. 1976. Hypersensitivity pneumonitis after exposure to isocyanates. *Thorax* 31:127–136.

Chen, S. E., and Bernstein, I. L. 1982. The guinea pig model of diisocyanate sensitization. I. Immunological studies. *J. Allergy Clin. Immunol.* 69(No. 1, part 2):123.

Close, L., et al. 1980. Acute and chronic effects of ammonia burns of the respiratory tract. *Arch. Otolaryngol.* 106:151–158.

Cockcroft, D. W., et al. 1982. Occupational asthma caused by cedar urea formaldehyde particle board. *Chest* 82:49–53.

Cockcroft, D. W., et al. 1983. To the editor. *Chest* 83:584–585.

Creasia, D. A., et al. 1977. Stimulation of DNA synthesis in the lungs of hamsters exposed intermittently to nitrogen dioxide. *J. Toxicol. Environ. Health* 2:1173–1181.

Cullen, M. H., et al. 1979. The effect of nitrous oxide on the cell cycle in human bone marrow. *Br. J. Haematol.* 42:527–534.

Dalton, M. L., and Bricker, D. L. 1978. Anhydrous ammonia burn of the respiratory tract. *Tex. Med.* 74:51–54.

Danks, J. M., et al. 1981. Toluene-diisocyanate induced asthma: Evaluation of antibodies in the serum of affected workers against a tolyl monoisocyanate protein conjugate. *Clin. Allergy* 11:161–168.

Davies, R. J., et al. 1977. The in vitro effect of toluene diisocyanate on lymphocyte cyclic adenosine monophosphate production of isoproterenol, prostaglandin and histamine. *J. Allergy Clin. Immunol.* 60:223–229.

DeNicola, D. B., et al. 1981. Early damage indicators in the lung, V. Biochemical and cytological response to N_2O inhalation. *Toxicol. Appl. Pharmacol.* 60:301–312.

Drozdz, M., et al. 1977. Effect of chronic exposure to nitrogen dioxide on collagen content in lung and skin of guinea pigs. *Environ. Res.* 13:369–377.

Dyck, P. J., et al. 1980. Nitrous oxide neurotoxicity studies in man and rat. *Anesthesiology* 53:205–209.

Ehrenberg, L., et al. 1974. Evaluation of genetic risks of alkylating agents: Tissue doses in the mouse from air contamination with ethylene oxide. *Mutat. Res.* 24:83–103.

Embree, J. W., et al. 1977. The mutagenic potential of ethylene oxide using the dominant-lethal assay on rats. *Toxicol. Appl. Pharmacol.* 40:261–267.

Ferguson, W. S., et al. 1977. Human physiological response and adaptation to ammonia. *J. Occup. Med.* 19:319–326.

Ficarra, B. J. 1980. Toxicologic states treated in the emergency room. *Clin. Toxicol.* 17:1–43.

Finelli, P. F. 1981. Changes in the basal ganglia following cyanide poisoning. *J. Comput. Assist. Tomogr.* 5:755–756.

Fleming, G. M., et al. 1979. Dysfunction of small airways following pulmonary injury due to nitrogen dioxide. *Chest* 75:720–721.

Galea, M. 1964. Fatal sulfur dioxide inhalation. *Can. Med. Assoc. J.* 91:345–347.

Gardner, D. E., et al. 1977. Role of time as a factor in the toxicity of chemical compounds in intermittent and continuous exposures. Part 1, Effects of continuous exposure. *J. Toxicol. Environ. Health* 3:811–820.

Garland, H., and Pearce, J. 1967. Neurological complications of carbon monoxide poisoning. *Q. J. Med.* 144:445–455.

Garry, V. F., et al. 1979. Ethylene oxide: Evidence of human chromosomal effects. *Environ. Mutagen.* 1:375–382.

Garvey, D. J., and Longo, L. D. 1978. Chronic low level maternal carbon monoxide exposure and fetal growth and development. *Biol. Reprod.* 19:8–14.

Ginsberg, M. D., and Myers, R. E. 1974. Fetal brain damage following maternal carbon monoxide intoxication: An experimental study. *Acta Obstet. Gynecol. Scand.* 53:309–317.

Glass, R. I., et al. 1980. Deaths from asphyxia among fisherman. *JAMA* 244:2193–2194.

Gooch, P. C., et al. 1977. Observations on mouse chromosomes following nitrogen dioxide inhalation. *Mutat. Res.* 48:117–120.

Goodman, A., et al. 1979. In vitro effects of nitrous oxide on bone marrow. *Blood* 54(No. 5, suppl. 1):38a.

Graham, D. L., et al. 1977. Acute cyanide poisoning complicated by lactic acidosis and pulmonary edema. *Arch. Int. Med.* 137:1051–1055.

Graham, J. A., et al. 1982. Influence of ozone and nitrogen dioxide on hepatic microsomal enzymes of mice. *J. Toxicol. Environ. Health* 9:849–856.

Gross, J. A., et al. 1978. Ethylene oxide neuropathy. *Neurology* 4:355.

Guidotti, T. E. 1980. Toxic inhalation of nitrogen dioxide: Morphologic and functional changes. *Exp. Molec. Pathol.* 33:90–103.

Haider, S. S., et al. 1981. Regional effects of sulfur dioxide exposure on the guinea pig brain lipids, lipid peroxidation and lipase activity. *Neurotoxicology* 2:443–450.

Haider, S. S., et al. 1982. Air pollutant sulfur dioxide-induced alterations on the levels of lipids, lipid peroxidation and lipid activity in various regions of the rat brain. *Acta Pharmacol. Toxicol.* 51:45–50.

Halperin, W. E., et al. 1983. Nasal cancer in a worker exposed to formaldehyde. *JAMA* 249:510–512.

Hamilton, A., and Hardy, H. L. 1974. *Industrial Toxicology,* 3d ed., pp. 229–233. Acton, Mass.: Publishing Sciences Group.

Harris, W. S. 1973. Toxic effects of aerosol propellants on the heart. *Arch. Int. Med.* 131:162–166.

Hatton, D. V., et al. 1977. Collagen breakdown and nitrogen dioxide inhalation. *Arch. Environ. Health* 32:33–36.

Hatton, D. V., et al. 1979. Collagen breakdown and ammonia inhalation. *Arch. Environ. health* 34:83–87.

Herrick, R. T., and Herrick, S. 1983. Allergic reaction to aromatic ammonia ampule. *Am. J. Sports Med.* 11:26.

Hidekazu, H. B., et al. 1981. Effects of acute exposure to nitrogen dioxide on primary antibody response. *Arch. Environ. Health* 36:114–2119.

Hoeffler, H. B., et al. 1982. Bronchiectasis following pulmonary ammonia burn. *Arch. Pathol. Lab Med.* 106:686–687.

Hong, K., et al. 1980. Metabolism of nitrous oxide by human and rat intestinal contents. *Anesthesiology* 52:16–19.

Jaeger, R. J., and Gearhart, J. M. 1982. Respiratory and metabolic response of rats and mice to formalin vapor. *Toxicology* 25:299–309.

Joel, D. D., et al. 1982. Effects of NO_2 on immune responses in pulmonary lymph of sheep. *J. Toxicol. Environ. Health* 10:341–348.

Johnson, W. K., et al. 1982. Lung function and morphology of dogs after sublethal exposure to nitrogen dioxide. *J. Toxicol. Environ. Health* 10:201–221.

Jones, G. R., et al. 1973. Pulmonary effects of acute exposure to nitrous fumes. *Thorax* 28:61–65.

Juhos, L. T., et al. 1980. A quantitative study of stenosis in the respiratory bronchiole of the rat in NO_2-induced emphysema. *Am. Rev. Respir. Dis.* 121:541–549.

Kapeghian, J. C., et al. 1982. Acute inhalation toxicity of ammonia in mice. *Bull. Environ. Contam. Toxicol.* 29:371–378.

Karol, M. H. 1983. Concentration-dependent immunological response to toluene diisocyanate (TDI) following inhalation exposure. *Toxicol. Appl. Pharmacol.* 68:229–241.

Karol, M. H., et al. 1979. Longitudinal study of tolyl-reactive IgE antibodies in workers hypersensitive to TDI. *J. Occup. Med.* 21:354–358.

Kaya, K., and Miura, T. 1982. Effects of nitrogen dioxide on fatty acid compositions of red cell membranes, sera, and livers in rats. *Environ. Res.* 27:24–35.

Klaassen, C. D. 1980a. In *The Pharmacological Basis of Therapeutics,* 6th ed., eds. A. G. Gilman, L. S. Goodman, and A. Gilman, p. 1643. New York: Macmillan.

Klaassen, C. D. 1980b. In *The Pharmacological Basis of Therapeutics,* 6th ed., eds. A. G. Gilman, L. S. Goodman, and A. Gilman, p. 1651. New York: Macmillan.

Kleinerman, J. 1979. Effects of nitrogen dioxide on elastin and collagen contents of lung. *Arch. Environ. Health* 34:228–232.

Koblin, D. D., et al. 1981. Inactivation of methionine synthetase by nitrous oxide in mice. *Anesthesiology* 54:318–324.

Koenig, J. Q., et al. 1980. Acute effects of inhaled SO_2 plus NaCl droplet aerosol on pulmonary function in asthmatic adolescents. *Environ. Res.* 22:145–153.

Kondo, H., et al. 1979. Nitrous oxide (N_2O) has multiple effects on cobalamin. *Blood* 54(no. 5, suppl. 1):41a.

Kondo, H., et al. 1981. Nitrous oxide has multiple deleterious effects on cobalamin metabolism and causes decreases of both mammalian cobalamin-dependent enzymes in rats. *J. Clin. Invest.* 67:1270–1283.

Korttila, K., et al. 1981. Time course of mental and psychomotor effects of 30 percent nitrous oxide during inhalation and recovery. *Anesthesiology* 54:220–226.

Kreiger, N. 1983. Formaldehyde and nasal cancer mortality. *Can. Med. Assoc. J.* 128:248.

Kreiger, R. A., and Garry, V. F. 1983. Formaldehyde-induced cytotoxicity and sister-chromatid exchange in human lymphocyte cultures. *Mutat. Res.* 120:51–55.

Kripke, B. J., et al. 1976. Testicular reaction to prolonged exposure to nitrous oxide. *Anesthesiology* 44:104–113.

Kripke, B. J., et al. 1977. Hematologic reaction to prolonged exposure to nitrous oxide. *Anesthesiology* 47:343–348.

Kuraitis, K. V., et al. 1981. Spleen changes in animals inhaling ambient levels of nitrogen dioxide. *J. Toxicol. Environ. Health* 7:851–859.

Lane, G. A., et al. 1980. Anesthetics as teratogens: Nitrous oxide is fetotoxic, xenon is not. *Science* 210:899–901.

Larkin, J. M., et al. 1976. Treatment of carbon monoxide poisoning: Prognostic factors. *J. Trauma* 16:111–114.

Lassen, H. C. A., et al. 1956. Treatment of tetanus. Severe bone-marrow depression after prolonged nitrous-oxide anaestheisa. *Lancet* 1:527–530.

Layzer, R. B. 1978. Myeloneuropathy after prolonged exposure to nitrous oxide. *Lancet* 2:1227–1230.

Layzer, R. B. 1978. Neuropathy following abuse of nitrous oxide. *Neurology* 28:504–506.

Lehninger, A. L. 1982a. *Principles of Biochemistry,* p. 171. New York: Worth.

Lehninger, A. L. 1982b. *Principles of Biochemistry,* p. 483. New York: Worth.

Longo, L. D. 1970. Carbon monoxide in the pregnant mother and fetus and its exchange across the placenta. *Ann. NY Acad. Sci.* 174:313–340.

Loughridge, L. W., et al. 1958. Acute renal failure due to muscle necrosis in carbon-monoxide poisoning. *Lancet* 2:349–351.

Malo, J., and Zeiss, R. 1982. Occupational hypersensitivity pneumonitis after exposure to idphenylmethane diisocyanate. *Am. Rev. Respir. Dis.* 125:113–116.

Mannix, R. C., et al. 1982. Effect of sulfur dioxide-sulfate exposure on rat respiratory tract clearance. *Am. Ind. Hyg. Assoc. J.* 43:679–685.

Marsh, G. M. 1982. Proportional mortality patterns among chemical plant workers exposed to formaldehyde. *Br. J. Ind. Med.* 39:313–322.

Marshall, B. E., and Wollman, H. 1980. General anesthetics. In *The Pharmaccological Basis of Therapeutics,* 6th ed., eds. Goodman and Gilman, pp. 280–291. New York: Macmillan.

McCabe, W. O. 1977. Silo fillers disease. *Clin. Med.* 84:15–16.

McKay, R. T., and Brooks, S. M. 1983. Effect of toluene diisocyanate in beta adrenergic receptor function. *Am. Rev. Respir. Dis.* 128:50–53.

McKay, R. T., et al. 1981. Isocyanate-induced abnormality of beta-adrenergic receptor function. *Chest* 80(no. 1, suppl.):61s-63s.

Merck. 1976. Merck Index, 9th ed. Rahway, N.J.: Merck.

Montague, T. J., and Macneil, A. B.1980. Mass ammonia inhalation. *Chest* 77:496-498.

Morse, D. L., et al. 1981. Death caused by fermenting manure. *JAMA* 245:63-64.

National Institute for Occupational Safety and Health. 1978a. Occupational health guideline for carbon monoxide. National Institute for Occupational Safety and Health, Public Health Service, Washington, D.C.

National Institute for Occupational Safety and Health. 1978b. Occupational health guideline for cyanide. National Institute for Occupational Safety and Health, Public Health Service, Washington, D.C.

National Institute for Occupational Safety and Health. 1978c. Occupational health guideline for hydrogen sulfide. National Institute for Occupational Safety and Health, Public Health Service, Washington, D.C.

National Institute for Occupational Safety and Health. 1978d. Occupational health guideline for nitrogen dioxide. National Institute for Occupational Safety and Health, Public Health Service, Washington, D.C.

National Research Council. 1981. *Formaldehyde and Other Aldehydes,* pp. 185-186. Washington, D. C.: National Academy Press.

Nethercott, J. R., et al. 1982. Erythema multiforme exudativum linked to the manufacture of printed circuit boards. *Contact Dermatitis* 8:314-322.

Nunn, J. F., and Chanarin, I. 1978. Editorial, nitrous oxide and vitamin B12. *Br. J. Anaesth.* 50:1089-1090.

O'Brien, I. M., et al. 1979. Toluene di-isocyanate-induced asthma. *Clin. Allergy* 9:1-6.

Olsen, J. H., and Dossing, M. 1982. Formaldehyde induced symptoms in a day care center. *Am. Ind. Hyg. Assoc. J.* 43:366-370.

Orehek, J., et al. 1976. Effect of short-term, low-level nitrogen dioxide exposure on bronchial sensitivity of asthmatic patients. *J. Clin. Invest.* 57:301-307.

Osbern, L. N., and Crapo, R. O. 1981. A report of toxic exposure to liquid manure. *Ann. Int. Med.* 95:312-314.

Paulet, G., et al. 1975a. Fluorocarbons and general metabolism in the rat, rabbit, and dog. *Toxicol. Appl. Pharmacol.* 34:197-203.

Paulet, G., et al. 1975b. Fate of fluorocarbons in the dog and rabbit after inhalation. *Toxicol. Appl. Pharmacol.* 34:204-213.

Peters, J. W. 1981. Hydrogen sulfide poisoning in a hospital setting. *JAMA* 246:1588-1589.

Ravizzo, A. G., et al. 1982. The treatment of hydrogen sulfide intoxication: Oxygen versus nitrates. *Vet. Hum. Toxicol.* 24:241-242.

Reinhardt, C. F., et al. 1971. Cardiac arrhythmias and aerosol "sniffing." *Arch. Environ. Health* 22:265-279.

Rogers, R. E., and Ferin, J. 1981. Effect of hydrogen sulfide on bacterial inactivation in the rat lung. *Arch. Environ. Health* 36:261-264.

Sahenk, Z., et al. 1978. Polyneuropathy from inhalation of N_2O cartridges through a whipped-cream dispenser. *Neurology* 28:485-487.

Sakata, M., et al. 1981. Acute toxicity of fluorocarbon-22: Toxic symptoms, lethal concentration, its fate in rabbit and mouse. *Toxicol. Appl. Pharmacol.* 59:64-70.

Sando, M. J. W., and Lawrence, J. R. 1958. Bone marrow depression following treatment of tetanus with protracted nitrous-oxide anaesthesia. *Lancet* 1:588.

Sangha, G. K., and Alarie, Y. 1979. Sensory irritation by toluene diisocyanate in single and repeated exposure. *Toxicol. Appl. Pharmacol.* 50:533-547.

Sangha, G. K., et al. 1981. Comparison of some mono- and diisocyanates as sensory irritants. *Toxicol. Appl. Pharmacol.* 57:241–246.

Scott, E. G., and Hunt, W. B. 1973. Silo fillers disease. *Chest* 63:701–706.

Sega, G. A., et al. 1981. Alkylation patter in developing mouse sperm, sperm DNA and protamine after inhalation of ethylene oxide. *Environ. Mutagen.* 3:371.

Shafer, N., et al. 1965. Primary myocardial disease in man resulting from acute carbon monoxide poisoning. *Am. J. Med.* 38:316–320.

Sheppard, D., et al. 1980. Lower threshold and greater bronchomotor responsiveness of asthmatic subjects to sulfur dioxide. *Am. Rev. Respir. Dis.* 122:873–878.

Sheppard, D., et al. 1981a. Exercise increases sulfur dioxide-induced bronchoconstriction in asthmatic subjects. *Am. Rev. Respir. Dis.* 123:486–491.

Sheppard, D., et al. 1981b. Inhibition of sulfur dioxide-induced bronchoconstriction by disodium cromoglycate in asthma patients. *Am. Rev. Respir. Dis.* 124:257–259.

Sherwin, R. P., and Richters, V. 1982. Hyperplasia of type 2 pneumocyte following 0.34 ppm nitrogen dioxide exposure: Quantitation by image analysis. *Arch. Environ. Health* 37:306–315.

Shragg, T. A., et al. 1982. Cyanide poisoning after bitter almond ingestion. *Western J. Med.* 136:65–69.

Sittig, M. 1981. *Handbook of Toxic and Hazardous Chemicals,* pp. 615–617. Park Ridge, N.J.: Noyes.

Skacel, P. O., et al. 1983. Studies on the haemopoietic toxicity of nitrous oxide in man. *Br. J. Haematol.* 53:189–200.

Smith, G. 1965. Carbon monoxide poisoning. *Ann. NY Acad. Sci.* 117:684–687.

Smith, R. P. 1980. Toxic responses of the blood. In *Toxicology* (2nd ed.), eds. Casarett and Doull, pp. 328–329. New York: Macmillan.

Smith, R. P., and Gosselin, R. E. 1964. The influence of methemoglobinemia on the lethality of some toxic anions II sulfide. *Toxicol. Appl. Pharmacol.* 6:584–592.

Smith, R. P., and Gosselin, R. E. 1966. On the mechanism of sulfide inactivation by methemoglobin. *Toxicol. Appl. Pharmacol.* 8:159–172.

Smith, R. P., et al. 1976. Management of acute sulfide poisoning. *Arch. Environ. Health* 31:166–169.

Snashall, P. D., and Baldwin, C. 1982. Mechanisms of sulfur dioxide induced bronchoconstriction in normal and asthmatic man. *Thorax* 37:118–123.

Snelling, W. M., et al. 1982. Teratology study in Fischer 344 rats exposed to ethylene oxide by inhalation. *Toxicol. Appl. Pharmacol.* 64:476–481.

Sobonya, R. 1977. Fatal anhydrous ammonia inhalation. *Hum. Pathol.* 8:293–299.

Sone, S., et al. 1974. Pulmonary manifestations in acute carbon monoxide poisoning. *Am. J. Roentgenol. Radium Ther. Nucl. Med.* 120:865–871.

Speizer, F. E., and Frank, N. R. 1966. The uptake and release of SO_2 by the human nose. *Arch. Environ. Health* 12:725–728.

Stine, R. J., et al. 1976. Hydrogen sulfide intoxication—A case report and discussion of treatment. *Ann. Int. Med.* 85:756–758.

Strohl, et al. 1980. Carbon monoxide poisoning in fire victims: A reappraisal of prognosis. *J. Trauma* 20:78–80.

Stryer, L. 1981. *Biochemistry,* 2nd ed., pp. 317–318. San Francisco, Calif.: Freeman.

Suzuki, A. K., et al. 1982. Changes of gaseous exchange in the lungs of mice exposed to nitrogen dioxide and their recovery process. *Toxicol. Lett.* 13:71–79.

Taylor, G. J., and Harris, W. S. 1970. Cardiac toxicity of aerosol propellants. *JAMA* 214:81–85.

Taylor, G. J., et al. 1971. Ventricular arrhythmias induced in monkeys by the inhalation of aerosol propellants. *J. Clin. Invest.* 50:1546–1550.

Temcharoen, P., and Thilly, W. g. 1983. Toxic and mutagenic effects of formaldehyde in *Salmonella typhimurium. Mutat. Res.* 119:89–93.

Treitman, R. D., et al. 1980. Air contaminants encountered by firefighters. *Am. Ind. Hyg. Assoc. J.* 41:796–802.

Van Der Westhuyzen, J., et al. 1982. Cobalamin (vitamin B_{12}) analogs are absent in plasma of fruit bats exposed to nitrous oxide. *Proc. Soc. Exp. Biol. Med.* 171:88–91.

VanErt, M., and Battigelli, M. C. 1975. Mechanism of respiratory injury by TDI (toluene diisocyanate). *Ann. Allergy* 35:142–147.

Vierra, E., et al. 1983. Effects of low intermittent concentrations of nitrous oxide on the developing rat fetus. *Br. J. Anaesth.* 55:67–69.

Walrath, J., and Fraumeni, J. F. 1983. Mortality patterns among embalmers. *Int. J. Cancer* 31:407–411.

Walton, M. 1973. Industrial ammonia gassing. *Br. J. Ind. Med.* 30:78–86.

White, E. S. 1971. A case of near fatal ammonia gas poisoning. *J. Occup. Med.* 13:549–550.

Wilson, P., et al. 1956. Bone-marrow depression in tetanus—Report of a fatal case. *Lancet* 2:442–443.

Winter, P. M., and Miller, J. N. 1976. Carbon monoxide poisoning. *JAMA* 236:1502–1504.

Woodford, et al. 1979. Obstructive lung disease from acute sulfur dioxide exposure. *Respiration* 38:238–245.

Wright, E. S., et al. 1982. Changes in phospholipid biosynthetic enzymes in type II cells and alveolar macrophages isolated from rat lungs after NO_2 exposure. *Toxicol. Appl. Pharmacol.* 66:305–311.

Yager, J. W., and Benz, R. d. 1982. Sister chromatid exchanges induced in rabbit lymphocytes by ethylene oxide after inhalation exposure. *Environ. Mutagen.* 4:121–134.

Zimmerman, S. S., and Truxal, B. 1981. Carbon monoxide poisoning. *Pediatrics* 68:215–224.

Chapter 14

Solvents and Chemical Intermediates

Thomas J. Haley

INTRODUCTION

Exposure to solvents and their vapors usually occurs in an occupational environment, but their injudicious use in the home has resulted in poisoning, which in some cases has resulted in fatalities. the usual home exposure agents include gasoline, lighter fluids, spot removers, and kitchen cleaners. Paint removers, tile cleaners, and solvents usually cause serious home exposures, while solvents and chemical intermediates are involved in occupational exposures. Another serious source of exposure involves chemical dumps where containers decay, causing contamination of the air and domestic water supplies. Browning (1953) and Patty (1963) give lists of solvent and vapors involved in industrial exposures, while Hanrahan (1979) has listed the types of exposures caused by dump sites or improper disposal of solvents and chemical intermediates in sewer systems.

The main goal of industrial hygiene and its practitioners is the prevention of exposure to toxic levels of solvents and vapors; thus the American Conference of Governmental Industrial Hygienists (ACGIH) has established threshold limit values (TLVs) to set safe levels for human exposure in industry (ACGIH, 1971, 1976a, 1977). As new information becomes available, the TLVs are revised upward or downward and new chemicals are added to the list. The TLVs are air concentrations of a chemical to which a given individual can be repeatedly exposed for 8 h/day, 5 days/week. The TLVs are time-weighted values, and limited exposures above them may be permitted but they must be compensated for by equivalent reductions below the limit during the working period.

The TLVs for solvents and vapors are expressed in parts per million (ppm) which means parts of solvents or vapors per million parts of air. The TLVs for fumes or mists are given as milligrams per cubic meter (mg/m^3) and the following formula converts these units;

$$ppm = \frac{(mg/m^3) \times 24.45}{\text{molecular weight of the chemical}}$$

The American Standards Association (ASA) has established a set of limits to prevent undesirable functional reactions that may have no discernable health effect, undesirable changes in body biochemistry or structure, or irritation or other adverse sensory effects.

After absorption, chemicals can be converted to less toxic, nontoxic, or more toxic derivatives by the P-450 monooxygenases located in the liver microsomal smooth endoplasmic reticulum (Hucker, 1973). Arene oxides are intermediates in the biotransformation of phenols, trans-dihydrodiols, and premercapturic acids, and their steady-state concentrations are related to rates of formation and to ability to isomerize to phenols, react with glutathione, and undergo enzymatic hydration. Cytotoxicity is caused by these intermediates, which covalently bind to tissue macromolecules. Epoxide hydrases are involved in the transformation of arene oxides to potent epoxides. Glutathione conjugation of arene oxides is a major pathway that significantly affects their tissue concentration, and any process that depletes liver glutatione concentrations can produce serious toxic effects. Glutathione reacts with arene oxides enzymatically and nonenzymatically via soluble glutathione-S-epoxide transferases (Jerina and Aly, 1974). The monooxygenases can be induced by prior administration of phenobarbital or 3-methylcholanthrene, causing an increase in biotransformation of xenobiotics. Another biotransformation process whereby many carbon–oxygen bonds are formed is the "NIH shift." In this phenomenon, the intramolecular migration of a ring substituent takes place during aromatic hydroxylation of the ring (Schreiber, 1974). Inducibility of skin hydroxylase in human neonates is related to genetic differences and the exposure of the mother to xenobiotics during pregnancy (Alvares et al., 1973). The placenta also contains biotransformation enzymes with a limited capacity to biotransform xenobiotics. This limitation is related to the quantity of enzymes and the number and variety of enzymes present (Juchau, 1978). Adult humans have a polymorphic acetylation pattern involving the enzyme acetylcoenzyme A, which transfers acetyl groups to the acceptor chemical molecule (Price Evans and White, 1964). Human studies have shown a biomodal acetylation pattern, with 61% fast acetylators and 39% slow acetylators (Parker, 1969; White and Price Evans, 1968). Such effects can greatly affect the ultimate excretion of xenobiotics.

With this introduction, a discussion of representative examples of solvents and intermediatives will be undertaken.

GASOLINE AND KEROSENE

Environmental   The products contain aliphatic hydrocarbons, hexane, heptane, pentane, octane, a variety of unsaturated aliphatic and aromatic hydrocarbons, and in nonleaded gasoline a large amount of benzene. These mixtures are used in the rubber industry, motor and engineering works, electrical works, paint and varnish industry, glue works, shoe industry, degreasing of leather, manufacturing of adhesive tape, and cleaning in the printing industry (Browning, 1953). Media reports, unsubstantiated but scientific evidence, have discussed ground and well-water contamination from gasoline and kerosene. These chemical mixtures have not been identified in U.S. water supplies (Environmental Protection Agency, 1976), and industrial effluent discharges (Perry et al., 1970).

Tissue Distribution   Gasoline and kerosene and their components distributed in all body tissues following ingestion or inhalation (Browning, 1953; Gerlowski and Jain, 1983).

Biotransformation   Gasoline contains a wide variety of aliphatic and aromatic hydrocarbons, and the metabolism of selected examples will be discussed. The new nonleaded variety contains a larger proportion of benzene, and its metabolism is discussed in the next section.

n-Hexane is widely used in glues and has produced polyneuropathy in workers (Yamamura, 1969). This chemical is metabolized to 2-hexanol (Perbellini et al., 1978), 2,5-hexanediol (Spencer et al., 1978), 5-hydroxy-2-hexanone (Krasavage et al., 1980) and 2,5-hexanediol (Spencer and Schaumberg, 1975). In shoe-industry workers using *n*-hexane, 2,5-hexanedione, 0.5–26 mg/l has been isolated from their urine (Perbellini et al., 1981). *n*-Hexane also produces central–peripheral neuropathy (Schaumberg and Spencer, 1976).

Toxicology   Acute exposure to high concentrations of gasoline vapor produces dizziness, coma, collapse, and death, and even in nonfatal cases, permanent brain damage has been reported (Machle, 1941). Atmospheric concentrations of 2000 ppm are not safe and can produce death (Gerarde, 1963a). In nonfatal cases, symptoms include unconsciousness, delirium, cyanosis, shallow or stertorous respiration, thready pulse, vomiting, inward strabismus, contracted pupils, and loss of reflexes (Plummer, 1913).

In less severe exposures, the symptoms include restlessness, mental excitement, rapid, irrational, and incoherent speech, flushed face, rapid pulse, and amnesia, but no staggering or incoordination (Elliott, 1913). Upon recovery, the patient has the following symptoms: irritability, violent headache, disturbances of speech, cyanosis, gastrointestinal disturbances, loss of sensitivity, and neuritis (Flury and Zernik, 1931; Sterner, 1941).

Symptoms of chronic gasoline intoxication include headache, giddiness, neuralgia, lack of concentration, respiratory disorders, disturbances of sensibility, loss of corneal reflex, tremor of the eyelids, paresthesia of the hands, increased knee jerks, and chronic polyneuritis (Flury and Zernik, 1931), as well as eye irritation, drowsiness, fatigue, anorexia, nausea, dizziness, and throat irritation (Drinker et al., 1943).

Inadvertent or intentional ingestion of gasoline, kerosene, and paint thinner can lead to pneumonitis, pulmonary edema, and hemorrhage when attempts to remove the solvent by emesis or gastric lavage, because small amounts may be aspirated into the lungs, causing rapid and severe irritation (Gerarde, 1963b).

AROMATIC HYDROCARBONS

Benzene

Environmental Evaporation losses of benzene from chemical plants, tank cars, gasoline spills, coke ovens, and automobiles contribute to the environmental contamination from this chemical, which in 1975 approximated 17.5 million gallons (Haley, 1977). Routine tanker discharges, port accidents, oceanic exploration and production, discarded lubricants, pipeline breakages, incomplete combustion of fuel, and untreated industrial and domestic sewage adds 11,000–12,000 million pounds per year of oil to the ocean (Blumer et al., 1971). It is estimated that crude oil contains 0.2% benzene, which upon release adds 22–24 million pounds of benzene to the seaway (Green and Morrell, 1973). About 122 million pounds of benzene are released by coke production (Faith et al., 1965). Gasoline evaporation from filler tubes, carburetors, and exhaust contributes 20% to urban hydrocarbon emissions, not counting the exhaust (Wendell et al., 1973). In 1971, it was estimated that transportation sources added 29.4 billion pounds of hydrocarbons to the atmosphere (Council on Environmental Quality, 1973). Benzene makes up 4% of automative emissions (Schofield, 1974). With the advent of nonleaded gasoline, the exposure to atmospheric benzene has increased for bulk loaders, service-station attendants, and the general public because the aromatic content of gasoline will increase to 48–50% (Berlin et al., 1974). Benzene exposure also occurred in a Swedish raincoat plant (Helmer, 1944), in two shoe factories (Savilahti, 1956; Juzwiak, 1969), in a rubber-coating company (Hardy and Elkins, 1948), in the leatherette industry (Kozlova and Volkova, 1960), and in rotogravure plants (Greenberg et al., 1939). Upon analyzing the detrimental effects of benzene on the working population, the National Institute for Occupational Health and Safety (NIOSH) recommended that the TLV of benzene be reduced from 10 ppm to 1 ppm as determined by an air sample collected at 1 l/min for 2 h (NIOSH, 1976).

Tissue Distribution When 23 human volunteers inhaled 47,110 ppm benzene for 2–3 h, the greatest absorption occurred in the first 5 min and approximately 50%

of the inhaled chemical was absorbed in 1 h. Postexposure, 30–50% was eliminated via the lungs and 0.1–0.2% was eliminated via the kidneys. No equilibrium was established between the air and the blood. In 10 subjects, 16.4–41.6% of inhaled benzene was eliminated via the lungs in 5–7 h, with the greatest amount being excreted in the first hour (Srobova et al., 1950). Exposure of 15 humans to 100 ppm of benzene showed retention of 46%, followed by pulmonary elimination of 12% and urinary elimination of 0.1–0.2% (Teisinger et al., 1952). Subjects exposed to 6000 ppm benzene retained 28–34% in the blood, and of this amount 55–60% was fixed in the bone marrow, fat depots, and liver, with the balance being excreted via the pulmonary route (Durior et al., 1946). Inhalation of 35 ppm benzene produced a steady state within 5–7 min and 47% was absorbed (Hunter, 1966). Benzene saturation of the blood occurs rapidly, reaching 70–80% within 30 min, but it requires 2–3 days to produce relative saturation because transfer of the chemical to fatty tissue is slow (Gerarde, 1963b). Six humans exposed to 52–60 ppm benzene for 4 h had a constant retention concentration of 30% at 3 h with a respiratory uptake of 46.9% and an excretion of 16.8% (Nomiyama and Nomiyama, 1974a). Pulmonary benzene decreased from 10 ppm to 0.5 ppm in 17 h (Nomiyama and Nomiyama, 1974b). After exposure to 80–100 mg/l for 6 h, humans retained 230 mg benzene and the lungs eliminated only 12% of the retained chemical (Hunter and Blair, 1972).

Biotransformation In animals, benzene is metabolized to phenol, hydroquinone, catechol, hydroxyhydroquinone, transmuconic acid, and L-phenylmercapturic acid, and excreted as free metabolites or conjugated with glucuronic or sulfuric acids. With the exception of the cat and pig, 17 other species use these processes to eliminate benzene metabolites. The cat excreted a total dose of [^{14}C]benzene as 87% phenylsulfate and 13% hydroquinone sulfate, whereas the pig excreted only phenylglucuronide (Snyder and Kocsism, 1975). In vitro cytochrome P-450 and mixed-function oxidases hydroxylate benzene via an arene intermediate, which can be inhibited by 3-amino-1,2,4-triazole (Snyder and Kocsism, 1975). Phenobarbital pretreatment of rats produces a three- to fourfold increase in aromatic hydroxylase in vitro and enhances phenol excretion in vivo (Ikeda and Ohtsuji, 1971). Pretreatment with hydroquinone, pyrogallol, or phenol enhances rat liver microsomal metabolism of benzene, but pyrocatechol decreases such metabolism in vitro (Saito et al., 1973). Phenobarbital and 3-methylcholanthrene induce rat liver benzene hydroxylase, but only chlorpromazine induces this enzyme in rat lung and the effect is minimal (Drew and Routs, 1974). It has been suggested that bone-marrow homogenates be utilized rather than liver homogenates to determine whether benzene acts directly or through its metabolites to cause aplastic anemia (Snyder and Kocsism, 1975). However, administration of phenol, catechol, or hydroquinone for 1 week did not induce aplastic anemia (Mitchell, 1972). The addition of fluoride to microsomal incubations stimulates benzene metabolism, producing phenol plus some highly polar unidentified metabolites (Post and Synder, 1983).

In humans, inhaled benzene was metabolized to 29% phenol, 2.9% pyrocatechol, and 1% hydroquinone (Teisinger et al., 1952). Metabolism of inhaled benzene produced phenols and diphenols, which were excreted as esters of glucuronic and sulfuric acids. The body sulfate pool was decreased (Durior et al., 1946). The urinary phenols derived from benzene metabolism were conjugated with glycine and with glucuronic and sulfuric acids (Hunter, 1966).

Toxicology   In humans, severe acute benzene exposure in enclosed spaces produces convulsions, paralysis, unconsciousness, and death. Lower benzene exposures cause euphoria, giddiness, headache, nausea, staggering gait, and unconsciousness (Browning, 1965). Acute benzene poisoning caused petechial hemorrhages of the brain, pleura, pericardium, urinary tract, mucous membranes, and skin. Breathlessness, nervous irritability, and unsteady gait persist for several weeks during recovery (Gerarde, 1960). Inhalation of 3000 ppm benzene can be tolerated for 0.5–1 h; 7500 ppm causes toxic effects in 0.5–1 h; and 20,000 ppm is fatal in 5–10 min (Flury, 1928). Respiratory-tract infection, hypo- and hyperplasia of sternal bone marrow, congested kidneys, and cerebral edema have been found at autopsy following acute benzene intoxication (Greenberg et al., 1939; Erf and Roades, 1939). At nonlethal concentrations, exposure time and concentration determine the extent of the effect on the central nervous system and hematopoietic system. Clinical symptoms include insomnia, agitation, headache, heaviness in the head, dizziness, drowsiness, breathlessness, unsteadiness, irritability, vertigo, nausea, and anorexia (Gerarde, 1960; Averill, 1899; Imamiya, 1973). Exposure to the odor threshold of benezene, 0.875 ppm, enhances the brain electropotential, but no changes occur at 0.469 ppm (Gusev, 1968). Sometimes, none of the above symptoms are present in clinically detectable benzene intoxications (Hardy and Elkins, 1948).

In chronic benzene intoxication in humans, mild poisonings produce headache, dizziness, nausea, vertigo, stomach pains, anorexia, and hypothermia. In severe intoxications, pale skin and mucous membranes, weakness, blurred vision, and dypsnea occur on exertion. Hemorrhagic tendencies include petechia, easy bruising, epitaxis, bleeding gums, and menorrhagia. Bone-marrow depression causes decreases in circulating peripheral erythrocytes and leukocytes. A normochromic or mild hyperchromic anemia results from a decrease in hemoglobin. Macrocytosis is observed. Neutrophils decrease and there is a relative lymphocytosis. A shift to the right in the differential count is seen, and the reduced numbers of platelets show anisocytosis, staining defects, and pyknosis of the chromomere. Red-cell fragility remains normal, but serum iron increases due to decreased utilization. Low serum bilirubin and reduced urobiligen are observed. Bone marrow has a decreased number of cells, no megakaryocytes, and immature forms of erythrocytes and leukocytes are present. Few intermediate or late normablasts, myelocytes, or metamyelocytes are found because of the shift in maturation. Chronic pancytopenia occurs with continuing exposure to benzene. There is no guarantee that the condition will not become irreversible when benzene exposure is terminated. The leukocyte defects may require several years to rectify. The severe thrombocytopenia produces hemorrhages often complicated by hypoprothrombinemia and hypofibrinogenemia. With the occurrence of acute pancytopenia, there is pyrexia with toxemia and a precipitous fall in blood elements. Hyperchromic, macrocytic anemia and severe hemorrhages occur. Blood culture may show *Escherichia coli*, staphylococci, or streptococci. A fatal outcome can occur in a few days to weeks

(Saita, 1973). Benzene is a powerful leukotoxin, destroying circulating leukocytes and damaging the bone marrow (Selling, 1916).

Studies on 217 workers exposed to 30–210 ppm benzene for 3 months to 17 years showed hematologic abnormalities. Blood changes were leukopenia, 9.7%; thrombocytopenia, 1.84%; leukopenia plus thrombocytopenia, 2.76%; leukocyte count of less than 4000/mm^3, 17.5%; hemoglobin less than 12 g/100 ml, 33%; packed cell volume less than 40%; and mild to moderate hypochromic or normochromic anemia, 33%. This latter condition was also found in 21% of 100 control subjects. Oral iron corrected the anemia (Aksoy et al., 1971). Further studies allowed a bone-marrow classification in four different ways: hypoplastic or acellular, hyperplastic, normoblast, or large erythrocyte precursors. Clinical signs were macrocytic anemia, mild reticulocytosis, hyperbilirubinemia, erythroblastemia, increased red blood cell (RBC) osmotic fragility, and elevated lactate dehydrogenase levels. Fetal hemoglobin was increased in 20 of 24 patients, while hemoglobin A$_2$ was increased in 21 of 24 (Aksoy et al., 1972a, b).

In a Swedish rubber raincoat factory, 60 workers exposed to 5320 ppm benzene developed chronic poisoning (Helmer, 1944). Depending on the job being done, the degree of benzene exposure in three rotogravure plants varied from 11 to over 1000 ppm. Chronic intoxication was found in 130 of 332 patients, with 22 very severe cases. Clinical symptoms included erythrocyte count less than 4.5 million, 48%; thrombocytes less than 100,000, 33%; leukocyte count less than 5000, 86%; and hemoglobin less than 13 g/100 ml, 15%. It has been suggested that chronic benzene intoxication is most easily detected by using RBC reduction and increased mean corpuscular volume, but other hematological parameters increase the diagnostic accuracy (Greenberg et al., 1939).

Workers in a shoe factory were exposed to 318,433 or 470 ppm benzene, and hematological abnormalities were found in 73%, thrombocytopenia in 62%, leukopenia in 32%, and anemia in 35%. All 3 abnormalities occurred in 31 patients and 1 in 147 patients while 27 had some defects 1 year later (Savilahti, 1956). Although no benzene measurements were made, 73% of 585 workers got benzene poisoning from the glue used in a shoe factory (Juzwiak, 1969). A report from the leather industry showed that 18.6% of 350 female workers had hematological changes that were caused by a glue containing benzene (Butareqiez et al., 1969). After exposure to 40–80 ppm, 16–52 rubber coating workers had deviations in more than one blood element (Hardy and Elkins, 1948). Substitution of naphtha for benzene still resulted in exposure of workers to 40 ppm benzene, and 8 of 68 workers showed mild hematological deviations. Measurement of urinary phenol concentrations in 162 workers indicated that this was good measure of benzene exposure, as there was a good correlation between atmospheric benzene and urinary phenol (Pagnotto et al., 1961).

A 5-year study of workers in the leatherette industry exposed to 25–78 ppm benzene suggested that the phagocytic index, which decreased earlier than blood morphological changes, was a better indication of chronic benzene poisoning (Kozlova and Volkova, 1960). A study of the health of 373 male workers in 14 paint workshops included CBC, specific gravity of whole blood and serum, urinary coproporphyrin and total sulfate ratio, and subjective clinical signs. Benzene concentrations varied by group: I, 6.6–68.5 ppm; II, 3.4–35.9 ppm; III, 0.3–22.1 ppm; and IV, 1.8 ppm. Due to the frequency of unspecified abnormal findings in groups I and II compared with group III, it was suggested that the maximum allowable concentration be set at 20 ppm (Horiuchi et al., 1973). It has been suggested that females and pregnant females are more susceptible than males to benzene poisoning (Cassan and Baron, 1956), but other investigators do not support this idea (Savilahti, 1956; Hunter, 1936; Smith, 1928; Mallory et al., 1939). Age is not involved.

Exposure to benzene produces significant increases in unstable and stable chromosome aberrations in both peripheral blood lymphocytes and bone marrow that persist for several years after cessation of exposure (Pollini and Colombi, 1964; Tough and Court-Brown, 1965; Forni and Moreo, 1969a,b; Tough et al., 1970; Forni et al., 1971a,b; Hartwich and Schwanitz, 1972). The stable changes persist or increase, while the unstable ones decrease. In a pregnant subject with pancytopenia and severe hemorragic problems, it was shown that her chromosome aberrations were not transmitted to her offspring (Forni et al., 1971a,b). In benzene-induced aplastic anemia, mutagenic effects may occur in blood cells (Vigliani and Saita, 1964). Human lymphocytes in culture show chromosome aberrations consisting of breaks and gaps after exposure to 2.2×10^{-3} M benzene (Koisumi et al., 1974).

With exposure to 0.11–0.158 mg/l, 35 workers caused changes in sera immunoglobulins as compared to 42 controls. IgG and IgA levels decreased significantly, whereas IgM levels increased. The fall in IgG reflects suppression of immunoglobulin-producing cells by benzene with inhibition of DNA synthesis, increasing the IgM level due to impairment of the feedback control of IgM synthesis by the decreased level of IgG (Lange et al., 1973). Because these workers showed autoleukocyte agglutinins, leukoagglutination and cytotoxic tests were given 76 workers exposed to benzene. While 10–35 exposed workers had leukocyte agglutinins reacting with autoleukoyctes from "O" Rh-negative blood, only 1 of 41 controls reacted. None of the sera was positive in the Gorer–O'Gorman cytotoxic test. This suggests the occurrence of an allergic component in benzene-induced blood dyscerasias (Lange et al., 1973). Lowered complement levels were found in 62 of 79 solvent-exposed workers, suggesting an involvement of immunological factors in chronic benzene intoxication (Smolik et al., 1973).

Benzene is known to produce hypoplasia of the bone marrow, causing aplastic anemia, but it was only in 1928 that the chemical induced leukemia (Delore and Borgomaho, 1928). Leukemia from chronic benzene exposure was reported in 250 cases in Germany (Boldt, 1974). In a case of heavy exposure for 4 years at 200 ppm, and lighter exposure for 6 years, typical myeloid leukemia with diffuse myeloid infiltration of the liver, spleen, and bone marrow was reported (Hunter, 1936). In a child exposed to benzene, sternal biopsy showed infiltration of the bone marrow with undifferentiated lymphoblasts (Hunter, 1936). Another study reported 10 cases of leukemia from chronic benzene exposure (Mallory et al., 1936). It is impossible, in most cases, to determine the incidence of benzene leukemias in the general population or to develop a relationship between the concentration and duration of exposure and the development of leukemia, because there is a lack of exposure data (Boldt, 1974). In a patient who showed hypocellular bone marrow after a 13-year benzene exposure, an apparent recovery was followed by leukemia in 15 years (DeGowin, 1963). French studies reported 14.7% chronic lymphocytic leukemia and 12.1% acute leukemia in people exposed to benzene. There were 31 occupational cases and 15 domestic cases (Girard et al., 1971). Chronic exposure to benzene at 150–200 ppm in the shoe industry resulted in the development of leukemia without prior aplastic anemia (Aksoy et al., 1972a,b,c). Following a mean benzene exposure time of 9.7 years, 26 shoe-industry workers out of 28,500 developed preleukemia or leukemia. Acute myeloblastic leukemia was observed in 14 (Aksoy et al., 1974a,b,c). Thus, benzene has been definitely established as an industrial leukemogenic agent (Eckardt, 1973).

An epidemiological survey of workers in the rubber industry demonstrated that chronic benzene exposure leads to lymphatic leukemia (McMichael et al., 1974, 1975). Another study of this same cohort associated lymphatic leukemia with the chemical intermediates styrene-butadiene and neoprene (McMichael et al., 1976). An additional study found excess mortality in both active and retired workers from neoplasms of the lymphatic and hematopoietic tissues (Andjelkovic et al., 1976). A study of a cohort of 13,571 rubber workers showed that in 5079 deceased employees there was an excess death rate from leukemia in tire workers, in processing, in the chemical division, in shops, in elevator areas, and with cleaning and industrial products from exposure to benzene (Monson and Nakano, 1976).

A survey of 17 refineries showed an increase in deaths from lymphomas (American Petroleum Institute, 1974). A previous study encountered difficulty with data collection in petroleum and the petrochemical industry, thus preventing correlation between benzene exposure and leukemia (Thorpe, 1974).

Occupational exposure to benzene has been directly associated with 50 cases of leukemia in France (Goguel et al., 1967), and in 13 new cases of chronic myelocytic leukemia and 23 acute leukemias along with 9 cases of chronic lymphocytic leukemia in 1970 (Girard and Revol, 1970). In the Soviet Union, printers, primers, apparatus men, and chemists developed leukemia from exposure to benzene (Tareeff et al., 1963). Similar results have been reported in Turkey (Aksoy et al., 1971, 1972a,b,c, 1975), in Italy (Vigliani and Forni, 1976), in Spain (Rozman et al., 1968), and in Scandinavia (Nissen and Soeborg Ohlsen, 1953). The report of 20 cases of acute erythroleukemia, a rare disease, is considered significant (Vigliani and Forni, 1976). Recently it has been suggested that chronic exposure to benzene may lead to the development of Hodgkin's disease (Aksoy et al., 1974a,b,c).

Consistent observations of chromosome aberrations associated with benzene exposure have been reported (Wurster-Hill et al., 1974; Stieglitz et al., 1974; Erdogan and Aksoy, 1973), and this genetic possibility is supported by the report of leukemia in a nephew and his paternal uncle (Aksoy et al., 1974b).

Toluene

Environmental   Environmental contamination with toluene reuslts from its use as a solvent in the rotogravure process, in the rubber industry, in linoleum industry, in dyeing, in the cleaning industry, in the impregnation of cartridge paper, in the production of paints, varnishes, glues, enamels, and lacquers, in the production of explosives, and as a chemical intermediative (Browning, 1953). Toluene is present in U.S. drinking water (Environmental Protection Agency, 1976; Perry et al., 1970). Glue sniffing also causes contamination (O'Brene et al., 1971).

Tissue Distribution   After inhalation, toluene is found in the lungs, blood, liver, and kidneys (Greenberg et al., 1942). The blood concentration increases with increased environment contamination (von Oettigen, 1942). Absorption of toluene by the lungs is rapid but then slows as excretion occurs (Jost, 1932).

Biotransformation   Toluene is converted to benzoic acid, conjugated with glycine, and excreted in the urine as hippuric acid (Williams, 1959). The excretion of hippuric acid in the urine is proportional to toluene exposure (Ogata et al., 1970). With voluntary exposures of humans to 200 ppm toluene, 68% of the calculated dose was excreted as hippuric acid (Ogata et al., 1971). The administration of 2 g glycine markedly increased urinary hippuric acid excretion (von Oettingen et al., 1942a).

Toxicology   Acute human exposure to toluene at 200–300 ppm for 8 h causes fatigue, weakness, and confusion (von Oettingen et al., 1942a). Loss of consciousness and vertigo have also been reported (Sack, 1941).

Chronic exposure to toluene at 600–800 ppm causes mental confusion, staggering gait, nausea, vomiting, anorexia, and severe headache (von Oettingen et al., 1942b). Pharyngitis and skin irritation has also been reported (Litzner and Edlich, 1934). A palpable enlargement of the liver occurred in a painter exposed to toluene (Greenberg et al., 1942). In contrast to benzene, toluene has not been linked to hematological diseases such as aplastic anemia or leukemia.

Ethylbenzene

Environmental   Environmental contamination with ethylbenzene results from its use as a solvent, antiknock agent in gasoline, and intermediate in gasoline (Proctor and Hughes, 1978). The U.S. production of ethylbenzene is 2.7–3.1×10^9 kg, from petroleum cracking. Gasoline contains 2–3%, 2.4–4.2×10^8 kg; residues in polystyrene are 8.4×10^7 kg; and motor vehicle exhaust contains 1.2×10^7 kg. However, the exact amount in the environment is known (International Trade Commission, 1976). Alkylated benzenes are present in U.S. drinking water at 10^{-6} g/l (Perry et al., 1970; Haley, 1981). This chemical has been found in river water, chemical-plant effluents, raw water, textile-plant effluents, and well water at 15 ppb (Barnham et al., 1972). It has also been detected in roasted filberts (Kinlin et al., 1972) and in cigarette smoke (Conkle et al., 1975).

Tissue Distribution   Ethylbenzene is widely distributed in human tissues after dermal or inhalation exposure. Furthermore, considerable more of this chemical is absorbed than toluene, styrene, or xylene (Dutkiewicz and Tyras, 1967, 1968). Ethyl benzene at $0.78-14 \times 10^{-6}$ g/h has been found in air from cigarette smokers (Conkle et al., 1975), in cord and maternal blood of humans (Dowty et al., 1976), and in subcutaneous fat from exposed humans (Wolff et al., 1977). Ethylbenzene persists in humans for days after exposure (Wolff, 1977).

Biotransformation Dogs and rabbits metabolize ethyl benzene to phenaceturic acid, mandelic acid, p-hydroxyacetophenone, m-hydroxyacetophenone, 2-hydroxyacetophenone, hippuric acid, and 1-phenylethanol (Kiese and Lenk, 1974). The same metabolic pattern is seen with rat liver microsomes in vitro (McMahon and Sullivan, 1966; McMahon et al., 1969).

Human dermal exposure to 112–156 mg/l of ethylbenzene resulted in a 4% per 24 h mandelic acid excretion when the rate of absorption was $0.11-0.12$ mg/cm^3·h; also, more ethylbenzene than toluene, styrene, or xylene was absorbed (Dutkiewicz and Tyras, 1967, 1968). Human gastrointestinal absorption produced the following urinary metabolites as a percent of the administered dose: phenaceturic acid, 10–20; mandelic acid, 1–2; p-hydroxyacetophenone, 13; m-hydroxyacetophenone, 0.3; 2-hydroxyacetophenone, 0.1; hippuric acid, 22–41; and 1-phenylethanol, 75 D(+) and 25 L(−) (Kiese and Lenk, 1974; Logemann et al., 1968; Bardodev and Bardojeva, 1970).

Human volunteers receiving an inhalation exposure to ethylbenzene at concentrations of 23, 43, 46, and 86 ppm retained 64% in their respiratory tract and excreted phenaceturic acid, mandelic acid, and 1-phenylethanol in their urine (Bardodev and Bardojeva, 1970).

Toxicology The oral LD50 of ethylbenzene in rats is 3.5 g/kg or 5.46 ml/kg (Wolf et al., 1956); the dermal LD50 is 17.8 m/kg and the inhalation LD50 in rats is 4000 ppm $\times$ 4 h (Smyth et al., 1962). Application of the chemical to rabbit's eye caused a slight conjunctival irritation but no corneal damage. When ethylbenzene was applied 10 to 20 times to rabbit's ear or shaved abdomen, moderate edema, superficial necrosis, chapped appearance, blistering, and exfoliation of large patches of skin were observed (Wolf et al., 1956).

Chronic oral administration of ethylbenzene for 6 months at doses of 408 to 680 mg/kg to rats caused cloudy swelling of the liver parenchymal cells and the tubular epithelium of the kidney but no hemopoietic effects (Wolf et al., 1956). Slight changes in liver and kidney weights occurred in rats and guinea pigs and slight testicular histopathology occurred in rabbits and monkeys inhaling 600 ppm ethylbenzene for 186 days (Wolf et al., 1956). Exposure of rabbits to 230 ppm of this chemical for 4 h/day for 7 months produced changes in blood cholinesterase activity, decreased plasma albumin, increased plasma globulins, leukocytosis, reticulocytosis, cellular infiltration, and lipid dystrophy of the liver, and dystrophic changes in the kidney and muscle chronaxia (Ivanov, 1964).

Human inhalation of 85 ppm ethylbenzene produced fatigue, insomnia, headache, and mild irritation of the eyes and respiratory tract (Bardodev and Bardojeva, 1970). When the chemical concentration was increased to 1000–5000 ppm, eye, nose, throat, and mucous-membrane irritation, lacrimation, dizziness, and central nervous system effects occurred (Gerarde, 1963b).

A study of 494 polymerization workers in styrene production reported prenarcotic symptoms, incoordination, dizziness, headache, and nausea (13%) and decreased radial and perineal nerve-conduction velocity (19%). Distalhypoasthenia involving the lower limbs was seen in 50% of the workers (Lilis et al., 1978). Workers in a baseball-bat plant exposed to ethylbenzene and other solvents reported mucous-membrane irritation and contact dermatitis (Rivera and Rostand, 1975). The number of individuals exposed to atmospheric ethylbenzene chronically is unknown, but the air of the Los Angeles basin contains 0.006–0.01 ppm of it, and five other sites in California have 0.01 ppm of the compound (Looneman, 1968; Neligan et al., 1965).

Methanol

Environmental Methanol is used in the manufacture of varnishes, shellac, and nitrocellulose lacquers, in the dye industry, in dry cleaning, in the hat industry, in manufacturing of artificial flowers, in boat and shoe manufacturing, as a solvent and intermediate in the chemical industry, in printing and lithography, as an antifreeze, for blending motor fuel, in manufacturing photographic films, as an alcohol denaturant, in manufacturing safety glass, in the manufacturing of artificial silk and patent leather, and in the manufacturing of xylonite (Browning, 1953). Methanol has been found in U.S. industrial effluent discharges (Perry et al., 1970).

Tissue Distribution Methanol is widely distributed in body tissues after absorption from ingestion, inhalation, or dermal exposure. The concentration in the cerebrospinal fluid is greater than in the blood. A metabolite of methanol, formaldehyde, has been found in the aqueous humour, cerebrospinal fluid, and abdominal fluid of rabbits. Urinary excretion is slow, and methanol and formic acid are found in the urine (Browning, 1953).

Biotransformation Hepatic alcohol dehydrogenase converts methanol into formaldehyde (Cooper and Kini, 1962), but hepatic catalase is also important in the oxidation of methanol (M. E. Smith, 1961; Tephly et al., 1961). Oxidation of methanol requires several days and occurs mainly in the liver and kidneys (Bartlett, 1950). Blood and urine concentrations of formic acid are directly related to the amount of methanol ingested (Bastrup, 1947; Lund, 1948). The metabolite, formaldehyde, damages the retinal cells, causing blindness (Kini and Cooper, 1962; Kini et al., 1962). The hepatic microsomal oxidizing system can oxidize methanol (Lieber and DeCarli, 1968).

Toxicology Symptoms of acute toxicity from exposure to methanol include minor central nervous system (CNS) depression, acidosis from production of formic acid, specific toxicity to retinal cells, headache, vertigo, vomiting, severe upper-abdominal pain, back pain, dyspnea, motor restlessness, cold clammy extremities, blurring vision, hyperemia of the optic disc, and diarrhea. In severe cases, symptoms include bradycardia, restlessness, delirium, slow shallow respiration, blindness, coma, and death (Harger and Forney, 1967).

Ethanol

Environmental Ethanol is used in the manufacturing of ether, collodion, artificial vinegar, explosives, pharmaceutical products, and as a gasoline additive; it is also used in the photographic, artificial silk, chemical, and varnish and lacquer industries (Browning, 1953). The largest exposure to ethanol occurs from the consumption of alcoholic beverages. Ethanol has been found in U.S. drinking-water supplies (Environmental Protection Agency, 1976) but not in U.S. industrial effluent discharges (Perry et al., 1970).

Tissue Distribution Upon absorption, ethanol is uniformly distributed in all body tissues and fluids. Concentration in the erythrocytes is less than in the plasma. Concentration is the brain rapidly approaches that in the blood. Cerebrospinal fluid concentration follows the blood concentration.

Biotransformation Ethanol is oxidized to acetaldehyde by hepatic alcohol dehydrogenase, a zinc-containing enzyme that utilizes nicotinamide dinucleotide (NAD) as the hydrogen acceptor and depends on free surfhydryl groups in the protein for activity (Westerfield, 1961). The acetaldehyde is converted by hepatic and renal aldehyde dehydrogenase into acetyl coenzyme A (CoA), which is oxidized through the citric acid cycle or utilized in anabolic processes involved in synthesis of cholesterol, fatty acids, and other tissue constitutents (Buttner, 1965). There are other hepatic enzymes capable of metabolizing ethanol (Hawkins and Kalant, 1972). The increased ratio of NADH:NAD induced by oxidation of ethanol results in increased lactate and fatty acid synthesis and decreases in the hepatic citric acid cycle activity and fatty acid oxidation. The causes of decreased uric acid excretion and increased urinary loss of magnesium are unknown (Lieber and Davidson, 1962). Human ingestion of ethanol results in hyperglycemia followed by hypoglycemia (Vartia et al., 1960), and it has been suggested that the initial glycogenolysis followed by hypoglycemia is a result of depletion of glycogen stores. Ganglionic blockade prevents the hyperglycemia, suggesting an adrenomedullary origin (Perman, 1962). Ethanol also acts as an inducer or inhibitor of the hepatic microsomal enzyme system, thus affecting the metabolism of drugs and other chemicals (Rubin and Lieber, 1971). Ethanol ingestion affects lipid metabolism, resulting in accumulation of triglycerides in the liver (Lieber, 1967). Catecholamines and corticosteroids released by ethanol (Ellis, 1966) cause increased mobilization from body fat depots (Poggi and DiLuzio, 1964), thus elevating plasma fatty acids (Mallov, 1961) with increased hepatic storage of triglycerides.

Ingested ethanol escaping oxidation varies between 2 and 10%, depending on the dose. Although most of the ingested ethanol is excreted via the kidney and lungs, small amounts have been found in sweat, tears, bile, gastric juice, saliva, and other secretions.

Toxicology Acute ethanol intoxication displays the following symptoms: talkativeness, boisterous behavior, delayed reflexes, minor muscular incoordination, nystagmus, loss of muscular control, decreased mental activity, cutaneous vasodilation, blurring of vision, lack of acuity for color, conjunctival reddening, pupillodilation, diplopia, difficulty in focusing, slurred speech, hand and lips tremor, loss of tone of facial muscles, incoordinate gait, complete loss of motor activity, stupor or coma, shallow slow respiration, heat loss, and cyanosis. On recovery, there is acidosis, brain edema, and cloudy swelling of the liver and kidneys. Unusual reactions include amnesia and mania. Blood concentration of 200 mg% is association with mild to moderate intoxication, of 300 mg% is definitely intoxicated, of 400 mg% is a state of advanced drunkness, and between 500 and 800 mg% is fatal (Thienes and Haley, 1972). When the blood concentration of ethanol reaches 150 mg%, a driver is more likely to have an accident (Holcomb, 1938).

Symptoms of chronic alcoholism include chronic hepatic cirrhosis, malnutrition, myocardial loss and fragmentation of large, swollen mitochondria, increased deposition of glycogen, dilatation of the sarcoplasmic reticulum, marked degeneration of the granular layer of the cerebellum, and ataxia (Thienes and Haley, 1972).

GLYCOLS AND GLYCOL ETHERS

Ethylene Glycol

Environmental Ethylene glycol is used as a solvent for dyes and for cellulose nitrate, as ethylene glycol electrolyte for electrolytic condensers, in skin lotions, as an antifreeze component, and in flavoring essenses (Browning, 1953). Ethylene glycol has not been found in U.S. drinking-water supplies (Environmental Protection Agency, 1976) or in U.S. industrial effluent discharges (Perry et al., 1970).

Tissue Distribution Ethylene glycol and its metabolites have been found in the liver, in the proximal and distal renal tubules and urinary bladder (Bove, 1966), and in the brain (Pons and Custer, 1946).

Biotransformation Ethylene glycol is metabolized in rabbits to CO_2, oxalic acid, and glycolic acid (Gessner et al., 1961). In liver slices, glycolaldehyde and glyoxylic acid were also detected. In the rat, the following metabolites were found: glycolaldehyde, glycolic acid, glyoxylic acid, and oxalic acid (Bove, 1966). The dog and human excreted unchanged ethylene glycol and oxalic acid (Gressner et al., 1961). Ethylene glycol is metabolized by alcohol dehydrogenase to produce severe metabolic acidosis via its metabolites in human, dog, and pigtail monkey (Clay and Murphy, 1977). The inhibition of alcohol dehydrogenase by ethanol prevents the metabolic acidosis (Wacker et al., 1965), and this competition causes inhibition of ethylene glycol metabolism (von Wartburg et al., 1964). In vivo studies in animals showed that the presence of ethanol markedly reduced the LD50 of ethylene glocol (Peterson et al., 1963), and giving pyridoxine and magnesium could prevent renal lesions (Gershoff and Andrus, 1962). Ethylene glycol also affects the mitochondria (Bachmann and Bulberg, 1971).

Toxicology Toxic doses of ethylene glycol in animals produced sluggish depressed functioning, some digestive-tract irritation, gross pathological changes in the kidneys with bloody urine and free blood under the capsule, and slight liver pathology with orange or reddish bile (Smyth et al., 1941). Another study reported focal necorsis of the liver, hemorrhagic areas in the stomach, lung congestion with hemorrhage, and hydropic degeneration of the cells lining the cortical convulted tubules (Laug et al., 1939). Women workers exposed to 40% ethylene glycol, 55% boric acid, and 5% ammonia had symptoms of loss of consciousness and absolute lymphocytosis, and nystagmus was observed in other workers in the plant (Troisi, 1950). Interpretation of these results is complicated by the presence of other components in the mixture. Two individuals who ingested 250–1000 ml ethylene glycol antifreeze were treated with ethanol infusions and enjoyed uneventful recoveries (Wacker et al., 1965). Human symptoms from ingestion of ethylene glycol antifreeze included vomiting, cyanosis, extreme prostration and coma, convulsions, and death from respiratory paralysis. Pathological examination showed severe renal epithelial damage, oxalate crystals in the tubules, congestion and edema of the central nervous system, and exudative meningoencephalitis (Pons and Custer, 1946).

Diethylene Glycol

Environmental Diethylene glycol is used in lacquers, cosmetics, antifreeze formulations, as a plasticizer, and as a softening agent, and only presents a hazard where mists are created or high temperatures cause it to vaporize (Rowe, 1963). This chemical has not been found in U.S. drinking water supplies (Environmental Protection Agency, 1976) or industrial effluents (Perry et al., 1970).

Tissue Distribution Diethylene glycol distributes into the lungs, intestine, kidneys, and liver (Laug et al., 1939).

Biotransformation Diethylene glycol is metabolized in oxalate, but not to the same extent as its ethylene congener (Fitzhugh and Nelson, 1946; Weil et al., 1967). Metabolism of the chemical should be reinvestigated.

Toxicology The acute toxic syndrome from diethylene glycol ingestion in mice, rats, rabbits, guinea pigs, and dogs is similar to that in humans. Symptoms include thirst, diuresis, suppression of urine with proteinuria, prostration, dyspnea, bloated appearance, pronounced hypothermia, coma, and death. Pathological changes include generalized edema; hemorrhagic lungs, intestines, and kidneys; pneumonia; soft, fragile liver; swollen, pale, and flabby kidneys; and the spleen containing blood pigment. Histological examination revealed degeneration of the renal cortex with hydropic degeneration of the central portion of the liver lobule, and extensive lung damage with pneumonia. The heart, stomach, intestine, brain, and bladder were essentially normal (Laug et al., 1939).

Propylene Glycol

Environmental Propylene glycol is used as a solvent in pharmaceuticals, cosmetics, foodstuffs, as a plasticizer, in antifreeze products, and in heat exchangers and hydraulic fluids. This chemical has not been found in U.S. drinking-water (Environmental Protection Agency, 1976) or in U.S. industrial effluent discharges (Perry et al., 1970).

Tissue Distribution Propylene glycol is distributed in the brain, liver, and kidneys (Laug et al., 1939).

Biotransformation Propylene glycol is rapidly combusted and excreted (Sollmann, 1957). The chick and rat metabolize propylene glycol to lactate and/or pyruvate (Ruddick, 1971). Two daily intraperitoneneal injections of 4 ml/kg of the chemical induced the microsomal enzymes involved in metabolizing aniline and p-nitroanisole and inhibited demethylation of aminopyrine without reducing the cytochrome P-450 levels (Dean and Stock, 1974).

Toxicology Large doses of propylene glycol administered to rats produced loss of equilibrium, marked depression, analgesia, coma, and death. Hemorrhagic areas in the small intestine were the only signs of gross pathology, and there were minimal microscopic changes in the liver and kidneys (Laug et al.,1939). No toxicity in humans has been reported.

Ethylene Glycol Monomethyl Ether

Environmental This chemical is used in manufacturing white lacquers, as a stiffener for shirt collars, and as a solvent for rotogravure inks (Browning, 1953). Ambient air concentrations in a shirt-collar factory varied from 25 to 76 ppm, depending on the amount of ventilation (Greenberg et al., 1938). Ambient air concentration in printing and cement spraying were 20 to 25 ppm, respectively (Elkings et al., 1942). Ethylene glycol monomethyl ether has not been found in U.S. drinking-water supplies (Environmental Protection Agency, 1976) or in industrial effluent discharges (Perry et al., 1970).

Tissue Distribution Ethylene glycol monomethyl ether is distributed in the cornea and lens, lungs, heart, liver, kidneys, and spleen after inhalation (Werner et al., 1943a).

Biotransformation This chemical is metabolized to methanol, formic acid, and oxalic acid by rabbits (Werner et al., 1943b) and by humans.

Toxicology Acute vapor exposure of mice to ethylene glycol monomethyl ether produced dypsnea, analgesia, and weakness (Werner et al., 1943a). Pathological changes consisted of follicular phagocytosis in the spleen, interstitial nephritis, and lung congestion with hemorrhage into the alveoli, but there were no changes in the other tissues. Chronic vapor exposure of rats to this chemical produced hemosiderosis and fatty infiltration of the bone marrow but no other significant changes (Werner et al., 1943b). Chronic vapor exposure of dogs resulted in increased secretion from the eyes and nose, hematuria, macrocytic anemia, decreased hematocrit, hypochromia, polychromatophilia, a marked increase in circulating immature granulocytes, oxaluria, increased blood urea, and increased erythrocyte fragility. Histological examination of the tissues revealed marked congestion of the blood vessels of the urinary bladder, pulmonary congestion, and hemosiderosis. There were no changes in the kidneys, adrenals, pancreas, and large and small intestines (Werner et al., 1943c).

Two patients exposed to vapors of ethylene glycol monomethyl ether in a shirt factory developed the following symptoms: personality change, dizziness, fainting spells, sleepiness, general hypertonicity, all reflexes hyperactive, transitory right-ankle clonus, persistent dilation of the pupils, moderate ataxia and positive Rhomberg sign, anemia, granulopenia, red blood cells with a high color index, vomiting; acidosis, loss of body weight, consistent nocturia, renal irritation, and a profound depression of the bone marrow (Parsons and Parsons, 1938). Examination of workers in a shirt factory revealed two workers with severe anemia, one worker with an abnormal leucocyte picture and neurological findings, and all of the workers showed macrocytic anemia associated with thrombocytopenia, disturbances in erythropoiesis, shift to the left in the granulocytes, and abnormal neurological findings (Greenberg et al., 1938). Five recent cases from a printing plant showed ataxia, tremors, slurred speech, personality changes, variable degrees of anemia, and erythrocyte counts below 4 million (Zavon, 1963).

Ethylene Glycol Monobutyl Ether

Environmental Ethylene glycol monobutyl ether is used for reducing viscosity of brushing lacquers and as a wetting-out solution for cotton thread (Browning, 1953). This chemical has not been found in U.S. drinking-water supplies (Environmental Protection Agency, 1976) or in industrial effluents (Perry et al., 1970).

Tissue Distribution Ethylene glycol monobutyl ether distributes in the cornea and lens, lungs, heart, liver, kidneys, and spleen after inhalation (Werner et al., 1943b).

Biotransformation The rat, rabbit, guinea pig, dog, rhesus monkey, and human metabolize ethylene glycol monobutyl ether to butoxyacetic acid (Carpenter et al., 1956).

Toxicology Symptoms of toxicity from this chemical in mice include dyspnea, corneal and lens opacity, marked follicular phagocytosis in the spleen, marked congestion of the cavernous veins of the spleen, and bronchiopneumonia (Werner et al., 1943a). Chronic vapor exposure of rats produced hemosiderosis, decreased hemoglobin, reticulocytosis, depressed erythrocyte counts, hemolysis, and suppression of the bone marrow. There was also damage to the lungs and kidneys (Werner et al., 1943b). Dogs showed similar symptoms, and histological examination showed pulmonary congestion, marked congestion of the alveolar airways, interstitial fibrosis, inflammatory changes in the bronchi, and necrosis of the liver (Werner et al., 1943c).

Human studies showed headache, eye and nose irritation, and hematuria (Browning, 1953).

CHLORINATED HYDROCARBONS

Chloroform

Environmental Chloroform has been used as an anesthetic, solvent for extraction of alkaloids, solvent for cellulose acetate, laquer coatings, sterilizant for catgut, and in floor polishes (Browning, 1953). This chemical has been found in drinking water up to 890 mg/l in private wells in Hardeman County, Tenn. (Clark et al., 1982). Chloroform has been found in U.S. drinking-water supplies and in industrial effluent discharges (Environmental Protection Agency, 1976; Perry et al., 1970). It has recently been banned in medicinal products in the United States (Anonymous, 1976). Chlorination of water supplies produces $CHCl_3$ (Maugh, 1981).

Tissue Distribution Chloroform is distributed in the brain, brainstem, cerebellum, pneumogastric and sciatic nerves, arterial and venous blood, liver, kidneys, spleen, heart, muscle, and subcutaneous fat (von Oettingen, 1937). Excretion is mainly through the lungs, 90%, and in the urine and milk. This compound is absorbed via the lungs, skin, and gastroinestinal tract (von Oettingen, 1955).

Biotransformation It has been shown that CO_2, 4–5%, and ^{14}C-labeled inorganic constituents, 2%, appeared in the urine (Van Dyke et al., 1964). The microsomal drug-metabolizing enzyme activity of rats is inhibited 40% by premedication with chloroform (Dingell and Heimberg, 1968), and giving the enzyme inducer phenobarbital causes increased hepatotoxicity (Scholler, 1970). Further investigation of the metabolism of $CHCl_3$ must be undertaken to establish the identity of its unknown metabolites. Chloroform depletes hepatic glutathione (Docks and Krishna, 1976).

Toxicology Symptoms of toxicity from ingestion of chloroform include severe gastrointestinal irritation, vomiting, colic, diarrhea, drowsiness, loss of consciousness, coma, and death (Tomb and Helmy, 1933). Inhalation of $CHCl_3$ causes headache, intoxication, salivation, mental unbalance, and sensitization of the heart to catecholamines, resulting in ventricular fibrillation (von Oettinger, 1937).

Subchronic and chronic toxicity from overexposure or abuse of chloroform produces similar symptoms, coupled with degenerative changes in the heart, liver, and kidneys, with albumin and casts in the urine. The chemical interferes with blood clotting by reducing the fibrinogen content, and there is a leucocytosis and changes in the ratio of polynuclears to mononuclears (von Oettingen, 1937).

The most important toxic effect of chloroform is its induction of centrizonal hepatic necrosis and steatosis accompanied by renal and myocardial injury (von Oettingen, 1964). The steatosis involves impaired exit of lipids from the liver and mobilization of lipids from body depots, causing accumulation of lipid in the myocardium and other organs (Stiles and McDonald, 1904). Dietary manipulation has different effects on hepatotoxicity. High calcium and low meat intake protects (Minot and Cutler, 1928), as does a high-protein diet (Goldschmidt et al., 1939); high carbohydrate is protective, while high fat is deleterious (Opie and Alford, 1915); fasting is dangerous (Davis and Whipple, 1919); and protein depletion is deleterious (Miller and Whipple, 1940). Chloroform also cause renal dysfunction in mice (Klassen and Plaa, 1966).

Carbon Tetrachloride

Environmental In the past, carbon tetrachloride was used as an anesthetic, as a shampoo, an anthelmintic, and as a dry cleaner, but these uses have been banned because they caused numerous cases of poisoning (Moller, 1933; Hardin, 1954). In industry, it is used as a solvent for oil, grease, fats, waxes, rubber, paint, lacquer, asphalt, gums, and resins (Hardin, 1954). Another use, since banned, was in fire extinguishers, and here the chemical was thermally degraded to phosgene, a deadly gas (Hardin, 1954). In industry, exposures to carbon tetrachloride vapor were dry cleaning, 29–1230 ppm; cleaning filters and centrifuges, 62–2050 ppm; and other workplaces, 1000 ppm (H. F. Smyth et al., 1936). Recent human exposures have resulted from leakage from landfills from improper disposal procedures (Hanrahan, 1979). The well water in Hardeman County, Tenn., had concentrations of carbon tetrachloride as high as 18,700 mg/l, and air in homes reached concentrations as high as 3600 mg/m^3 (Clark et al., 1982). In contrast, the Ohio River release in 1977 only reached a high of 340 mg/l (Anonymous, 1977). This chemical has also been found in other sources of U.S. drinking water (Environmental Protection Agency, 1976) and in industrial effluent discharges (Perry et al., 1970). The TLV for carbon tetrachloride is 10 ppm (ACGIH, 1976b), but NIOSH has recommended that the ceiling be dropped to 2 ppm (OSHA, 1978).

Tissue Distribution   When administered to dogs via the intestinal tract, carbon tetrachloride has been found in the brain, portal blood, kidney, body fat depots, liver, lungs, muscle, pancreas, spleen, and bone marrow, with the highest concentration in the last (Robbins, 1929). The rate of absorption is increased in the presence of fat and ethanol (Robbins, 1929). Monkeys inhaling [^{14}C]carbon tetrachloride readily absorbed the compound, and the principle route of excretion was the lungs, with smaller amounts in the urine and feces. The radiolabel was found in blood carbonate, in exhaled CO_2, and in urinary urea and carbonate. There were also unidentified metabolites (McCollister et al., 1951).

Biotransformation   Carbon tetrachloride is metabolized to CO_2 in experimental animals (McCollister et al., 1951; Rubinstein and Kanics, 1964). It has been shown that carbon tetrachloride is converted to chloroform by the rat liver (Butler, 1961). It has been suggested that it converts to the free radical CCl_3 (Rechnagel, 1967) and this is supported by the observation of morphological alteration of the liver endoplasmic reticulum (Bassi, 1960; Ashworth et al., 1963) and an effect on drug-metabolizing enzymes (Dingell and Heimberger, 1968; Sasame et al., 1968; David et al., 1971). The split products of carbon tetrachloride biotransformation attack glucose 6-phosphate (Recknagel and Lombarid, 1961) and protein synthesis (Smuckler et al., 1962) by affecting the lipoidal elements of the endoplasmic reticulum. The discovery of CCl_3CCl_3, a new CCl_4 metabolite, suggests the condensation of two CCl_3 free radicals (Fowler and Alexander, 1969). Low doses of carbon tetrachloride cause inhibition of activity of the microsomal aminopyrine demethylase enzyme system (Glende, 1972) and the ethylmorphine demethylase enzyme system (David et al., 1971). It has been suggested that CCl_4 toxicity is the result of free-radical metabolites causing lipid peroxidation, because antioxidants protect against CCl_4 toxicity (Gallagher, 1962) and peroxidation of lipid has been reported (Recknagel and Ghoshal, 1966; Klaassen and Plaa, 1969), but new data indicated that a better correlation exists with irreversible $^{14}CCl_4$ binding to cellular constitutents than to peroxidation (Diaz Gomez et al., 1975). Pretreatment of rats with CCl_4 caused serum pseudocholinesterase levels to be reduced to 50% (Kay, 1969).

Carbon tetrachloride exposure at 1500 ppm of rats caused marked changes in serum esterase, xanthine oxidase, and glutamic–oxaloacetic transaminease (GOT) activities (Block and Cornish, 1958). Exposure to 6000 ppm CCl_4 for 4 h caused an increase in these enzyme activities, followed by a marked drop in such activities. Liver esterase and xanthine oxidase activities were both depressed (Cornish and Block, 1960). Human exposure to CCl_4 results in a striking elevation in SGOT activity, which returns to normal when exposure is terminated (Wroblewski et al., 1956). Serum SGOT levels return to normal in 9 days, but liver histology requires 70 days after CCl_4 ingestion (Dawborn et al., 1961). Elevation in lactic dehydrogenase peaks

at 12 h, serum (SGOT) and malic dehydrogenase at 24 h, and glutamate dehydrogenase at 36 h. Depression of glucose 6-phosphatase, NADPH reductase, aminopyrine demethylase, aniline demethylase, and cytochrome P-450 activities occurs within
1 h. AT 10–20 h postexposure to CCl_4, the mitochondria show increased membrane
permeability, disorganization of the tricarboxylic acid cycle, abnormality of ATPase,
loss of respiratory control, and impairment of fatty acid oxidation (Zimmerman,
1979).

Toxicology Symptoms of acute carbon tetrachloride toxicity include nausea,
vomiting, abdominal pain, edema, jaundice, headache, fever, diarrhea, anorexia, dizziness, nose bleeds, convulsions, dyspnea, ambylopia, hematemesis, coma, flank
pain, chills, hiccough, and rash (Hardin, 1954). Subacute effects were albuminuria,
nitrogen retention, hematuria, oliguria, pulmonary edema, hypertension, hepatomegaly, leucocytosis, high icterus index, delayed diuresis, subconjunctival hemorrhage,
pneumonia, congestive heart failure, ascites, and electrocardiographic changes (Hardin, 1954).

Symptoms of chronic intoxication include all those seen with acute toxicity, along
with increased nonprotein nitrogen and blood potassium, hepatitis, and renal failure
(Smyth et al., 1936; von Oettingen, 1937). The severe hepatitis can produce an
extremely high fat content of the blood in the heart and large pulmonary arteries
(MacMahon and Weiss, 1929).

Carbon tetrachloride when used as an anthelminitic (Docherty and Burgess,
1922) has produced rapid lesions in the liver, consisting of fatty degeneration (Docherty and Nicholls, 1923). This chemical causes gastrointestinal irritation, nervous
hyperexcitability followed by depression, bilirubinemia, hypoglycemia, retention of
guanidine in the blood, and severe central necrosis of the liver (Minot and Cutler,
1928). Inhalation of large amounts of CCl_4 produces chronic cirrhosis of the liver
(Butsch, 1932). It has been shown that intermittent exposure to this chemical results
in development of hepatic cells resistant to its toxic effects (Smyth and Smyth, 1936).
In dogs, the Bromsulphalein retention time was the most sensitive test for hepatotoxicity following ingestion of CCl_4, followed by the serum phosphatase level, which
rose, while prothrombin time and galactose tolerance were of little use (Drill and Ivy,
1944). Vapor exposure to CCl_4 caused typical cirrhosis with hepatomegaly, splenomegaly, and ascites (Hardin, 1954). The mechanism of such damage is related to
alteration of the plasma membrane, with subsequent release of intracellular potassium, proteins, cytoplasmic enzymes, coenzymes, and intracellular accumulation of
water and Ca^{2+}. Effects on the mitochondrial membrane result in disruption of oxidative phosphorylation process (Zimmerman, 1979). Concomitant with these hepatic
effects is the development of kidney failure (Selman and Wirtschafter, 1937; Gray,
1947).

Carbon tetrachloride is extremely nephrotoxic and is the commonest cause of
acute renal failure (Jordan et al., 1957). Ingestion of alcoholic beverages greatly
increases the development of CCl_4-induced anuria and a fatal outcome (Farrier and
Smith, 1950). It is essential in acute renal failure from CCl_4 that the agent be identified along with the route of exposure, coupled with gastrointestinal manifestations,

hemorrhagic phenomena, and possibly the delayed onset of oliguira (New et al., 1962). It is necessary in cases presenting concomitant gastrointestinal, hepatic, and renal symptoms of uncertain origin to establish a possible CCl_4 exposure (Nielsen and Larsen, 1965). The anuria develops in 1-7 days and persists for 15 days, and urinary sediments contain protein, red and white blood cells, and hyaline, granular, and red-cell casts (Guild et al., 1958). In acute renal failure, there is a marked reduction in renal plasma flow and p-aminohippurate renal extraction ratio. There is a marked reduction in glomerular filtration, along with abnormal tubular back-diffusion of the filtrate. The latter plays a most important role in the early oliguira, while decreased renal blood flow is important during late oliguria and early diuresis. Recovery occurs, with gradual improvement in renal blood flow and glomerular filtration being reached at day 100 and 200 (Sirota, 1949). In the rat kidney, CCl_4 causes a reversible lesion limited to the proximal tubule with changes in the mitochondria, followed by cell swelling and proliferation of the smooth-surfaced endoplasmic reticulum (Striker et al., 1968). Carbon tetrachloride becomes concentrated in the kidney; it contact with the tubular cell wall destroys the cell, and the inflammatory process extends from living tubular cells into the interstitial surrounding areas, producing kidney edema, aggravating the nephrosis by inducing anoxia (Hardin, 1954).

Carbon tetrachloride has several effects on the nervous system. This chemical causes toxic amblyopia and can affect the optic nerve, causing blindness in some cases (Gocher, 1936). This toxic amblyopia is characterized by concentric constriction of all the color fields without central scotomata (Wirtschafter, 1933). Acute carbon tetrachloride toxicity causes headache, diplopia, incoordination, paresthesias, impaired vision, confusion, and coma (Stevens and Foster, 1953).

Trichloroethylene

Environmental Trichloroethylene is used as a degreaser in solvent soaps, in painting and enamelling, as a solvent for tar and pitch, in dyeing and dry cleaning, as an extractant for fixed oils, in recovery of wax and paraffin in refuse, in rubber cement in the boot and shoe industry, in the textile and printing industries, in cleaning films and photographic plates, for impregnating and cleaning artificial silk and leather, in optical grinding pastes, in chemical processing, as a solvent for sulfur and phosphorus, and as an anesthetic (Browning, 1953). Trichloraethylene has been found in U.S. drinking-water supplies (Environmental Protection Agency, 1976) and in U.S. industrial effluent discharges (Perry et al., 1970). It has been used by "glue sniffers" to obtain a high (Litt and Cohen, 1969).

Tissue Distribution Trichloroethylene is widely distributed in body tissues, including brain, heart, liver, and kidneys (Browning, 1953). It also has been observed to attack the central and peripheral nervous system (Feldman and Mayer, 1968).

Biotransformation Trichloroethylene is converted into a carcinogenic epoxide by hepatic microsomal enzymes (Van Duuren and Banerjee, 1976). This chemical is converted into trichloroacetic acid and trichloroethanol with small amounts of chloroform and monochloroacetic acid and is excreted in the urine (Butler, 1949). Rats excrete five to seven times more of trichlorethanol than trichloroacetic acid (Ikeda and Ohtsuji, 1972), and the former has been related to pronounced central nervous system depression (Mikishava and Mikisha, 1966). This compound accumulates in the body because daily exposure to 100 ppm results in only one-third being excreted as metabolites in the urine during the workday (Ikeda et al., 1972) and it has been shown that metabolite excretion gradually increases after repeated daily exposures (Stewart et al., 1970a). It has also been reported that trichloroethanol urinary excretion is proportional to ambient trichloroethylene concentration (Ikeda et al., 1972).

Toxicology Symptoms of acute toxicity from ingestion or inhalation of trichloroethylene include lethargy, confusion, headache, palsies of the II, III, V, VI, and VII cranial nerves, and increased theta-wave activity and slow alpha-wave frequencies in the electroencephalogram. There are also prolonged conduction times in the facial nerve, slowed conduction velocity in the ulnar nerve, bilateral dysfunction of the nasociliary nerve affecting mainly the longer myelinated fibers, but no involvement of the descending trigeminal nucleus (Feldman and Mayer, 1968). Inhalation ("glue sniffing") causes liver dysfunction, jaundice, nausea, paresthesias, tinnitus, ataxia, headache, hepatitis, and acute renal failure (Litt and Cohen, 1969). In mice, mild hepatic dysfunction was observed following median effective doses of trichloroethylene (Klaassen and Plaa, 1966). Death is caused by respiratory failure or ventricular fibrillation induced by adrenergic discharge of catecholamines (Browning, 1953).

Chronic exposure to trichloroethylene produces the following symptoms: sleepiness, giddiness, headaches, fatigue, indigestion, vertigo, leucopenia, anemia, retrobulbar neuritis, polyneuritis, tremor, spastic ataxia, chronic eczema, and corneal inflammation (Browning, 1953). Hepatitis and cirrhosis of the liver are rarely caused by trichloroethylene, in contrast to chloroform, carbon tetrachloride, and tetrachloroethane (Browning, 1953). In dogs, chronic inhalation of trichlorethylene, 500–750 ppm, caused glycogen depletion and hydropic parenchymatous degeneration in the liver (Seifter, 1944). Addiction to trichloroethylene has been reported (Baader, 1927).

Tetrachloroethylene

Environmental Tetrachloroethylene is used for dry cleaning and as a fat solvent in duplicating operations, constituent in solvent soaps, and degreaser and reinsolvent for fabric and fiber impregnation (Browning, 1953). This chemical has been found in U.S. drinking-water supplies (Environmental Protection Agency, 1976) but not in industrial effluent discharges in the United States (Perry et al., 1970). Tetrachloroethylene has been found in well water in Hardeman County, Tenn., at 2405 mg/l (Clark et al., 1982).

Tissue Distribution Tetrachloroethylene has been found in the lungs, liver, and kidneys. The chemical is largely excreted via the lungs (Stewart et al., 1970b).

Biotransformation Tetrachloroethylene is slowly metabolized, and only a small amount is excreted as metabolites principally as trichloroacetic acid (Ikeda and Ohtsuji, 1972) and inorganic chloride (Utzinger, 1977).

Toxicology Symptoms of acute toxicity from exposure to tetrachloroethylene included narcosis, slight fatty infiltration of the liver, and kidney congestion (Browning, 1953). Central nervous system effects and hepatotoxicity have also been reported (Irish, 1962). Moderate hepatic dysfunction was observed in mice (Klaassen and Plaa, 1966).

In animals, chronic exposure produced fatty infiltration of the liver but no cirrhosis in rats. With a concentration of 2300 ppm, slight nonprogressive changes in the liver, kidney, and spleen have been reported (Browning, 1953).

CHEMICAL INTERMEDIATES

Hexachlorocyclopentadiene

Environmental Hexachlorocyclopentadiene is produced by light chlorination of natural gas rich in pentane, neopentane, and cyclopentane, with the product then subjected to high-temperature chlorination at temperatures of 450–480 °C with excess chlorine. In the hypochlorite process, dicyclopentadiene is thermally depolymerized with alkali hypochlorite in organic solvents (Reimschneider, 1963). The resultant product is the starting material for synthesis of the diene group of pesticides produced by the Diels–Alder reaction with suitable unsaturated compounds. Further information on these processes is given in the review by Ungnade and McBee (1958).

Disposal of residues from these syntheses have caused environmental contamination of the aquifer supplying water to the residents of Hardeman County, Tenn., "the valley of the drums." Both hexachlorocyclopentadiene and hexachlorobicycloheptadiene were found in air, waste water, and urine of the population (Clark et al., 1982). Indoor air samples had concentrations ranging from 0.06 to 0.1 mg/m^3. Hexachlorocyclopentadiene, 0.3–4 ppb, has also been found in waste water of the North Wastewater Treatment Plant at Memphis, Tenn. (Elia et al., 1980), and in the waste in the Morris Foreman Wastewater Treatment Plant at Louisville, Ky., where the waste was illegally dumped into the municipal sewer system (Morse et al., 1979).

Tissue Distribution Using a model ecosystem, it was shown that hexachlorocyclopentadiene was stored in alga 33%, snail 50%, misquito 46%, and fish 41% (Lu et al., 1975). With a 30-day study of the effect of this chemical in larval and juvenile flathead minnows, it was shown that concentrations of 7.3, 38.4, and 40 mg/l were detrimental to this species. The residues in the fish were less than 0.1 mg/l in all tanks, giving a biological concentration factor of less than 11. It was concluded that hexachlorocyclopentadiene did not accumulate in this fish (Spehar et al., 1979). Exposure of sea lamprey, rainbow trout, and bluegill to concentrations of hexachlorocyclopentadiene of 1000 and 5000 mg/l caused rapid distress and death (Applegate et al., 1957). Similar results were reported in bluegill sunfish and largemouth bass (Davis and Hardcastle, 1959). Injection of 38.4 mg/fish of hexachlorocyclopentadiene into goldfish with sacrifice time of 2, 4, 6, and 8 days showed constant residue levels in the gills and spinal cord and marked increase with time in the kidney and bile attributed to conversion to more polar derivatives. Other tissues showed reduced residue levels (Podowski and Khan, 1979). All of these studies measured the ^{14}C label in hexachlorocyclopentadiene but did not not identify either the parent compound or its metabolites, thus making interpretation of the significance of the results difficult.

Studies of [^{14}C]hexachlorocyclopentadiene in rats showed that 33% of the administered dose appeared in the urine in 7 days and 10% appeared in the feces, while the tissues showed only traces, with the kidney retaining 0.5% and the liver less than 0.5% of the dose. Subcellularly, hexachlorocyclopentadiene was associated with the kidney and liver cytosol fractions (Mehendale, 1977).

In another study, mice and rats of both sexes were given [^{14}C]hexachlorocyclopentadiene orally and their urine and feces were collected for 7 days. No real differences were found between species and sexes. At a dose of 2.5 mg/kg, 83.4% was found in the feces by day 3, and at a dose of 25 mg/kg, 85.5% was found at the same time interval. At sacrifice of the animals, rats had maximum ^{14}C residues in the kidneys, while mice had their maximum in the liver. In a 30-day feeding experiment utilizing 1, 5, or 25 ppm, both species has the highest residues in kidney, liver, and adipose tissue. It was also shown that the chemical was not appreciably eliminated via the pulmonary route (Dorough, 1979).

Biotransformation   Mehendale (1977) reported that hexachlorocyclopentadiene was metabolized to four polar unidentified metabolites.

Toxicology   Treon et al. (1955) administered hexachlorocyclopentadiene to rats and rabbits and induced diarrhea, lethargy, and decreased rate of respiration. At autopsy, the rabbits showed diffuse degenerative changes in the brain, heart, liver, and adrenal glands, degeneration and necrosis of the epithelium of the renal tubules, and severe hyperemic and edematous lungs. In rats, similar changes were observed, along with liver necrosis and necrotizing gastritis of the proximal segment of the stomach. Dermal application of the chemical in rabbits produced a purplish-black local discoloration, subcutaneous edema, acanthosis, hyperkeratosis, epilation, and chronic inflammation, and, in those that died, visceral changes like those seen after oral administration. Three-day dermal application in two monkeys produced severe irritation, necrosis, dirty brown discoloration, edema, sensitivity to touch, blisters with serum oozing, and finally hard encrustations, fissuring, necrosis, and hemorrhaging. Similar results were obtained after dermal application in the guinea pig.

In another study of acute oral toxicity of hexachlorocyclopentadiene in rats, Kommineni (1978) observed brown discoloration around the nostrils and anus and brown fluid in the urinary bladder. Histopathological examination revealed atelectasis with moderate thickening of the alveolar walls of the lungs with macrophages and neutrophils; denuded epithelium of the bronchi but no edema; coagulative necrosis of the gastric squamous epithelium; neutrophilic infiltration of the submucosa of the nonglandular stomach; moderate edema of the submucosa, submuscularis, and muscularis; and in some cases ulcers of the nonglandular stomach. Skin painting in rabbits produced subcutaneous edema from the sternum to the inguinal region, and the histopathological changes in internal tissue were similar to those previously reported for rabbits.

Further dermal studies in rabbits showed weight loss, cachexia, marked dermal irritation, and hypoactivity (IRDC, 1972).

Exposure to a concentration of 13 ppm hexachlorocyclopentadiene for $1/4$ h was fatal to rats, mice, and rabbits, but guinea pigs survived (Treon et al., 1955). Symptoms included closure of the eyes, reddening of the lids, sneezing and runny nose, lacrimation, salivation, retraction of the head, and irregular breathing in all species studies. Diffuse degeneration of the brain, heart, and adrenal glands, and degeneration and necrosis of the liver and renal tubules, together with severe lung hyperemia, edema, acute bronchitis, interstitial pneumonitis, obliterative bronchitis and bronchiolitis, and necrotic bronchial epithelium infiltrated with neutrophils, erythrocytes, fibrin, and reacting inflammatory cells in the alveolar tissues were also found. Prolonged intermittent exposure of all species to 0.15 ppm hexachlorocyclopentadiene caused degenerative changes in the liver and kidneys. With exposure to 17,624 ppm of the chemical for 4 h, rats died after exhibiting the following signs: eye squint, dyspnea, cyanosis, salivation, lacrimation, nasal discharge, gray coloration of the skin, severe lung hemorrhage, and hydrothorax (IRDC, 1972).

Instillation of 09.1 ml hexachlorocyclopentadiene into rabbit eyes resulted in severe ocular irritation and death (IRDC, 1972).

A 6-month study of chronic oral administration of low doses of hexachlorocyclopentadiene to rats by Soviet investigators showed no changes in behavior, conditional reflexes, hemoglobin, erythrocytes, leukocytes, peripheral reticulocytes, ascorbic acid content, or histological structure of the organs (Naishstein and Lisovskaya, 1965).

A electromicroscopic study of the lungs of rats and monkeys exposed to concentration of 0.01–0.2 ppm hexachlorocyclopentadiene showed electron-lucent inclusion bodies in bronchiolar Clara cells of the rats but not in monkeys (Prentice et al., 1980).

Exposure of laboratory personnel to vapors of hexachlorocyclopentadiene while cleaning equipment resulted in headache (Treon et al., 1955). Exposure of humans to hexachlorocyclopentadiene-contaminated sewage sludge in a wastewater treatment plant caused the following symptoms: respiratory distress, dizziness, headache, and irritation of the eyes, throat, nose, lungs, and skin but no fatalities (Elia et al., 1980).

Vinyl Chloride

Environmental The main use of vinyl chloride is in the production of polyvinylchloride polymer, of which 2,428,000 kg were produced in the United States in 1973 (Haley, 1975b). Unreacted monomer is found in the polymer, PVC. PVC floor coverings continuously release vinyl chloride, which is hazardous to health (Dya-chuk, 1970a,b). PVC has been recommended for areas of short-time residence (bath-tubs, corridors, or railway coaches) but not for homes or offices (Stankevich et al., 1968). When PVC is used as a floor converting, the area should be well ventilated for at least 1 month after laying to reduce vinyl chloride exposure (Kalmanovich, 1968a,b). Similar precautions must be followed where PVC is used in upholstery and interior trims in automobiles (Slepak and Teplyakova, 1974). The use of PVC wallpa-per, upholstery, etc. in homes presents a toxic gas hazard of HCl and CO in case of fire (Stark, 1969).

In vinyl chloride and polyvinyl chloride plants, respiratory protection must in-clude gas masks, chemical cartridge, and powered air-purifying respirators to prevent vinyl chloride exposure (Carlson, 1974). Concentrations of vinyl chloride, 10–40 mg/l have caused toxic angioneurosis in Soviet PVC plants (Filatova et al., 1965), and it has been suggested that remote-control automated equipment and mechaniza-tion of operations in the work area will decrease environmental contamination from vinyl chloride (Filatova, 1966).

Vinyl chloride causes a problem in waste water, but pH adjustment and coagula-tion allows the solids to be incinerated (Morris, 1954). Coagulation with lime is more efficient than salt, allowing various PVC polymers to be disposed of in sewage (Ko-tulski, 1965). Soviet plants utilize waste recycling (Arkhipov et al., 1973). Vacuum rabble, atomized, and drum-type driers are recommended for PVC plants to trap gases and prevent environmental contamination (Gauruseyka and Filatova, 1959)

Migration of vinyl chloride from PVC bottles and films into food or beverages depends on its initial concentration of the product, and heat sealing and cutting of PVC food packaging films results in local environmental contamination of HCl, 0.2–2.3 mg/m^3, and particulates, 7.5–19 mg/m^3 (Van Houten et al., 1974).

The public at large is exposed to vinyl chloride from its use as a propellant for hair sprays, pesticides, and room deodorants (Kuebler, 1958; Iosaki, 1958). Newer propellant mixtures of vinyl chloride and fluorocarbons contain 22% more vinyl chloride than previously, and such blends in home products are less corrosive to container, have good flammability characteristics, have a low tendency to fractionate, and are safe for both pressure- and cold-filling (Scott and Terrill, 1962). The extent of products in aerosol containers include deodorants, hair sprays, cosmetics, cleaners, paints, laundry aids, polishes, room deodorants, coatings, finishings, insect sprays, food, and automotive and industrial products (Anonymous, 1974). With the identifi-cation of vinyl chloride as a carcinogen, its use in pesticide products was banned (Agee, 1975; Quarles, 1974; Train, 1974). The degree of exposure to vinyl chloride in the breathing zone from spraying hair spray, pesticide, deodorants, disinfectant or furniture polish inside a room varies from 35 to 245 ppm/h·week (B. W. Gay, W. A. Lonneman, K. Bribord, and J. Moran, unpublished data, April 1974). The extent of effect from such vinyl chloride exposures is unknown, but other ingredients have been shown to cause thesaurosis, sudden death from cardiac failure, allergies, asth-matic attacks, oropharyngeal irritation, dermatitis, bronchioconstriction, hypersensi-tivity reactions, and granulomatous lung disease. This latter condition has been asso-ciated with aerosol deodorants containing zirconium salts (Bernstein, 1972).

Tissue Distribution Vinyl chloride has a local irritating effect on skin and mucous membranes. It readily distributes in blood and is 82% eliminated in 10 min. Low concentrations have no effect on heart rate or blood pressure, but high concentrations cause hypertension. At a concentration of 20 vol%, respiratory paralysis, salivation, and emesis occur in dogs but there is no liver or kidney pathological changes. These effects also occur in mice, rats, guinea pigs, and rabbits (Lehmann and Flury, 1938). Vinyl chloride anesthesia in the dog causes muscle incoordination and serious cardiac arrhythmias (Carr et al., 1947). Death by respiratory paralysis was produced in guinea pigs inhaling 2.5–40% vinyl chloride. The chemical caused unsteadiness and ataxia, rapid jerky respiration followed by shallow respiration, and surgical anesthesia. Gross pathological findings included congestion and edema of the lungs and hyperemia of the liver and kidneys (Patty et al., 1930). At 10 vol%, dogs showed cardiac irregularities, including tachycardia, bradycardia, inversion of the R wave, abnormalities in the QRS interval, sinus arrhythmia, transitory left-axis deviation, AV block, ventricular tachycardia, ventricular multiform extrasystoles, and inversion of the T wave with an elevated ST segment (von Oettingen, 1955). Repeated exposures to 200–500 ppm vinyl chloride for 7 h daily for 4.5 months had no effect in guinea pigs and dogs but cause histological changes in the liver and kidneys of rats and rabbits (Torkelson et al., 1961). When rats were exposed to 2% vinyl chloride for 8 h/day for 3 months, there were changes in liver and spleen weights and a decrease in leukocytes, an increase in erythrocytes, but no effect on growth rate, hemoglobin, hematocrit, or prothrombin time (Lester et al., 1963). Liver and kidney changes caused by vinyl chloride have been reported from Germany (Schotter, 1969), and Soviet investigators observed cardiac arrhythmias, bradycardia, and changes in the phonocardiogram in rats exposed to 0.03–0.05 mg/l of vinyl chloride for 5 months (Vazin and Plokhova, 1969b). Such exposures increased secretion of catecholamines and changes in the biopotential in the posterior hypothalamus in rabbits (Vazin and Plokhova, 1969a). No compound-related symptoms or pathology were observed in rats, rabbits, or monkeys exposed to 250–500 ppm vinyl bromide for 6 months, but at levels of 10,000 ppm there was a decrease in body weight and activity in male rats (Leong and Torkelson, 1970). Central nervous system and cardiac dysfunction, bone resorption, and osteoporosis were found in rats and rabbits exposed to 0.03–0.04 mg/l vinyl chloride for 6 months (Basalaev et al., 1972). Vinyl chloride changes the bioelectrical activity in cortex and the anterior and posterior hypothalamic nuclei of rabbits (Vazin and Polkhova, 1968). Exposure of rats to vinyl chloride at 30,000 ppm for 4 h/day for 1 year produced degeneration of the brain, liver, and kidneys and the development of a histopathological condition in the skeleton and connective tissue similar to human acroosteolysis. Bones undergo processes of intense periosteal growth and diffuse, chondrial metaplasia. Connective tissue dissociates into collagen bundles with reduced numbers of cells, the elastic reticulum is markedly reduced and fragmentary, and lumen of the dermal vessels is hypertrophied. Fibrous tissue even surrounds and infiltrates the nerve endings (Viola, 1970).

Biotransformation It has been postulated that vinyl chloride is converted into ethylene monochlorohydrin by the hepatocyte enzymes, with further conversion to chloral and chloroacetic acid. The latter has been found in workers exposed to vinyl chloride (Gregorescu and Tiba, 1966). Exposure of cell-free liver microsomal preparation to vinyl chloride produces chloroethylene oxide and chloroacetylaldehyde, which has been trapped with 3,4-dichlorobenzenethiol with the metabolites identified by gas chromatography–mass spectrometry (Gothe et al., 1974). In vivo, the reactions may involve the glutathione S-transferases, which catalyze the reaction of glutathione with β-unsaturated compounds (Clapp et al., 1969).

Toxicology Vinyl chloride has anesthetic properties but causes respiratory irritation with dryness and mucous-membrane atrophy, followed by chronic bronchitis. It also causes hepatitis (Tribukh et al., 1949). Toxicity symptoms from exposure to vinyl chloride include euphoria, intoxication, skin sensations of formication, heat, dyspeptic disturbances, epigastric pain with swelling of the hypochrondrium, anorexia, hepatomegaly, splenomegaly, hepatitis without jaundice, ulcers, Raynaud's syndrome, allergic dermatitis, and scleroderma. Hypersomnia persists even after leaving the contaminated environment, and repeated exposures leads to neurological asthenia (Suciu et al., 1963). Vinyl chloride poisoning is progressive even in the absence of further exposure (Antonyuzhenko, 1968). Long-term adverse reactions include functional disturbances of the CNS with adrenergic sensory polyneuritis (Smirnova and Granik, 1970). ECG recordings showed changes in rhythm, conductance, and repolarization processes and an increased systolic index (Kudryavtseva, 1970). German investigations reported Raynaud's syndrome, skin disease, osteolytic syndrome, and thrombocytopenia (Juhe et al., 1973).

Thermoregulation is disturbed in chronic vinyl chloride poisoning, with body temperature increasing $1-2\,°C$ as a result of peripheral changes in the visual, auditory, taste, and olfactory analyzers referable to effects of vinyl chloride on the brainstem reticular formation (Antonyuzhenko et al., 1972a,b). Chronic vinyl chloride exposure, 1.75–18 years, caused scleroderma with thickening and homogenization of collagen bundles and fragmentation and rarefaction of elastic fibers. Finger clubbing, osteolysis of the distal phalanges, and Raynaud's syndrome were also observed. Thrombocytopenia, splenomegaly, and liver dysfunction with marked fibrosis in the portal areas, and pulmonary insufficiency with restrictive changes in the lungs were also reported (Lange et al., 1974). Similar changes in workers' health have been reported from the U.S.S.R. (Filatova et al., 1965). Visual and vestibular malfunction has been found in chronic vinyl chloride poisoning (Antonyuzhenko et al., 1972a,b). Correlations of clinical and environmental measurements for workers exposed to vinyl chloride have been made, including blood pressure, bromsulfalein retention, icterus index, hemoglobin, and beta-protein, along with ambient air samples of vinyl chloride (Kramer and Mutchler, 1972). Two accidental deaths from acute vinyl chloride intoxication showed the following: cyanosis, local burns of the conjuctiva and cornea, congestion of the lungs and kidney, and failure of the blood to clot. Blood levels of vinyl chloride were not obtained (Danziger, 1960).

Clinical symptoms of chronically poisoned vinyl chloride workers include headache, dizziness, heightened fatigue, sleep disorders, decreased memory capacity, diaphoresis, paresthesia, pain in the extremities, paling of fingers and toes, edema of these extremities, and pain and unfavorable sensation in the region of the heart. An adrenacorticotropin (ACTH) test correlated these changes with modification in adrenal–cortical function (Rumyantseva and Goryacheva, 1968). Increased urinary excretion of monochloracetic acid has been correlated with ambient vinyl chloride and the duration of exposure (Gregorescu and Tiba, 1966). There is a decrease in blood catalase activity and an increase in peroxidase, indophenoploxidase, and glutathione content after 1 year of vinyl chloride exposure (Gabor et al., 1962). Romanian investigators found no change in blood catalase or serum and pyruvic acid activity in vinyl chloride workers. However, serum albumin, serum cholinesterase, and pseudoesterase decreased. The beta- and gamma-globulins increased, but the beta-to-alpha lipoprotein ratio decreased (Gabor et al., 1964). Thyroid impairment and skin and muscle collagenosis has been reported (Suciu et al., 1967).

Vinyl chloride and its polymers cause many allergic manifestations. Vinyl chloride, PVC, and vinyl acetate produce a sensitization dermatitis in workers (Morris, 1953). This effect has been attributed to the plasticizers used (Key, 1968). The use of epoxy resins used as plasticizers–stabilizers in PVC products has caused hypersensitivity in consumers (Fregert and Rorsman, 1963). Contact dermatitis has been reported from the use of tricresylphosphate as a plasticizer–stabilizer for PVC plastics (Pegum, 1966). Vinyl chloride and dibutylphthalate released from floor coverings have produced eczematous dermatitis in children (Kalmanovich, 1968a,b). Liberation of volatile materials from PVC flood tile has caused mucosal irritation of the eyes and respiratory tract of infants and adults (Dyachuk, 1970a,b). It has been shown that the plasticizer di-2-ethylhexylphthalate migrates from PVC blood bags into stored blood, and then into body tissue. The toxicological implications of this migration are unknown, but the plasticizer is lethal to the embryonic chick heart in culture. It has been suggested that other plastics should be used for storing blood (Jaeger and Rubin, 1972). In contrast to vinyl chloride, vinyl acetate does not appear to cause contact dermatitis (Deese and Joyner, 1969).

One of the worst toxicological manifestations of vinyl chloride is the development of acroosteolysis with dissolution of the bones of the terminal phalanges of the fingers and sacroiliac joints. The patella and the phalanges of the feet may also be involved. This condition is accompanied by Raynaud's phenomena and skin lesions (Harris and Adams, 1967). Thirty-one cases of the disease were reported from one American company. The disorder could have been related to physical or chemical injury or a personal idiosyncrasy, because there is no known specific cause (Wilson et al., 1967). French PVC workers also had the disease (Chatelain and Motillon, 1967). Progression of the bone lesion can lead to fragmentation of the distal phalange (Anghelescu et al., 1969). After examination of 20 PVC workers, Italian investigators attributed this lesion to sympathetic neurocirculatory dystonia connected with an identified pathogenic cofactor (Nitti et al., 1970). A Soviet scientist suggested the involvement of higher centers in the hypothalamus in acroosteolysis (Basalaev, 1970). The latent period for the development of acroosteolysis can be 5 days or 30 days. Furthermore, it is not known if the portal of entry is the skin or lungs (McCord, 1970). An epidemiological survey of 5011 workers in 32 vinyl chloride and PVC plants in the United States and Canada discovered 25 cases of acroosteolysis. The condition was associated with hand cleaning of polymerizers and appeared to be a systemic rather than a local disease (Dinman et al., 1971). There was a strong association between development of the condition and manual cleaning of reactors (Cook et al., 1971). Clinical study of four cases of the disease showed that Raynaud's phenomena preceded the osteolytic lesions. Negative Ca and PO$_4$ balance could be present, and ^{18}F scintiscans revealed variable fluoride uptakes correlated with the radiographic lesions. A wide variety of clinical parameters were normal (Dodson et al., 1971). Industrial hygiene precautions to reduce exposure and prevent the disease include water wash and reduction of ambient vinyl chloride to 50 ppm, gloves, a yearly physical examination, and X-ray examination of the hands (Gitsios, 1971). German experience with long-term vinyl chloride exposure, 1–3.5 years, not only showed circulatory, skin, and bone disorders but also deafness, vision failure, giddiness, and liver dysfunction (Juhe and Lange, 1972). It has been suggested that 3% or less of the workers engaged in PVC production are affected by the disease (Markowitz et al., 1972). The occurrence of idiopathic acroosteolysis with papular skin lesions makes it essential that vinyl chloride and PVC exposure be determined in all cases diagnosed as acroosteolysis (Meyerson and Meier, 1972). It must be remembered that the bone lesions can progress even after vinyl chloride exposure has been terminated, then recovery can occur (Misgeld et al., 1973). Rapid diagnosis to prevent progression of vinyl chloride produced scleroderma, Raynaud's syndrome, and acroosteolysis is necessary if mortality, now at least 10%, is to be reduced. Periodic thrombocyte counts have been suggested as the diagnostic tool, because thrombocytopenia occurs much earlier than other signs of vinyl chloride poisoning (Juhe et al., 1973).

The most disastrous effect of chronic vinyl chloride exposure is the development of hepatic angiosarcoma. A Soviet survey of 350 workers covering the years 1957–1960 discovered epithelial hepatitis in 15% of PVC workers but no cancer (Pushkin, 1965). A German survey of 120 PVC workers in 1973 found hepatic dysfunction but no cancer (Marsteller et al., 1973). The first hepatic angiosarcoma cases in PVC workers were reported in the United States in 1974, but retrospective studies showed one case in 1968, one in 1971, and one in 1973. Death occurred within 14 months of diagnosis, regardless of the treatment instituted (Creech and Johnson, 1974). Clinical and pathological studies should be instituted among vinyl chloride and PVC workers to develop better diagnostic methods for liver cirrhosis and angiosarcoma because the usual battery of liver function tests does not detect the periportal fibrosis that precedes sarcoma development (Manucuso, 1974). Diagnostic difficulties in vinyl chloride-induced angiosarcoma are illustrated by three cases in which the primary diagnosis was gastric ulcers. A more precise diagnosis recommends the use of serum alkaline phosphatase and serum glutamic–oxaloacetic transaminase (SGOT) determinations coupled with hepatic photoscans using ^{131}I, rose bengal, and ^{198}Au. Needle biopsy, while useful, can result in an exsanguinating hemorrhage because of the vascular nature of the tumor (Block, 1974). A recent epidemiological survey showed that vinyl chloride and PVC workers may develop cancers at multiple sites, further complicating the problem (Tabershaw and Gaffey, 1974). A systemic detection program for surveillance of PVC workers suggests the use of laboratory tests, roentgenographic examinations, and clinical evaluations to detect hepatic damage in an early and possible reversible or curable state. The α-glutamic transpeptidase test was the most useful for detecting abnormalities and reflecting the extent of liver damage (Makk et al., 1974). A survey of workers in a PVC plant revealed 11 cases of hepatic disease, including 7 cases of angiosarcoma. Ages at diagnosis ranged from 28 to 56 years in hepatic disease cases and 36 to 58 years in those with angiosarcoma. The range of exposure periods was 5–29 years. Portal fibrosis and portal hypertension characterized nonmalignant liver disease (Falk et al., 1974). Liver angiosarcoma has been found in one British PVC worker (Lee and Harry, 1974).

Vinylidene Chloride

Environmental Vinylidene chloride, either liquid or vapor, is highly irritating to the eyes and skin but is most dangerous by the inhalation route. To prevent exposure, the chemical should be handled in a closed system with adequate ventilation being provided in the working area (Anonymous, 1966). The TLV for vinylidene chloride is 5 mg/m^3 (MCA, 1972). Exposures of 2 ppm vinylidene chloride have occurred in spacecraft and nuclear submarines (Altman and Dittmer, 1966). Employee health may be affected by the widespread use of vinylidene chloride polymers in food wrappings, which could release unreacted monomer into the food chain (Lehman, 1951). Vinylidene chloride copolymers containing a minimum of 85% vinylidene chloride have been approved for use with irradiate foods, and such uses could result in migration of free radicals as well as unreacted monomer (Anonymous, 1968). Vinylidene chloride has not been found in U.S. drinking water (Environmental Protection Agency, 1976) or in industrial effluent discharges (Environmental Protection Agency, 1979).

Tissue Distribution Vinylidene chloride is widely distributed to body tissues, causing hepatic midzonal necrosis. damaged parenchyma, and thrombosis, but no fatty infiltration. Electron-microscopic changes include cytoplasmic changes in the parenchymal cells with loss of their microvilli and fibrin deposits on the plasma membrane, delamination and vacuolation of the Golgi cisternae, and an increase in the electron lucency of the mitochondria, but no degranulation of the cisternae of the rough endoplasmic reticulum (Jaeger et al., 1976). The chemical causes eye and skin irritation in rabbits (Rylova, 1953). Inhalation exposure to 61–189 mg/m^3 for 90 days caused mortality and hepatic damage but had no effect on hematological parameters in rats, guinea pigs, dogs, rabbits, and monkeys (Pendergast et al., 1967). Inhalation of vinylidene chloride for 20 6-h exposures at 500 ppm caused nose irritation, weight loss, and liver damage (Gage, 1970). Aqueous extracts of vinylidene chloride polymer caused no changes in adrenal ascorbic acid or the hemogram (Sporn et al., 1970). Similar Soviet studies based on 10-month feeding to mice and rats showed decreased weight gain, increased mortality, and cardiac, liver, and kidney lesions (Kovalev et al., 1970).

Biotransformation   Oral administration of 2 mg/kg of vinylidene chloride to rats decreased liver glucose 6-phosphatase (G-6-Pase) and increased alkaline phosphatase (AP), tyrosine transaminase (TT), plasma alkaline phosphatase, and alanine transaminase. Females were more susceptible than males. Phenobarbital enzyme induction reduced hepatic G-6-Pase, AP, and TT, as well as plasma alanine transaminase (Jenkins et al., 1972). Inhalation studies showed no change in hepatotoxicity as measured in terms of serum serum glutamic–pyruvic transaminase (SGPT) or SGOT of liver G-6-Pase. The microsomal enzyme inducers phenobarbital and 3-methylcholanthrene and the inhibitors 2-diethylaminoethyl-2,2-diphenyl valerate and 2,4-dichloro-6-phenyl-phenoxyethyldiethylamine all increased lethality (Carlson and Fuller, 1972). Both in vivo and in vitro, vinylidene chloride did not increase either lipoperoxidation or conjugated dienes in the liver (Jaeger et al., 1973b), nor did it decrease hepatic glutathione or increase lethality and hepatotoxicity (Jaeger et al., 1973a). Administration of vinylidene chloride to fasted rats increased lethality and SAKT, and diethylmaleate-induced reduction in liver glutathione potentiated hepatotoxicity (Jaeger et al., 1974).

The biotransformation pathway of vinylidene chloride, including serum and urinary metabolites, is unavailable, but the presence of the double bond in this chemical could lead to free-radical formation with the resultant product acting as an alkylating agent (Van Each and Van Logten, 1975). It has been suggested that hepatotoxicity from unsaturated compounds is related to conversion to epoxides, which are more toxic and act as alkylating agents. Their interaction with glutathione depletes this vital material in the liver (Brodie et al., 1971). If vinylidene chloride follows a biotransformation pathway similar to vinyl chloride (Gothe et al., 1974), then the chemical is converted to dichloroethylene oxide and then to dichloroacetylaldehyde, which under the influence of glutathione epoxytransferase combines with glutathione and is finally converted to a mercapturic acid derivative and dichloroacetic acid (Haley, 1975a). Covalent binding probably plays a prominent role in the development of the necrosis of the centroblobular hepatocytes (Reid and Kirshna, 1973).

Toxicology   It has been suggested that human exposure to vinylidene chloride results, within 8–30 h, in irreversible damage to the trigeminal nerve. In the beginning, sensory disturbances involve the face, mouth, and tongue, then spread to the second and third cervical segments. One subject showed motor weakness of the jaw muscles, the lateral recti of the eyes, and the tongue muscles. Electromyographic examination of the trigemino–facial reflexes revealed a functional disturbance of the interneuronal system (Brosner et al., 1970). Further studies of these patients suggested that the toxic agent was either mono-ordi-chloroacetylene, which appeared during production or storage of the vinylidene chloride copolymer (Henschler et al., 1970). By environmental surveillance, the Dow Chemical Co. polymerization processes showed vinylidene chloride concentrations of 5 ppm or less. Worker clinical parameters studies were systolic and diastolic blood pressure, timed vital capacity, bromsulfalein retention, icterus index, alkaline phosphatase, SGOT, thymol turbidity, serum protein, AG ratio, hemoglobin, hematocrit, erythrocytes, leukocytes, prothrombin time, and urine specific gravity. All data were examined by a statistical matrix, and only the liver-function tests gave any evidence of impairment. However, these data are difficult to evaluate because the environment also contained vinyl chloride, a known hepatic toxicant (Kramer and Mutchler, 1972). By using a gas-chromatographic or infrared analysis, a more definite diagnosis of the degree of environmental exposure to vinylidene chloride can be made (Stewart et al., 1965). Exposure to a multiplicity of chemicals at levels far below their TLVs (e.g., on spacecraft or nuclear submarines) presents a toxicologic problem complicated by potentiation and antagonism of noxious effects. Moreover, the time-concentration coupled with long latency may make diagnosis of acute effects impossible (Anderson and Saunders, 1963). Inhalation of vinylidene chloride produces varying degrees of narcosis, depending on the amount inhaled. Chronic inhalation of small quantities causes chronic hepatic and renal dysfunction. Ocular contact produces pain, conjunctivitis, transient corneal injury, and iritis, but usually no permanent injury. Dermal contact causes irritation. Removal from the area and washing with water usually counteracts the injurious effect of vinylidene chloride (Wessling and Edwards, 1970).

Dermal contact with inhibited vinylidene chloride causes irritation that is partially related to the inhibitor, monomethyl ether of hydroquinone. This chemical has also produced occupational leucoderma and skin depigmentation of the forearms and head from local contact. The occupational aspects must always be considered, otherwise and erroneous diagnosis of vitiligo will be made (Chivers, 1972).

REFERENCES

ACGIH. 1971. 1976a, 1977. *Threshold Limit Values of Airborne Contaminants.* Cincinnati, Ohio.

ACGIH. 1976b. *Carbon Tetrachloride. Documentation of the TLV's for Substances in Workroom Air,* ed ed., pp. 43–44. Cincinnati, Ohio: ACGIH.

Agee, J.L. 1975. Vinyl chloride. Pesticide products containing vinyl chloride. *Fed. Reg.* 40:3494.

Aksoy, M., Dincol, K., Akgun, T., Erdem, S., and Dincol, G. 1971. Haematological effects of chronic benzene poisoning in 217 workers. *Br. J. Ind. Med.* 28:296–302.

Aksoy, M., Dincol, D., Erdem, S., Akgun, T., and Dincol, G. 1972a. Details of blood changes in 32 patients with pancytopenia associated with long-term exposure to benzene. *Br. J. Ind. Med.* 29:54–56.

Aksoy, M., Dincol, K., Erdem, S., Akgun, T., and Dincol, G. 1972b. Details of blood changes in 32 patients with pancytopenia associated with long-term exposure to benzene. *Br. J. Ind. Med.* 29:56–64.

Aksoy, M., Erdem, S., and Dincol, G. 1974a. Leukemia in shoe-workers exposed chronically to benzene. *Blood* 44:837–841.

Aksoy, M., Erdem, S., Erdogan, G., and Dincol, G. 1974b. Acute leukemia in two generations following chronic exposure to benzene. *Hum. Hered.* 24:70–74.

Aksoy, M., Dincol, K., Erdems, J., and Dincol, G. 1972c. Acute leukemia due to chronic exposure to benzene. *Am. J. Med.* 52:160–166.

Aksoy, M., Erdem, S., Dincol, K., Hepyuksel, T., and Dincol, G. 1974c. Chronic exposure to benzene as a possible contributory etiologic factor in Hodgkin's disease. *Blut* 28:293–298.

Aksoy, M., Erdem, S., and Dincol, G. 1975. Two rare complications of chronic benzene poisoning—Myeloid metaplasia and paroxymal nocturnal hemoglobinuria. *Blut* 30:255–260.

Altman, P. L., and Dittmer, D. S. 1966. *Environmental Biology*, pp. 326, 328. Bethesda, Md.: Federation of the American Society for Experimental Biology.

Alvares, A. P., Leigh, S., Kappas, A., Levin, W., and Conney, A. H. 1973. Induction of aryl hydrocarbon hydroxylase in human skin. *Drug Metab. Dispos.* 1:386–390.

American Petroleum Institute. 1974. A mortality study of petroleum refinery workers, p. 41. Medical research report EA 7402. American Petroleum Institute, Washington, D.C.

Anderson, W. L., and Saunders, R. A. 1963. Evolution of materials in the closed system. In *Symposium on Toxicity in the Closed Ecological System*, eds., M. Honma and H. J. Crosby, pp. 9–18. Palo Alto, Calif.: Lockheed Missiles and Space Co.

Andjeikovic, D., Taulbee, J., and Symons, M. 1976. Mortality experience of a cohort of rubber workers, 1964–1973. *J. Occup. Med.* 18:387–394.

Anghelescu, M. O., Dobrinescu, E., Hagi-Paraschiv-Dossios, L., Dobrinescu, G., and Ganea, V. 1969. Clinico-pathogenic considerations of Raynaud's phenomenon in the employees of the vinyl polychloride industry. *Med. Int.* 21:473.

Anonymous. 1966. Vinylidene chloride monomer. Plastics Dept., The Dow Chemical Co., Midland, Mich.

Anonymous. 1968. Food additives. Packaging materials for use during irradiation of prepackaged foods. *Fed. Reg.* 33:4659.

Anonymous. 1974. Aerosol products growth rate slumps. *C & E News*, May 20.

Anonymous. 1976. Chloroform banned from drugs, other uses. *C & E News*, April 12.

Anonymous. 1977. Carbon tetrachloride spill causes stir along the Ohio River. *C & E News* 55:7.

Antonyuzhenko, V. A. 1968. Occupational poisoning by vinyl chloride. *Gig. Tr. Prof. Zabol.* 12:50.

Antonyuzhenko, V. A., Golva, I. A., and Aliyeva, N. K., 1972a. The state of the analyzer functions during chronic occupational intoxication with certain substances having a narcotic effect. *Gig. Truda* 9:19.

Antonyuzhenko, V. A., Golva, I. A., and Aliyera, N. K. 1972b. The state of analyzer functions in chronic occupational poisoning with some narcotic substances. *Gig. Truda* 16:19.

Applegate, V. C., Howell, J. H., and Hall, A. E., Jr. 1957. Toxicity of 4326 chemicals to larval lampreys and fishes. *U.S. Fish. Wild. Serv. Spec. Sci. Rep. Fish.* 207. U.S. Department of the Interior, Washington, D.C.

Arkhipov, A. S., Marchenko, E. N., Filatova, V. S., Egorov, Y. L., Novoselova, T. I., and Martynova, A. P. 1973. Technical progress in the chemical industry and industrial hygiene. *Gig. Tr. Prof. Zabol.* 8:1.

Ashworth, C. T., Luibel, F. J., Sanders, E., and Arnold, N. 1963. Hepatic cell degeneration. Correlation of fine structure with chemicals and histochemical changes in hepatic cell injury produced by carbon tetrachloride in rats. *Arch. Pathol.* 75:212–225.

Averill, C. 1899. Benzole poisoning. *Br. Med. J.* 1:709.

Baader, E. W. 1927. Tatigkeitsbericht der abteilung fur gewerbekrankheiten des kaiserin Auguste-Victoria-Krankenhaus in Berlin-Lichtenberg. *Zentralbl. Gew. Hyg.* 14:385.

Bachmann, E., and Golberg, L. 1971. Reappraisal of the toxicity of ethylene glycol. 3. Mitochondrial effects. *Food Cosmet. Toxicol.* 9:39–55.

Bardodev, A., and Bardojeva, E. 1970. Biotransformation of ethylbenzene, styrene and alpha-methylstyrene in man. *Am. Ind. Hyg. Assoc.* 31:206.

Barnham, A. K., Caldy, G. V., Fritzx, V. S., Junk, G. A., Suec, H. J., and Willis, R. 1972.

Identification and estimation of neutral organic contaminants in potable water. *Anal. Chem.* 44:139.

Bartlett, G. R. 1950. Combustion of C^{14} labeled methanol in intact rat and its isolated tissues. *Am. J. Physiol.* 163:614–618.

Baselaev, A. V. 1970. Experience with the use of large-frame photo-fluorography in examining skeletal bone of persons occupationally dealing with unsaturated hydrocarbons of the ethylene series (olefins) and their chlorine derivatives (vinyl chloride, trichlorethylene). *Gig. Tr. Prof. Zabol.* 14:34.

Basalaev, A. V., Vazin, A. N., and Kochetkov, A. G. 1972. On the pathogenesis of changes developing due to long-term exposure to the effect of vinyl chloride. *Gig. Truda* 16:24.

Bassi, M. 1960. Electron microscopy of rat liver after carbon tetrachloride poisoning. *Exp. Cell Res* 20:313–323.

Bastrup, J. T. 1947. On the excretion of formic acid in experimental poisoning with methylalcohol. *Acta Pharmacol. Toxicol.* 3:312–322.

Benzene in the work environment. 1974. Considerations bearing on the question of safe concentrations of benzene in the work environment (MAK-Wert). Communication of the working group "Establishment of Mak-Wert" of the Senate Commission for the Examination of Hazardous Industrial Materials, prepared in cooperation with Dr. Gerund Buttner, Harold Boldt Verlag, Boppard, Germany.

Berlin, M., Gage, J., and Johnson, E. 1974. Increased aromatics in motor fuels: A review of the environmental and health effects. *Work Environ. Health* 11:1.

Bernstein, I. L. 1972. Medical hazards of aerosols. *Postgrad. Med.* 25:62.

Block, J. B. 1974. Angiosarcoma of the liver following vinyl chloride exposure. *JAMA* 229:53.

Block, W. A., and Cornish, H. H. 1958. Effects of carbon tetrachloride inhalation on rat serum enzymes. *Proc. Soc. Exp. Biol. Med.* 97:178–180.

Blumer, M., Sanders, H. L., Grassle, J. F., and Hampson, G. R. 1971. A small oil spill. *Environment* 13:2.

Bove, K. E. 1966. Ethyleneglycol toxicity. *Am. J. Clin. Pathol.* 45:46–50.

Brodie, B. B., Reid, W. D., Cho, A. K., Sipes, G., Kirshna, G., and Gillette, J. R. 1971. Possible mechanism of liver necrosis caused by aromatic organic compounds. *Proc. Natl. Acad. Sci. USA* 68:160.

Brosner, F., Henschler, D., and Hopf, H. C. 1970. Chlorierte acetylene als ursache einer irreparablen trigeminusstorung bei zwei patienten. *Dtsch. Z. Nervenheilk.* 197:163.

Browning, E. 1953. *Toxicity of Industrial Organic Solvents,* p. 411. New York: Chemical Publishing.

Browning, E. 1965. *Toxicity and Metabolism of Industrial Solvents,* pp. 3–65. New York: Elsevier.

Butareqiez, L., Gosk, S., and Gluszczowa, M. 1969. Examination of the state of health of women workers in the leather industry especially form the gynecological point of view. *Med. Przemysolwa* 20:67.

Butler, T. C. 1949. Metabolic transformation of trichloroethylene. *J. Pharmacol. Exp. Ther.* 97:84–92.

Butler, T. C. 1961. Reduction of carbon tetrachloride in vivo and reduction of carbon tetrachloride and chloroform in vitro by tissues and tissue constituents. *J. Pharmacol. Exp. Ther.* 134:311–319.

Butsch, W. L. 1932. Cirrhosis of the liver caused by carbon tetrachloride. *JAMA* 99:728–729.

Buttner, H. 1965. Aldehyde und alkolhydrogenase-aktivitat in leber und niere der rata. *Biochem. Z.* 341:300–314.

Carlson, G. P., and Fuller, G. C. 1972. Interaction of modifiers of hepatic microsomal drug metabolism and the inhalation toxicity of 1,1-dichloroethylene. *Res. Commun. Chem. Pathol. Pharmacol.* 4:553.

Carlson, J. W. 1974. Respiratory protection against exposure to vinyl chloride. *Fed. Reg.* 39:45012.

Carpenter, C. P., Pozzani, V. C., Weil, C. S., Nair, J. H., Keck, C. A., and Smyth, H. F. 1956. The toxicity of butyl cellosolve solvent. *Arch. Ind. Health* 14:114-131.

Carr, C. J., Krantz, J. C., Jr., and Sauerwald, M. D. 1947. Anesthesia 27. Narcosis with vinyl chloride. *Anesthesia* 8:359.

Carr, C. J., Burgison, R. M., Vitch, J. R., and Krantz, J. C., Jr., 1949. Anesthesia 34. Chemical constitution of hydro-carbons and cardiac automaticity. *J. Pharmacol. Exp. Ther.* 97:1.

Cassan, G., and Baron, J. 1956. Usefulness of blood tests in workers exposed to benzene. *Arch. Mal. Prof. Med. Trav. Secur. Soc.* 17:602.

Chatelain, A., and Motillon, P. 1967. An acroosteolysis syndrome of occupational origin and of recent verification in France. *J. Radiol. Electrol.* 48:277.

Chivers, C. P. 1972. Two cases of occupational leucoderma following contact with hydroquinone monomethyl ether. *Br. J. Ind. Med.* 29:105.

Clapp, J. J., Kay, C. M., and young, L. 1969. Observations on the metabolism of allyl compounds in the rat. *Biochem. J.* 114:6P.

Clark, C. S., Meyer, C. R., Gartside, P. A., Majeti, V. A., Specker, B., Balistreri, W. F., and Elia, V. J. 1982. An environmental health survey of drinking water contamination by leechate from a pesticide waste dump in Hardeman County, TN. *Arch. Environ. Hlth.* 37:9-18.

Clay, K. L., and Murphy, R. C. 1977. On the metabolic acidosis of ethylene glycol intoxication. *Toxicol. Appl. Pharmacol.* 39:39-49.

Conkle, J. P., Camp, B. J., and Welch, B. E. 1975. Trace composition of human respiratory gas. *Arch. Environ. Health* 30:290.

Cook, W. A., Giever, P. M., Dinman, B. D., and Magnuson, H. J. 1971. Occupational acroosteolysis. 2. An industrial hygiene study. *Arch. Environ. Health* 22:74.

Cooper, J. R., and Kini, M. M. 1962. Biochemical aspects of nethanol poisoning. *Biochem. Pharmacol.* 11:405-416.

Cornish, H. H., and Block, W. D. 1960. A study of carbon tetrachloride. II. The effect of carbon tetrachloride inhalation on serum and tissue enzymes. *Arch. Environ. Health* 1:18-22.

Council on Environmental Quality. 1973. Fourth Annual Report of the Council on Environmental Quality, p. 266. Government Printing Office, Washington, D.C.

Creech, J. L., Jr., and Johnson, M. N. 1974. Angiosarcoma of the liver in the manufacture of polyvinyl chloride. *J. Occup. Med.* 16:150.

Danziger, H. 1960. Accidental poisoning by vinyl chloride. *Can. Med. Assoc.* 82:828.

David, D. C., Schoreder, D. H., Gram, T. E., Regan, R. L., and Gillette, J.R. 1971. A comparison of the effects of halothane and carbon tetrachloride on the hepatic drug metabolizing system. *J. Pharmacol. Exp. Ther.* 177:556-566.

Davis, J. T., and Hardcastle, W. S. 1959. Biological asay of herbicides for fish toxicity. *Weeds* 7:397-404.

Davis, N. C., and Whipple, g. H. 1919. The influence of fasting and various diets on the liver injury effect by chloroform anesthesia. *Arch. Ind. Med.* 23:612-635.

Dawborn, J.K., Ralston, M., and Weiden, S. 1961. Acute carbon tetrachloride poisoning. Transaminase and biopsy studies. *Br. Med. J.* 1:493-494.

Dean, M. E., and Stock, B. H. 1974. Propylene glycol as a drug solvent in the study of hepatic microsomal metabolism in the rat. *Toxicol. Appl. Pharmacol.* 28:44–52.

Deese, D. E., and Joyner, R. E. 1969. Vinyl acetate. A study of chronic human exposure. *Am. Ind. Hyg. Ass. J.* 30:449.

DeGowin, R. L. 1963. Benzene exposure and aplastic anemia followed by leukemia 15 years later. *JAMA* 185:748–751.

Delore, P., and Borgomaho, C. 1928. Leucemia aigue au cours de l'intoxication benzenique. Sur l'origine toxique de certaines leucemies aigues et leur relations avec les anemies graves. *J. Med. Lyon* 9:227–233.

Diaz Gomez, M. I., DeCastro, C. R., D'Acosta, N., DeFenos, O. M., DeFerreya, E. C., and Castro, A. J. 1975. Species differences in carbon tetrachloride-induced hepatotoxicity: The role of CCl₄ activation and of lipid peroxidation. *Toxicol. Appl. Pharmacol.* 34:102–114.

Dingell, J. V., and Heimberg, M. 1968. The effects of aliphatic halogenated hydrocarbons on hepatic drug metabolism. *Biochem. Pharmacol.* 17:1269–1278.

Dinman, B. D., Cook, W. A., Whitehouse, W. M., Magnuson, H. J., and Ditcheck, T. 1971. Occupational acroosteolysis. 1. An epidemiological study. *Arch. Environ. Health* 22:61.

Docherty, J. R., and Burgess, E. 1922. The action of carbon tetrachloride on the liver. *Br. Med. J.* ii:907–908.

Docherty, J. F., and Nicholls, L. 1923. Report of three autopsies following carbon tetrachloride treatment. *Br. Med. J.* ii:753.

Docks, E. L., and Kirshna, G. 1976. The role of glutathione in chloroform-induced hepatotoxicity. *Exp. Mol. Pathol.* 24:13.

Dodson, V. N., Dinmanm, B. D., Whitehouse, W. M., Nasar, A. N. M., and Magnuson, H. J. 1971. Occupational acroosteolysis. 3. A clinical study. *Arch. Environ. Health* 22:83.

Dorough, H. W. 1979. The accumulation, distribution and dissipation of hexachlorocyclopentadiene (C56) in tissues of rats and mice. Unpublished report to the Velsicol Chemical Corp.

Dowty, B. J., Laseter, J. L., and Storer, J. 1976. The transplacental migration and accumulation in blood of volatile organic constituents. *Pediatr. Res.* 10:696.

Drew, R. T., and Fouts, J. R. 1974. The lack of effects of pretreatment with phenobarbital and chlorpromazine on the acute toxicity of benzene in rats. *Toxicol. Appl. Pharmacol.* 27:183–193.

Drill, V. A., and Ivy, A. c. 1944. Comparative value of Bromsulphalein, serum phosphatase, prothrombin time and intravenous galactose tolerance tests in detecting hepatic damage produced by carbon tetrachloride. *J. Clin. Invest.* 23:209–216.

Drinker, P., Yaglou, C. P., and Warren, M. R. 1943. The threshold toxicity of gasoline. *J. Ind. Hyg.* 15:225.

Durior, M. R., Fabre, A., and Derobert, L. 1946. The significance of benzene in the bone marrow in the course of benzene blood diseases. *Arch. Mal. Prof. Med. Trav. Secur. Soc.* 7:77.

Dutkiewicz, T., and Tyras, H. 1967. Skin absorption of ethylbenzene in man. *Br. J. Ind. Med.* 34:330.

Dutkiewicz, T., and Tyras, H. 1968. Skin absorption of toluene, styrene and xylene in man. *Br. J. Ind. Med.* 35:248.

Dyachuk, I. A. 1970a. Hygienic assessment of polyvinyl chloride tiles for covering floors in apartments. *Gig. Sanit.* 35:91.

Dyachuk, I. A. 1970b. A contribution to the hygienic evaluation of PVC floor tiles for apartments. *Gig. Sanit.* 35:424.

Eckardt, R. E. 1973. Recent developments in industrial carcinogens. *J. Occup. Med.* 15:904.

Elia, V. J., Clark, C. S.,Majeti, V. A., Macdonald, T., and Richdale, N. 1980. Worker exposure to organic chemicals at an activated sludge wastewater treatment plant, pp. 265–273. Wastewater and Aerosols Diseases, EPA-600/9-80-028.

Elkings, H. B., Stort, E. D., and Hammond, J. W. 1942. Determination of atmospheric contaminants. II. Methyl cellosolve. *J. Ind. Hyg. Toxicol.* 24:229.

Elliott, M. S. 1913. Poisoning by petroleum spirits. *Nav. Med. Bull. Washington* 7:416.

Ellis, F. W. 1966. Effects of ethanol on plasma corticosterone levels. *J. Pharmacol. Exp. Ther.* 153:121–127.

Environmental Protection Agency. 1976. Organic compounds identified in drinking water in the United States. Health Effects Research Laboratory, Environmental Protection Agency, Cincinnati, Ohio.

Environmental Protection Agency, 1979. Identification of Organic Compounds in Industrial Effluent Discharges, Environmental Research Laboratory, Athens, GA (EPA-600/5/79/016).

Erdogan, G., and Aksoy, M. 1973. Cytogenetic studies in thirteen patients with pancytopenia and leukaemia associated with long-term exposure to benzene. *New Istanbul. Contrib. Clin. Sci.* 10:230–247.

Erf, L. A., and Roades, C. P. 1939. The hematological effects of benzene (benzol) poisoning. *J. Ind. Hyg. Toxicol.* 21:421.

Faith, W. L., Keyes, D. B., and Clark, R. L. 1965. *Industrial Chemicals,* pp. 125–127.

Falk, H., Creech, J. L., Jr., Heath, C. W., Jr., Johnson, M. N., and Key, M. M. 1974. Hepatic disease among workers at a vinyl chloride polymerization plant. *JAMA* 230:59.

Farrier, R. M., and Smith, R. H. 1950. Carbontetrachloride nephrosis. A frequently undiagnosed cause of death. *JAMA* 143:965–967.

Feldman, R. G., and Mayer, R. F. 1968. Studies of trichloraethylene intoxication in man. *Neurology* 18:309.

Filatova, V. A. 1966. Hygienic evaluation of new technological problems in chemical industries. *Gig. Sanit.* 10:3.

Filatova, V. S., Gronsberg, E. Shi, Amirnova, N. A., Stulova, E. A., and Oreshkevich, I. V. 1965. Occupational hygiene and health condition of workers engaged in the production of latex polyvinyl chloride. *Gig. Truda* 9:9.

Fitzhugh, O. G., and Nelson, A. A. 1946. Comparison of the chronic toxicity of triethylene glycol with that of diethylene glycol. *J. Ind. Hyg. Toxicol.* 28:40–43.

Flury, E. 1928. IIa. modern occupational intoxications from the aspects of pharmacology and toxicology. *Arch. Exp. Pathol. Pharmakol.* 138:65.

Flury, F., and Zernik, F. 1931. *Schadliche Gase, Dampfe, Nebel, Rauch- und Staubarten.* Berlin: Springer.

Forni, A., and Moreo, L. 1969a. Cytogenetic studies in a case of benzene leukemia. *Eur. J. Cancer* 5:459.

Forni, A., and Moreo, L. 1969b. Chromosome studies in a case of benzene induced erythroleukemia. *Eur. J. Cancer* 5:459.

Forni, A., Pacifico, E., and Limoto, A. 1971a. Chromosome studies in workers exposed to benzene or toluene or both. *Arch. Environ. Health* 22:373.

Forni, A., Cappellini, A., Pacifico, E., and Vigliani, E. C. 1971b. Chromosome changes and their evolution in subjects with past exposure to benzene. *Arch. Environ. Health* 23:385.

Fowler, J. S., and Alexander, F. 1969. A new metabolite of carbon tetrachloride. *Br. J. Pharmacol.* 36:181P.

Fregert, S., and Rosman, H. 1963. Hypersensitivity to epoxy resins used as plasticizers and stabilizers in polyvinyl chloride (PVC) resins. *Acta Dermatol-Venereol.* 43:10.

Gabor, S., Lecca-Radu, M., and Manta, I. 1962. Certain biochemical indexes of the blood in workers exposed to toxic substances (benzene, chlorobenzene, vinylchloride). *Prom. To-kiskol. Klishiska Prof. Zabolevanii Khim. Etiol. Sb.* 221–223.

Gabor, S., Lecca-Radu, M., Perda, N., Abrudean, S., Ivanof, L., Anea, Z., and Valaczkay, C. 1964. Biochemical changes in workers occupied in vinyl chloride synthesis and polymerization. *Igiena (Buchar.)* 13:409.

Gage, J. C. 1970. The subacute inhalation of 109 industrial chemicals. *Br. J. Ind. Med.* 27:1.

Gallagher, C. H. 1962. The effect of antioxidants on poisoning by carbon tetrachloride. *Aust. J. Exp. Biol. Med. Sci.* 40:241–254.

Gauruseyka, O. M., and Filatova, V. S. 1959. Hygienic evaluation of certain types of drying units used in chemical industry. *Gig. Tr. Prof. Zabol.* 2:32.

Gerarde, H. W. 1960. *Toxicology and Biochemistry of Aromatic Hydrocarbons,* pp. 97–108. New York: Elsevier.

Gerarde, H. W. 1963a. The aliphatic (open chain, acyclic) hydrocarbons. In *Industrial Hygiene and Toxicology,* 2nd ed., ed. F. A. Patty, vol. II. New York: Interscience.

Gerarde, H. W. 1963b. The aromatic hydrocarbons. In *Industrial Hygiene and Toxicology,* 2nd ed., ed. F. A. Patty, pp. 1219–1240. New York: Interscience.

Gerlowski, L. E., and Jain, R. K. 1983. Physiologically based pharmacokinetic modeling: Principles and applications. *J. Pharm. Sci.* 72:1103–1128.

Gershoff, S. N., and Andrus, S.B. 1962. Effect of vitamin B_6 and magnesium on renal deposition of calicum oxalate by ethylene glycol administration. *Proc. Soc. Exp. Biol. Med.* 109:99–102.

Gessner, P. K., Parke, D. V., and Williams, R. T. 1961. Studies in detoxication. *Biochem. J.* 79:482–489.

Girard, R., and Revol, L. 1970. Frequency of benzene exposure in the course of acute hemopathies. *Nouv. Rev. Fr. Hematol.* 10:477–484.

Girard, R., Tolot, F., and Bourrett, J. 1971. Malignant haemopathies and benzene poisoning. *Med. Lav.* 62:71.

Gitsios, C. T. 1971. Acroosteoylsis in PCV workers. *Med. Bull. (Esso)*31:49.

Glende, E. A., Jr. 1972. Carbon tetrachloride induced protection against carbon tetrachloride toxicity. *Biochem. Pharmacol.* 21:1697–1702.

Gocher, T. E. P. 1936. Carbon tetrachloride poisoning. *Northwest Med.* 43:228–230.

Goguel, A., Cavigneaux, A., and Bernard, J. 1967. Benzene leukemia in the Paris region between 1950 and 1965 (a study of 50 cases). *Nouv. Rev. Fr. Hematol.* 7:465–480.

Goldschmidt, S., Vars, H. M., and Ravdin, I. S. 1939. The influence of the foodstuffs upon the susceptibility of the liver to injury by chloroform, and the probable mechanism of their action. *J. Clin. Invest.* 18:277–289.

Gothe, R., Calleman, C. J., Ehrenberg, L., and Wachmeister, C. A. 1974. Trapping with 3,4-dichlorobenzenethiol of reactive metabolites formed in vitro from the carcinogen vinyl chloride. *Ambio* 3:234.

Gray, I. 1947. Carbon tetrachloride poisoning. Report of seven cases with two deaths. *NY State J. Med.* 47:2311–2315.

Green, A. D., and Morrell, C. E. 1973. Petroleum chemicals. In *Kirk-Othmer Encyclopedia of Chemical Technology,* vol. 10, pp. 177–210. New York: Wiley.

Greenberg, L., Mayer, M. R., Goldwater, L. J., Burke, W. J., and Moskowitz, S. 1938. Health hazards in the manufacture of "fuzed collars." I. Exposure to ethylene glycol monomethyl ether. *J. Ind. Hyg. Toxicol.* 20:134–147.

Greenberg, L., Mayers, M. R., Goldwater, L., and Smith, A. R. 1939. Benzene (Benzol) poisoning in the rotogravure printing industry in New York City. *J. Ind. Hyg. Toxicol.* 21:395–420.

Greenberg, L. M., Mayer, M. R., Heinmann, H., and Moskowitz, S. 1942. Effects of exposure to toluene in industry. *JAMA* 118:573.

Gregorescu, I., and Tiba, G. 1966. Vinyl chloride: Industrial toxicological aspects. *Rev. Chim. (Buchar.)* 17:499.

Guild, W. R., Young, J. V., and Merrill, J. P. 1958. Anuria due to carbon tetrachloride intoxication. *Ann. Int. Med.* 48:1221–1227.

Gusev, I. S. 1968. Comparative toxicity studies of benzene, toluol, and zylol by the reflex activity methods in biological effects and hygienic importance of atmospheric pollutants, book 10. *U.S.S.R. Lit. Air Pollut. Occup.* 17:60.

Haley, T. J. 1975a. Vinylidene chloride: A review of the literature. *Clin. Toxicol.* 8:633–643.

Haley, T. J. 1975b. Vinyl chloride: How many unknown problems? *J. Toxicol. Environ. Health* 1:531–548.

Haley, T. J. 1977. Evaluation of the health effects of benzene inhalation. *Clinical Toxicology* 11:531–548.

Haley, T. J. 1981. Review of the literature on ethylbenzene. Dang. Prop. Ind. Material Rept. 1,2–4, July/Aug.

Hanrahan, D. 1979. Hazardous wastes: Current problems and near-term solutions. *Technol. Rev.* 81:21–31.

Hardin, B. L., Jr. 1954. Carbon tetrachloride poisoning—A review. *Ind. Med. Surg.* 23:93–105.

Hardy, H. L., and Elkins, H. B. 1948. Medical aspects of maximum allowable concentrations—Benzene. *J. Ind. Hyg. Toxicol.* 30:196–200.

Harger, R. N., and Forney, R. B. 1967. Aliphatic alcohols. In *Progress in Chemical Toxicology,* ed. A. Stolman, vol. 3, pp. 20–21. New York: Academic.

Harris, D. K., and Adams, W. G. F. 1967. Acroosteolysis occurring in men engaged in the polymerization of vinyl chloride. *Br. Med. J.* 2:712.

Hartwich, G., and Schwanitz, G. 1972. Chromosome studies after chronic exposure to benzol. *Dtsch. Med. Wochenschr.* 97:45.

Hawkins, R. D., and Kalant, H. 1972. The metabolism of ethanol and its metabolic effect. *Pharmacol. Rev.* 24:67–157.

Helmer, K. J. 1944. Accumulated cases of chronic benzene poisoning in the rubber industry. *Acta Med. Scand.* 118:354.

Henschler, D., Brosner, F., and Hopf, H. C. 1970. "Polyneuritis cranialis" durch vergiftung mit chlorierten acetylenen bein umgang mit vinylidene chlorid-copolymeren. *Arch. Toxikol.* 26:62.

Holcomb, R. L. 1938. Alcohol in relation to traffic accidents. *JAMA* 111:1076–1085.

Horiuchi, K., Horguichi, S., and Aratake, K. 1973. Studies on the maximum allowable concentration of benzene in the air of workshops. *Osaka City Med. J.* 9:79.

Hucker, H. B. 1973. Intermediates in drug metabolism reactions. *Drug. Metab. Rev.* 2:33–56.

Hunter, C. G. 1966. Aromatic solvents. *Ann. Occup. Hyg.* 9:191.

Hunter, C. G., and Blair, D. 1972. Benzene. Pharmacokinetic studies inman. *Ann. Occup. Hyg.* 15:193.

Hunter, F. T. 1936. Chronic exposure to benzene (benzol). II. The clinical effects. *J. Ind. Hyg. Toxicol.* 21:331.

Ikeda, M., and Ohtsuji, H. 1971. Phenobarbital-induced protection against toxicity of toluene and benzene in the rat. *Toxicol. Appl. Pharmacol.* 20:30–43.

Ikeda, M., and Ohtsuji, H. 1972. A comparative study on the excretion of Fujiwara reaction-positive substances in the urine of humans and rodents given trichloro- or tetrachloro-derivatives of ethane and ethylene. *Br. J. Ind. Med.* 29:94–104.

Ikeda, M., Hatsue, O., Imamura, T., and Komoikey, Y. 1972. Urinary excretion of total trichloro-compounds, trichloroethanol, and trichloroacetic acid as a measure of exposure to trichloroethylene and tetrachloroethylene. *Br. J. Ind. Med.* 29:328–333.

Imamiya, S. 1973. The effects of hydrocarbons in human bodies in work environments. *Kankojo Sozo* 3:62.

Iosaki, H. 1958. Vinyl chloride finding increased use in Japanese aerosols. *Aerosol Age* 3:22.

IRDC. 1972. Acute toxicity studies in rats and rabbits. International Research and Development Corp. Unpublished report prepared for Velsicol Chemical Corp.

Irish, D. D. 1962. Halogenated hydrocarbons. I. Aliphatic. In *Industrial Hygiene and Toxicology*, ed. F. A. Patty, 2nd ed., vol. II. New York: Interscience.

Ivanov, S. V. 1964. Toxicology and hygienic rating of ethylbenzene content in the atmosphere of industrial areas. *Gig. Tr. Prof. Zabol.* 8:9.

Jaeger, R. J., and Rubin, R. J. 1972. Migration of a phthalate ester plasticizer from polyvinyl chloride blood bags into stored human blood and its localization in human tissues. *N. Engl. J. Med.* 287:1114.

Jaeger, R. J., Conolly, R. B., and Murphy, S. D. 1973a. Diurinal variation of hepatic glutathione concentration and its correlation with 1,1-dichloroethylene inhalation toxicity in rats. *Res. Commun. Chem. Pathol. Pharmacol.* 6:465–471.

Jaeger, R. J., Trabulus, M. J., and Murphy, S. D. 1973b. Biochemical effects of 1,1-dichloroethylene in rats: Dissociation of its hepatotoxicity from lipoperoxidative mechanism. *Toxicol. Appl. Pharmacol.* 24:457.

Jaeger, R. J., Conolly, R. B., and Murphy, S. D. 1974. Effect of 18 hr. fast and glutathione depletion of 1,1-dichloroethylene-induced hepatotoxicity and lethality in rats. *Exp. Mol. Pathol.* 20:187–198.

Klaassen, C. D., and Plaa, G. L. 1966. Relative effects of various chlorinated hydrocarbons on liver and kidney function in mice. *Toxicol. Appl. Pharmacol.* 9:139–151.

Klaassen, C. D., and Plaa, G. L. 1969. Comparison of the biochemical alterations elicited in livers from rats treated with carbon tetrachloride, chloroform, 1,1,2-trichloroethane and 1,1,-trichloroethane. *Biochem. Pharmacol.* 18:2019–2027.

Koizumi, A., Dobashi, Y., Tachibana, Y., Tsuda, K., and Katsunuma, H. 1974. Cytokinetic and cytogenetic changes in cultured human leukocytes and HeLa induced by benzene. *Ind. Health (Japan)* 12:23.

Kommineni, C. 1978. Pathology report on rats exposed to hexachlorocyclopentadiene. Internal memo dated Feb. 14. U.S. Department of Health, Education and Welfare, Public Health Service Center for Disease Control, NIOSH, Washington, D.C.

Kotulski, B. 1965. Characteristics and purification of waste waters from production of vinyl resins. *Gaz. Woda. Tech. Sanit.* 39:46.

Kovalev, O. A., Blinova, T. S., Severovostokov, V. I., and Broitman, A. Y. 1970. Hygienic assessment of some coatings for concrete tubs. *Gig. Sanit.* 35:35.

Kozlova, T. A., and Volkova, A. P. 1960. The blood picture and phagocytic activity of workers in worker having contact with benzol. *Gig. Sanit.* 25:29.

Kramer, C. G., and Mutchler, J.E. 1972. The correlation of clinical and environmental measurements for workers exposed to vinyl chloride. *Am. Ind. Hyg. Assoc. J.* 33:19.

Krasavage, W. J., O'Donoghue, J. L., DiVincenzo, G. D., and Terhaar, C. J. 1980. The relative neurotoxicity of methyl-*n*-butyl ketone and its metabolites. *Toxicol. Appl. Pharmacol.* 57:433–444.

Kudryavtseva, O. F. 1970. Characteristics of electrocardiographic changes in patients with vinyl chloride poisoning. *Gig. Tr. Prof. Zabol.* 14:54.

Kuebler, H. 1958. Vinyl chloride as an aerosol propellant. *Aerosol Age* 3:26.

Lange, A., Smalik, R., Zatonski, W., and Glazman, H. 1973. Leukocyte agglutinins in workers exposed to benzene, toluene and xylene. *Int. Arch.Arbeitsmed.* 31:243.

Lange, C.-E., Jube, S., Stein, G., and Veltman, G. 1974. Die sogenannte vinylehlorid-krankheit-eine berufsbedingte systemsklerose? (The so-called vinyl chloride sickness—an occupational-related systemic sclerosis?) *Int. Arch. Arbeitsmed.* 32:1.

Laug, E. P., Calvery, H. O., Morris, H. J., and Woodward, G. 1939. The toxicology of some glycols and derivatives. *J. Ind. Hyg. Toxicol.* 21:173-201.

Lee, F. I., and Harry, D.S. 1974. Angiosarcoma of the liver in a vinyl-chloride worker. *Lancet* 1:1316.

Lehman, A. J. 1951. Chemicals in foods: A report to the association of Food and Drug Officials on current developments. *Assoc. Food & Drug Officials U.S. Q. Bull.* 15:82.

Lehmann, K. B., and Flury, F. 1938. *Toxicology and Hygiene of Industrial Solvents,* part 1, pp. 1–166. Baltimore: Williams & Wilkins.

Leong, B. K. J., and Torkelson, T. R. 1970. Effects of repeated inhalation of vinyl bromide in laboratory animals with recommendations for industrial handling. *Am. Ind. Hyg. Assoc. J.* 31:1.

Lester, D., Greenberg, L. A., and Adams, W. R. 1963. Effects of single and repeated exposure of humans and rats to vinyl chloride. *Am. Ind. Hyg. Assoc. J.* 24:265.

Lieber, C. S. 1967. Metabolic derangement induced by alcohol. *Annu. Rev. Med.* 18:35-54.

Lieber, C. S., and Davidson, C. S. 1962. Some metabolic effects of ethyl alcohol. *Am. J. Med.* 33:319-327.

Lieber, C. S., and DeCarli, l. M. 1968. Ethanol oxidation by hepatic microsomes: Adaptive increase after ethanol feeding. *Science* 162:917-918.

Lilis, R., Lorimer, W. V., Diamond, S., and Selikoff, I. J. 1978. Neurotoxicity of styrene in production and polymerization workers. *Environ. Res.* 15:133.

Litt, I. F., and Cohen, M. I. 1969. "Danger—Vapor Harmful": Spot-remover sniffing. *N. Engl. J. Med.* 281:543-544.

Litzner, S., and Edlich, W. 1934. Toluuol-vergiftungen, chronische, gewerbliche. *Samml. Vergiftungsf.* 5:9.

Logemann, W. A., Gellar, T. A., and Altschuller, A. P. 1968. Aromatic hydrocarbon in the atmosphere of the Los Angeles basin. *Environ. Sci.* 2:1017.

Looneman, W. A. 1968. Aromatic hydrocarbon in the atmosphere of the Los Angeles basin. *Environ. Sci. Technol.* 2:117.

Lu, P.-Y., Metcalf, R. L., Hirwe, A. S., and Williams, J. W. 1975. Evaluation of environmental distribution and fate of hexachlorocyclopentadiene, chlordene, heptachlor and heptachlor epoxide in a laboratory model ecosystem. *J. Agric. Food Chem.* 23:867-873.

Lund, A. 1948. Excretion of methanol and formic acid in man after methanol consumption. *Acta Pharmacol. Toxicol.* 4:205-212.

Machle, W. 1941. Gasoline intoxication. *JAMA* 117:1965-1971.

MacMahon, H. E., and Weiss, S. 1929. Carbon tetrachloride poisoning with macroscopic fat in the pulmonary artery. *Am. J. Pathol.* 5:623-630.

Makk, L., Creech, J. L., Jr., Whelan, J. G., and Johnson, M. N. 1974. Liver damage and angiosarcoma in vinyl chloride workers. *JAMA* 230:64.

Markowitz, S. S., McDonald, C. J., Fethiere, W., and Kerzner, M. S. 1972. Occupational acroosteolysis. *Arch. Dermatol.* 106:224.

Marsteller, H. J., Lelbach, W. K., Mueller, R., Jube, S., Roher, H. G., and Veltman, G. 1973.

Chronic-toxic liver damage in PVC production workers. *Dtsch. Med. Wochenschr.* 98:2311.

Maugh, T. H., III. 1981. New study links chlorination and cancer. *Science* 211:694.

Mallory, T. B., Gall, E. A., and Brickley, W. J. 1939. Chronic exposure to benzene(benzol)—III. The pathologic results. *J. Ind. Hyg. Toxicol.* 21:355.

Mallov, S. 1961. Effect of ethanol intoxication on plasma free fatty acids in the rat. *Q. J. Stud. Alcohol* 22:250–253.

Manucuso, T. F. 1974. Cancer and vinyl chloride—Polymerization implications, problems and uses. Presentation to the Industrial Union Dept. AFL-CIO, February.

Manufacturing Chemists Association. 1972. *Gudie for Safety in the Chemical Laboratory,* 2d ed., app. 4, pp. 441. New York: Van Nostrand-Reinhold.

McMahon, R. E., and Sullivan, H. R. 1966. Microsomal hydroxylation of ethylbenzene. Stereospecificity and the effect of phenobarbital induction. *Life Sci.* 7:921.

McMahon, R. E., Sullivan, H. R., Craig, J. C., and Pereira, W. E., Jr. 1969. The microsomal oxidation of ethylbenzene: Isotopic, stereochemical and induction studies. *Arch. Biochem. Biophys.* 132:575.

McMichael, A. J., Spirtas, R., and Kupper, L. L. 1974. An epidemiologic study of mortality within a cohort of rubber workers. *J. Occup. Med.* 16:458–464.

McMichael, A. J., Spirtas, R., Kupper, L. L., and Gamble, J.F. 1975. Solvent exposure and leukemias among rubber workers—An epidemiologic study. *J. Occup. Med.* 17:234–239.

McMichael, A. J., Spirtas, R., Gamble, J. R., and Tousey, P. M. 1976. Mortality among rubber workers—Relationship to specific jobs. *J. Occup. Med.* 18:178–185.

McCord, C. P. 1970. A new occupational disease in born. *J. Occup. Med.* 12:234.

McCollister, D. D., Beamer, W. H., Atchison, G. J., and Spencer, H. C. 1951. The absorption, distribution and elimination of radioactive carbon tetrachloride by monkeys upon exposure to low vapor concentrations. *J. Pharmacol. Exp. Ther.* 102:112–124.

Mehendale, H. M. 1977. Chemical reactivity—Absorption, retention, metabolism and elimination of hexachlorocyclopentadiene. *Environ. Health Perspect.* 21:275–278.

Meyerson, L. B., and Meier, G. C. 1972. Cutaneous lesions of acroosteolysis. *Arch. Dermatol.* 106:224.

Mikiskava, H., and Mikisha, A. 1966. Trichlorethanol in trichloroethylene poisoning. *Br. J. Ind. Med.* 23:116–125.

Miller, L. L., and Whipple, G. H. 1940. Chloroform liver injury increases as protein stores decrease. Studies in nitrogen metabolism in these dogs. *Am. J. Med. Sci.* 199:204–216.

Minot, A. S., and Cutler, J. T. 1928. Guanidine retention and calcium reserve as antagonistic factors in carbon tetrachloride and chloroform poisoning. *J. Clin. Invest.* 6:369–401.

Misgeld, V., Stolpmann, H. J., and Schulte, S. 1973. Intoxication by vinyl chloride polymers and/or their additives. *Z. Haut-Geschl. Kv.* 48:425.

Mitchell, J. R. 1972. Mechanisms of benzene-induced aplastic anemia. *Fed. Proc.* 30:561.

Moller, K. D. 1933. Some cases of carbon tetrachloride poisoning in connection with dry shampooing and dry cleaning with as survey of the use and action of the substance. *J. Ind. Hyg.* 15:418–432.

Monson, R., and Nakano, K. K. 1976. Mortality among rubber workers.—I. White male union employees in Akron, Ohio. *Am. J. Epidemiol.* 103:284–296.

Morris, G. E. 1953. Vinyl plastics. Their dermatological and chemical aspects. *Arch. Ind. Occup. Med.* 8:535.

Morris, H. E. 1954. Integrated pollution control. *Petro. Refiner.* 33:229.

Morse, D. L., Kandusky, J. R., Weiseman, C. L., and Landrigen, P. J. 1979. Occupational exposure to hexachlorocyclopentadiene: How safe is sewage. *JAMA* 241:2177–2179.

Naishstein, S. Y., and Lisovskaya, E. V. 1965. Maximum permissible concentration of hexach-lorocyclopentadiene in water bodies. *Gig. Sanit.* 30:177.

Neligan, R. E., Leonard, M. J., and Bryan, R. J. 1965. The gas chromatographic determination of a aromatic hydrocarbons in the atmosphere. American Chemical Society, Division of Water Waste Chemicals, preprint 5, p. 118. Washington, D.C.

New, P. S., Lubash, G. D., Sheer, L., and Rubin, A. L. 1962. Acute renal failure associated with carbon tetrachloride intoxication. *JAMA* 181:903–906.

Nielsen, V. K., and Larsen, J. 1965. Acute renal failure due to carbon tetrachloride poisoning. *Acta Med. Scand.* 178:363–374.

NIOSH. 1976. NIOSH revised recommendation for an occupational exposure standard for benzene. U.S. Department of Health, Education and Welfare, Public Health Service, Center for Disease Control, Cincinnati, Ohio.

Nissen, N. I., and Soeborg Ohlsen, A. 1953. Review and report of a case in a benzene (Benzol) worker. *Acta Med. Scand.* 145:56–71.

Nitti, G., Petruzzellis, V., and Fasano, V. 1970. Reographic observations on workers belonging to the plastic materials industry. *Securitas* 55:683.

Nomiyama, K., and Nomiyama, H. 1974a. Respiratory retention, uptake and excretion or organic solvents in man. Benzene, toluene, *n*-hexane, trichloroethylene, acetone, ethyl acetate and ethyl alcohol. *Int. Arch. Arbeitsmed.* 32:75.

Nomiyama, K., and Nomiyama, H. 1974b. Respiratory elimination of organic solvents in man. Benzene, toluene, *n*-hexane, trichloroethylene, acetone, ethyl acetate and ethyl alcohol. *Int. Arch. Arbeitsmed.* 32:85.

O'Brene, E. T., Yeoman, W. B., and Hobby, J. A. 1971. Hepatorenal damage from toluene in a "glue sniffer." *Br. Med. J.* 3:29–30.

Ogata, M., Tomokuni, K., and Takatsuka, Y. 1970. Urinary excretion of hippuric acid and *m*- and *p*-methylhippuric acid in the urine of persons exposed to vapours of toluene and *m*- and *p*-xylene as a test exposure. *Br. J. Med.* 27:43–50.

Ogata, M., Takatsuka, Y., and Tomokuni, K. 1971. Excretion of hippuric acid and *m*- and *p*-methylhippuric acid in the urine of persons exposed to vapours of toluene and *m*- and *p*-xylene in an exposure chamber and in workshops, with specific reference to repeated exposures. *Br. J. Ind. Med.* 28:383–385.

Opie, E. L., and Alford, L. B. 1915. The influence of diet upon necrosis caused by hepatic and renal poisons. Part I, Diet and the hepatic lesions of chloroform, phosphorus or alcohol. *J. Exp. Med.* 21:1–37.

OSHA. 1978. Occupational health guideline for carbon tetrachloride, pp. 1–5, U.S. Department of Labor, Washington, D. C.

Pagnatto, L. D., Elkins, H.B., Burgsh, H. G., and Walkley, E. J. 1961. Industrial benzene exposure from petroleum naphtha—I. Rubber coating industry. *Am. Ind. Hyg. Assoc. J.* 22:417.

Parker, J. M. 1969. Human variability in the metabolism of sulfamethazine. *Hum. Hered.* 19:402.

Parsons, C. E., and Parsons, M. E. M. 1938. Toxic encephalopathy and "granulopenic anemia" due to volitile solvents in industry: Report of two cases. *J. Ind. Hyg. Toxicol.* 20:124–133.

Patty, F. A. 1963. *Industrial Hygiene and Toxicology,* vol. II, 2d ed. New York: Interscience.

Patty, F. A., Yabnt, W. P., and Waite, C. P. 1930. Acute response of guinea pigs to vapors of some new commercial organic compounds. 5. Vinyl chloride. *Publ. Health Rep.* 45:1963.

Pegum, J. S. 1966. Contact dermatitis from plastics containing triaryl phosphates. *Br. J. Dermatol.* 78:626.

Pendergast, J. A., Jones, R. A., Jenkins, L. J., Jr., and Seigel, J. 1967. Effects on experimental animals of long-term inhalation of trichloroethylene, carbon tetrachloride, 1,1,1-trichloroethane and dichlorodifluoromethane. *Toxicol. Appl. Pharmacol.* 10:270.

Perbellini, L., DeGrandis, D., Semenzato, F., Rizzuto, N., and Simonati, A. 1978. An experimental study on the neurotoxicity of *n*-hexane metabolites: Hexanol-1 and hexanol-2. *Toxicol. Appl. Pharmacol.* 46:421–427.

Perbellini, L., Brugnone, F., and Faffuri, E. 1981. Neurotoxic metabolites of "commercial hexane" in the urine of shoe factory workers. *Clin. Toxicol.* 18:1377–1384.

Perman, E. S. 1962. Effect of ethanol on oxygen uptake and on blood glucose concentration in anaesthetized rabbits. *Acta Physiol. Scand.* 55:189–202.

Perry, D. L., Chuang, C. C., Jungclaus, G. A., and Warner, J. S. 1970. Identification of organic compounds in industrial discharges, p. 42. U.S. Environmental Research Laboratory, Athens, Ga. EPX-60014-79-016.

Peterson, D. I., Peterson, J. R., Hardinge, M. D., and Wacker, E. C. 1963. Experimental treatment of ethylene glycol poisoning. *JAMA* 186:955–957.

Plummer, S. W. 1913. Case of petrol intoxication. *Br. Med. J.* i:661.

Podowski, A., and Khan, M. A. Q. 1979. Fate of hexachlorocyclopentadiene in goldfish (*Carassius auratus*), p. 25. Unpublished report to the Velsicol Chemical Corp. Chicago, Il.

Poggi, M., and Diluzio, H. R. 1964. The role of liver and adipose tissue in the pathogenesis of the ethanol-induced fatty liver. *J. Lipid Res.* 5:437–441.

Pollini, G., and Colombi, R. 1964. Medullary chromosome damage in aplastic anemia caused by benzol. *Med. Lavoro* 55:241.

Pons, C. A., and Custer, R. P. 1946. Acute ethylene glycol poisoning. *Am. J. Med. Sci.* 211:544–552.

Post, G. B., and Snyder, R. 1983. Fluoride stimulation of microsomal benzene metabolism. *J. Toxicol. Environ. Health* 11:799–810.

Prentice, D. E., Edmondson, N. A., and Lewis, D. J. 1980. Toxicity of hexachlorocyclopentadiene after 14 weeks inhalation in rats and cynomolgus monkeys. Electron microscopy of terminal bronchioles. Unpublished report to Velsicol Chemical Corp. Chicago, Il.

Price Evans, D. A., and White, T. A. 1964. Human acetylation polymorphism. *J. Lab. Clin. Med.* 63:394.

Proctor, N. H., and Hughes, M. P. 1978. *Chemical Hazards in the Workplace*, pp. 251–252. Philadelphia: Lippincott.

Pushkin, G. A. 1965. Lesions of the liver and bile ducts of workers producing some kinds of plastics. *Sov. Med.* 28:132.

Quarles, J. 1974. Vinyl chloride. *Fed. Reg.* 39:26480.

Rechnagel, R. O. 1967. Carbon tetrachloride hepatotoxicity. *Pharmacol. Rev.* 19:145–208.

Recknagel, R. O., and Ghoshal, A. K. 1966. Quantitative estimation of peroxidative degeneration of rat liver microsomal and mitochondrial lipids after carbon tetrachloride poisoning. *Exp. Mol. Pathol.* 5:413–426.

Recknagel, R. O., and Lombardi, B. 1961. Studies of biochemical changes in subcellular particles of rat liver and their relationship to a new hypothesis regarding the pathogenesis of carbon tetrachloride fat accumulation. *J. Biol. Chem.* 236:564–569.

Reid, W. D., and Kirshna, G. 1973. Centrolobular hepatic necrosis related to covalent binding of metabolites of halogenated aromatic hydrocarbons. *Exp. Mol. Pathol.* 18:80.

Riemschneider, R. 1963. The chemistry of the insecticides of the diene group. *World Rev. Pest. Control.* 2:29–61.

Rivera, R. A., and Rostand, R. a. 1975. Health hazard evaluation/toxicity determination report. National Institute for Occupational Safety and Health, Washington, D.C. NIOSH 74-121-203.

Robbins, B. H. 1929. The absorption, distribution and excretion of carbon tetrachloride in dogs under various conditions. *J. Pharmacol. Exp. Ther.* 37:203–216.

Rowe, V. K. 1963. Glycols. In *Industrial Hygiene and Toxicology,* 2d ed., ed. F. A. Patty, vol. II. New York: Interscience.

Rozman, C., Woessner, S., and Saez-Serrania, J. 1968. Acute erythromyelosis after benzene poisoning. *Acta Haematol. (Basel)* 40:234–237.

Rubin, E., and Lieber, C. S. 1971. Alcoholism, alcohol, and drugs. *Science* 172:1097–1102.

Rubinstein, D., and Kanics, L. 1964. The conversion of carbon tetrachloride and chloroform to carbon dioxide by rat liver homogenates. *Can. J. Biochem. Physiol.* 42:1577–1585.

Ruddick, J. a. 1971. Toxicology, metabolism and biochemistry of 1,2-propanediol. *Toxicol. Appl. Pharmacol.* 21:102–111.

Rumyantseva, Y. P., and Goryacheva, L. A. 1968. Glucocorticoid function of the adrenal cortex in patients with chronic intoxication with certain unsaturated chlorinated hydrocarbons. *Gig. Truda* 12:16.

Rylova, M. L. 1953. Toxicity of 1,1-ethene dichloride. *Farmakol. Toksikol. (Mosc.)* 16:47.

Sack, G. 1941. Ein fall von toluol-vergiftung. *Samml. Vergiftungsf.* 10:41.

Saita, G. 1973. Benzene induced anaemias and leukaemias. In *Blood Disorders Due to Drugs and Other Agents,* pp. 127–146, ed. R. H. Girdwood. Amsterdam: Excerpta Medica.

Saito, F. U., Kocsis, J. J., and Snyder, R. 1973. Effect of benzene on hepatic drug metabolism and ultrastructure. *Toxicol. Appl. Pharmacol.* 26:209–217.

Sasame, H. A., Castro, J. A., and Gillette, J. R. 1968. Studies on the destruction of liver microsomal cytochrome P-450 by carbon tetrachloride administration. *Biochem. Pharmacol.* 17:1759–1768.

Savilahti, M. 1956. More than 100 cases of benzene poisoning in a shoe factory. *Arch. Gewerbepathol. Gewerbehyg.* 15:147.

Schaumberg, H. H., and Spencer, P. S. 1976. Degeneration in central and peripheral neurvous systems produced by pure n-hexane: An experimental study. *Brain* 99:183–192.

Schofield, K. 1974. Problems with flame ionization detector in automotive exhaust measurement. *Environ. Sci. Technol.* 8:826.

Scholler, K. I. 1970. Modification of the effects of chloroform on the rat liver. *Br. J. Anaesth.* 42:603–605.

Schotter, W. 1969. Toxicology of vinyl chloride. *Chem. Technol. (Leipzig)* 21:708.

Schreiber, E. C. 1974. Metabolically oxygenated compounds: Formation, conjugation and possible biological implications. *J. Pharm. Sci.* 63:1177–1190.

Scott, R. J., and Terrill, R. R. 1962. Vinyl chloride–fluorocarbon mixtures as aerosol propellants. *Aerosol Age* 7:18.

Seifter, J. 1944. Liver injury in dogs exposed to trichloroethylene. *J. Ind. Hyg.* 26:250.

Selling, L. 1916. Benzol as a leukotoxin. Studies on the degeneration and regeneration of the blood and haematopoietic organs. *Johns Hopkins Hosp. Rep.* 17:83.

Selman, J. J., and Wirtschafter, Z. T. 1937. Ingestion of carbon tetrachloride: A public health hazard. *Ohio State Med. J.* 33:167–170.

Sirota, J. H. 1949. Carbon tetrachloride poisoning in man. I. The mechanisms of renal failure and recovery. *J. Clin. Invest.* 28:1412–1422.

Slepak, N. I., and Teplyakova, R. V. 1974. Hygienic assessment of artificial leather upholstery made of polyvinyl. *Gig. Sanit.* 29:17.

Smirnova, N. A., and Granik, N. P. 1970. Long-term side effects of acute occupational poisoning by certain hydrocarbons and their derivatives. *Gig. Tr. Prof. Zabol.* 14:50.

Smith, A. R. 1928. Chronic benzol poisoning among women industrial workers. A study of the women exposed to benzol fumes in six factories. *J. Ind. Hyg.* 10:73.

Smith, M. E. 1961. Interrelationships in ethanol and methanol metabolism. *J. Pharmacol. Exp. Ther.* 134:233–237.

Smolik, R., Grzybek-Hryncewica, K., Lange, A., and Zatonski, W. 1973. Serum complement level in workers exposed to benzene, toluene and xylene. *Int. Arch. Arbeitsmed.* 31: 243.

Smuckler, E. A., Iseri, O. A., and Benditt, E.P. 1962. An intracellular defect in protein synthesis induced by carbon tetrachloride. *J. Exp. Med.* 116:55–72.

Smyth, H. F., Jr., Carpenter, C. A., Weil, C. S., Pozzani, U. C., and Striegel, J. A. 1962. Range-finding toxicity data, List VI. *Am. Ind. Hyg. Assoc. J.* 23:95.

Smyth, H. r., and Smyth, H. F., Jr. 1936. Safe practices in the industrial use of carbon tetrachloride. *JAM* 107:1683–1687.

Smyth, H. F., Jr., Seaton, J., and Fischer, L. 1941. The single dose toxicity of some glycols and derivatives. *J. Ind. Hyg. Toxicol.* 23:259–268.

Smyth, H. F., Smyth, H. F., Jr., and Carpenter, C. P. 1936. The chronic toxicity of carbon tetrachloride; animal exposures and field studies. *J. Ind. Hyg. Toxicol.* 18:277–298.

Snyder, R., and Kocsism, J. J. 1975. Current concepts of benzene toxicity. *CRC Crit. Rev. Toxicol.* 3:265–288.

Sollmann, T. 1957. *A Manuel of Pharmacology* 8th ed, p. 129. Philadelphia: Saunders.

Spehar, R. L., Vieth, G. D., DeFoe, D. L., and Bergstedt, B. V. 1979. Toxicity and bioaccumulation of hexachlorocyclopentadiene, hexachloronorbornadiene and heptachloronorbornene in larval and early juvenile flathead minnows, *Pimephales promelas*. *Bull. Environ. Contam. Toxicol.* 21:576–583.

Spencer, P. S., and Schaumberg, H. H. 1975. Experimental neuropathy produced by 2,5-hexanedione, a major metabolite of the neurotoxic industrial solvent methyl-*n*-butylketone. *J. Neurol. Neurosurg. Psychiatry* 8:771–775.

Spencer, P. S., Bischoff, M.C., and Schaumberg, H. H. 1978. On the specific molecular configuration of neurotoxic aliphatic hydrocarbons causing central–peripheral axonopathy. *Toxicol. Appl. Pharmacol.* 44:17–28.

Sporn, A., Cristea, A., Ilean, D., Ghizelea, L. D., and Stoenescu, L. 1970. Contributions to investigations on the toxicity of vinylidene chloride polymer extracts. *Igiena (Buchar)* 19:587.

Srobova, J., Teisinger, J., and Skramousky, S. 1950. Absorption and elimination of inhaled benzene in man. *Arch. Ind. Hyg. Occup. Med.* 2:1.

Stalova, E. A. 1973. Characteristics of the state of termoregulation in chronic vinyl chloride poisoning. *Gig. Tr. Prof. Zabol.* 17:53.

Stankevich, K. I., Oudienko, T. L., Tomachevskay, L. A., Fainzilber, I. D., and Rozhko, G. M. 1968. Hygienic aspects of some polymeric materials used in housing construction. *Vreach. Delo* 5:105.

Stark, G. W. V. 1969. Toxic gases from PVC in household fires. *Rubber Plastic Age* 50:283.

Sterner, J. H. 1941. Study of hazards in spray painting with gasoline as a diluent. *J. Ind. Hyg.* 23:437.

Stevens, H., and Foster, F. M. 1953. Effect of carbon tetrachloride on the nervous system. *Arch. Neurol. Psychiatry* 70:635–649.

Stewart, R. D., Dodd, H. C., Gay, H. H., and Erley, D. S. 1970a. Experimental human exposure to trichlorethylene. *Arch. Environ. Health* 20:64–71.

Stewart, R. D., Baretta, E. D., Dodd, H. C., and Torkelson, T. R. 1970b. Experimental human exposure to tetrachloroethylene. *Arch. Environ. Health* 20:224–229.

Stewart, R. D., Dodd, H. C., Erley, D. S., and Holder, B. B. 1965. Diagnosis of solvent poisoning. *JAMA* 193:1097.

Stieglitz, R., Stobbe, H., and Schuttmann, W. 1974. Leukosis induced by benzene. *Arch. Geschwulstforsch.* 44:145–148.

Stiles, H., and McDonald, S. 1904. Delayed chloroform poisoning. *Scot. Med. Surg. J.* 15:97.

Striker, G. E., Smuckler, E. A., Kohnen, P. W., and Nagle, R. B. 1968. Structural and functional changes in rat kidney during CCl_4 intoxication. *Am. J. Pathol.* 53:769–789.

Suciu, I., Drejman, I., and Valaskai, M. 1963. Investigation of the diseases produced by vinyl chloride. *Med. Intern.* 15:967.

Suciu, I., Drejman, I., and Valaskai, M. 1967. A study of diseases caused by vinyl chloride. *Med. Lavoro* 56:261.

Tabershaw, I. R., and Gaffey, W.R. 1974. Mortality study of workers in the manufacture of vinyl chloride and its polymers. *J. Occup. Med.* 16:509.

Tareeff, E. M., Kontchalovskaya, N. M., and Zorina, L. A. 1963. Benzene leukemias. *Acta Unio Int. Contra Cancrum* 19:751–755.

Teisinger, J., Bergernova-Fiserova, V., and Kudrna, J. 1952. The metabolism of benzene in man. *Procounti Lekarstui* 4:175.

Tephly, T. R., Parks, R. E., and Mannering, G. J. 1961. The effects of 3-amino-1,2,4 triazole (AT) and sodium tungstate on the peroxidative metabolism of methanol. *J. Pharmacol. Exp. Ther.* 131:147–151.

Thienes, C. H., and Haley, T. J. 1972. *Clinical Toxicology,* 5th ed., pp. 41–46. Philadelphia: Lea and Febiger.

Thorpe, J. J. 1974. Epidemiologic survey of leukemia in persons potentially exposed to benzene. *J. Occup. Med.* 16:375–382.

Tomb, J.W., and Helmy, M. M. 1933. The toxicity of carbon tetrachloride and its allied halogen compounds. *J. Trop. Med. Hyg.* 36:265–270.

Torkelson, T. R., Oyen, F., and Rowe, V. K. 1961. The toxicity of vinyl chloride as determined by repeated exposures of laboratory animals. *Am. Ind. Hyg. Assoc. J.* 22:354.

Tough, I. M., and Court-Brown, W. M. 1965. Chromosome aberrations and exposure to ambient benzene. *Lancet* 1:684.

Tough, I. M., Smith, P. G., Court-Brown, W. M., and Harnden, D.G. 1970. Chromosome studies of workers exposed to atmospheric benzene. *Eur. J. Cancer* 6:49.

Train, R. E. 1974. Vinyl chloride. *Fed. Reg.* 39:14753.

Treon, J. F., Cleveland, F. P., and Cappel, J. 1955. The toxicity of hexachlorocyclopentadiene. *AMA Arch. Ind. Health* 11:459–472.

Tribukh, S. L., Tikhomirova, N. P., Levin, S. V., and Kozlov, L. A. 1949. Working conditions and measures for their sanitation in the production and utilization of vinyl chloride plastics. *Gig. Sanit.* 10:38.

Troisi, F. M. 1950. Chronic intoxication by ethylene glycol vapour. *Br. J. Ind. Med.* 7:65–69.

Ungnade, H. E., and McBee, E. T. 1958. The chemistry of perchlorocyclopentenes and cyclopentadienes. *Chem. Rev.* 52:249–320.

U.S. International Trade Commission. 1976. *Synthetic Chemicals, U.S. Production and Sales,* p. 27. U.S. Government Printing Office, Washington, D.C.

Utzinger, R. 1977. A review on the toxicity of trace amounts of tetrachloroethylene in water. *Chemosphere* 9:517–524.

Van Duuren, G. L., and Banerjee, S. 1976. Covalent interaction of metabolites of the carcinogen trichloroethylene in rat hepatic microsomes. *Cancer Res.* 36:2419.

Van Dyke, R. A., Chenoweth, M. B., and Poznak, A. V. 1964. Metabolism of volatile anesthetics. I. Conversion in vivo of several anesthetics to $^{14}CO_2$ and chloride. *Biochem. Pharmacol.* 13:1239–1247.

Van Each, G. J., and Van Logten, M. J. 1975. Vinyl chloride: A report of a European assessment. *Toxicology* 4:1.

Van Houten, R. W., Cutworth, A. L., and Irvine, C. H. 1974. Evaluation and reduction of air contamination produced by thermal cutting and sealing of PCV packaging material. *Am. Ind. Hyg. Assoc. J.* 35:218.

Vartia, O. K., Forsander, O. A., and Krusius, F. E. 1960. Blood sugar values in hangover. *Q. J. Stud. Alcohol.* 21:577–604.

Vazin, A. N., and Plokhova, E. T. 1968. On the pathogenesis of an infection developing secondarily to a chronic exposure of the organism to the action of vinyl chloride. *Farmakol. Toksikol. (Mosc.)* 31:369.

Vazin, A. N., and Plokhova, E. I. 1969a. Changes in adrenaline-like substances in rabbit blood following chronic exposure to vinyl chloride fumes. *Gig. Tr. Prof. Zabol.* 13:46.

Vazin, A. N., and Plokhova, E. I. 1969b. Changes of cardiac activity in rats chronically exposed to the effect of vinyl chloride, vapours. *Farmakol. Toksikol. (Mosc.)* 32:220.

Vigliani, E. C., and Forni, A. 1976. Benzene and leukemia. *Environ. Res.* 11:122–127.

Vigliani, E. D., and Saita, G. 1964. Benzene and leukemia. *N. Engl. J. Med.* 271:872–876.

Viola, P. L. 1970. Pathology of vinyl chloride. *Med. Lavoro* 61:174.

von Oettingen, W. F. 1937. The halogenated hydrocarbons: Their toxicity and potential dangers. *J. Ind. Hyg. Toxicol.* 19:349–448.

von Oettingen, W. F. 1955. The halogenated aliphatic, olefinic, cyclic, aromatic and aliphatic–aromatic hydrocarbons including the halogenated insecticides, their toxicity and potential dangers, pp. 195–197. Public Health Service publication 144, U.S. Government Printing Office, Washington, D.C.

von Oettingen, W. F. 1964. *The Halogenated Hydrocarbons of Industrial and Toxicological Importance.* Amsterdam: Elsevier.

von Oettingen, W. F., Neal, P. A., and Donahue, D. D. 1942a. Toxicity and potential dangers of toluene: A preliminary report. *JAMA* 118:579.

von Oettingen, W. F., Neal, P. A., Donahue, D. D., Svirbely, J. L., Baernstein, H. D., Monaco, A. R., Valaer, P. J., and Mitchell, J. L. 1942b. Toxicity and potential dangers of toluene, with special reference to its maximum permissible concentration. Public Health Bulletin 279, U.S. Government Printing Office, Washington, D.C.

von Wartburg, J. P., Bethune, J. L., and Vallee, B. L. 1964. Human liver-alcohol dehydrogenase. Kinetic and physiochemical properties. Biochemistry 3:1775–1782.

Wacker, E. C., Haynes, H., Cruyan, R., Fisher, W., and Coleman, J. 1965. Treatment of ethylene glycol poisoning with ethyl alcohol. *JAMA* 194:1231–1233.

Weil, C. S., Carpenter, C. P., and Smyth, H. F., Jr. 1967. Urinary bladder calculus and tumor response following either feeding of diethylene glycol or calcium stone implantation. *Ind. Med. Surg.* 36:55–57.

Wendell, R. E., Narco, J. E., and Croke, K. g. 1973. Emission prediction and control strategy: Evaluation of pollution from transportation systems. *J. Air Pollut. Control Assoc.* 23:91.

Werner, H. W., Mitchell, J. L., Miller, J. W., and von Oettingen, W. F. 1943a. The acute toxicity of vapors of several monoalkyl ethers of ethylene glycol. *J. Ind. Hyg. Toxicol.* 25:157–163.

Werner, H. W., Zawrocki, C. Z., Mitchell, J. L., Miller, J. W., and von Oettingen, W. F. 1943b. Effects of repeated exposures of rats to vapors of monoalkyl ethylene glycol ethers. *J. Ind. Hyg. Toxicol.* 25:374–379.

Werner, H. W., Mitchell, J. L., Miller, J. W., and von Oettingen, W. F. 1943c. Effects of repeated exposure of dogs to monoalkyl ethylene glycol ether vapors. *J. Ind. Hyg. Toxicol.* 25:409–414.

Wessling, R., and Edwards, F. g. 9170. Poly(vinylidene chloride). In *Kirk-Othmer Encyclopedia of Chemical Technology,* eds. H. F. Mark, J. J. McKetta, Jr., and D. F. Othmer, vol. 21, pp. 275–303. New York: Wiley.

Westerfield, W. W. 1961. The intermediary metabolism of alcohol. *Am. J. Clin. Nutr.* 9:426–431.

White, T. A., and Price Evans, D. A. 1968. The acetylation of sulfamethazine and sulfamethoxypridazin in human subjects. *Clin. Pharmacol. Ther.* 9:80.

Williams, R. T. 1959. *Detoxication Mechanisms.* New York: Wiley.

Wilson, R. H., McCormick, W. E., Tatum, C. F., and Creech, J. F. 1967. Occupational acroosteolysis. Report of 31 cases. *JAMA* 201:577.

Wirtschafter, Z. T. 1933. Toxic amblyopia and accompanying physiological disturbances in carbon tetrachloride intoxication. *Am. J. Public Health* 23:1035–1038.

Wolf, M. A., Rowe, V. K., Collister, D. D., Hollingsworth, R. L., and Oyen, E. 1956. Toxicological studies of certain alkylated benzenes and benzene. *Arch. Ind. Health* 14:387.

Wolff, M. S. 1977. Evidence for existence in human tissues for plastic and rubber manufacture. *Environ. Health Perspect.* 17:183.

Wolff, M. S., Daum, S. M., Lorimer, W. V., and Seiphikoff, I. M. 1977. Styrene and related hydrocarbons in subcutaneous fat from polymerization workers. *J. Toxicol. Environ. Health* 2:997.

Wroblewski, F., Jervis, G., and LaDue, J. S. 1956. The diagnostic, prognostic and epidemiologic significance of serum glutamic oxaloacetic transaminase (SGO-T) alterations in acute hepatitis. *Ann. Intern. Med.* 45:782–811.

Wurster-Hill, D. H., Cornwell, G. G., III, and McIntyre, O. R. 1974. Chromosomal aberrations and neoplasm—A family study. *Cancer* 33:72–81.

Yamamura, Y. 1969. *N*-Hexane polyneuropathy. *Folia Psychiatr. Neurol. Jpn.* 23:45–57.

Zavon, M. R. 1963. Methyl cellosolve intoxication. *Am. Ind. Hyg. Assoc. J.* 24:36–41.

Zimmerman, H. J. 1979. Direct (toxipathic) hepatotoxins: Haloalkanes and elemental phosphorus. In *Hepatotoxicity,* chap. 9, ed. H. J. Zimmerman, pp. 198–219. New York: Appleton-Century-Crofts.

Chapter 15

Toxic Effects of Chemicals on the Immune System

R. P. Sharma

R. V. Reddy

INTRODUCTION

The immunotoxic potential of chemicals has only recently received attention in safety evaluation and toxicology. The subspeciality of immunotoxicology has become recognized in toxicological sciences because of rapid advancements of research in this area. Primary emphasis on the immunotoxicity studies has been with chemicals that have a potential for long-term exposure or persistence in the environment. Most early studies have been limited to pesticides, metals, and persistent synthetic chemicals like polychlorinated biphenyls (PCB). Additionally, as toxicity evaluation is becoming more thorough and an increasing number of organs are examined microscopically in chronic toxicity studies, the effect of chemicals on primary organs of the immune system (e.g., thymus, spleen, bone marrow) is more obvious.

The general concepts of immunology are ancient and were derived primarily from the study of resistance to infection. Many basic theories in immunology preceded the development of microbiology and at times even contributed to it. Contributions to immunology were made by anthropologists, anatomists, biologists, chemists, and geneticists.

Higher organisms have developed defense mechanisms that protect them from external invaders of biological origin. This protection is carried out by a highly evolved and complex immune system. The immune system responds to various macromolecules that are termed antigenic, and that are generally the components of invading organisms. Proteins and other large biological molecules are antigenic in nature because an immunologic defense can be experimentally elicited against them. Many small molecules, although not antigenic by themselves, elicit a specific immune reactivity if they are linked to large molecules (e.g., proteins). Such small molecules thus conjugated to proteins are termed *haptens*.

Immune reactions can be produced against molecules that are foreign to the host, including the cellular components of allogeneic organisms. The reactions may be elicited in response to an altered host tissue protein, as in the case of damage of organs or tissues, leading to an autoimmune reaction. The presence of a macromolecule where it is not supposed to be can also initiate an immune response. For example, an immune response can be mounted against nervous tissue from an otherwise compatible donor if the tissue is injected systemically.

There is growing evidence that various chemicals possess immunotoxic properties. A chemical may be either immunosuppressive or immunostimulatory; sometimes the same chemical exhibits both of these properties, depending on the dose regimen, type, and protocol of the tests employed. Immune responses are considered to be sensitive in relation to other toxic injury produced by chemicals. This is not always true, however; often a chemical may have an indirect effect on the immune system, that is, via a primary toxic effect on another organ or tissue. Some chemicals possess selective immunotoxic properties exhibited at dose levels at which no other toxicity is evident.

A number of environmental chemicals and drugs have been investigated for their immunotoxic potential. The immunotoxicity studies are particularly important for a variety of food additives and contaminants. Exposure to such chemicals is unavoidable and often continues for long periods—perhaps a lifetime. Accidental contamination of food has been reported, such as polybrominated biphenyl (PBB) contamination of food animals in Michigan (Kay, 1977). Some investigators have emphasized the immunotoxic effects of food constituents on local immune mechanisms such as the response of gut-associated lymphatic tissue, since this tissue may be in contact with relatively high concentrations of the food chemicals during the absorption process (Archer, 1978).

ANATOMICAL ORGANIZATION
OF THE IMMUNE SYSTEM

The general functions of immunity are administered by the lymphoreticular system. The cellular elements of this system are distributed throughout the body tissues, as well as in blood and lymphatic channels. The cells are also found in body tracts exposed to the external environment: respiratory, gastrointestinal, and genitourinary.

The nonspecific reticular system consisting of reticular cells (free and fixed macrophages and histiocytes) is distributed throughout the lymphatic organs and also in liver. In various capsulated lymphatic organs, the reticular network is attached to the internal surface of the capsule, whereas in noncapsulated organs it is coextensive with the tissues. The reticular network provides the fixed or stable element of the lymphatic organs and somehow provides for the selective accumulation of a different population of lymphoid cells.

The Lymphatic System

It is well established that the lymphatic system is the main unit of immune responses, together with the macrophages and the reticuloendothelial system present in many organs. The lymphatic system consists of primary lymphatic organs, where differentiation of lymphocytes occurs, such as thymus and bursa (in birds) or its mammalian equivalent—fetal liver and later perhaps bone marrow, and secondary or peripheral organs to which lymphocytes migrate. The secondary organs include the spleen and lymph nodes, as well as the peritoneal cavity and lymphatic ducts. The lymphatic ducts connect various lymphoid organs with the general circulation. Birds do not have well-defined lymph nodes, and the primary lymphoid organs are connected to circulation by lymphatic ducts. Various parenchymatous organs in birds have a diffuse lymphatic channel system.

The basic cellular unit of the lymphatic system are lymphocytes present both in peripheral circulation and different lymphoid organs. These cells, along with other differential cells such as plasma cells, macrophages, polymorphonuclear (PMN) leukocytes, and blast cells, are involved in the responses that collectively characterize the immune function (see Fig. 1).

Like other cells of the hematopoietic system, the different immunocytes are produced in the bone marrow. The stem cells, which originate in the bone marrow and are further differentiated into various hemotologic components, cannot be distinguished from each other. The precursors of lymphocytes originate in the bone marrow of adults or in the fetal liver (or yolk sac in birds) of the prenatal organism. These stem cells then migrate either to thymus or to the bursa of Fabricius or its mammalian equivalent. Following the differentiation in the primary lymphoid organs, the immunocompetent cells leave their differentiating organs and do not return there in appreciable numbers. A number of stem cells produced in the bone marrow in adult mammals, however, acquire surface immunoglobulins and migrate to the spleen; others normally home to various lymph nodes.

In the cortical region of the thymus, the residential cells undergo constant divisions with a complete turnover of cells in 3–4 days. Only a fraction of these, however, leave the organ to enter circulation. Others are destroyed in the thymus itself. In lymph nodes, a small number of cells are derived from cell division; others enter from the circulating pool, mostly from blood and a small fraction through afferent lymphatic channels. In most mammalian species, the lymphocytes leave the lymph node via efferent channels and enter the circulation through the thoracic duct. Although both B- and T-lymphocytes (named after bursa and thymus, respectively) enter the lymph node together, the B-cells preferentially migrate toward the cortex and form the germinal centers. The T-cells remain primarily in the paracortical area. Plasma cells, however, are found generally in the medullary region, suggesting that the B-cells have to migrate through a T-cell-dependent area. The transit time of T-

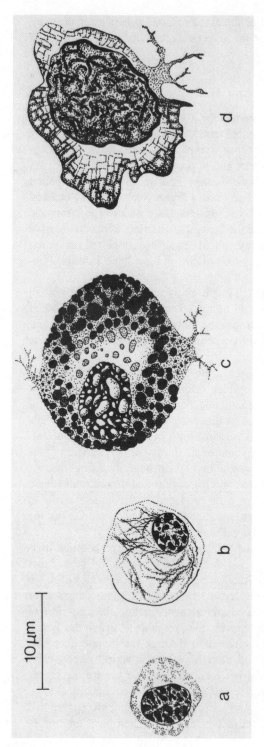

Figure 1 Various cells important in immunologic functions. The cells are drawn to indicate their relative size: (a) lymphocyte; (b) plasma cell; (c) macrophage; and (d) blast cell.

lymphocytes from circulation through the lymph node and back to the thoracic duct has been estimated to be 18–24 h. The B-cells have a slightly longer retention time in lymph nodes, approximately 30 h. The longer transit time of B-cells is not dependent on their splenic retention. Rabbits and sheep have virtually no B-cells in their peripheral circulation.

In spleen, both B- and T-cells enter from the arterial circulation in the periarterial lymphatic zone and migrate peripherally. The B-lymphocytes accumulate to form germinal centers that do not have T-cells. Both B- and T-cells leave the spleen via the marginal zone channels leading to the red pulp, and from there may leave this organ via the splenic vein.

Major Lymphatic Organs

Other than bone marrow, which is the principal site of hematopoiesis and production of stem cells, the major lymphatic organs are thymus, spleen, and lymph nodes. Lymphatic vessels carry materials from connective-tissue spaces into the blood. Lymphatic capillary networks lie in the connective tissue underneath most external or internal body surfaces. These capillaries drain into larger collecting vessels, which ultimately drain into the thoracic duct or the right lymphatic trunk. These large lymphatic vessels then drain lymph into the venous circulation.

Lymph nodes are complex chambers through which the lymph flows enroute to the blood. Lymph nodes filter lymph, provide for phagocytosis, support the proliferation of lymphocytes, and house plasma cells that produce antibodies.

The thymus is distinct among the lymphatic organs. It is fully developed before birth and undergoes a marked but gradual atrophy with age. It is the principal source of long-lived circulating T-lymphocytes. In the thymus, the entrance and exit and proliferation and differentiation of lymphocytes and the death of cells are carried out. The gland has distinct cortical and medullary regions.

The spleen is a large discriminating filter interposed in the blood stream. It also plays a role in erythrocyte destruction. It stores and produces erythrocytes, platelets, granulocytes, and lymphocytes. The organ is grossly divided into white pulp, consisting of diffuse and nodular lymphatic tissue, and red pulp, which contains erythrocyte-rich blood.

Somewhat nonspecific collections of germinal centers are found throughout the gastrointestinal mucosa and are called *gut-associated lymphoid tissue* (GALT). In some areas the collection is large enough to be identified. These specific areas are tonsils, appendix, Peyer's patches, and in birds the bursa of Fabricius.

Abundant lymphoid tissue is found in association with the large airways in lungs. Well-organized lymph nodes are present at all branch points of bronchi. Lymphoid tissue is also found accompanying smaller airways, with collections of lymphoid cells in the walls of airway branches, down to the level of respiratory bronchioles. Pulmonary alveoli contain large numbers of pulmonary alveolar macrophages that are free to move about as scavangers of foreign materials. The lung and other epithelial secretory organ systems in the body are equipped with a secretory immune system

LYMPHOCYTE DIFFERENTIATION AND FUNCTION

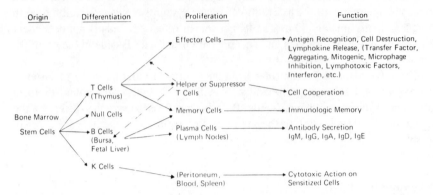

Figure 2   Scheme of production and function of various cells important in immunlogic function. In addition, there are also natural killer (NK) cells that are present in the organism. *(From Sharma, 1981a.)*

that is capable of responding to foreign agents by the production of specific humoral antibodies, IgA.

CELLULAR COMPONENTS OF THE IMMUNE SYSTEM

Various cells that are involved in immunologic mechanisms and their related functions are indicated in Fig. 2. In addition to the expression of immunity (e.g., antibody production, cytotoxicity, and the release of various lymphokines), a variety of cells are involved in cell–cell interactions. These interactions are generally characterized as macrophage processing of antigen and interaction with B-cells, T-cell–B-cell interactions, and macrophage–T-cell–B-cell interactions.

Humoral versus Cellular Immunity

Two separate types of immune responses can be mounted against antigenic invaders; the two mechanisms are mediated through different populations of lymphocytes. The humoral mechanisms, mediated through the production of antigen-specific antibodies, are carried out by B-lymphocytes. The B-cells are named after the discovery that the bursa of Fabricius in the chicken was responsible for the differentiating cells involved in the production of antibodies. Cell-mediated immunity depends on T-cells, which are thymus-dependent and can be abolished by thymic irradiation or neonatal thymectomy. The cellular immune responses are absent in athymic animals (e.g., nude mice). Although the two mechanisms are largely different, the different types of cells cooperate with each other. For example, T-cells are important in influencing the ultimate expression of humoral immunity. A simplified diagrammatic representation of lymphocyte differentiation is presented in Fig. 2. Descriptions of the two types of immunologically distinct lymphocytes are further elaborated as follows.

The B- and T-cells are structurally indistinguishable from each other in their size and shape when observed under a conventional microscope. Scanning electron microscopy, however, has provided valuable distinguishing features in these two types of cells. The B-cell surfaces are covered with microvilli or fingerlike projections, which are rare or scanty on the T-cells. The surfaces of the two types of cells are functionally different as they contain molecules for different types of receptors. The T-lymphocytes from certain inbred mice strains (for example C3H, CBA) contain lymphocyte alloantigens (called θ or Thy 1 antigen) on their surface, while these antigens are absent on B-cells. These alloantigens are present on other cells such as those of brain, skin and fibroblasts. Anti-θ sera can be prepared to neutralize the functional characters of T-lymphocytes and for their recognition. Another series of alloantigens, called Ly alloantigens (Ly 1, 2, 3, and 5), are restricted to T-lymphocyte surfaces, but Ly 4 is present both on T- and B-cells. The T-cells can be distinguished in a population by the heterosera prepared against thymus or brain (heteroantigens), which can be made specific by absorption with B-cells. Similarly, B-cell-specific antisera can be prepared from the homogeneous population of B-cells, such as from human chronic lymphocytic leukemia.

Surface Receptors on Lymphocytes

In addition to the alloantigens present on lymphocyte surfaces as mentioned above, there are other receptors that distinguish the cell populations. The T-lymphocytes of certain species contain specific receptors for erythrocytes of other species. For example, T-cells from human and pig have receptors for sheep erythrocytes, whereas guinea pig T-cells have those for rabbit red blood cells. These receptors provide an easy approach for differentiating the T-lymphocytes by the technique of rosette formation. If human lymphocytes are gently mixed with sheep erythrocytes and centrifuged, the T-cells will appear under a microscope as a rosette of erythrocytes aggregated around the cells. These heterologous erythrocyte receptors are different from the antigen receptors and do not require the presence of immunoglobulin on the T-cell surface. The lymphocytes involved in humoral immunity (B-cells) have surface receptors for active fixed complement (C3b). Red cells coated with such complement will form rosettes with B-cells and also with macrophages or other cells (PMN leukocytes, platelets). Primate erythrocytes have similar receptors. The lymphoid cells other than T-cells also have receptors for the Fc portion of IgG. These receptors can play a valuable role in the techniques used for characterizing different types of cells in immunology and immunotoxicology. A number of lymphocytes have specific receptors for viruses, specific antigens, and macromolecules that elicit the mitogenic transformation of immune-competent cells.

Lymphokines

A variety of soluble factors, called lymphokines, are released by T-lymphocytes and macrophages; these factors have important biologic actions on other cells. Many lymphokines are not fully characterized and possibly involve several components. Most of the lymphokines are heat-stable and effectively degraded by chymotrypsin.

The lymphokines may affect other lymphocytes or macrophages or even other cells of the body. Table 1 lists various lymphokines that have been described. Interferon, considered as a lymphokine since it is produced by T-cells, protects body cells from viral antigens. It is possible that several different lymphokines indicated in Table 1 may be identical factors possessing different functions, and perhaps more such factors will be discovered in the future possessing other lymphokine activities. Levels of lymphokines have been estimated in immunotoxicologic evaluations.

Immunoglobulins

Immunoglobulins (Ig) or antibodies are a group of glycoproteins closely related by structure and function. These have been identified in five major subclasses: IgM, IgG, IgA, IgE, and IgD. The basic structure of an immunoglobulin molecule consists of two identical light and two identical heavy polypeptide chains, held together by disulfide bonds. The basic antibody unit consists of a distinct constant region (Fc portion) and a variable region (Fab). The amino acid sequences of several antibodies have been determined. The Fab portion of the antibody is specific for and selectively binds an antigen determinant. The Fc region is involved in complement fixation and binds antibody to cell surfaces (e.g., binding of IgE to mast cells or immunoglobulin binding to cells in antibody-dependent cytotoxicity).

The immunoglobulins IgM and IgG are the main circulating antibodies. Produced by plasma (antibody-producing) cells in lymph nodes, IgM is the first type of antibody produced after an antigenic challenge, whereas IgG appears a few days later when the production of IgM is gradually declining. In case of a secondary immune response caused by reexposure to the same antigen, an amplified and a persistent production of IgG is observed; the IgM response is similar to the primary one. The secondary enhanced response is due to the presence of antigen-sensitive *memory* cells. IgA is the secretory immunoglobulin found in external secretions such as saliva, tears, and secretions of the gastrointestinal, urogenital, and respiratory tracts. Only a small portion (15%) of the circulating immunoglobulins are IgA type. The other immunoglobulin, IgE is involved in allergic reactions. The IgE binds to mast cells or basophils, which then degranulate upon interaction with antigens and release biologically active substances (histamine, serotonin, etc.) to mediate a hypersensitivity reaction. The IgD is primarily associated with the B-cell surface-membrane-bound receptors for antigens.

The quantitation of either total or specific globulins is one of the common tests employed in immunotoxicity evaluations. The production of antibodies can be induced in vivo by antigenic administration or the lymphocytes can be stimulated in vitro by antigens to become antibody-secreting plasma cells (Archer, 1978). The antibody level can be determined by routine titration techniques (hemagglutination, precipitation), or by measuring the antibody levels by radioimmunoassay (RIA) or enzyme-linked immunosorbent assay (ELISA). Electrophoretic quantitation, including immunoelectrophoresis, is also a useful analytical technique. The number of antibody-producing cells can be determined by fluorescent staining (Street and

Table 1   Factors Produced by Lymphocytes That Have Effects on Other Cells

Agents	Functions
Chemotactic factors	
CFM	Aggregation of macrophages
CFL	Aggregation of lymphocytes
CFP	Aggregation of PMN leukocytes
Migration inhibition factors for macrophage (MIF)	Antigen-independent inhibition
Mitogenic factors	
SMIF	Antigen-specific inhibition
MF or LTF	Lymphocyte transformation
LMF or NSF	Antigen-dependent B-cell mitosis or nonspecific factor
Macrophage stimulating factors	
MAF	Activation of macrophages
SMAF	Specific factor
Lymphocyte maturation factors	
IgT	Specific (thymus-replacing)
NSF	Nonspecific for B-cell maturation
Lymphotoxin (LT)	Cytostatic
Proliferation inhibitory (PIF)	Prevents transformation
Skin reactive factor (SRF)	Causes skin reaction
Interferon (IF)	Protects cells from viruses
Transfer factor (TF)	Transfer of immunity
Complement inhibitor (CI)	Prevents complement-dependent cytotoxicity
Interleukin 1 (IL-1)[a]	T-cell activation
Interleukin 2 (IL-2)	T-cell growth
Interleukin 3 (IL-3)	T-cell growth
Colony-stimulating factor (CSF)	Stimulation of granulocytes and macrophages
B-Cell growth factor (BCGF)	Growth of B-cells

[a]Produced by macrophages.

Sharma, 1975) or by a commonly used plaque-forming-cell assay (Mishell and Dutton, 1967).

Complement

A complex system consisting of 11 serum proteins, mostly of the β-class globulins, is present in most vertebrates. The function of this system is to enhance the action of antibody by causing a cell–membrane alteration, often cytolysis. The complement combines with the Fc receptors of an antibody molecule and is enzymatically activated to a cytotoxic membrane attack complex. Immunotoxic chemicals can modify the function of complement and thus alter the inflammatory process. Complement factors have been evaluated in immunotoxicologic testing (Olenchock et al., 1983).

Table 2   Mitogenic Agents Used for Lymphocyte Proliferation in Cell Cultures[a]

Mitogen (source)	Abbreviation	General use or target cells
Phytohemagglutinin (*Phaseolus vulgaris*)	PHA	Indicative of T-cell function; mature thymus cells are more responsive than immature ones
Concanavalin A (*Canavalis ensiformis*)	Con A	Indicative of immature T-cell reactivity
Pokeweed mitogen (*Phytolocca americana*)	PWM	Nonspecific lymphocyte stimulant; generally used to indicate B-cell responsiveness
Bacterial lipopolysaccharide (*Escherichia coli*)	LPS	Specific for B-cell response
Purified protein derivative (*Mycobacterium tuberculosis*)	PPD	Stimulates B-cells but also a T-cell stimulant in tuberculin-sensitized individuals or animals
Specific antigen or hapten	—	Can be employed to evaluate the specific response, e.g., in case of allergy
Lymphokines (mixed cell cultures	MLC	To evaluate the general responsiveness of lymphocytes as stimulated by the presence of allogeneic cells; process believed to be macrophage-dependent

[a]Reproduced from Sharma (1981a) with permission of the publisher.

Responsiveness of Lymphocytes to Mitogens

In the body, specific subpopulations of B- and T-lymphocytes undergo clonal division when there is an antigen challenge. This division is preceded by the formation of blast cells that ultimately divide into clones. The sensitized cells often respond to a subsequent challenge of the same antigen at an amplified level. The process of cell division is simulated in an in vitro system if the lymphocytes sensitized in vivo are treated with the same antigen in a culture. A similar phenomenon is observed when the lymphocytes are incubated in the presence of certain lectins derived from plants. Different populations of cells have different types of receptors (for glycoproteins) that can be distinguished by mitogenic stimulation in cultures. The molecules that initiate the transformation of lymphocytes are called mitogens or blastogens. Some mitogens bind with both types of cells; however, they can be selective in blast formation of lymphocyte subpopulations.

The response of lymphocytes to different mitogens has been used to evaluate the functional ability of lymphocytes or their subpopulations. It has also provided a diagnostic tool for identifying certain diseases. Table 2 includes a listing of selected mitogens, their sources, and the cells that are affected. Although the exact implications of mitogenic stimulation are not well understood, lymphocyte transformation techniques have been employed in immunotoxicological assessment of chemicals and drugs. Incorporation of labeled thymidine is easily quantitated in lymphocytic cultures undergoing blast formation.

FACTORS INFLUENCING IMMUNE RESPONSES

A variety of physiological and environmental factors are known to cause modifications of the immune reactions (Vos, 1977). Some of these may be hormonal factors, such as thymosin, which is required for the maturation of thymocytes. Steroid hormones and their various synthetic analogs have immunosuppressant properties. A number of drugs have been used to either cause suppression of immune reactions or stimulate responses. Use of adjuvant materials (e.g., bacterial cell-wall preparations) in conjunction with various antigens has been recognized to enhance immunity against the antigen used. Some of these factors have been discussed below.

A soluble product derived from the thymus, called thymosin, has been shown to affect the maturation of thymocytes. However, the injection of thymosin does not always reverse the effects of neonatal thymectomy. The passage of soluble factors from thymus implants within a diffusion chamber (that does not allow migration of living cells) repairs the immunological defects produced by thymectomy. Cells devoid of the Thy antigen can be converted to competent thymic cells when incubated with thymus extracts, even though the extract does not contain any detectable Thy antigen.

Corticosteroids have long been recognized as possessing lympholytic properties. Natural adrenocorticosteroids as well as their synthetic analogs reduce the size and lymphoid contents of the lymph nodes and spleen, although they do not produce any affect on proliferating stem cells of bone marrow. The mechanism of action of these chemicals is not well understood; they are believed to interfere with the cell cycle of activated lymphocytes. Both cellular and humoral immune responses are suppressed by the glucocorticoids; the effects may be different at different stages of cell differentiation. These chemicals have gained popularity in their clinical use as immunosuppressants in conditions like organ transplant or in the management of autoimmune diseases.

Different types of stress are known to alter an individual's sensitivity to infection. Adverse physical stimuli cause a physiological stress exemplified by the general adaptation syndrome. Among the somatic characteristics of the general adaptation syndrome are hypertrophy of the adrenal cortex and atrophy of lymphatic tissue. Environmental stress has been shown to cause an increase in the amount of circulating glucocorticoids.

A number of other cytotoxic alkylating agents, such as 6-mercaptopurine and cyclophosphamide, are clinically used as immunosuppressants in conjunction with the glucocorticoids. These chemicals are potent inhibitors of protein synthesis and are employed in autoimmune disorders or in organ-transplantation patients to prevent graft rejection. The environmental chemicals that are of concern in immunotoxicology are nowhere similar to these chemicals in their potency.

A potent alkaline phosphate inhibitor, levamisole, has been used as an immunostimulant or antianergic agent in humans and experimental animals. It has been investigated for its possible therapeutic applications in diseases associated with the impairment of cellular immunity. In cancer patients, treatment with levamisole after surgery or radiation therapy, either alone or in conjunction with other antimetabolites, has been known to prolong the disease-free interval. In an experimental situation, this chemical promoted the rejection of isograft in mice and produced an enhancement of the delayed-type hypersensitivity (Renoux et al., 1976). It has been proposed that the efficacy of levamisole in stimulating immune responses is greater in individuals that have depressed immune functions.

Individuals and animals can be made unresponsive to an antigenic stimulation. This phenomenon has been referred to as immunotolerance or immune paralysis. Generalized immune tolerance may occur by genetic defects or may be produced by the destruction or elimination of primary lymphoid organs. Damage to the lymphatic system by X-rays or immunotherapy leads to a general immunotolerance. Specific immunotolerance can be produced either by antigens or antibodies to the antigen receptors on the immunocompetent cells. The agents that lead to immunotolerance are called tolerogens; the phenomenon is often dose-dependent. Immunologic unresponsiveness can be exhibited to a different antigen after a challenge with another antigen; this usually persists for several days after the first challenge. Several models of specific immunotolerance produced by antigens or antibodies have been proposed. The exact mechanism of tolerance is not well understood; it may involve several different pathways, either at the specific cellular level or at the level of the antigen or both, that ultimately produce immune effects.

IMMUNE FUNCTIONS

The system consists of two distinct but not independent entities, commonly referred to as humoral immunity (involving the production of antibodies) and the cell-mediate immune response. Cells like macrophages and granulocytes are part of a rather nonspecific immune mechanism, whereas specific responses are carried out by lymphocytes. Table 3 presents a general description of the various cell types involved in immune responses. Functional properties of the immune system are best measured when the system is challenged by a stimulus, such as an antigenic substance or a parasitic organism capable of mounting a defense within the host. The response can vary depending on the stimulus used, the dose and time regimen of antigenic challenge, and the dose and time consideration of the chemical being evaluated. In most cases a single evaluation technique or even a battery of tests may not be adequate to fully define the immunotoxic potential of a chemical.

It is often contended that immunologic responses are more sensitive than other toxic effects produced by a chemical. A chemical should be considered immunotoxic only if it produces its effects on the immune system in doses considerably less than those capable of producing other systemic damage. In most cases, however, an effect on the immune system is observed at exposure levels that induce stress in the test organism via other toxic mechanisms. Since immune responses depend largely on the

Table 3 Primary Components of the Immune System and Various Types of Immune Functions

Types of cells	Functions
T-Lymphocytes	Antigen recognition, delayed hypersensitivity, retention of immunologic information (memory cells), regulation of immune functions (cell cooperation–helper and suppressor cells), cytotoxicity (tissue damage), autoantigenic recognition and control, production of lymphokines
B-Lymphocytes	Production of antibodies, antigen specificity, antibodies may cause complement activation, immunologic memory
Macrophages	Antigen processing, phagocytosis, lysosomal enzyme release
Other blood cells (platelets, mast cells, heterophils, eosinophils, basophils)	Interaction with antibodies, release of biologically active substances, phagocytosis, lysosomal reactions

proliferation of cells and on synthesis of proteins (antibodies or other lymphocytic factors) and other metabolic intermediates, the chemicals that are capable of inhibiting macromolecular synthesis will likely have an effect on the immunologic responses as well.

APPROACHES IN EVALUATING IMMUNOTOXIC EFFECTS OF CHEMICALS

There is no single or simple test that can be used for the evaluation of either immunosuppressive or immune-enhancing effects of test chemicals. Various plans and models proposed by different workers are summarized in Table 4. A list of tests that have been used in the evaluation of generalized immune responses by environmental chemicals is presented. Specific tests employed for the testing of humoral and cell-mediated immunity are indicated. The picture is not complete until the important interacting cells in various immune functions (i.e., macrophages) are also considered. The macrophages play an important role in both humoral and cellular immune responses by cooperating with selective immunocytes. Little emphasis has been placed on studying these cells in various immunotoxicologic evaluations. The awareness of the role of macrophages in immunotoxicity is becoming more important and interesting. Undoubtedly, more tests of different kinds have been performed and will be added to these lists as more data on immunologic testing become available and more is known about the immunologic mechanisms governing the activities of various cells and their subpopulations.

In vitro tests using heterogeneous mixtures of cells or their isolated subpopulations are becoming more useful. In many cases the reactivity of specific cells to surface-acting agents can be readily evaluated in vitro by using the mitogens. Direct effects of chemicals can be evaluated by their addition to cultures but should be viewed with caution. A number of chemicals decrease the response of lymphocytes to blastogenic agents by virtue of being cytotoxic. On the other hand, some chemicals may have nonspecific mitogenic properties themselves. Interaction of chemicals with mitogens in the medium may modify their function. Similar effects can be produced if the interfering molecules in the medium, such as specific fractions of serum proteins, are neutralized or altered by the presence of test chemicals.

Lymphocyte cultures in vitro are useful when carried out after administering the test chemicals to the animals and then looking for the mitogenic responsiveness of cells harvested from major lymphatic organs. In this case the test chemical can be transformed in the body if its action is dependent on the formation of reactive metabolite. Direct addition of metabolizing systems (i.e., mixed-function oxidases of liver microsomal systems) have not been of value, since their presence may modify lymphocyte transformation in vitro. At the same time, chemicals that modify the immunologic mechanisms indirectly (i.e., through alteration of other systems like steroid levels) can be suitably evaluated by in vivo administration of chemicals. Various immunotolerant mechanisms require specific T-suppressor cells or macrophages at other locations than from where the lymphocytes are harvested, or may involve autoimmunologic responses through haptenic conjugations; these may be detected only by the administration of test chemicals in the intact animal.

Table 4   Examples of Various Tests Employed in Immunotoxicologic Testing

General	Cell-mediated immunity
Lymphatic organ weights	Delayed hypersensitivity (PPD)
Lymphatic organ lesions	Adjuvant-induced arthritis
Peripheral leucocyte counts	Host-versus-graft assay
Infectivity	T-Dependent antigens
Tumor or graft survival	T-Cell Markers (rosette formation
Lymphocyte transformation (MLC)	or specific mitogens)
Presence of immune complex	Tests for lymphokines
Epidemiological survey	Macrophage tests
Humoral immunity	Disposal of bacteria in lymph organs
Globulin levels	Nonspecific phagocytosis
Complement levels	(carbon clearance)
Specific antibody titers	Metabolic activity of cells
(T-dependent or independent	(nitro blue tetrazolium reduction,
antigens)	oxygen consumption)
Evaluation of plasma cells	Enzyme assay (lysosomal)
B-Cell markers	
(antimicroglobulins or mitogens)	

[a]A variety of tests employing different protocols and analytical techniques have been employed for various types as listed here. Reproduced from Sharma and Zeeman (1980), with permission.

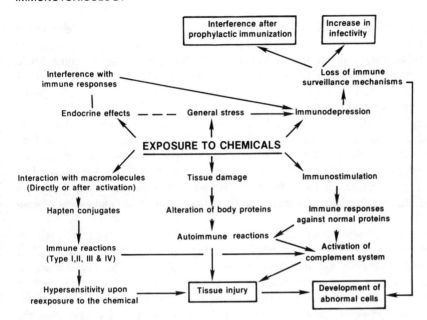

Figure 3 A general scheme of various types of toxicologic responses in the immune system produced by chemicals. For various cellular or biochemical steps of actions, see Fig. 4. *(From Sharma, 1984a.)*

MECHANISMS INVOLVED IN IMMUNOTOXICITY

The effects of immunotoxic chemicals are produced by a variety of ways, such as via producing damage to organs or tissue and then exhibiting an immune response to the altered tissue component, or via cellular or molecular inhibition of the expression of immune responses against antigens. There are limited studies with toxic chemicals dealing with the exact location or mechanisms of immunotoxic effects.

Immune mechanisms are highly complex and, in spite of the fact that the purpose of the immune system has been known for a long time, the exact functions of each of its components are still not fully understood. The system has remarkable amplification and feedback steps. The lymphoid system is the primary component of immune functions, and various lymphocytes or immunocompetent cells have been recognized. The two main populations of lymphocytes, T-cells and B-cells, are responsible for cell-mediated and antibody-type immune mechanisms, respectively. The T-cells further appear in a number of subpopulations, that is, antigen recognition cells, effector cells, helper cells, and suppressor cells. The B-cells are believed to appear in an infinite number of subsets, since specific cell clones are capable of producing specific antibodies against only one antigen.

Such variety and complexity make it difficult to evaluate the effects of chemicals on the immune system in a simplistic way. Figure 3 illustrates the general scheme of immunotoxicity by various chemicals. A single chemical may exert different effects on various steps in the immune system. For example, an antibiotic may possess a sensitizing potential and thus trigger the immune response, while simultaneously depressing protein synthesis, which has opposite effects. Based on the dose level of the chemical being tested and the duration of treatment, paradoxical effects can often be observed. In addition, the variety of procedures employed in testing the immunotoxic potential of chemicals may lead to a chemical showing no effect, a positive effect, or even an inhibitory effect, depending on the type of test used. Some of these complexities have been described recently (Sharma and Zeeman, 1980).

Allergic sensitization to chemicals is well known. Most chemicals, although not antigenic in nature by themselves, can bind with host proteins and then elicit an immune response. Both cell-mediated and antibody-type responses may be evoked and, based on the way they produce tissue injury, they have been characterized as type I–IV mechanisms (Burrell, 1976). Reexposure to a chemical may lead to a localized or generalized toxicity phenomenon, based on the route and extent of contact.

Chemicals can also affect the immune system and produce subsequent toxic injury through the development of autoimmunity. Immune responses are normally not elicited against the body's own proteins; however, chemical damage to certain organs or tissues may alter the precise regulatory mechanisms. Either an alteration in protein structure or a sudden appearance of the proteins at abnormal location can induce the production of antibodies against body proteins. These antibodies will then damage the tissues to which they are specific. Autoimmunity mechanisms as a cause of tissue damage have been characterized in a number of immunodeficiency diseases, which might be genetic in origin. Chemically induced autoimmunologic disorders are often difficult to characterize.

One effect of environmental chemicals that has received much attention is the stimulation or depression of immune responses against known natural antigens. These chemicals are present in the ambient environment or may be introduced into the body via the food chain. Some chemicals have an adjuvant-like action. Stimulation of immunity is not necessarily harmful in itself, but can increase the probability of hypersensitivity reactions or the development of autoimmunologic phenomena. Suppression of immune responses, however, can be deleterious to the well-being of the host. It may increase the occurrence of common infections by lowering the natural resistance of the individual. Such suppression may lead to an interference with prophylactic immunization. Hypersensitivity to other toxic materials, such as endotoxins, has been suggested as a result of an immunosuppression (Vos et al., 1978). There is growing evidence that immune-surveillance mechanisms are important in the survival of altered cells; immune suppression may favor the existence and growth of tumor cells. Although still open to skepticism in the case of occupational or environmental chemicals, reports have indicated that prolonged depression of immune responses can increase the cancer rate in patients (Penn, 1974).

Figure 4 illustrates a number of possible sites that are vulnerable to the effects of immunototoxic chemicals. A parameter of all cell types that can easily be evaluated is clonal proliferation. Sensitized cells are capable of multiplying themselves and require cell cooperation, that is, involvement of helper or suppressor T-cells. Alteration of such proliferation can be hypothetically achieved by general inhibitors of protein

STEPS   **IMMUNE PATHWAYS**

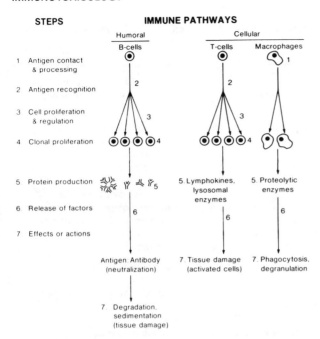

Figure 4 Schematic plan of steps during manifestation of immunologic responses that are likely to be affected by chemical toxicants. *(From Sharma and Zeeman, 1980.)*

and nucleic acid synthesis, or alteration of cell surface receptors, such as lack of stimulus or the presence of tolerogens. Modification of cellular membranes or receptors is a possible mechanism of immunototoxic effects. A number of chemicals are believed to influence selective lymphocyte populations; however, little conclusive information is available to indicate such effects (Table 5).

Chemicals that inhibit the synthesis of proteins or nucleic acids (e.g., cyclophosphamide, actinomycin D) can also prevent or modify the synthesis of antibodies, lymphokines, or various enzymes that are important for the expression of immunity. Release of pharmacologically important factors is the basis of tissue reaction or damage, or neutralization of the antigen itself. Additional factors like the complement system can further modify the antigen–antibody reactions.

Tissue responses subsequent to the expression of the immune system can also be modified by chemical treatments. This effect may lead to protection from injury as well as increased injury. For example, short-term DDT exposure in mice protected them from endotoxin-produced lung edema by decreasing the histamine content of the lungs (Gabliks and McLean, 1979). A long-term exposure to DDT caused increased pulmonary edema and mortality after challenge to influenza A_2 virus, even though the viral replication in the lungs was not altered by the pesticide treatment (Gabliks and Utz, 1979). In the latter case, DDT caused depletion of histamine from mast cells, with a consequent increase in the synthesis of this potent substance by the same cells.

Table 5   Some Possible Immunotoxicological Mechanisms and Associated Effects and Conditions

Immunologic nature	Effect or mechanisms	Chemical agent or associated condition
General	Damage to primary lymphoid organs	Radiation, TCDD, organotins
	Effect on stem-cell-producing site	Chloramphenicol, benzene, radiation
	Deficiency of polymorphonuclear leukocytes	Infections, chronic glomerulomatous disease, myeloperoxidase deficiency
	Inhibition of protein or nucleic acid synthesis	Antimetabolites, alkylating agents (cyclophosphamide)
	General stress mechanisms	Lack of nutrients, steroid hormones
Specific cellular	Interference with interactions between T-cell and antigen	Cancer antigens, chronic infections
	Lack of specific lymphocytes (selective destruction)	Thymic aplastia, antilymphocytic serum
	Defective lymphocyte proliferation	Chronic infection
	Defective lymphokine production	Chronic mucocutaneous candidiasis
	Stimulation of T-cells	Levamisole
Nonspecific cellular	Maturation defect	(Hypothetical)
	Lack of lysozymes	Acute viral infection, steroids, phenothiazines
	Alteration of lymphocyte receptors	Alkylating agents
Humoral	Absence of B-lymphocytes	Specific antibodies to B-cells; Bruton's sex-linked agamma-globulinemia
	Failure of differentiation to plasma cells	Defective antigen presentation macrophage depression, lack of IgG and IgA with raised IgM
Complement related	Deficiency of complement (notably C3)	Vinyl chloride, infections, tumors
	Complement activation	Transfusion reactions, erythro-blastosis fetalis, hemolytic reactions to drugs or chemicals
Macrophage	Blockade of reticuloendothelial system	Saturating dose of carbon
	Macrophage stimulation	Adjuvant, endotoxin, *Listeria monocytogenes*
Enzyme inhibition	Inhibition of esterases	Organophosphates
	Stabilization of lysosomal membrane	(Hypothetical), metals?

(See footnote on page 573.)

Table 5   Some Possible Immunotoxicological Mechanisms and Associated Effects and Conditions (*Continued*)

Immunologic nature	Effect or mechanisms	Chemical agent or associated condition
Immunotolerance or cellular anergy	Antigen-induced competition with recognition receptors	High dose of monomeric flagellin, tolerance to thyroglobulin
	Immune complex blocking factors	Certain tumor immunity
Autoimmunologic	Antibody induced immuno-suppression	SRBC antibodies
	Production of antibodies or specific cells against normal tissues	Allergic encephalomyelitis, organ damage with specific antibodies

[a]Reproduced from Sharma (1981b), with permission from the publisher.

IMMUNOTOXIC CHEMICALS

A number of industrial and environmental chemicals and drugs have been investigated for their immunotoxic potential. It is difficult to even briefly summarize all the chemicals that have been shown to produce effects on the immune system. Therefore only a few representative chemicals will be discussed here. Table 6 lists some of the chemicals that have been shown to have adverse effects on the immune system.

Table 6   Important Chemical and Physical Agents That Have Been Shown to Influence the Immune System[a]

Types	Selected examples
Dusts and fibers	Cotton dust, coal dust, silica, asbestos
Halogenated hydrocarbons	Polychlorinated biphenyls, polybrominated biphenyls, pesticides, dioxins, benzofurans
Organophosphorus pesticides	Parathion, methylparathion
Plasticizers and plastic monomers	Diisocyanates, organotin compounds, vinyl chloride, styrene, formaldehyde
Metals	Mercury, lead, cadmium, nickel, arsenic, chromium, selenium, zinc
Electromagnetic radiation	X-ray, microwave, ionizing radiation
Food additives and contaminants	Antioxidants, antibiotics, endotoxins, mycotoxins, pesticides
Drugs	Alkylating agents, antibiotics, cyclo-phosphamide, anesthetics, diethylstilbestrol
Biological antigens	Organic dusts, venoms, bacterial toxins
Miscellaneous	Cigarette smoking, marijuana

[a]Reproduced from Sharma (1984b).

Immunotoxic Effects of Metals

Of the various classes of chemicals, different heavy metals, both in their inorganic and organic forms, and various oxidation states, have been studied, and indeed several of these elicit toxic responses on the immune system. Toxic metals such as lead, cadmium, and mercury may possess immunotoxic properties at exposure levels that may not produce effects on other systems of the organism. In general, studies by various investigators have found lead, mercury, and nickel to be immunosuppressive, whereas low doses of selenium, zinc, and mangnese are immunostimulant. Organic tin compounds are highly thymotoxic (Seinen, 1981). Cadmium has been reported to have mixed effects, showing suppressive effects in certain test situations but either no effect or stimulation of the immune system in others. The immunotoxic effects of heavy metals have been reviewed in detail (Koller, 1980; Koller and Vos, 1981). Table 7 lists the effects of selected metals and their related compounds employed in recent studies on immune system toxicity.

The immunotoxic effects of metals are believed to be mediated by a variety of mechanisms. Metals form complexes with biological macromolecules, forming chelates, sometimes replacing essential metals in the process. Protein synthesis, membrane integrity, and/or nucleic acid replication are often affected by metals. The in vitro and in vivo effects of the same metal are sometimes opposite. For example, lead produces immunosuppression when administered internally, whereas it will act as a mitogenic agent in lymphocyte cultures, thus increasing the proliferation activity of these cells. A few reports dealing with heavy metal action on the cells of immune system in vitro are indicated in Table 8. In vitro studies have promise for discerning cellular and molecular mechanisms involved; however, they offer little value in predicting the in vivo immunotoxic potential of a chemical.

Several heavy metals and their compounds are likely to cause allergic sensitivity. Nickel dermatitis is a well-recognized problem in workers associated with processing of this metal and its alloys. Sensitivity to nickel has been reported in approximately 12% of the people showing skin diseases. Housewives handling nickel-based utensils or wearing nickel-containing jewelry and others handling nickel coins have been reported to develop nickel dermatitis. In a grouping of 24 most common allergens, nickel was ranked sixth (Baer et al., 1973). Women show a higher incidence of nickel sensitization than do men (National Academy of Sciences, 1975). Nickel sensitivity can be determined by patch test, with susceptible patients frequently not responding to other metals such as chromium. Occupational exposure to nickel occurs in electroplating shops, nickel refineries, and in businesses that require handling of articles made of nickel (hairdressers, waitresses, and jewelry manufacturing).

A number of patients showing "chrome-ulcers" have shown sensitivity reactions to chromium(VI) (National Institute for Occupational Safety and Health, 1975). The incidence of positive responses, however, is much less than for nickel. Exposure to chromium has occurred in dyers, painters, printers, and chrome-plant workers (electroplating). A large number of toxic reactions to chromium seem due to a direct effect of the metal, although immune mechanisms may complicate the effects in some individuals.

Table 7 Heavy Metals and Their Compounds Tested for Immunotoxic Potential

Metals or compounds	Effects
Immunosuppressive	
Lead (acetate or nitrate)	Generally affects thymus-dependent antibody production, lymphocyte blastogenesis, increased mortality when challenged to infection, increased viral tumor growth, decreased macrophage function and interferon production, and no effect on natural killer cell activity. Many studies were conducted using toxic levels of lead exposure (Gaworski and Sharma, 1978; Blakely et al., 1980; Blakely and Archer, 1981, 1982; Lawrence, 1981a; Kirkvliet and Steppan, 1982; Neilan et al., 1983).
Cadmium (chlorides)	Decrease in antibody-forming cells and in ratio of cytotoxic to phagocytic cells, affects hemotopoisis, decreases lymphocyte blast formation, and increases susceptibility to infection. Some studies, however, have shown either opposite or no effects (Koller et al., 1975; Gaworski and Sharma, 1978; Loose et al., 1978; Gallagher and Gray, 1982; Nelson et al., 1982; Bozelka and Burkholder, 1982; Shippel et al., 1983; Stelzer and Pazdernik, 1983; Romsten-Wesenberg and Wesenberg, 1983).
Arsenic	Increased infectivity, decreased antibody formation (Gainer and Pry, 1972; Blakely et al., 1980).
Mercury (inorganic or methylmercury)	Both organic and inorganic form of mercury suppress immune responses. Decreased antibody formation, lymphocyte function and increased infectivity have been reported (Dieter et al., 1983; Blakely et al., 1980).
Nickel (inorganic; sulfide and chloride)	Reduces lymphatic organ weights, decreases formation of interferon, decreases cell-mediated immunity and lymphocyte blast formation (Sonnenfeld et al., 1983; Smialowicz et al., 1984).
Tin (di-*n*-octyltin dichloride and di-*n*-butyltin dichloride)	Reduction in thymus weight and other lymphoid organs, damage to lymphocyte nuclear DNA (Seinen, 1981; McLean et al., 1983).
Immunostimulants	
Zinc	Stimulation at low dose followed by a depression at higher doses. At high doses, decreased antibody production and blastogenesis of splenic cells were reported (Gaworski and Sharma, 1978).
Manganese	Dose-related increase in natural killer cell activity (Rogers et al., 1983).
Selenium	Stimulation of antibody-forming cells (Koller et al., 1979).

Table 8   Representative In Vitro Effects of Metals on Immune-Complement Cells

Effects	Metals
Stimulation of mitogen-stimulated lymphocyte transformation	Zinc, iron, lead, nickel, mercury (Gaworski and Sharma, 1978; Lawrence, 1981b; Blakely and Archer, 1982; Treagan, 1979)
Inhibition of lymphocyte proliferation	Cadmium, mercury, zinc, tin (Gaworski and Sharma, 1978; Lawrence, 1981b; Loose et al., 1978; Gallagher and Gray, 1982; Nelson et al., 1982)
Metals acting as mitogens	Mercury, cadmium, lead, zinc, chromium, arsenic (Treagan, 1979)

Occupational exposure to beryllium causes severe respiratory complications, often persistent. The onset of symptoms may be delayed from 5 to 10 years after a known exposure to this metal. Remissions may be precipitated by stresses such as illness, surgery, or pregnancy. The respiratory problems have been considered to be mediated via sensitized lymphocytes similar to the pattern in delayed hypersensitivity reactions (Marx and Burrell, 1973). Sensitivity is transferable by lymphocytes and can be alleviated to some extent by antilymphocyte serum. Various chemical mediators characteristic of delayed-type hypersensitivity reactions have been observed in patients with berylliosis. It has been postulated that the metal acts as an antigen after complexing with host proteins, and also acts as an adjuvant for the immune responses against other antigens.

Immune suppression has also been suggested to be caused by certain chemically inert metal compounds. Carbon particles and silicones suppress antibody synthesis and also impair lymphocyte function. The action of such insoluble particles depends largely on their physical shape, just as physical shape is responsible for other types of occupational lung damage.

Effects of Pesticides on the Immune System

Pesticides represent a diverse group of chemicals used to control pests, in both agricultural and public-health applications. Most of these are intended for deliberate release into the environment. Their presence is ubiquitous in air, soil, food, and water. Increased risk of exposure to these biologically active chemicals occurs at various stages of formulation, manufacture, transportation, and application.

Because of the widespread use of these chemicals, many have been investigated for their immunotoxic potential. Many studies, however, employed otherwise toxic doses of the chemical. In some cases the results reported are in contradiction to each other and depend on either the test method employed or the exposure regime used (Sharma and Zeeman, 1980). Various studies of pesticide effects on the immune system have been discussed recently by Street (1981) and have been summarized in Table 9.

Table 9 Pesticides Causing Immunologic Problems[a]

Immunotoxic response	Class of chemical	Examples
Dermal sensitivity (allergic response)	Insecticides	BHC
		Butyphos
		Cartap
		Chlorfenvinphos
		Chlorobenzilate
		Chlorophos
		Cyanox
		Cyanphenphos
		DDT
		Diazinon
		Dichlorvos
		Dicofol
		Dimite
		Dinofen
		Fenitrothion
		Formothion
		Karathane
		Leptophos
		Lindane
		Malathion
		Methomyl
		Methyl mercaptophos
		Naled
		Nicotine sulfate
		Nitrofen
		Omite
		Ovex
		Phenthoate
		Pirimiphos-methyl
		Salithion
		Schradan
		Thiometon
		Thiophanate
	Fungicides	Benomyl
		Captan
		Difolatan
		Dinofen
		Mancozeb
		Maneb
		Nematin
		PCNB
		Thiram
		Zineb
	Herbicides	CDAA
		Chlorothalonil

(See footnote on page 579.)

Table 9   Pesticides Causing Immunologic Problems[a](Continued)

Immunotoxic response	Class of chemical	Examples
Dermal sensitivity (allergic response) (Cont.)	Herbicides (Cont.)	2,4-D Daconil Paraquat 2,4,5-T Trifluralin
	Rodenticides	Phosphine
Pesticides altering host defense mechanisms	Chlorinated insecticides	Chlordane p,p'-DDT Dieldrin Endrin Heptachlor Hexachlorobenzene Lindane Mirex Toxaphene
	Organophosphorus insecticides	Carbophenothion Crufomate DEP Diazinon Dichlorvos Dimethoate Leptophos Malathion Methylmercaptophos Methylparathion Ronnel Trichlorofon Triisopropylphosphate
	Carbamate insecticides	Carbaryl Carbofuran Dicresyl
	Miticides	Chlorobenzilate Milbex
	Herbicides	Barban Diquat Fluometuron Linuron Molinate Monum Paraquat Propham Tillam

(See footnote on page 579.)

Table 9 Pesticides Causing Immunologic Problems[a](Continued)

Immunotoxic response	Class of chemical	Examples
Pesticides altering host defense mechanisms (Cont.)	Fungicides	Eptam
		Maneb
		Thiram
		Triphenyltin acetate
		Zineb
		Ziram
Pesticides eliciting autoimmune antibodies	Insecticides	Aldrin
		Anthio
		Caprolactam
		Carbon tetrachloride
		Chlorophos
		DDT
		Fenthion
		Hexachlorocyclohexane
		Lindane
		Methaphenylamine diamine
		Methylmercaptophos
		Milbex
		Phosphamide
		Polychloropinene
	Herbicides	2,4-D
		Monouron
	Fungicides	Mercurials
		Thiram

[a]Adapted from Street (1981).

A concern often expressed regarding occupational exposure to pesticides is the development of hypersensitivity. The response is often cutaneous, perhaps because of the mode of exposure to these chemicals. Many of the reports indicated were clinical observations; other unknown factors may also be involved. Only recently has experimental production of allergy to some of the conjugated insecticides have been demonstrated via the production of specific antibodies (Cushman and Street, 1983). Pesticides do alter the host defense mechanisms, but it is questionable if many of these will produce an alteration of immunological responses at very low levels of exposure. Accidental contamination indeed may produce immunosuppression but is associated with other major toxic effects in the exposed individual. As is evident from Table 9, a large number of pesticides have been found to possess immunosuppressive properties.

Many cases have been reported where exposure, to either a single or a group of pesticides, is shown to cause development of immune responses to normal body tissues of their components [see Street (1981) for a comprehensive discussion]. Limited experimental observations suggest the same; it is possible that such autoimmune reactions follow substantial tissue pathology. This is an area of research that is quite neglected, even though some of the autoimmune reactions are considered dose-dependent and hence likely to be manifested at low levels of exposure.

Other Environmental Chemicals

Some synthetic halogenated chemicals are very persistent in the environment and have been reported to cause contamination of animal feeds, thus entering the human food chain. The persistence, ubiquitous nature, similarity to certain pesticides in terms of biologic effects, and incidences of mass human poisoning via food have led to vigorous investigations of the immunologic effects of polychlorinated biphenyls (PCB). Vos and Driel-Grootenhuis (1972) reported that suppression of both cell-mediate and humoral immunity occurred in guinea pigs given Aroclor 1260 (a PCB mixture) in their diet. Street and Sharma (1975) investigated the dose-related aspects of immunosuppression by Aroclor 1254 in rabbits. Aroclor 1254 caused an enlargement of the spleen and atrophy of the thymic cortex. Other parameters of immune reactivity were not consistently affected in a dose-dependent manner; these included antibodies against sheep red blood cells (SRBC) and delayed-type hypersensitivity. Another consistent effect observed was on total serum immunoglobulins, which decreased at all dose levels and at all time points, although the decline was not significant.

In a similar study, in mice given Aroclor 1248 in their diet, a reduction in both primary and secondary plaque-forming cells (PFC) was observed (Loose et al., 1977). Thomas and Hinsdill (1978) concluded that an occasional ingestion of a moderate amount of PCB-contaminated food would not cause appreciable immunosuppression in humans. In the studies reported by these authors, low levels of Aroclor 1248 in the diet caused clinically observable effects in monkeys but the immune responses were decreased only in a relatively high dose group and the effects were not consistent. The contact hypersensitivity to 2,4-dinitro-1-fluorobenzene (DNFB) was altered in offspring from rabbits treated with Aroclor 1248, but only when the dietary levels were 250 ppm (Thomas and Hinsdill, 1980).

Epidemics of PCB poisoning have occurred in Japan (Yusho disease) in 1968 and in Taiwan (Yu-Cheng disease) in 1979. In both cases the poisoning was via adulterated cooking oil. Chang and co-workers reported on the immune status of patients showing chloracne in the Taiwan episode. The levels of IgA and IgM were significantly depressed in these patients (Chang et al., 1981). The phagocytic leucocytes obtained from the exposed individuals lacked membrane receptors having immunoglobulins and also complement receptors (Chang et al., 1982a). Cell-mediated immunity was also depressed (Chang et al., 1982b). Although the exact intake of PCB in these patients was unknown, Kashimoto et al. (1981) suggested dibenzofurans (potent immunosuppressant contaminants in PCB mixtures) as a major causative agent for problems in Yusho disease.

Contamination of cattle feed by a fire-retardant, Firemaster (a polybrominated biphenyl mixture, PBB), in Michigan in 1973 prompted several investigations on the immunotoxic potential of this compound. In cattle, small amounts of PBB did not induce alteration of immune functions (Kateley et al., 1982). In swine, however, Howard et al. (1980) reported a decreased responsiveness of peripheral lymphocytes to mitogenic stimulation when animals were given relatively large doses (200 ppm) of PBB. In mice, PBB at doses of 10 ppm or higher caused decreased thymus weight and diminished PFC in splenic cells, but no effect on delayed-type hypersensitivity (Fraker, 1980). High doses of Firemaster (167 ppm) in mice caused a similar reduction after 3 weeks, with a recovery at 6 weeks of treatment (Loose et al., 1981). The sensitivity of mice to endotoxin when the animals were treated with PBB was also increased.

The effects of PBB-contaminated meat on Michigan farmers have been reported by Bekesi et al. (1978). A population of these people indicated altered lymphoblastogenesis that was not related to serum PBB levels.

Various chlorinated phenols have been found in a variety of foods and have been evaluated for their immunotoxic potential. The results reported have been conflicting and in some instances were suggested to be due to the impurities present in commercial products. Many studies have focused on pentachlorophenol, a widely used wood preservative and pesticide. Prompted by an episode of suspected poisoning in dairy cattle by pentachlorophenol, Forsell et al. (1981) investigated the immunologic profile of cattle given a commercial grade of this chemical and indicated no effect in treated animals.

Large doses (500 ppm) of technical-grade pentachlorophenol in mice caused increased survival of tumors after syngeneic transplant (Kerkvliet et al., 1982a). Similar effects were reported for viral-induced tumors. A depressed cytotoxic T-cell activity and increased phagocytosis of peritoneal macrophages were observed at this treatment level. In another study, Kerkvliet et al. (1982b) reported a delayed and suppressed antibody response. None of the effects were noticed with a similar dose of purified pentachlorophenol; it appears that the effects were caused by dioxin (a highly toxic impurity well known for its immunosuppressive effect) present in the technical grade. Purified pentachlorophenol, however, was reported to be immunosuppressive in growing chickens (Prescott et al., 1982) and neonatal mice (Exon and Koller, 1983).

It appears that in most cases of chlorinated organic chemicals associated with environmental contamination, the immunotoxic effects are caused by dioxin or dibenzofuran impurities. Toxic dioxins, particularly 2,3,7,8-tetrachlorodibenzo-p-dioxin (TCDD), are highly toxic and immunosuppressive. Similar toxicity is also indicated for the analog 2,3,7,8-tetrachlorodibenzofuran (TCDF); however, these chemicals produce immunotoxic effects discernible only at levels that induce other pathologic lesions. The immunotoxic effects of TCDD have been reviewed (Sharma, 1981c). The sensitive immune responses are very likely T-cell mechanisms and are species-dependent; the effects are known to be reversible. Epidemiologic studies, however, failed to indicate immunotoxic effects of TCDD in individuals showing other clinical symptoms.

Industrial Chemicals

Exposure to chemicals in an occupational environment is a concern in industrial medicine. Yet only a few studies have been reported dealing with such chemicals. A major health concern in this situation is the allergic response of exposed individuals. Both cutaneous and respiratory-type syndromes of hypersensitivity have been reported. Two of the chemicals that are well-known for their allergic effects are described here.

Formaldehyde produces both primary and allergic irritation of exposed skin and the respiratory tract. Although the potential of sensitization due to formaldehyde has been recognized for a long time (Horsefall, 1934), the current practice of incorporating this chemical into polymers used for domestic insulation has increased the number of people exposed to it. Allergic reactions to formaldehyde have been reported among textile workers, resin and glue production personnel, and in other plastic-manufacturing and -handling operations. Hospitals and laboratories also use this chemical. Although allergic effects due to formaldehyde have been documented by several reports, no definite estimates of their incidence in either total numbers of exposed people or in those suffering with dermatitis or eczema are available.

Bronchial hypersensitivity to toluene diisocyanate (TDI) has been recognized for several years. Exposure to any of a variety of diisocyanates, such as TDI, methylene diphenyl diisocyanate (MDI), and hexamethylene diiscoyanate (HDI), used in the manufacturing of polyurethane foams, coatings, elastomers, and spandex fibers, has been reported to cause similar effects (National Institute for Occupational Safety and Health, 1978). Experimental investigations of TDI hypersensitivity have led to a better understanding of the immunologic mechanisms underlying the allergic phenomenon. Hypersensitivity reactions to diisocyanates involve reagin-type antibody (IgE), which is largely localized in the organs of production (i.e., lungs) and gives rise to pulmonary reactions. As high as 20% of exposed personnel may develop an allergy to TDI (Bruckner et al., 1968).

A number of industrial diseases exhibit sequelae that are likely to involve the development of autoimmunity. The role of autoimmune mechanisms is difficult to prove. The lesions are highly variable from individual to individual, and only a fraction of the exposed population may be affected. The disease can be produced in few experimental animal species; however, there is a lack of a definite dose–response relationship. In many cases a characteristic delay occurs between exposure and onset of symptoms; often the lesions are accompanied by other allergic reactions.

A more convincing role of autoimmune mechanisms has been described in solvent-induced nephrotoxicity (Beirne et al., 1972). In a study involving eight patients with progressive nephritis and the presence of antiglomerular basement membrane antibody, an extensive exposure to hydrocarbon solvents was apparently related to the problem in six individuals. It was suggested that the interaction of solvents with the basement membrane was responsible for producing the antibodies and subsequent renal and pulmonary damage. Similarly, in another report, circulating immune complexes were present in 19 out of 28 patients suffering with vinyl chloride disease

(Ward et al., 1976). Several individuals suffering with this disorder have had antitissue antibodies against nuclei, smooth muscle, gastric parietal cells, and thyroid.

A number of other industrial chemicals, primarily those used in the manufacture of plastics, have been studied for their effects on parameters of immune system (Sharma, 1981d). Toluene diisocyanate stimulated lymphocytes in vitro; vinyl chloride and styrene produced a similar effect only if animals were exposed in vivo (Sharma and Gehring, 1979). Dioxane depressed T-cell while stimulating B-cell responses. In other studies, benzene, vinylidene chloride, ethylenimine, and epichlorohydrin did not produce any consistent in vitro effects on the immunocompetent cells, although many of these chemicals were cytotoxic in high concentrations (Thurman et al., 1978).

Recently, immunosuppressive effects of benzene (Wierda et al., 1981) and of trichloroethylene (Sanders et al., 1982) have been described. Several other studies involving industrial chemicals do not suggest the effects on the immune responses as a potential toxicological problem.

Immunotoxic Effects of Drugs

A number of drugs indeed have the capability of altering the function of the immune system and for that reason are used therapeutically. If the chemicals are developed and used for this purpose, then their effect is not necessarily toxic, it is desirable. On the other hand, several drugs have been known to have side effects involving the immune system or its functions.

Diethylstilbestrol (DES) is a synthetic estrogen used in therapy for several purposes. The immunosuppressive potential of this drug has been studied since the chemical has been used as a growth promotor in animals and is a known carcinogen. Luster et al. (1981) reported DES to be a suppressor of both cell-mediated and humoral immunity, but it was found to be a potent stimulant of macrophage function. Diethylstilbestrol increased tumor susceptibility and increased mortality against parasitic infection (Dean et al., 1980). Offspring from mice dosed with DES showed suppressed cell-mediated immune function, but the humoral activity was enhanced in males, with no alteration in female offspring (Luster et al., 1979). Archer et al. (1982) reported that lymphoproliferation caused by in vivo administration of staphylococcal enterotoxin A was enhanced by a simultaneous treatment with DES.

Cyclophosphamide is a potent immunosuppressive agent that is an inhibitor of protein synthesis. Both T-cell and humoral functions are impaired. For its potent immunosuppressive effect it is often used as a positive control in evaluation of other chemicals for their immunotoxic activity. The effect of cyclophosphamide is reportedly selective for B-cell responses (Smith et al., 1981; Noble and Norbury, 1983). In mammals, cyclophosphamide suppressed systemic and local graft (-versus-) host reaction, caused depletion of various leucocyte elements, and interfered with the mitogen-induced lymphocyte transformation, in addition to having a marked inhibitory effect on antibody synthesis.

Other drugs that have also been reported to have immunosuppressive properties include dexamethasone (Noble and Nobury, 1983), azathiopurine (Smith et al.,

Table 10   Immunotoxic Effects of Selected Mycotoxins

Toxin	Effects	Reference
Aflatoxin	Decreased humoral response to T-cell-dependent antigen	Thaxton et al. (1974)
	Suppression of phagocytosis by heterophils	Chang and Hamilton (1979)
	Increased mortality to infection	Boonchuvit and Hamilton (1975)
	Decreased lymphoproliferation	Reddy et al. (1983a), Miller et al. (1978)
Citrinin	Stimulation of B- and T-cell responses	Reddy et al. (1983b)
Fusarium T-2 toxin	Increased infectivity	Boonchuvit et al. (1975)
	Increased viral reactivation	Friend et al. (1983)
	Decreased lymphoproliferation, depression of B- and T-cell responses	Rosenstein and Lafarge-Frayssinet (1983)
	Decreased antibody responses	Jagadeesan et al. (1982), Rosenstein et al. (1981)
Ochratoxin A	Decreased phagocytosis by heterophils	Chang and Hamilton (1980)
	Inhibition of IgG response	Creppy et al. (1982)
Rubratoxin B	Decreased lymphoproliferation	Taylor et al. (1983)

1981), chlorpromazine (Elferink, 9179), and chloral hydrate (Kauffmann et al., 1982). Several other drugs may indeed have similar properties, but it does not appear that therapeutic doses of these in most instances will cause alteration of immunologic functions to any appreciable extent. Some hallucinogens like Δ^9-tetrahydrocannabinol (in marijuana) have a distinct potential of causing immunosuppression if used repeatedly (Desoize et al., 1981; Nahas et al., 1981). Recently, phencyclidine has also been reported to be immunosuppressive (Khansari et al., 1984).

Mycotoxins

Various mycotoxins are sometimes encountered as food contaminants. Various studies using mycotoxins have been conducted primarily because of their potential implication in livestock health; animal feed is frequently contaminated with mycotoxins. The immunosuppressive effects of aflatoxin have been investigated. Studies with several mycotoxins are summarized in Table 10. All mycotoxins are not necessarily immunosuppressive. It would not be surprising if more than one mycotoxin were simultaneously present in foods. Currently there is no information available on the possible synergistic or antagonistic effects of mycotoxins on immune function.

INTERACTIONS BETWEEN CHEMICALS
WITH REGARD TO THEIR ACTION
ON IMMUNE SYSTEM

Sharma (1984b) has recently discussed the scant information available on chemical interactions in relations to their effect on the immune system. Very few investigations have actually dealt with interactions between chemicals in relation to their effects in modifying immune functions. In many cases the exact site of chemical immunotoxicity is not well understood because immune functions are highly complex and multifaceted. In some cases studies were undertaken to elucidate the mechanisms or site of immunotoxic action. The immunotoxicity of one chemical can be modified by a second chemical that alters xenobiotic metabolism. Immunomodulation by drugs having opposite effects on the immune system was shown. Metals can either enhance or suppress immune responses; studies involving interactions of metals suggest both synergistic and antagonistic effects on immune responses. Various environmental chemicals that modify the immune functions may also interact with chemical carcinogens, especially since several carcinogens are also immunosuppressive.

CONCLUSION

A number of chemicals can alter immune functions or have toxic effects that involve immune mechanisms. Available information on the role of immune mechanisms in the manifestation of toxicity by various chemicals is inadequate. More experimental and epidemiological studies need to be performed, particularly when the chemicals produce allergic sensitization or may lead to autoimmune diseases. Immune suppression is sufficiently important to toxicology work that more studies relating dose and effect need to be conducted. Immunosuppressive potentials of chemicals are of little importance if the effects occur only with exposure levels that equal or exceed those that directly affect health. Predicting the immunotoxicology effects of chemicals requires more information. Defining the mechanisms of action and the structure–activity relationships must await additional data.

REFERENCES

Archer, D. L. 1978. Immunotoxicology of foodborne substances: An overview. *J. Food Protect.* 41:983–988.

Archer, D. L., Smith, B., and Peeler, J. T. 1982. Analysis of in vivo and in vitro mitogen-induced T-cell activation: 1. Disparate effects of diethylstilbestrol. *J. Environ. Pathol. Toxicol.* 5:445–453.

Baer, R. L., Ramsey, D. L., and Biondi, E. 1973. The most common contact allergens 1968–1970. *Arch. Dermatol.* 108:74–78.

Beirne, G. J., Brennen, J. T., and Madison, M. D. 1972. Glomerulonephritis associated with hydrocarbon solvents mediated by antiglomerular basement membrane antibody. *Arch. Environ. Health* 25:365–369.

Bekesi, J. G., Holland, J. F., Anderson, H. A., Fischbein, A. F., Rom, W., Wolff, M. S., and

Selikoff, I. J. 1978. Lymphocyte function of Michigan dairy farmers exposed to poly-brominated biphenyls. *Science* 119:1207–1209.

Blakely, B. R., and Archer, D. L. 1981. The effect of lead acetate on the immune response in mice. *Toxicol. Appl. Pharmacol.* 61:18–26.

Blakely, B. R., and Archer, D. L. 1982. Mitogen stimulation of lymphocytes exposed to lead. *Toxicol. Appl. Pharmacol.* 62:183–189.

Blakely, B. R., Sisodia, C. S., and Mukkur, T. K. 1980. The effect of methyl mercury, tetraethyl lead and sodium arsenite on the humoral immune response in mice. *Toxicol. Appl. Pharmacol.* 52:245–254.

Boonchuvit, B., and Hamilton, P. b. 1975. Interaction of aflatoxin and paratyphoid infections in broker chickens. *Poult. Sci.* 54:1567–1573.

Boonchuvit, B., Hamilton, P. B., and Burmeister, H. R. 1975. Interaction of T-2 toxin with salmonella infections of chickens. *Poult. Sci.* 54:1693–1696.

Bozelka, B. E., and Burkholder, P. M. 1982. Inhibition of mixed leukocyte culture responses in cadmium-treated mice. *Environ. Res.* 27:421–432.

Bruckner, H. C., Avery, S. B., Stetson, D. M., and Dodson, V. N. 1968. Clinical and immu-nological appraisal of workers exposed to diisocyanates. *Arch. Environ. Health* 16:619–625.

Burrell, R. 1976. Immunologic reactions to inhaled physical and chemical agents. In *Hand-book of Physiology, Reactions to Environmental Agents*, eds. D. H. Lee and S. D. Mur-phy, pp. 285–298. Bethesda, Md.: American Physiological Society.

Chang, C., and Hamilton, P. B. 1979. Impaired phagocytosis by heterophils from chickens during aflatoxicosis. *Toxicol. Appl. Pharmacol.* 48:459–466.

Chang, C., and Hamilton, P. B. 1980. Impairment of phagocytosis by heterophils from chick-ens during ochratoxicosis. *Appl. Environ. Microbiol.* 39:572–575.

Chang, K., Hsieh, K., Lee, T., Tang, S., and Tung, T. 1981. Immunologic evaluation of patients with polychlorinated biphenyl poisoning: Determination of lymphocyte subpopu-lations. *Toxicol. Appl. Pharmacol.* 61:58–63.

Chang, K., Hsieh, K., Lee, T., and Tung, T. 1982a. Immunologic evaluation of patients with polychlorinated biphenyl poisoning: Determination of phagocyte Fc and complement re-ceptors. *Environ. Res.* 28:329–334.

Chang, K., Hsieh, K., Tang, S., Tung, T., and Lee, T. 1982b. Immunologic evaluation of patients with polychlorinated biphenyl poisoning: Evaluation of delayed type skin hyper-sensitive response and its relation to clinical studies. *J. Toxicol. Environ. Health* 9:217–223.

Creppy, E. D., Stomer, F. O., Roschenthatler, R., and Dirheimer, G. 1982. Effect of two metabolites of ochratoxin A (4R)-4-hydroxyochratoxin A and ochratoxin on immune re-sponse in mice. *Infect. Immun.* 39:1015–1018.

Cushman, J. R., and Street, J. C. 1983. Allergic hypersensitivity to the insecticide malathion in BALB/c mice. *Toxicol. Appl. Pharmacol.* 70:29–42.

Dean, J. H., Luster, M. I., Boorman, J. A., Luebke, R. W., and Lauer, L. D. 1980. The effect of adult exposure to diethylstilbestrol in the mouse: Alteration in tumor susceptibility and host resistance parameters. *J. Reticuloendothel. Soc.* 28:571–582.

Desoize, B., Nahas, G. G.,Leger, C., and Banchereau, J. 1981. Cannabinoids and the immu-nity system. In *Immunologic Consideration in Toxicology*, ed. R. P. Sharma, vol. II, pp. 61–82. Boca Raton, Fla.: CRC.

Dieter, M. P., Luster, M. I., Boorman, G. A., Jameson, G. W., Dean, J. H., and Cox, J. W. 1983. Immunological and biochemical responses in mice treated with mercuric chloride. *Toxicol. Appl. Pharmacol.* 68:218–228.

Elferink, J. G. R. 1979. Chlorpromazine inhibits phagocytosis and exocytosis in rabbit poly-morphonuclear leukoyctes. *Biochem. Pharmacol.* 28:965–968.

Exon, J. H., and Koller, L. D. 1983. Effects of chlorinated phenols on immunity in rats. *Int. J. Immunopharmacol.* 5:131–136.

Forsell, J. H., Shull, L. R., and Kateley, J. R. 1981. Subchronic administration of technical pentachlorophenol to lactating dairy cattle: Immunotoxicologic evaluation. *J. Toxicol. Environ. Health* 8:543–558.

Fraker, P. J. 1980. The antibody mediated and delayed type hypersensitivity response of mice exposed to polybrominated biphenyls. *Toxicol. Appl. Pharmacol.* 53:1–7.

Friend, S. C. E., Bebiuk, L. A., and Schiefer, H. B. 1983. The effects of dietary T-2 toxin on immunological function and herpes simplex reactivation in Swiss mice. *Toxicol. Appl. Pharmacol.* 69:234–244.

Gabliks, J., and McLean, S. 1979. DDT and inflammatory responses. 2. Bacterial endotoxin induced pulmonary edema in mice and rats. *Pestic. Biochem. Physiol.* 12:264–268.

Gabliks, J., and Utz, C. 1979. DDT and inflammatory responses. 1. Influenza infection in mice fed DDT. *Pestic. Biochem. Physiol.* 12:257–263.

Gainer, J. H., and Pry, T. W. 1972. Effects of arsenicals on viral infections in mice. *Am. J. Vet. Res.* 33:2299–2308.

Gallagher, K. E., and Gray, I. 1982. Cadmium inhibition of RNA metabolism in murine lymphocytes. *J. Pharmacol.* 3:339–361.

Gaworski, C. L., and Sharma, R. P. 1978. The effects of heavy metals on [^{3}H]thymidine uptake in lymphocytes. *Toxicol. Appl. Pharmacol.* 46:305–313.

Horsfall, F. L. 1934. Formaldehyde hypersensitiveness—An experimental study. *J. Immunol.* 27:569–581.

Howard, S. K., Werner, P. R., and Sleight, S. D. 1980. Polybrominated biphenyl toxicosis in swine: Effects of some aspects of the immune system in lactating sows and their offspring. *Toxicol. Appl. Pharmacol.* 55:146–153.

Jagadeesan, V., Rukmini, C., Vijayaraghavan, M., and Tulpule, P. G. 1982. Immune studies with T-2 toxin: Effect of feeding and withdrawal in monkeys. *Food Chem. Toxicol.* 20:83–87.

Kashimoto, T., Miyata, H., Kunita, S., Tung, T., Hsu, S., Chang, K., Tang, S., Ohi, G., Nakagawa, J., and Yamamoto, S. 1981. Role of polychlorinated dibenzofuran in Yusho (PCB poisoning). *Arch. Environ. Health* 36:321–326.

Kateley, J. R., Insalaco, R., Codere, S., Willett, L. B., and Schambacher, F. L. 1982. Host defense system in cattle exposed to polybrominated biphenyl. *Am. J. Vet. Res.* 43:1288–1295.

Kauffmann, B. M., White, K. L., Sanders, V. M., Douglas, K. A., Sain, L. C., Borzelleca, J. F., and Munson, A. E. 1982. Humoral and cell mediated immune status in mice exposed to chloral hydrate. *Environ. Health Perspect.* 44:147–151.

Kay, K. 1977. Polybrominated biphenyls (PBB) environmental contamination in Michigan. *Environ. Res.* 13:74–93.

Kerkvliet, N. I., and Steppan, L. B. 1982. Immunotoxicology studies on lead: Effects of exposure on tumor growth and cell-mediated tumor immunity after syngeneic or alloge-neic stimulation. *Immunopharmacology* 4:213–224.

Kerkvliet, N. I., Baecher-Steppan, L., and Schmitz, J. A. 1982a. Immunotoxicity of pentach-lorophenol (PCP) increased susceptibility to tumor growth in adult mice fed technical PCP-contaminated diet. *Toxicol. Appl. Pharmacol.* 62:55–64.

Kerkvliet, N. I., Baecher-Steppan, L., Claycomb, A. T., Craig, A. M., and Sheggeby, G. C. 1982b. Immunotoxicity of technical pentachlorophenol (PCP-T): Depressed humoral immune responses to T-dependent and T-independent antigen stimulation in PCP-T exposed mice. *Fundam. Appl. Toxicol.* 2:90–99.

Khansari, K., Whitten, H. D., and Fudenberg, H. H. 1984. Phencyclidine-induced immunodepression. *Science* 225:76–78.

Koller, L. D. 1980. Immunotoxicology of heavy metals. *Int. J. Immunopharmacol.* 2:269–279.

Koller, L. D., and Vos, J. G. 1981. Immunologic effects of metals. In *Immunologic Considerations in Toxicology,* ed. R. P. Sharma, vol. 1, pp. 67–78. Boca Raton, Fla.: CRC.

Koller, L. D., Exon, J. H., and Roan, J. G. 1975. Antibody suppression by cadmium. *Arch. Environ. Health* 30:598–601.

Koller, L. D., Kerkvliet, N. I., Exon, J. H., Brauner, J. A., and Patton, N. M. 1979. Synergism of methylmercury and selenium producing enhanced antibody formation in mice. *Arch. Environ. Health* 34:248–252.

Lawrence, D. A. 1981a. In vivo and in vitro effects by lead on humoral and cell mediated immunity. *Infect. Immun.* 31:136–143.

Lawrence, D. A. 1981b. Heavy metal modulation of lymphocyte activities. 1. In vitro effects of heavy metals on primary humoral immune responses. *Toxicol. Appl. Pharmacol.* 57:439–451.

Loose, L. D., Pittmann, K. A., Benitz, K., and Silkworth, J. B. 1977. Polychlorinated biphenyl and hexachlorobenzene induced humoral immunosuppression. *J. Reticuloendothel. Soc.* 22:253–271.

Loose, L. D., Silkworth, J. B., and Warrington, D. 1978. Cadmium-induced phagocyte cytotoxicity. *Bull. Environ. Contam. Toxicol.* 20:582–588.

Loose, L. D., Mudzinski, S. P., and Silkworth, J. B. 1981. Influence of dietary polybrominated biphenyl on antibody and host defense responses in mice. *Toxicol. Appl. Pharmacol.* 59:25–39.

Luster, M. I., Faith, R. E., McLachlan, J. A., and Clark, G. C. 1979. Effect of in utero exposure to diethylstilbestrol on the immune response in mice. *Toxicol. Appl. Pharmacol.* 47:279–285.

Luster, M. I., Boorman, G. A., Dean, J. H., Lawson, L. D., Wilson, R., and Haseman, J. 1981. Immunological alterations in mice following acute exposure to diethylstilbestrol. In *Biological Relevance of Immune Suppression,* eds. J. H. Dean and M. Padarathsingh, pp. 153–171. New York: Van Nostrand.

Marx, J. J., and Burrell, R. 1973. Delayed hypersensitivity to beryllium compounds. *J. Immunol.* 111:590–598.

McLean, J. R. N., Birnboim, H. C., Pontefat, R., and Kaplan, J. G. 1983. The effect of tin chloride on the structure and function of DNA in human white blood cells. *Chem. Biol. Interact.* 46:189–200.

Miller, D. M., Stuart, B. P., Crowell, W. A., Cole, R. J., Goven, A. J., and Brown, J. 1978. Aflatoxicosis in swine. Its effects on immunity and relationship to salmonellosis. *Am. Assoc. Vet. Lab. Diagn.* 21:135–146.

Mishell, R. I., and Dutton, R. W. 1967. Immunization of mouse spleen cell cultures from normal mice. *J. Exp. Med.* 126:423–442.

Nahas, G., Leger, L., Desoize, B., and Banchereau, J. 1981. Inhibitory effects of psychotropic drugs on blastogenesis of cultured lymphocytes. In *Immunologic Considerations in Toxicology,* ed. R. P. Sharma, vol. II, pp. 83–91. Baco Raton, Fla.: CRC.

National Academy of Sciences. 1975. Medical and biological effects of environmental pollutants—Nickel, pp. 129–143. National Academy of Sciences, Washington, D.C.

National Institute for Occupational Safety and Health. 1975. Criteria for a recommended standard—Occupational exposure to chromium (VI), pp. 46–57. U.S. Government Printing Office, Washington, D.C.

National Institute for Occupational Safety and Health. 1978. Criteria for a recommended standard—Occupational exposure to diisocyanates, pp. 26–36. U.S. Government Printing Office, Washington, D.C.

Neilan, B. A., O'Neill, K., and Handwerger, B. S. 1983. Effect of low-level lead exposure on antibody-dependent and natural killer cell-mediated cytotoxicity. *Toxicol. Appl. Pharmacol.* 69:272–275.

Nelson, D. J., Schumacher, L. K., and Stotsky, G. 1982. Effects of cadmium, lead and zinc on macrophage-mediated cytotoxicity toward tumor cells. *Environ. Res.* 28:154–163.

Noble, C., and Norbury, K. C. 1983. The differential sensitivity of rat peripheral blood T cells to immunosuppressants: Cyclophosphamide and dexamethasone. *J. Immunopharmacol.* 5:341–358.

Olenchock, S. A., Mull, J. C., Mentnech, M. S., Lewis, D. M., and Bernstein, R. S. 1983. Changes in humoral immunological parameters after exposure to volcanic ash. *J. Toxicol. Environ. Health* 11:395–404.

Penn, I. 1974. Clinical immunosuppression and human cancer. *Cancer* 34:1474–1480.

Prescott, C. A., Wilkie, B. N., Hunter, B., and Julian, R. J. 1982. Influence of a purified grade of pentachlorophenol on the immune response of chickens. *Am. J. Vet. Res.* 43:481–487.

Reddy, R. V., Sharma, R. P., and Taylor, M. J. 1983a. Dose and time related response of immunologic functions to aflatoxin B_1 in mice. In *Development in the Science and Practice of Toxicology,* eds. A. W. Hayes, R. C. Schnell, and T. S. Miya, pp. 431–434. Amsterdam: Elsevier Science.

Reddy, R. V., Taylor, M. J., and Sharma, R. P. 1983b. Evaluation of citrinin toxicity on the immune system in mice. *Toxicologist* 3:341.

Renoux, G., Renoux, M., Teller, M. N., McMahon, S., and Buillaumin, J. M. 1976. Potentiation of T cell mediated immunity by levamisole. *Clin. Exp. Immunol.* 25:288–296.

Rogers, R. R., Garner, R. J., Riddle, M. M., Leubke, R. W., and Smialowicz, R. J. 1983. Augmentation of murine natural killer cell activity by manganese chloride. *Toxicol. Appl. Pharmacol.* 70:7–17.

Romsten-Wesenberg, G. B., and Wesenberg, F. 1983. Effect of cadmium on the immune response in rats. *Environ. Res.* 31:413–419.

Rosenstein, Y., and Lafarge-Frayssinet, C. 1983. Inhibitory effect of fusarium T2 toxin on lymphoid DNA and protein synthesis. *Toxicol. Appl. Pharmacol.* 70:283–288.

Rosenstein, Y., Kretschmer, R. R., and Lafarge-Frayssinet, C. 1981. Effect of fusarium toxins, T-2 toxin and diacetoxyscirpenol on murine T-independent immune responses. *Immunology* 44:555–560.

Sanders, V. M., Tucker, A. N., White, K. L., Kauffmann, B. M., Hallett, P., Carchman, R. A., Borzelleca, J. F., and Monson, A. E. 1982. Humoral and cell-mediated immune status in mice exposed to trichloroethylene in the drinking water. *Toxicol. Appl. Pharmacol.* 62:358–368.

Seinen, W. 1981. Immunotoxicity of alkylatin compounds. In *Immunologic Considerations in Toxicology,* ed. R. P. Sharma, vol. 1, pp. 103–119. Boca Raton, Fla.: CRC.

Sharma, R. P. 1981a. Immunity and the immune system. In *Immunologic Considerations in Toxicology,* ed. R. P. Sharma, vol. 1, pp. 9–18. Boca Raton, Fla.: CRC.

Sharma, R. P. 1981b. Tissue or cell injury in immune mechanisms. In *Immunologic Considerations in Toxicology,* ed. R. P. Sharma, vol. I, pp. 37–44. Boca Raton, Fla.: CRC.

Sharma, R. P. 1981c. Effects of tetrachlorodibenzo-*p*-dioxin (TCDD) on immunologic system.

In *Immunologic Considerations in Toxicology,* ed. R. P. Sharma, vol. I, pp. 89–102. Boca Raton, Fla.: CRC.

Sharma, R. P. 1981d. Industrial compounds and modification of immune responses: Studies with vinyl chloride. In *Immunologic Considerations in Toxicology,* ed. R. P. Sharma, vol. I, pp. 79–88. Boca Ration, Fla.: CRC.

Sharma, R. P. 1984a. Chemical interactions and compromised immune system. *Fundam. Appl. Toxicol.* 4:345–351.

Sharma, R. P. 1984b. Overview of known chemical immunotoxicants. In *Chemical Regulation of Immunity in Veterinary Medicine,* eds. M. Kende, J. Gainer, and M. Chirigos, pp. 313–318. New York: Liss.

Sharma, R. P., and Gehring, P. J. 1979. Immunologic effects of vinyl chloride in mice. *Ann. NY Acad. Sci.* 320:551–563.

Sharma, R. P., and Zeeman, M. G. 1980. Immunologic alterations by environmental chemicals: Relevance of studying mechanisms versus effects. *J. Immunopharmacol.* 2:285–307.

Shippel, R. L., Burgess, D. H., Ciavarra, R. P., Dicapua, R. A., and Stake, P. E. 1983. Cadmium-induced suppression of the primary immune response and acute toxicity in mice: Differential interaction of zinc. *Toxicol. Appl. Pharmacol.* 71:303–306.

Smialowicz, R. J., Rogers, R. R., Riddle, M. M., and Stott, G. A. 1984. Immunologic effects of nickel: 1. Suppression of cellular and humoral immunity. *Environ. Res.* 33:413–427.

Smith, S. R., Terminelli, C., Kipilman, C. T., and Smith, Y. 1981. Comparative effects of azathioprine, cyclophosphamide and frentizole on cellular immunity in mice. *J. Immunopharmacol.* 3:133–170.

Sonnenfeld, G., Sterps, U. N., and Costa, M. 1983. Differential effects of amorphous and crystalline nickel sulfide on murine/interferon production. *Environ. Res.* 32:474–479.

Stelzer, K. J., and Pazdernik, T. L. 1983. Cadmium-induced immunotoxicity. *Int. J. Immunopharmacol.* 5:541–548.

Street, J. C. 1981. Pesticides and the immune system. In *Immunologic Considerations in Toxicology,* ed. R. P. Sharma, vol. 1, pp. 45–66. Boca Raton, Fla.: CRC.

Street, J. C., and Sharma, R. P. 1975. Alteration of induced cellular and humoral immune responses by pesticides and chemicals of environmental concern: Quantitative studies of immunosuppression by DDT, Aroclor 1254, carbaryl, carbofuran and methylparathion. *Toxicol. Appl. Pharmacol.* 32:587–602.

Taylor, M. J., Reddy, R. V., and Sharma, R. P. 1983. Immunotoxicologic evaluation of rubratoxin B in male CD-1 mice. *Toxicologist* 3:1, 341.

Thaxton, J. P., Tung, H. T., and Hamilton, P. B. 1974. Immunosuppression in chickens by aflatoxin. *Poult. Sci.* 53:721–725.

Thomas, P. T., and Hinsdill, R. D. 1978. Effect of polychlorinated biphenyls on the immune response of rhesus monkeys and mice. *Toxicol. Appl. Pharmacol.* 44:41–51.

Thomas, P. T., and Hinsdill, R. D. 1980. Perinatal PCB exposure and its effect on the immune system of young rabbits. *Drug. Chem. Toxicol.* 3:173–184.

Thurman, G. B., Simms, B. G., Goldstein, A. L., and Kilian, D. F. 1978. The effects of organic compounds used in the manufacture of plastics on the responsivity of murine and human lymphocytes. *Toxicol. Appl. Pharmacol.* 44:617–641.

Treagan, L. 1979. A survey of the effects of metals on the immune response. *Biol. Trace Elem. Res.* 1:141–148.

Vos, J. G. 1977. Immune suppression as related to toxicology. *CRC Crit. Rev. Toxicol.* 5:67–101.

Vos, J. G., and Driel-Grootenhuis, L. V. 1972. PCB induced suppression of the humoral and cell-mediated immunity in guinea pigs. *Sci. Total Environ.* 1:298–302, 1972.

Vos, J. G., Kreeftenberg, J. G., Engel, H. W. B., Minderhoud, A., and Van Noorle-Jansen, L. M. 1978. Studies on 2,3,7,8-tetrachlorodibenzo-*p*-dioxin induced immune suppression and decreased resistance to infection: Endotoxin hypersensitivity, serum zinc concentrations and effect of thymosin treatment. *Toxicology* 9:75–86.

Ward, A. M., Udnoon, S., Watkins, J., Walker, A. E., and Darke, C. S. 1976. Immunological mechanisms in the pathogenesis of vinyl chloride disease. *Br. Med. J.* 1:936–938.

Wierda, D., Irons, R. D., and Greenlee, W. F. 1981. Immunotoxicity in $C_{57}BL/6$ mice exposed to benzene and Aroclor 1254. *Toxicol. Appl. Pharmacol.* 60:410–417.

Chapter 16

Clinical Toxicology

Thomas J. Haley

INTRODUCTION

Clinical toxicology is the branch of medical science that covers poisoning from various xenobiotics and chemical and physical means for counteracting the deleterious effects of such chemicals or natural products.

The home presents the greatest potential for poisoning, because of the availability of detergents, lye, bleaches, cleaners, pesticides, and other chemicals. In rural settings the large volume of agricultural chemicals constitutes additional hazards. Table 1 shows deaths from ingestion of various chemicals readily available in the home. Table 2 lists the types of materials either accidentally ingested or inhaled or used with suicidal intent. This table illustrates the extent of the problem and points out the problem engendered when the exact poison is unknown. Table 3 gives the actual deaths in children under 5 years of age for the period 1973–1976 and indicates the lack of parental control over such chemicals. Household or yard plants constitute another source of poisoning in children under 5 years of age, and there is a general lack of understanding by parents of the chance for poisoning of their children (see Table 4). Drug abuse, particularly in a social setting with one's peers, has become a real problem in the 14- to 30–year–old group, where many legitimate useful drugs are taken just for kicks.

Table 1   Total Deaths from Accidental Poisonings[a]

Poison	1973	1974	1975	1976
Antibiotics and other anti-infectives	21	9	27	20
Hormones and synthetic substitutes	23	28	32	26
Systemic and hematologic agents	44	53	61	58
Analgesics and antipyretics	827	967	1275	1067
(Salicylate and congeners)	(95)	(83)	(98)	(79)
Sedatives and hypnotics	596	620	557	508
(Barbiturates)	(362)	(330)	(266)	(224)
Autonomic nervous system and psychotherapeutic drugs	139	165	178	190
(Tranquilizers)	(87)	(106)	(103)	(92)
Central nervous system depressants and stimulants	36	40	37	36
(Amphetamines)	(21)	(18)	(11)	(11)
Cardiovascular drugs	123	143	158	138
Gastrointestinal drugs	9	6	3	4
Other and unspecified drugs and medicants	626	711	804	792
Total drugs	2444	2742	3132	2839
Alcohol	333	370	391	337
Cleaning and polishing agents	10	13	12	14
Disinfectants	2	8	6	6
Paints and varnishes	1	1	5	0
Petroleum products and other solvents	41	54	54	45
Pesticides, fertilizers, or plant foods	32	35	30	31
Heavy metals (and their fumes)	21	23	13	15
Corrosives and caustics	15	13	16	22
Noxious foodstuffs and poisonous plants	3	5	6	6
Other and unspecified solid and liquid substances	781	752	1029	846
Total other substances	1239	1274	1562	1322
Total	3683	5016	4694	4161

[a]Adapted from Mortality Statistics (1978).

Table 2 Type of Poisoning—General Categories

Product	Total cases	Accidental ingestion	Kicks, trip	Inhalation	Other	Unknown	Self-poisoning			
							Self-poisoning	Unknown intent	Gesture	Suicide intent
Medicines	71,495	42,118	2,811	68	1,061	6,537	18,900	7,600	5,102	6,198
Internal[b]	60,398	32,143	2,703	28	903	5,953	18,668	7,468	5,056	6,144
Aspirin[b]	5,234	4,039	13	1	21	316	844	339	304	201
Other[b]	55,164	28,104	2,690	27	882	5,637	17,824	7,129	4,752	5,943
External[b]	11,097	9,975	108	40	158	584	232	132	46	54
Cleaning and polishing agents	18,050	16,093	31	610	52	952	312	157	57	98
Petroleum products	4,659	4,021	24	117	24	427	46	21	9	16
Cosmetics	10,908	10,492	26	15	293	56	30	9	17	
Pesticides	8,836	6,527	6	958	517	626	202	97	24	81
Gases and vapors	1,418	171	4	1,219	—	17	7	1	1	5
Plants	12,946	11,627	552	4	24	687	52	33	7	12
Turpentine, paint, etc.	5,899	5,010	79	395	24	340	51	23	9	19
Miscellaneous	11,780	7,943	465	459	1,980	802	131	79	19	41
Unknown	1,286	420	59	11	14	338	444	259	58	127
Total	147,277	104,422	4,057	3,867	3,711	11,019	20,201	8,292	5,295	6,614

[a]Adapted from listing by the National Clearinghouse for Poison Control Centers (1978).
[b]These totals are included in medicines.

Table 3   Deaths of Children under 5 Years of Age from Accidental Poisonings[a]

Poison	1973	1974	1975	1976
Antibiotics and other anti-infectives	4	0	3	3
Hormones and synthetic substitutes	0	0	0	1
Systemic and hematologic agents	14	7	6	10
Analgesics and antipyretics	37	32	24	29
(Salicylate and congeners)	(26)	(24)	(17)	(25)
Sedatives and hypnotics	6	3	3	1
(Barbiturates)	(5)	(2)	(2)	(1)
Autonomic nervous system and psychotherapeutic drugs	16	11	11	10
(Tranquilizers)	(3)	(6)	(1)	(1)
Central nervous system depressants and stimulants	3	1	0	0
(Amphetamines)	(0)	(0)	(0)	(0)
Cardiovascular drugs	3	5	4	4
Gastrointestinal drugs	6	6	3	1
Other and unspecified drugs and medicants	13	16	11	5
Total drugs	102	81	65	64
Alcohol	0	2	1	2
Cleaning and polishing agents	6	6	7	8
Disinfectants	0	0	0	0
Paints and varnishes	1	0	0	0
Petroleum products and other solvents	16	20	21	12
Pesticides, fertilizers, or plant foods	10	13	6	6
Heavy metals (and their fumes)	4	6	2	3
Corrosives and caustics	3	3	4	7
Noxious foodstuffs and poisonous plants	1	1	0	1
Other and unspecified solid and liquid substances	6	3	8	2
Total	149	1135	114	41

[a]Adapted from Mortality Statistics (1978).

Table 4   Plants (Excluding Mushrooms and Toadstools): Under 5 Years of Age, 1976

Name	Cases	Percent of total category	Symptom	Hospital-izations
Philodendron	740	8.1	45	1
Yew	359	4.0	8	1
Dieffenbachia	318	3.5	58	0
Holly berries	306	3.4	4	1
Pyracantha	260	2.9	7	0
Poinsettia	233	2.6	7	0
Pokeweed	222	2.4	13	1
Woody nightshade	183	2.0	5	2
African violets	178	2.0	2	0
Jerusalem cherry	174	1.9	3	1
Black elder	151	1.7	2	1
Begonia	128	1.4	5	0
Total plants in category	9085	100	417	35

[a]Adapted from listing by the National Clearinghouse of Poison Control Center (1978).

HOUSEHOLD CHEMICALS

Alkalies

Source of Exposure   Concentrated lye, sodium carbonate (washing soda), detergents, dishwashing products, and oven cleaners are available in the home (Durham, 1979; Temple and Veltri, 1979; Grant, 1983).

Acute Toxicity   Severe irritation of the eyes, mucous membranes, skin, various dermatoses. Eye irritation cause disintegration and sloughing of the conjunctival and corneal epithelium, corneal opacification, marked edema, ulceration, and symblepharon. Inhalation induces nasal irritation and severe pneumonitis. On the skin, severe burns, deep ulceration, and loss of hair occur. Ingestion produces severe abdominal pain, and corrosion of the lips, mouth, tongue, and pharynx, with vomiting of the mucosa. Absorbed via the eyes, skin, and intestinal tract.

Chronic Toxicity   Esophageal stricture, skin scarring, and permanent corneal opacification.

Duration of Symptoms   Usually lasts for 7–13 days when recovery begins.

Pathology   A distinctive liquifaction and dissolution of the tissue with subsequent scarring.

Diagnosis History of exposure with nasal irritation, pneumonitis, severe burns of the eyes and skin, with temporary loss of hair. Must be differentiated from other types of conjunctivitis, mucous-membrane irritation, allergies, viral or bacterial pneumonia, and cardiogenic pulmonary edema.

Treatment Removal from exposure, flushing eyes and skin with water, use of an antibiotic ointment to prevent ocular adhesions, pulmonary edema requires hospitalization. For ingestion use diluted vinegar or fruit juice, followed by a demulscent, milk, eggs, or gelatin, followed by stomach emptying where possible. A stomach tube is contraindicated because of the possibility of penetration of the abdomen.

Concentrated Acid

Source of Exposure Acid solutions used for cleaning brick or bathroom fixtures or industrially as a gas (Durham, 1979; Grant, 1983).

Acute Toxicity Ingestion causes burns in the mouth, esophagus, and stomach, with pain, nausea, and vomiting. Inhalation causes coughing, burning in the throat, choking sensation, inflammation of the nose, throat, and eyes, laryngeal spasm, and pulmonary edema. Skin exposure causes burns and possible dermatitis. Absorbed orally, by inhalation, and via the skin.

Chronic Toxicity Prolonged exposure to diluted solutions causes dermatitis and tooth erosion.

Duration of Symptoms From 7 to 14 days, depending on the route of exposure.

Pathology Dehydration of the tissue, yellowing of the skin with HNO_3, and charring with H_2SO_4.

Diagnosis History of exposure with skin, eye, and throat irritation, coughing, inflammation, and ulceration of the nose, throat, and larynx, burning in the throat, choking sensation, burning of the eyes and skin, dermatitis, laryngeal spasm, and pulmonary edema. Must be differentiated from upper-respiratory viral infection with fever, myalgias, and lymphocytosis; bronchiogenic pneumonia, cardiogenic pulmonary edema, and adult respiratory distress syndrome.

Treatment Flush eyes and skin with water and for pulmonary complications use 60–100% oxygen inhalation with intubation and mechanical ventilation and positive and expiratory pressure breathing. Inflammation of the lung is treated with a short course of steroids. For ingestion give milk of magnesia along with demulscents.

Fluorides

Source of Exposure   Sodium fluoride in pesticides and rodenticides and sodium fluosilicate and sodium fluoroacetate in rodenticides (Chenoweth et al., 1951; Lidbeck et al., 1943).

Acute Toxicity   Symptoms from fluoride include gastralia, nausea, vomiting, tetany, muscular weakness and fasciculations, collapse, and myocardial failure. Fluoroacetate cause hypoglycemia, restlessness, anxiety, nausea, vomiting, muscular spasms, pulsus alternans, premature systoles, epileptiform seizures, and death by ventricular fibrillation. Both fluoride and fluoroacetate are absorbed orally.

Chronic Toxicity   Fluoride symptoms include mottled and brittle teeth, anorexia, dense bones, loss of weight and strength, and pain in legs and back. Sensitive individuals have eczema, atopic dermatitis, and urticaria.

Duration of Symptoms   Death may occur in the first hour or after several hours.

Pathology   The blood fails to clot, fatty and parenchymatous degeneration of the liver and kidneys, ulcerated and inflammed gastric mucosa, lung congestion, premature rigor mortis, and hard bones.

Diagnosis   History of ingestion, chemical identification of the poison, check for increased fluoride in the tissues and increased density of the long bones.

Treatment   Cause emesis or do a gastric lavage, give milk or calcium salts to combine with the fluoride. In chronic poisoning, stop the ingestion of fluoride, use special care on the teeth, and give milk and calcium salts. In fluoroacetate poisoning, give sodium glycerol monoacetate at 0.15 g/lb body weight intramuscularly distributed over several injection sites and procainamide or phenytoin at 100–500 mg intravenously followed by 0.5–1 g orally every 4–6 h.

Oxalate

Source of Exposure   Oxalic acid-containing drain cleaners; ink and stain removers; rhubarb, spinach, sorrel, and other sour grasses (Thienes and Haley, 1972).

Acute Toxicity   Symptoms include gastric irritation, burning pain, nausea, vomiting, hypocalcemia, hyperirritability of the central nervous system and skeletal muscles, clonic seizures, fibrillary twitching, suppression of urine; oxalate crystals in the ureter and bladder cause hematuria and pain. Absorbed from the intestinal tract.

Chronic Toxicity   Stones in the urinary tract.

Duration of Symptoms Lasts as long as exposure continues.

Pathology Erosions in the mouth, esophagus, and stomach, with reddening of the mucosa, and oxalate crystals in the kidney tubules.

Diagnosis History of ingestion, presence of oxalate crystals in the urine, and hypocalcemia with its accompanying symptoms. Must be differentiated from idiopathic epilepsy, hypertensive encephalopathy, various causes of hypocalcemia, uremia, prophyria, hypoxic encephalopathy, viral encephalitis, various nephroses, intrinsic renal disease, toxic nephroses, glomerulonephritis, chronic pyelonephritis, allergic reactions, diabetes, collagen vascular disease, cancer, and diseases altering renal hemodynamics.

Treatment Give calcium-containing foods, various calcium salts, wash out the stomach or give an emetic to remove residural oxalate. Use diazepam or phenobarbital to counteract the convulsions, and maintain the fluid and electrolyte balance in the presence of oliguria and anuria.

Phenols

Sources of Exposure Disinfectants and cleaning solutions, skin medications, sera, vaccines, and inks (Deichmann et al., 1952).

Acute Toxicity Symptoms include dark-colored urine, mucous-membrane whitening; skin numbness followed by reddening and necrosis; vomiting, dizziness, delirium, convulsions, collapse, loss of consciousness, fever or hypothermia, labored breathing, oliguria, stimulation followed by depression of the central nervous system, myocardial depression, and glomerular and tubular degeneration in the kidney. Absorbed orally and via the skin and lungs.

Chronic Toxicity Similar to acute but caused by lesser amounts of phenols over extended periods; also causes deposition of a dark pigment in the skin.

Duration of Symptoms Death may occur early from seizures or respiratory or circulatory failure or may be delayed several days, resulting in hepatic and renal failure.

Pathology At point of application, irritation may vary from hyperemia to necrosis and sloughing; esophagus appears to be tanned; cerebral edema and cardiac dilatation. Glomerular and tubular degeneration and central hepatic necrosis result from systemic poisoning.

Diagnosis History of exposure with phenolic breath, whitening of oral cavity, oliguria, albuminura; eye, nose, and throat irritation; anorexia, weight loss, weakness, muscle ache and pain, dark urine, cyanosis, coma, seizures, hepatic and renal damage, skin burns, dermatitis, and ochrnosis. Must be differentiated from various other conditions causing seizures, jaundice, viral hepatitis, liver abscess, liver tumor, alcoholic liver disease, pancreatic tumors, gallstones, hemolytic anemia, and bile-duct carcinoma.

Treatment Flush skin and eyes with water to remove irritant; control seizures with diazepam or phenobarbital; use a demulscent in oral ingestions; wash stomach repeatedly with 25% bicarbonate solution to remove phenol. The use of ethanol is contraindicated, as it increases phenol absorption.

Bleaches

Source of Exposure Household bleach containing 5% sodium hypochlorite (Grant, 1983).

Acute Toxicity Symptoms include corrosion of the skin and mucous membranes, vomiting, coughing, choking, lethargy, coma, hyperthermia, rapid pulse and respiration, hypotension, audible rales and rhonchi, clonic seizures, cicatricial injury to the stomach, esophageal stricture, ulcerative esophagitis; pain and inflammation of the mouth, pharynx, esophagus and stomach; mucous-membrane erosion, cold and clammy skin, cyanosis, confusion, delirium; edema of the pharynx, glottis, and larynx, with stridor and obstruction, mediastinitis, or peritonitis. Inhalation of hypochlorous acid fumes causes respiratory-tract irritation and pulmonary edema. Skin contact results in vesicular eruptions and eczematoid dermatitis. Absorbed orally.

Chronic Toxicity Shows the above pulmonary and dermal reaction.

Duration of Symptoms From 19 h to several days.

Pathology Focal necrosis; hemorrhage and superfacial erosion of the gastric mucosa, acute tracheobronchitis, obstructive atelectasis, bronchial exudation, esophageal ulceration, and strictures of the esophagus and stomach.

Diagnosis History of exposure and an empty bleach bottle.

Treatment Wash the skin with large amounts of water. In cases of ingestion, give demulscents (milk, egg white, starch paste, milk of magnesia); 1% sodium thiosulfate will neutralize the hypochlorite, opiates will control the pain, and intravenous fluids will control shock. Under no circumstances should sodium bicarbonate solution be given, as it releases carbon dioxide, and acidic antidotes are also contraindicated.

Solvents

Source of Exposure Charcoal starter, lighter fluid, pain thinner, gasoline, and kerosene are available in most households (Gerarde, 1960).

Acute Toxicity Symptoms include skin and mucous-membrane irritation, transient euphoria, burning sensation in the chest, headache, tinnitus, nausea, weakness, restlessness, incoordination, confusion, disorientation, drowsiness, coma, seizures, cyanosis of the extremities, ventricular fibrillation, respiratory arrest; burning sensation in the mouth, esophagus, and stomach, vomiting, eructation, bloody diarrhea; with aspiration, rapid breathing, cyanosis, tachycardia, low-grade fever, basilar rales, massive pulmonary edema, pneumonic hemorrhage, infection, pneumonia, cardiac dilatation, hepatosplenomegaly, albuminuria with casts and cells, atrial fibrillation–flutter, and cardiac failure. Absorbed orally or by inhalation.

Chronic Toxicity See glue sniffing.

Duration of Symptoms From hours to weeks.

Pathology Degenerative lesions in the liver, kidneys, bone marrow, and spleen; fatty infiltration of the liver and myocardium, pulmonary lesions, and pulmonary edema.

Diagnosis History of exposure and a hydrocarbon breath along with symptoms described under acute toxicity.

Treatment Give activated charcoal or mineral oil to entrap the hydrocarbons; emetics and gastric lavage are contraindicated; central depression is treated with nikethamide; pulmonary bacterial invasion is treated with antibiotics and pulmonary edema with positive-pressure oxygen therapy.

Household Plants

Many household plants contain various alkaloids, glycosides, and neutral principles that are extremely toxic when ingested by young children. Symptoms produced by such agents will be discussed based on Table 4 from the Bulletin of Poison Control Centers (1978).

Cyanogenic Glycosides

Source of Exposure Ingestion of the berries of chokeberry. (*Prunus virginiana* or *caroliniana*) or the shoots, leaves, bark, or roots of black elder (*Sambucus canadensis*) (Radeleff, 1970; Thienes and Haley, 1972).

Acute Toxicity   These plants produce cyanide toxicity with the following symptoms: corrosion of the upper alimentary tract, especially the stomach, inactivation of oxidative enzymes, formation of cyanohemoglobin, reflex stimulation of respiration, headache, ataxia, mental confusion, cyanosis, coma, asphyxial seizures, involuntary micturition and defecation, mydriasis, vomiting, decreased then increased pulse rate, and death. Absorbed orally.

Chronic Toxicity   Seldom occurs because one exposure cause lack of interest in such plants.

Duration of Symptoms   Death can occur in the first half hour or recovery in a few hours.

Pathology   Marked irritation and reddening of the stomach, reddening of the lungs, and degeneration of the central nervous system, including the corpus callosum and substantia nigra.

Diagnosis   The plant parts must be identified to establish the causative agent; "peach-pit" odor of the vomitus, bright-red venous blood, and cyanosis. Must be differentiated from other forms of asphyxia and insulin poisoning.

Treatment   Gastric lavage or administration of an emetic to remove offending agent, inhalation of amyl nitrite, wash stomach with 5% sodium thiosulfate. In serious cases, give 0.2 g of sodium nitrite in 50 ml sterile distilled water intravenously over a 2- to 3-min period followed by 10–20 g of sodium thiosulfate in 50 ml water over a 5-min period (Chen and Rose, 1956).

Castor Beans

Source of Exposure   Ingestion of the beans of *Ricinus communis*, which contain the toxic protein ricin (Balint, 1974).

Acute Toxicity   Symptoms include nausea, headache, general malaise, somnolence, loss of consciousness, clonic seizures, bloody diarrhea with tenesmus, thirst, dehydration, cyanosis, hypotension, changes in the electrocardiogram (ECG), asthmatic symptoms, exanthema, liver necrosis, nephritis, proteinuria, rise in excretion of nonprotein nitrogen, conjuctivitis, mydriasis, optic-nerve lesion, changes in biological data and death. Absorbed orally.

Chronic Toxicity   None reported as death occurs acutely.

Duration of Symptoms   First symptoms appear in 12 h and death occurs after 48 h.

Pathology   Bleeding in serous membranes, hemorrhages in the stomach and intestine; degenerative changes in the heart, liver, and kidneys; infiltration of the lymph nodes, changes in the spleenic lymphoid elements, and extensive hemorrhages in the myocardium.

Diagnosis   History of seed ingestion and positive identification of seed parts and destruction of lymphoid cells. Effects on the intestine must be differentiated from typhoid fever and arsenic.

Treatment   Gastric lavage or use of an emetic to remove residual poison, followed by antiricin antiserum and symptomatic therapy.

Cardiac Glycosides

Source of Exposure   Ingestion of the flowers, leaves, or seeds of foxglove (*Digitalis purpurea*) or oleander (*Nerium oleander*) (Dimond, 1957; Dubnow and Burchell, 1965; Soderman, 1965).

Acute Toxicity   Symptoms include vomiting, bradycardia, heart block, inverted T-wave with a prolonged PR interval and depressed ST segment of the ECG, ventricular tachycardia with marked irregularity, extrasystoles, coupled rhythm and atrial tachycardia with block, purging, abdominal pain, yellow or green vision with an inability to see blue, central scotoma, depression, confusion, memory defects, delirium, psychosis, headache, drowiness, anorexia, rarely seizures, vertigo, muscular weakness, and death by ventricular fibrillation. Absorbed orally.

Chronic Toxicity   Same as acute.

Duration of Symptoms   Death can occur after 2 h or longer but recovery can occur in 24 h.

Pathology   Severe poisoning may cause myocardial hemorrhage, necrosis, fragmentation of heart muscle fibers, cellular infiltration, and fibrosis.

Diagnosis   History of plant ingestion with positive identification of plant parts. Vomiting, bradycardia, heartblock with inverted T-wave with prolonged PR interval and depressed ST segment of the ECG are pathognomic of cardiac glycoside poisoning. Must be differentiated from coronary artery obstruction.

Treatment Depletion of myocardial potassium may be counteracted by giving KCl orally in doses of 2 g 3–5 times daily or in severe case intravenously at doses of 40 mEq slowly over 1–2 h with ECG monitoring. When symptoms of digitalis intoxication cease or the T-waves peak, KCl administration must be stopped. Myocardial irritability can be reduced with oral or subcutaneous administration of 0.1–1g quinidine sulfate, or oral procainamide at 0.5–1 g every 4–6 h of intravenously at 100 mg/min or phenytoin at 25 mg/min until the arrhythmia is partially controlled, then orally at 100 mg at periods of 4–8 h.

Conine

Source of Exposure Ingestion of poison hemlock (*Conium maculatum*) or fool's parsley (*Ethusa cyanapium*) (Bowman and Sanghvi, 1963).

Acute Toxicity Symptoms include dizziness, nausea, cold perspiration, vomiting, pallor, excitement, general weakness, purging, bradycardia or tachycardia, increased cardiac output, mental confusion, seizures, pronounced paralysis of the motor nerve ends, and asphyxia from paralysis of both the central and peripheral nerves of respiration. Absorbed orally.

Chronic Toxicity Has not been reported.

Duration of Symptoms Death may occur with 0.5 h or in 3–12 h; severe symptoms disappear within 24 h.

Pathology Congestion of the brain and abdominal viscera as a result of asphyxia.

Diagnosis Difficult unless plant parts can be identified.

Treatment Gastric lavage with 1:1000 potassium permanganate, hot drinks, external heat, and symptomatic treatment with artificial respiration and oxygen.

Several other household and ornamental plants will be discussed briefly to call attention to their poisonous properties. Treatment is supportive (Wyeth Laboratories, 1966).

The juices of dumb cane (*Deffenbachia seguine*) and elephant's ear (*Colocasia antiquorum*) contain microscopic needles of calcium exalate, which cause dermatitis and, on ingestion, marked irritation and swelling of the tongue and oral mucosa and possible paralysis of the vocal cords.

Pyracantha has thorns whose tips break off upon penetrating the skin and cause festering wounds.

Poinsettia (*Euphorbis pulcherrima*) upon ingestion of the juice of the leaves, stems, or flowers, causes vomiting, diarrhea, abdominal cramps, and possibly delirium. The sap caused skin irritation and, if rubbed into the eyes, temporary blindness.

Pokeweed (*Phytolacca americana*) upon ingestion of the roots, leaves, fruit, or seeds, causes a burning sensation in the mouth, intestinal cramps, vomiting, diarrhea, visual disturbances, and weakened pulse and respiration.

Woody nightshade (various species of *Solanum*) contains the alkaloids solanidine and solaneine, which cause confusion, cardiac depression, clammy skin, and death if ingested.

Mistletoe (*Phoradendron flavescens*) upon ingestion of its berries, causes acute gastroenteritis and cardiovascular collapse.

Christmas rose (*Helleborus niger*) contains helleborin and helleborein, which cause a burning sensation in the mouth, throat, esophagus, and stomach; and nausea, vomiting, muscular weakness, bradycardia, hypotension, and a curare-like paralysis of skeletal muscle with respiratory failure.

Monkshood (*Aconitum napellus*) contains the alkaloid aconitine, which causes a numbing sensation of the lips and tongue, bradycardia, dimmed vision, irregular breathing, and death.

Autumn crocus (*Colchicum autumnale*) bulbs and seeds contain colchicine, which, upon ingestion, causes severe abdominal pain, nausea, vomiting, profuse watery bloody diarrhea, hematuria, oliguria, rapid and weak pulse, ascending paralysis of the central nervous system, and death by respiratory paralysis.

Larkspur (*Delphinium* sp.) young plants and seeds contain diterpenoid alkaloids, which produce digestive upset, excitement followed by depression of the central nervous system, and death.

Yew (various species of *Taxus*) contains alkaloids in the seed that cause nausea, vomiting, diarrhea, myocardial depression, difficult respiration, and circulatory failures.

AGRICULTURAL CHEMICALS

Cholinesterase Inhibitors

Source of Exposure   In formulation of sprays and dusts, inhalation of dusts and sprays, and by ingestion of chemicals used in the home and agriculture (Haley, 1956; DuBois, 1958; Holmstedt, 1959; Nishimura and Tamura, 1967; Hayes, 1975).

Acute Toxicity   Symptoms include inactivation of plasma, erythrocyte, and brain cholinesterase; cutaneous flushing, profuse sweating, colic, salivation, nausea, dizziness, bronchioconstriction, increased bronchial-gland secretion, increased respiration rates, asthma, lacrimation, vomiting, purging, intense noises, myopia, loss of accommodation for far vision, pain in the eyeballs, micturation, prostration, seizures, collapse, hypotension, bradycardia, and myocardia stoppage. Lowering of brain cholinesterase causes muscular weakness and paralysis of legs, arms, back, and diaphragm. The fluoridated antiesterases cause permanent brain damage. The carbamates are reversible anticholinesterases, whereas the phosphates are not. Absorbed by inhalation, ingestion, or via the skin.

Chronic Toxicity Causes disseminating demyelation of the motor nerves.

Duration of Symptoms Several hours to days, depending on regeneration of cholinesterases.

Pathology Findings of asphyxia, pulmonary edema, increased bronchial mucus, hemorrhagic bowels, miosis, and myocardial dilatation.

Diagnosis History of exposure, lowered blood cholinesterase coupled with the above acute symptoms.

Treatment Organophosphates require injection of atropine sulfate at 0.5 mg intravenously or 1 mg subcutaneously repeated every 15 min until pupils dilate, heart rate increases, and intestinal spasms cease. In addition, give 1 g pralidoxime in 200 ml saline repeated once in 3–6 h. This latter chemical is contraindicated in carbamate poisoning. General supportive measures include maintenance of body temperature, suction to remove bronchial secretions, and oxygen with positive-pressure breathing.

Triorthocresylphosphate

Source of Exposure Contaminated cooking oil, hydraulic fluid, lubricant additive, flame retardant, and plasticizer cause home and occupational exposure (Cavangagh, 1973; Ishikawa, 1973; Johnson, 1975).

Acute Toxicity After ingestion, symptoms include stomach irritation, burning and colicky pain in the abdomen, nausea, vomiting, and, after 3–4 days, tingling in the extremities, gradual motor paralysis of the legs, footdrop, wrist-drop, loss of plantar and Achilles reflexes, wasting of the interosseous muscles, and loss of ability to support the weight of the body. Absorbed orally and by inhalation.

Chronic Toxicity None reported because most exposures are acute.

Duration of Symptoms Usually from 3 to 4 days.

Pathology Degeneration of myelin sheaths of the motor nerve fibers, chromatolysis, and pyknotic changes in the anterior horn cells and degenerative changes in the affected muscles.

Diagnosis History of exposure; the acute toxic symptoms must be differentiated from the flaccid paralysis produced by ethanol, lead, arsenic, poliomyelitis, botulism, and other diseases of the nervous system.

Treatment The delay in symptoms results in damage long after absorption; thus only supportative treatment can be undertaken.

Rotenone

Source of Exposure   Spraying crops and living areas (Haley, 1978b).

Acute Toxicity   Symptoms include dermatitis, conjuctivitis, pharyngitis, rhinitis, numbness of mucous membranes, nausea, and vomiting in humans, and respiratory stimulation, seizures, respiratory depression, coma, and respiratory failure in animals. Absorbed orally.

Chronic Toxicity   None reported for humans, but causes central lobular hepatic necrosis, suppression of growth, and renal injury in animals.

Duration of Symptoms   As long as exposure continues.

Pathology   No information on humans, but animals show central lobular hepatic necrosis and renal damage.

Diagnosis   History of exposure with mucous-membrane numbness, nausea, vomiting, and tremors. Must be differentiated from other chemical intoxications and disease entities causing similar symptoms.

Treatment   Removal from contaminated area and clothing, thorough washing of the skin particularly the genital region and the use of antihistamines orally and as ointments.

Piperonyl Butoxide

Source of Exposure   From use as a pesticide on containers for foods and as a household spray (Haley, 1978a).

Acute Toxicity   Symptoms include ocular irritation with edema of the eyelids, lachrimation, hyperemia of the blood of the cornea, reddening of the skin with roughening, thickening, and cracking of the epidermis, temporary weight loss, pancytopenia, thrombocytopenia, leukopenia, polycythemia, and unspecified anemias. Absorbed orally, dermally, and by inhalation.

Chronic Toxicity   No information available.

Duration of Symptoms   From hours to 1 week.

Pathology   None reported for humans, but animals show gastrointestinal hemorrhages, bloody fluid in the thoracid cavity, and splenomegaly.

Diagnosis   History of exposure, but must be differentiated from other chemicals producing similar irritations and from allergies.

Treatment Nonspecific as condition clears spontaneously when exposure is terminated; however, antihistamines may be useful to counteract the skin problems.

Chlorophenothane or DDT

Source of Exposure From use as an agricultural and household pesticide by ingestion of concentrated solutions. Banned in the United States but still used for malarial control throughout the world (Haley, 1956; Princi, 1957; Hayes, 1975).

Acute Toxicity Symptoms include tiredness, heaviness, and aching of the limbs, headache, paresthesia of the tongue, lips, and face, nervous irritability, apprehension, mental sluggishness, dizziness, disturbance of equilibrium, confusion, mydriasis, loss of vibratory sense of fingers and toes, tremors, nausea, vomiting, muscle fibrillations, clonic and tonic seizures, coma, and fever. Solutions absorbed by ingestion, inhalation, and dermally.

Chronic Toxicity Causes anorexia, hepatic necrosis, and inanition.

Duration of Symptoms From several hours to days.

Pathology Central lobular hepatic necrosis and swelling, vacuolization, tigrolysis, renal degeneration, and fine basophilic reticulation of the cytoplasm of the cells of the brain and spinal cord.

Diagnosis History of exposure and identification of DDT and its metabolites in urine or tissues; must be differentiated from other chemicals causing hepatic and renal lesions and seizures.

Treatment For cutaneous exposure, remove contaminated clothing and wash skin with soap and water. For ingestion, give an emetic or lavage with saline followed by a saline cathartic. Convulsions should be controlled with diazepam or pentobarbital intravenously.

2,4-D or 2,4-Dichlorophenoxyacetic Acid

Source of Exposure Spraying operation or accidental or purposeful ingestion (Young and Haley, 1977; Hall, 1983).

Acute Toxicity Symptoms include peripheral neuropathy, ataxia, reflex disorders, damage to the peripheral and central nervous systems, fibrillary twitching, paralysis of the intercostal muscles, skeletal-muscle damage; elevated SGOT, SGPT, lactic dehydrogenase, aldolase, and creatine phosphokinase; hemaglobulinuria, myoglobulinuria, and death. Absorbed by ingestion, inhalation, or dermally.

Chronic Toxicity   Any of the acute symptoms, but mostly nervous system damage.

Duration of Symptoms   May persist for 3 months.

Diagnosis   History of exposure, fibrillary muscle twitching, and elevation of the above enzymes, but must be differentiated from other intoxications producing the same symptoms.

Treatment   Remove from the contaminated area, remove contaminated clothing, use gastric lavage to remove residue from the stomach, artificial respiration or oxygen to counteract intercostal muscle paralysis, then symptomatic therapy.

Paraquat

Source of Exposure   Ingestion of granulated or liquid formulations and inhalation of aerosols during spraying (Autor, 1977; Haley, 1979; Bismuth et al., 1982).

Acute Toxicity   Symptoms include ocular irritation followed in 1 week by extensive loss of the bulbar conjunctiva of the globe and tarsal conjunctiva of both eyelids, reactive anterior uveitis, corneal edema, stenosis of both lower puncta, obstruction of the canaliculi, and loss of visual activity. Effects of the finger nails consist of transverse white bands of discoloration, loss of surface, transverse ridging, gross deformity of the nail plate, and nail loss. Effects on the skin are contact dermatitis, erythema, violaceous erythema, encrustations, bullae, edema, and exudative intertrigo. Symptoms from ingestion include jaundice, epigastric pain; excoriation of the lips, mouth, and fauces, decreased urine output, pulmonary interstitial edema, respiratory distress, toxic myocarditis, and death from pulmonary fibrosis. Inhalation produces similar effects. Absorbed orally, dermally and by inhalation.

Chronic Toxicity   No reports because of acute fatalities.

Duration of Symptoms   From hours to weeks usually ending fatally.

Pathology   Inflammation of the larynx, trachea and bronchi, lungs voluminous and solid with hemorrhages and edema fluid, lungs airless with heavy fibroblastic proliferation in the alveolar walls; diffuse polymorphonuclear, mononuclear, macrophage and eosinophilic infiltration; gland-like structures in the epithelium of the terminal bronchi, centrolobular degeneration of the liver, tubular degeneration and ischemic glomerular degeneration in the kidney and myocarditis.

Diagnosis   History of exposure and the symptoms given under acute toxicity.

Treatment   Wash the eyes with water, use chloramphenical ointment and 1% atropine drops to permit ocular tissues and eyelids to heal and syringe lacrimal ducts to cure epiphora. After ingestion, use gastric lavage with repeated administration of suspensions of Fuller's earth or bentonite to reduce body burden of paraquat and forced diuresis with mannitol. Predinsone, 1 gm/day, has proved useful. Presently there is no antidote for the pulmonary complications of paraquat intoxication and peritoneal or hemodialysis or hemoperfusion have been unsuccessful. Oxygen therapy is contraindicated because this only increases the pulmonary production of hydrogen peroxide and a long-lived dihydroderivative of paraquat.

DRUGS OF ABUSE

Amphetamines

Source of Exposure   Prescription drugs and illicit street drugs (Connell, 1958; Costa and Garattini, 1970).

Acute Toxicity   Symptoms include restlessness, dizziness, tremor, hyperactive reflexes, talkativeness, tenseness, irritability, insomnia, confusion, assaultiveness, increased libido, anxiety, delirium, hallucinations, panic states, suicidal or homicidal tendencies occur, fatigue, central depression, headache, chilliness, pallor, flushing, palpitation, cardiac arrhythmias, anginal pain, hypertension, hypotension, circulatory collapse, sweating, dry mouth, metallic taste, anorexia, nausea, vomiting, diarrhea, abdominal cramps, seizures, and coma. Absorbed orally or intravenously.

Chronic Toxicity   All of the above with toxic psychoses, abnormal mental phenomena, marked weight loss and dermatitis.

Duration of Symptoms   Acute symptoms persist for 2 h or more and chronic symptoms persist for 2 or 3 weeks after withdrawal. The amphetamines cause physical and psychological addiction and show cross-tolerance to each other, and there is a withdrawal syndrome.

Pathology   Main finding is cerebral hemorrhages.

Diagnosis   History of amphetamine consumption; finding them and their metabolites in the urine; and any of the above acute symptoms, but they must be differentiated from cocaine poisoning.

Treatment   Gastric lavage or emetic to remove drug from the stomach; paraldehyde, barbiturates, or phenothiazine tranquilizers will counteract the central nervous system excitation, and nitroglycerine or sodium nitrite will reduce the hypertension.

Cocaine

Source of Exposure   Alkaloid extracted from *Erythoxylon coca* and sold in the illicit drug market (Goodman and Gilman, 1965).

Acute Toxicity   Symptoms include garrulousness, anxiety, nausea, vomiting, pallor, pupillary dilations, headache, tremors, clonic and tonic seizures, cold sweat, hypotension, weak and rapid pulse, and respiratory failure. Absorbed by insufflation and intravenously.

Chronic Toxicity   Symptoms include emaciation, facial pallor, sunken eyes, tremor, mydriasis, anorexia, and mental and moral deterioration. Sniffing cocaine causes ulceration and perforation of the nasal septum.

Duration of Symptoms   Death occurs within 2–30 min after acute symptoms develop. Recovery may occur in 1–2 h.

Pathology   Cardiac dilatation, signs of asphyxia and malnutrition.

Diagnosis   Evidence of taking the drug necessary; identification of the drug or its metabolites in the urine is of assistance. The seizure phase must be differentiated from epilepsy.

Treatment   Intravenous injection of a short-acting barbiturate to control the seizures and artificial respiration to maintain blood oxygenation. Speed is essential because cocaine can cause death from respiratory paralysis before the physician realizes what is happening.

Lysergic Acid Diethylamide, LSD-25

Source of Exposure   Ingestion of a street drug synthetized from ergot (Cohen, 1964; Eveloff, 1968).

Acute Toxicity   Symptoms include hallucinations of form, color, time, and space; depersonalization, restlessness, vertigo, nausea, sweating, hyperpyrexia, hypotension, paresthesia, increased rate of respiration, mydriasis, dryness of the mouth, and serious psychotic episodes. Absorbed via the intestinal tract.

Chronic Toxicity   An acute episode can recur many months afterward without taking another dose. There is cross-tolerance to mescaline.

Duration of Symptoms   Up to 24 h.

Pathology   None reported.

Diagnosis   History of taking the drug essential because symptoms are similar to those from other hallucinogens.

Treatment   No specific treatment available, but phenothiazine tranquilizers will control the excitement phases of the hallucination.

Mescaline, Mescal Buttons, Peyote

Source of Exposure   Ingestion of the dried tops of the cactus *Lophophora williamsii* or the pure alkaloid mescaline (Alles, 1959; Hock et al., 1952).

Acute Toxicity   Symptoms include nausea, vomiting, anxiety, a feeling of a fear of dissolution, loss of time sense, occipital headache, visual illusions and hallucinations associated with beautiful colors, mydriasis, muscular relaxation, bradycardia, and a feeling of peace and contentment. Large doses produce rapid and shallow breathing, loose bloody stools, anesthesia, depression of the central nervous system, and death from respiratory paralysis. Absorbed orally.

Chronic Toxicity   Similar to acute but no physical dependence occurs.

Duration of Symptoms   Effects last up to 12 h.

Pathology   Signs of asphyxia.

Diagnosis   History of ingestion of the drug essential, but hallucinations, mydriasis, heightened reflexes, followed by depression and rapid and shallow respiration are suggestive. Must be differentiated from other hallucinogens.

Treatment   Remove residual drug by gastric lavage or with an emetic and treat symptomatically.

Cannabis Sativa, Marijuana, Hashish, 1-*trans*-Δ^9-Tetrahydrocannabinol

Source of Exposure   Smoking marijuana cigarettes, ingestion of cannabis resin or tetrahydrocannabinol (Wolstenholme, 1965; Daqirmann and Boyd, 1962; Bloomquist, 1968; Kolansky and Moore, 1971).

Acute Toxicity   Symptoms include generalized depression of the brainstem reticular formation and the primary sensory pathways, disorientation, and dissociation of personality; euphoria, emotional excitement, uncontrolled laughter, hallucinations, illusions, distorted sense of time and space, increased sensitivity to sound, feeling of a profound understanding of the meaning of things, loss of motor control, paresthesia, disturbed preception, violent or aggressive behavior, tachycardia, slight hypertension, conjunctival injection, increased blood sugar and appetite, urinary frequency, dryness of the mouth and throat, nausea, vomiting, and diarrhea. Absorbed by ingestion or inhaling the smoke.

Chronic Toxicity Tolerance develops but not physical dependence. Stopping intake causes restlessness, insomnia, and anorexia.

Duration of Symptoms Effects occur rapidly from inhaling the smoke but are of short duration; on ingestion, 30–60 min passes before effects occur, and they last for 3–5 h.

Pathology No characteristic changes reported.

Diagnosis History of smoking or ingestion of the drug required. Urinary analysis for tetrahydrocannabinol and its 7-OH and 11-OH metabolites is of assistance. Must be differentiated from other hallucinogens.

Treatment Gastric lavage or an emetic to remove ingested drug, followed by symptomatic treatment.

Methaqualone

Source of Exposure Prescription drug and street drug (Inaba et al., 1973; Pascarelli, 1973).

Acute Toxicity Symptoms include delirium, coma, restlessness, hypertonia, seizures, vomiting, increased secretions, aspiration pneumonitis, respiratory obstruction, cutaneous edema, pulmonary edema, hepatic damage, renal insufficiency, bleeding, shock, aplastic enemia, headache, fatigue, dizziness, transient paresthesia of the extremities, dry mouth, epigastric distress, diarrhea, diaphoresis, bromhidrosis, exanthema, urticaria, and respiratory arrest. Absorbed orally.

Chronic Toxicity All of the above plus psychological and physical dependence.

Duration of Symptoms Several hours to day, depending on the total dose ingested.

Pathology Acute cardiac failure, pneumonia, and terminal shock.

Diagnosis History of drug taking, empty bottle, and any of the signs of acute toxicity, particularly restlessness, hypertonia, and seizures. Must be differentiated from sedation produced by other drugs and grand mal seizures.

Treatment Empty stomach by lavage or an emetic, maintain adequate ventilation, support the blood pressure and give succinylcholine chloride to control the seizures. Analeptics are contraindicated.

Nutmeg

Source of Exposure Ingestion of the dried ground seeds of *Myristica fragrans,* which contain a volotile oil, myristicin (Weiss, 1960; Payne, 1963).

Acute Toxicity Symptoms include euphoria, heaviness of the limbs, dreamlike state, tachycardia, palpitations, dry mouth, thirst, agitation, hyperactivity, incoherent speech, redness of the face and shoulders, and drowsiness. Absorbed orally.

Chronic Toxicity Similar to acute.

Duration of Symptoms Twelve to 24 h.

Pathology Possible hepatic necrosis.

Diagnosis History of taking the spice essential. Must be differentiated from other hallucinogens.

Treatment Gastric lavage or emetic to remove spice from stomach, then symptomatic treatment.

Phencyclidine, PCP

Source of Exposure Ingestion or smoking of an illicit street drug (Liden et al., 1975; Tong et al., 1976; Eastman and Cohen, 1975; Hoogwerf et al., 1978; Pearlson, 1981; Castellani et al., 1982).

Acute Toxicity Symptoms include increased respiratory rate, hypertension, tachycardia, slight hyperthermia, nonresponse to verbal stimuli, disorientation in time and place, confusion, fearful, amnesic, agitated, excitement, combative, irritable, emotional lability, dysarthria, vocalizing, eyes open with ptosis, roving eye movements, bilateral, horizontal, and vertical nystagmus; decreased or absent corneal reflexes, facial grimacing, muscle tremors and twitching, generalized seizures, vomiting, diaphoresis, lacrimation, salivation, bronchorrhea, and coma. Absorbed orally, by inhalation, insufflation, and occasionally intravenously.

Chronic Toxicity All of the above along with tolerance requiring increased dosage and psychological dependence.

Duration of Symptoms From several hours to 15 days, depending on the dose.

Pathology Intracerebral hemorrhage, hypertensive encephalopathy, myoglobinuria, renal failure, and cardiovascular and respiratory failure.

Diagnosis Disorientation, agitation or excitement, blank stare, uncommunicative, gross ataxia, muscle rigidity, horizontal and vertical nystagmus, stupor, coma, hypertension, tachycardia, increased secretions, diaphoresis, generalized motor seizures, muscle tremors and twitching, opisthotonic posturing, decerebrate rigidity, and the presence of phencyclidine in the urine make a positive diagnosis. The absence of mydriasis and the presence of ataxia and nystagmus rule out CNS stimulants and LSD, and the presence or absence of respiratory depression, systolic and diastolic hypertension, and increased deep tendon reflexes differentiate PCP coma and stupor from a sedative overdose.

Treatment No specific agent is available, but seizures can be controlled by diazepam, 10–15 mg intravenously, followed by phenytoin. Control motor restlessness and agitation with repeated doses of diazepam, 10–15 mg orally. Hypertension may be reduced with diazoxide. Recently it has been shown that physostigmine, meperidine, and haloperidol can control many of the symptoms of PCP intoxication. Phenothiazine tranquilizers are contraindicated in acute intoxications, but they can be used to treat persistent psychoses.

Asthma Powder

Source of Exposure Ingestion of a teaspoonful or a triple zero capsule containing a powder composed of *Atropa belladonna* or *Datura stramonium* with their alkaloids; atropine, scopolamine, or hyoscyamine; or consumption of the seeds and leaves of jimson weed (Weintraub, 1960; Mikolich et al., 1975).

Acute Toxicity Symptoms include dryness of the mouth and throat, mydriasis with loss of accommodation for near vision, increased intraoccular pressure, tachycardia, flushing of the skin, talkativeness, restlessness, mental confusion, delirium, mania, seizures, hallucinations, amnesia, depression, exhaustion, and coma. Absorbed via the intestinal tract.

Chronic Toxicity Symptoms include mental confusion and hallucinations followed by recovery.

Duration of Symptoms Symptoms develop rapidly and persist for 3–7 days.

Pathology Changes due to asphyxia.

Diagnosis History of taking the mixture or presence of dark-green filled capsules along with flushed face, mydriasis, dry mucous membranes, and cerebral excitement or depression. Urinary analysis will indicate the alkaloids present. Must be differentiated from other hallucinogens.

Treatment   Gastric lavage to remove poison followed by charcoal to reduce absorption; sedation with short-acting barbiturates, chloral hydrate, or paraldehyde to control excitement phase, artificial respiration with oxygen for the depressed respiration, and ice bag and alcohol sponges to reduce temperature.

Glue Sniffing

Source of Exposure   Sniffing glue containing amyl and ethyl acetate, paint in spray cans, paint thinner, gasoline, and other solvents (Lawton and Malmquist, 1961; Glaser and Massengale, 1962).

Acute Toxicity   Symptoms include pleasant exhilaration, euphoria, excitement, ataxia, slurred speech, diplopia, tinnitus, drowsiness, stupor, and unconsciousness. Absorbed via the lungs.

Chronic Toxicity   All of the acute symptoms, and damage to the liver, kidneys, and hematopoietic system. Can lead to habituations, tolerance, and psychological dependence.

Duration of Symptoms   Depends upon the dose and may be from 12–24 h.

Pathology   Damage to the liver, kidneys, and hematopoietic system.

Diagnosis   History of use along with breath odor of solvent or traces of paint around the nose and mouth coupled with the above symptoms.

Treatment   Nonspecific using symptomatic and supportive measures.

Tolatile Nitrites

Source of Exposure   Diversion of amyl nitrite pearls or use of butyl and isobutyl nitrites (Haley, 1980).

Acute Toxicity   Symptoms include peripheral vasodilatation, irritation of the upper respiratory tract, tachycardia, reduced pulse pressure, hypotension, hypertension, flushing of the face, pulsation in the head, cyanosis, confusion, vertigo, motor unrest, weakness, yellow vision, fainting, shallow respiration; weak, slow, and irregular pulse; clammy skin, ocular hyperemia, corneal erosion, methemoglobinemia, increased intestinal peristalis, ashen grey skin, drowsiness, mydriasis, vasomotor collapse, syncope, and death by cardiovascular collapse. Absorbed by ingestion and inhalation.

Chronic Toxicity   All of the acute symptoms plus hypertrophy of the left ventricle, shortness of breath on exertion, development of tolerance on repeated use, trapping of the blood in the veins of the lower extremities and death from anoxia.

Duration of Symptoms Effects begin 30–60 sec after inhalation and in 5 min after ingestion and continue until nitrite ion is destroyed. Methemoglobinemia persists until hemoglobin returns to oxyhemoglobin.

Pathology Brownish blood from methemoglobinemia, signs of asphyxia, and liver and kidney degeneration.

Diagnosis History of drug use, blood analysis to identify methemoglobin, and urine analysis to identify nitrate. Differential diagnosis requires elimination of exposure to other methemoglobin formers: shoe dye, stove polish, acetanilide, or acetophenetidin consumption and aniline derivatives.

Treatment Intravenous injection of 50 ml of 1% methylene blue in 1.8% sodium sulfate every hour until 200 ml have been given or oral sodium ascorbate, 100–500 mg, 2–3 times daily. In the acute phase, oxygen inhalation may be required.

Poisonous Mushrooms

Source of Exposure Ingestion of *Amanita muscaria* containing bufotenin and muscarine, *Amanita phalloides* containing psilocin and psilocybin (Grossman and Malbin, 1954; Wassen, 1959; Wieland and Wieland, 1959; Puharich, 1959; McCawley et al., 1962; Paaso and Harrison, 1975).

Acute Symptoms Symptoms produced by *A. muscaria* include marked lacrimation, salivation, sweating, miosis, dyspnea, severe abdominal pain, frequent watery and painful bowel movements, cardiovascular collapse, vertigo, weakness, confusion, coma, and seizures. Symptoms produced by *A. phalloides* include severe abdominal pain, nausea, vomiting, diarrhea, bloody vomitus and stools, marked dehydration and thirst, oliguria or anuria, cyanosis, hypotension, feeble heart action, and coma. Symptoms produced by *Psilocybe* species include hallucinations and are similar to atropine.

Chronic Toxicity None reported because of the rapid toxicity of mushrooms.

Duration of Symptoms *Amanita muscaria* and *Psilocybe* species act in a few minutes to 2 h, while *A. phalloides* acts in 6–15 h and further symptoms in 2–3 days with death in 50–100% of the cases.

Pathology *Amanita phalloides* produces jaundice, acute yellow atrophy, and other degenerative changes in the liver and kidney degeneration.

Diagnosis   History of mushroom consumption with possible identification of plant parts obtained by gastric lavage and symptoms of muscarinic poisoning by *A. muscaria* and *Psilocybe* species. Delayed death, 5–8 days, occurs with *A. phalloides*.

Treatment   Immediate gastric lavage, atropine injections for *A. muscaria* intoxication, tranquilizers to control *Psilocybe* intoxication, and systematic and supportive treatment in *A. phalloides* intoxication. Atropine is contraindicated in *Psilocybe* intoxication.

PRINCIPLES OF ANTIDOTAL THERAPY

Antidotal therapy is based on the principle that another chemical is given to remove a toxin from its site(s) of action, enhance its excretion, and prevent tissue destruction and death. However, antidotes have deleterious properties of their own that may contribute to a fatal outcome. Such chemicals will be discussed, pointing out their physiological effects.

Miscellaneous Antidotal Substances

Dimercaprol   Braun et al. (1946); Modell et al. (1946); Stevenson et al. (1948); Langcope and Leutscher (1949).

Symptoms of toxicity include hypertension with tachycardia, nausea, vomiting; burning sensation of the lips, mouth, and throat; constriction in the throat, chest, and hands; conjunctivitis, lacrimation, blepharal spasm, rhinorrhea, salivation, tingling of the hands, burning sensation of the penis, diaphoresis, abdominal pain, and occasionally a sterile abscess of the injection site.

Edetate   Foreman et al. (1956); Belknap (1961); Atlman et al. (1962).

Symptoms of toxicity include severe hydropic degeneration of the proximal tubules with destruction of the tubular epithelium, rapid onset of malaise, fatigue, excessive thirst, hyperthermia, chills, severe myalgia, frontal headache, anorexia, nausea, vomiting, urinary frequency and urgency, sneezing, nasal congestion, lacrimation, glycosuria, anemia, dermatitis, transitory lowering of systolic and diastolic blood pressure, prolonged prothrombin time and inversion of the T-wave of the ECG.

d-Pencillamine   Goldberg et al. (1963); Tu et al. (1963); Adams et al. (1964); Marcus (1982).

Symptoms of toxicity include hyperthermia; pruritic, morbilliform, and urticarial rashes; leukopenia, eosinophilia, thrombocytopenia, anorexia, nausea, vomiting, loss of salty and sweet taste, nephrotoxicity, optic neuritis, systemic lupus erythromatosus-like syndrome on prolonged use, and extravasation of blood into the skin over pressure points of the elbows, knees, and toes.

Deferrioxamine   Schafir (1961); Bannerman et al. (1962); Henderson et al. (1963); Santo and Piscotta (1964); McEnery and Greengaard (1966).

Symptoms of toxicity include hypotension, skin rashes, gastrointestinal irritation, occasional cataract formation, and renal damage.

Pralidoxime   Symptoms of toxicity include neuromuscular blockage, inhibition of acetylcholinesterase, mild weakness, blurred vision, diplopia, dizziness, headache, nausea, and tachycardia.

Atropine   Berger and Ballinger (1947); Cullumbine et al. (1955); Thienes and Haley (1972).

Symptoms of toxicity include tachycardia, palpitations, dry mouth, mydriasis, blurring of near vision, disturbed speech, difficulty in swallowing, restlessness, fatigue, headache, dry and hot skin, difficulty in micturition, reduced intestinal peristalsis, ataxia, excitement, hallucinations, delirium, and coma.

Barbiturates   Fisher (1949); Koppanyi (1957); Shubin and Weil (1965).

Symptoms of toxicity include coma, depression of reflexes, positive Babinski signs, ECG abnormalities, miosis, slow or rapid shallow respiration; Cheyne–Stokes rhythm, hypoxia, respiratory acidosis; hypotension from depression of the medullary vasomotor centers and by direct action on the myocardium, sympathetic ganglia, and vascular smooth muscle, and hypoxia; shock, tachycardia, cold and sweaty skin, rise in the hematocrit, atelectasis, pulmonary edema, bronchopneumonia, hypothermia, and renal failure.

Benzodiazepines   Kaelbling (1960); Zbinden et al. (1961).

Symptoms of toxicity include sedation, ataxia, incoordination, dysarthria, dizziness, inattention, hypotonia, excitement, acute psychotic episodes, increased appetite or anorexia, weight loss, increased salivary and bronchial secretions, cardiovascular and respiratory depression, skin rash, nausea, headache, sexual impotency, vertigo, light-headedness, agranulocytosis, and menstrual disorders.

DTPA (Diethylenetriaminepentaacetic Acid)   Nenot and Stather (1979).

Symptoms of toxicity similar to edetate from chelation of essential metals. Is not effective in removing polonium or other actinides when they are in extracellular fluids or deposited in bone, but if administered soon after intake will remove the actinides from blood, extracellular fluids, bone, and other tissues.

Arsenic

Source of Exposure   Ingestion of ant poison, reduction of iron pyrites, rodenticides, contaminated drinking water, herbicides, coloring materials, mordants, arsenious oxide, Fowler's solution, arsphenamine, acetarsone, tryparsamide, carbarsone, and cacodyl compounds (Vallee et al., 1960; Robson and Jelliffe, 1963; Kyle and Pease, 1965; Lander et al., 1975; Freeman and Couch, 1979; Gerhardt et al., 1978; Fernando, 1979; Morse et al., 1979).

Acute Toxicity Symptoms include metallic taste, dryness and irritation of the mouth and throat; difficulty in swallowing, vomiting, severe abdominal pain, profuse "rice water" bloody diarrhea, loud borborigmi, tender abdomen, body dehydration, hypotension, oliguria, albuminuria, cyanosis, cold extremities, edematous skin, flushed skin, pain in the limbs, headache, seizures, muscular weakness, unconsciousness, collapse, degeneration of the central nervous system and optic nerves, depression of the myocardium with prolonged QT interval and abnormal T-waves in the ECG, and increased permeability and dilation of the small arterioles and capillaries. On recovery, there is transverse striation of the nails. Not all of the above symptoms are seen in every case of arsenic poisoning, as they are compound- and dose-dependent. Absorbed orally, dermally, and by inhalation.

Chronic Toxicity Symptoms include vague malaise, abdominal complaints, pruritis, arthralgia, pains in the extremities with gradual loss of strength, diarrhea or constipation, albuminuria, flushed skin, edema of the skin and lower eyelids, marked emaciation, brownish skin, pigmentation of the clavicles and elbows, numbness, burning, tingling, itching, muscle fasciculation or gross tremors, muscular atropy, paralysis, fatty degeneration of the liver, aplastic anemia, palmar and plantar keratosis, arsenical cancer of the skin, liver, or lungs, exfoliative dermatitis, acute granulocytopenia, hairlessness, and death.

Duration of Symptoms In *acute poisoning*, death may occur in 24 h or in 3–7 days, and recovery requires weeks to months.

Pathology In acute poisoning, the intestinal tract is inflamed and ulcerated, the mucous membranes of the stomach and intestine are edematous, and the intestinal tract is filled with fluid and mucous shreds. At death, there is fatty degeneration or yellow atrophy of the liver, glomerular nephritis, endocardial petechiae, and fatty infiltration of the myocardium, edema of the brain with patchy necrosis of hemorrhagic encephalitis, and peripheral neuropathy characterized by demyelinization and degeneration of the axis cylinders. In *chronic poisoning*, the above changes occur along with basophilic stippling of the erythrocytes, eosinophilia, pancytopenia with neutropenia, thrombocytopenia, anemia, and anisopoikilocytosis.

Diagnosis A history of arsenic ingestion or identification of arsenic in excreta or tissues is imperative because bacterial dysentery, cholera, and acute encephalitis exhibit the same symptoms.

Treatment Gastric lavage or emesis to remove the residual arsenical should be done. Intramuscular injection of dimercaprol, 2.5 mg/kg repeated every 4 h for the first 2 days, followed by injections once or twice daily for 10 days or until symptoms disappear, is necessary to remove tissue-bound arsenic. Modified Ringer's solution should be utilized to combat fluid and ion loss and morphine to relieve the diarrhea. Bed rest and preservation of body heat are necessary to acute arsenisism.

Antimony

Source of Exposure Improper glazing of enamelware, medicinal antimony compounds, cough syrup containing tartar emetic, antimony-containing alloys and catalysts, smelting of ores, sulfides used in rubber compounding and pyrotechnics, coloring agents and compounds used in organic synthesis (Stevenson et al., 1948; Browning, 1969; Oehme, 1978, 1979).

Acute Toxicity Symptoms include pain in the mouth and stomach, colic, nausea, vomiting, meteorism, diarrhea, edema of the lips, chills, muscle cramps, hepatitis, jaundice, metallic taste, dysosmia, dermatitis, rhinitis, irritation of the eyes, sore throat, headache, pain or tightness in the chest, shortness of breath, and papules and pustules around sweat and sebaceous glands. Absorbed orally, dermally, and by inhalation.

Chronic Toxicity Same as arsenic.

Duration of Symptoms Same as arsenic.

Pathology Same as arsenic.

Diagnosis The gastrointestinal effects must be differentiated from arsenic poisoning and bacterial infections. Viral infections can cause the same ocular and mucous-membrane effects, and upper-respiratory infections and allergies must be ruled out. The tracheobronchial effects are similar to cardiogenic pulmonary edema and viral or bacterial pneumonia.

Treatment Remove ingested antimony compound by gastric lavage, and for eye and skin effects wash with warm water. Hospitalization with observation is necessary to determine delayed-onset pulmonary edema, which can be treated with positive-pressure breathing with oxygen, and the edema fluid can be removed by administration of diuretics. To hasten excretion of tissue antimony, use dimercaprol as under arsenic.

Barium Salts

Source of Exposure Electronic tubes, rodenticide, ceramics, paints, enamels, paper manufacturing, electrodes, optical glasses, pyrotechnics, explosives, mordants, synthetics rubber vulcanization, corrosion inhibitors, lubricants, drilling mud, water softeners, photographic papers, lithographic inks, and radiopaque medium (Dean, 1950; Kay, 1954; Burnibel, 1962; Browning, 1969).

Acute Toxicity Symptoms include tingling sensations in the neck and face, colic, burning in abdomen, vomiting, purging, fibrillary tremors, irregularity of the pulse with ectopic beats, hypertension, smooth-muscle contractions, skeletal-muscle fasciculations, myocardial arrhythmias, extreme systole and ventricular fibrillation, or respiratory-muscle paralysis. Absorbed orally or by inhalation.

Chronic Toxicity Symptoms include benign pneumoconiosis, mucous-membrane and skin irritation, anorectal granuloma, bronchial irritation, and pulmonary X-ray changes consisting of small, dense, circumscribed nodules.

Duration of Symptoms Death may occur early or only after 10–12 h. The pneumoconiosis is permanent.

Pathology Intestinal spasm with mucosal hemorrhages and myocardial dilatation.

Diagnosis Symptoms from ingestion include gastroenteritis, muscle spasm, bradycardia, extrasystoles, and hypokalemia; and from inhalation, bronchial irritation, pneumoconiosis, and eye and skin irritation. These must be differentiated from other pneumoconioses, miliary tuberculosis, berylliosis, Hodgkin's disease, lipoid pneumonitis, histoplasmosis, and actinomycosis.

Treatment Ingestion is treated with sodium or magnesium sulfate, 15 g in water, antispasmodies to reduce intestinal spasm, and phenytoin, 100 mg intravenously, to prevent ventricular fibrillation. There is no treatment for pneumoconiosis, but further exposure must be prevented.

Beryllium

Source of Exposure Hardening agent in alloys, source of neutrons, neutron reflector and moderator in atomic reactors, radio-tube parts, aerospace structures, and in inertial guidance systems (Tepper, 1972; Sprince et al., 1978.

Acute Toxicity Symptoms include allergic skin rash, granulomatous nodules, acute pneumonitis, conjuctivitis, nasopharyngitis, cough, fever, dyspnea, coarse and fine rales, and central necrosis of the liver, and X-rays show diffuse pulmonary infiltration. Absorbed by inhalation or penetrating wounds of the skin.

Chronic Toxicity Symptoms include chronic pneumonitis, cough, dyspnea, enlargement and failure of the right ventricle of the heart; X-rays reveal diffuse nodular mottling of the lungs; anorexia, weight loss, fever, hypercalcemia, inhibition of alkaline phosphatase, elevated gamma-globulin, pulmonary edema, spontaneous pneumothorax, and skin and lung granulomas.

Duration of Symptoms Death occurs from acute pulmonary involvement in 3–5 weeks and, in recovered cases, X-ray changes persist for 1 year. Chronic pulmonary symptoms occurs from several months to years and persist indefinitely.

Pathology Acute skin and pulmonary lesions show edema with polymorphonuclear and round-cell infiltration and hepatic necrosis. Chronic granulomatous lesions occur in the lung, skin, brain, and liver; there are numerous giant cells, decreased liver function, renal calculi are formed, and lymph nodes and other tissues contain beryllium.

Diagnosis Symptoms include conjuctivitis, periorbital edema, nasopharylngitis, tracheobronchitis, pneumonitis, pulmonary granulomatosis, cough, dyspnea, weakness, marked weight loss, hepatomegaly, skin ulcers, dermatitis, and granuloma. Must be differentiated from viral upper-respiratory-tract infection, cardiogenic pulmonary edema, bacterial and viral pneumonia, adult respiratory distress syndrome, sarcoidosis, primary irritant dermatitis, nummular eczema, atopic dermatitis, psoriasis, herpes infection, pustular eruptions of the hands and soles, and erythema multiforme.

Treatment Skin contamination should be removed by washing, and any beryllium entering the skin must be excised immediately. Steroid therapy should be employed in acute and chronic berylliosis. Hospitalization is advised with 72-h observation when large inhalation exposure occurs to check for delayed-onset pneumonitis.

Cadmium

Source of Exposure Battery manufacturing, pigments, electroplating, making alloys and solder, ceramics, vapor lamps, welding, and contaminated water or food (Friberg et al., 1974; Lauwerys et al., 1974; Gross et al., 1976; Brown, 1977; Cadmium 77, 1978).

Acute Toxicity Symptoms include marked gastroenteritis, nausea, vomiting, diarrhea, abdominal distress, and collapse. Inhalation of Cd dusts or fumes causes temporary pneumonitis, pulmonary edema; metal fume fever with chills, hyperthermia, and malaise lasting 24–48 h, retrosternal pain, and renal cortical necrosis. Absorbed orally and by the lungs.

Chronic Toxicity Symptoms include irreversible lung damage of the emphysematous type, abnormal pulmonary function, renal tubular necrosis, anemia, eosinophilia, yellow discoloration of the teeth, rhinitis, possible nasal-septum ulceration, olfactory nerve damage, anosmia, osteoporosis, osteomalacia, increased excretion of β_2-microglobulin, proteinuria, aminoaciduria, phosphaturia, glucosuria, increased urinary calcium, pain in the back and joints, waddly gait, bone fractures, crossstriation of the long bones, and fatal renal failure.

Duration of Symptoms Acute symptoms persist for 7–10 days, terminating in death or recovery, which requires weeks to months. Chronic symptoms persist for years consisting mainly of lung emphysema, liver damage, and kidney damage with proteinuria. Once absorbed, Cd is well retained with a half-life of 10–40 years. The level of urinary Cd is unrelated to the severity or duration of exposure but only indicates absorption. Blood Cd is only an indicator of recent exposure.

Pathology Renal tubular necrosis, congested lungs, intraalveolar fibrinous exudate, alveolar-cell metaplasia, renal calculi, bone fractures, and high Cd concentrations in the kidney.

Diagnosis Symptoms include delayed onset pulmonary edema, dyspenea, chest constriction, substernal pain, headache, chills, muscle aches, nausea, vomiting, diarrhea, emphysema, proteinuria, anosmia, mild anemia, glucosuria, hypercalcinuria, phosphaturia, aminoaciduria, and hypophosphatemia. It is essential to differentiate Cd intoxication form upper-respiratory-tract viral or bacterial infections, cardiogenic pulmonary edema, pneumonia, and adult respiratory distress syndrome.

Treatment There is no antidote for cadmium intoxication, and the use of dimercaprol or edetate only increases renal damage and thus they are contraindicated. Pulmonary complications may be treated with 60–100% oxygen, with or without positive-pressure breathing. Short-term steroid therapy will decrease pulmonary inflammation, and diuretics will reduce the edema.

Chromium Salts

Source of Exposure Manufacturing of chrome steel and chrome–nickel steel, electroplating, catalyst, mordant, leather tanning, green varnishes, paints, inks, and glazes for porcelain (Fregert and Rossman, 1964; Browning, 1969; Oehme, 1978, 1979; Friberg et al., 1979).

Acute Toxicity Symptoms include sensitivity dermatitis; on inhalation, pharyngitis, bronchitis, and perforated nasal septum; lung cancer, papillomas of the nose and throat; nausea, vomiting, ulcers of the stomach and bowel, renal damage, impairment of pulmonary function, pneumoconiosis, lung fibrosis, wheezing, chest pain, hepatic centralobular necrosis, Kupffer-cell proliferation, histiocytic infiltration of the portal areas, bile-pigment imbibition, decreased prothrombin activity, elevated icterus index, and an abnormal Bromsulphalein test. Absorbed orally, dermally, or by inhalation.

Chronic Toxicity Symptoms include ulcers of the nasal septum; irritation of the conjunctiva, pharynx, and larynx; asthmatic bronchitis, severe frontal headache, wheezing, dyspnea, cough, pain on inspiration, jaundice, impaired liver function, erythematous eruption, wheeping eczema, discoloration of the teeth, rhinitis, nose bleed, epigastric pain, skin ulceration, pulmonary edema, and kidney damage.

Duration of Symptoms Persist and become more severe as long as exposure continues.

Pathology Renal proximal convoluted tubular injury, progressing to entire nephron damage. Hepatic biopsy revealed centrolobular necrosis, Kupffer-cell proliferation, portal area infiltrated with lymphocytes and histiocytes, and bile-pigment imbibition. Local contact causes skin ulceration.

Diagnosis Symptoms of respiratory irritation, including cough, dypsnea, wheezing, and chest pain; irritation, ulceration, and perforation of the nasal septum; jaundice, renal damage, eye injury, and conjunctivitis from chromic acid or chromate; skin ulcers, dermatitis, and lung cancer. Must be differentiated from viral pneumonia, cardiogenic pulmonary edema, adult respiratory distress syndrome, primary irritant dermatitis, nummular eczema, atopic dermatitis, psoriasis, herpes infections, drug eruptions, erythema multiforme, and pustular eruptions of the palms and soles.

Treatment High-level inhalation requires hospitalization, chest X-rays, blood-gas analysis, oxygen administration, mechanical ventilation; fluid balance must be maintained; inflammatory reactions of the lungs can be controlled with short-term steroid medication and diuretics. Flushing eyes and skin with water will remove chromic acid contamination. Ingested chromium compounds should be removed by gastric lavage using water or soap solution. Hemodialysis may be necessary to remove chromium from the blood and tissues.

Cobalt Compounds

Source of Exposure In alloys, catalysts, enamels, semiconductors, grinding wheels, pigments, painting on glass or porcelain, coloring rubber, bleaching agents, lacquer driers, varnishes, hydrometers, printing inks, storage battery electrodes, powder metallurgy, plastic resins, electroplating baths, and as a hydrodesulfuration catalyst (Passow et al., 1961; Browning, 1969; Friberg et al., 1979).

Acute Toxicity Symptoms include interstitial pneumonitis, sensitization of the skin and respiratory tract; obstructive airways syndrome, cough, wheezing, shortness of breath; erythematous papular dermatitis of the ankles, elbow flexures, and side of the neck. Absorbed orally and by inhalation.

Chronic Toxicity An extension of acute toxicity.

Duration of Symptoms Continue until removal from contact with cobalt compounds.

Pathology Nothing distinctive.

Diagnosis Symptoms include cough, dyspnea, shortness of breath, decreased pulmonary function, and dermatitis. Must be differentiated from farmer's lung sensitivity pneumonitis, berylliosis, Hamman–Rich syndrome, Loeffler's syndrome, sarcoidosis, various diffuse interstitial fibroses, asthma of various causes, laryngeal edema, endobronchial disease, acute left ventricular failure, eosinophilic pneumonias, nummular eczema, atopic dermatitis, psoriasis, and various drug and viral eruptions.

Treatment Removal from exposure, wash eyes and skin, treat interstitial disease with steroids and dermatitis with antihistamines.

Iron Salts

Source of Exposure Alloyed with carbon, manganese, chromium, and nickel in steel; radionuclides for tracer studies and as a hematinic (Bannerman, 1962; Henderson et al., 1963; Santo and Piscotta, 1964; McEnery and Greengaard, 1966; Stein et al., 1976).

Acute Toxicity Symptoms include vomiting, weakness, pale face, coldness, restlessness, drowiness, backache, rapid respiration, tachycardia, muscle twitching and seizures, black or bloody diarrhea, gastroenteritis, and collapse from poisoning of the metallic enzyme of the central nervous system. Blood iron may reach 6 mg/dl. Absorbed orally.

Chronic Toxicity None reported.

Duration of Symptoms May persist for 4 days depending on the dose ingested.

Pathology Serum iron may be 100 times normal; centrolobular hepatic necrosis, increased urinary bilirubin, urobilinogen, bile salts, and albumin; jaundice, elevated serum transaminases, cloudy swelling and necrosis of gastric and upper-intestinal mucosa, pyloric stenosis, and death within 4 days.

Diagnosis Evidence of ingestion of iron tablets coupled with the above symptoms. Must be differentiated from salicylate poisoning, which produces similar gastrointestinal symptoms.

Treatment Gastric lavage or give an emetic to remove residual iron salt and prevent further absorption. Deferrioxamine, 2–3 g orally and 1–2 g intravenously, to chelate the iron and increase urinary excretion. Shock symptoms should be treated with 50 mg methoxamine in 200 ml dextrose solution intravenously.

Lead

Source of Exposure Tank linings, pipes, equipment for handling corrosive gases and liquids, X-ray and atomic shielding, manufacturing of lead alkyls, pigments, organic and inorganic lead compounds, bearing metal and alloys, storage batteries, ceramics, plastic, electronic devices, building construction, solder, metallurgy of steel and other metals, water supplies and pesticides (Goldbert et al., 1963; Haley, 1969, 1971; Seppalainen et al., 1975).

Acute Toxicity Symptoms include acute gastroenteritis, burning in the pharynx, pain in the epigastrium, vomiting, diarrhea, shock, and death. Absorbed orally, dermally, and by inhalation.

Chronic Toxicity Symptoms include delirium, mania, colic, facial pallor, mild anemia, basophilic stippling of the erythrocytes, lead line on the gums, antithrombin effect, lead palsy, arteriosclerosis, chronic arteriosclerotic nephritis, impaired heme synthesis, blocking of delta-aminolevulinic acid dehydrogenase, retinal stippling about the optic disc, increased erythrocyte fragility, hemolysis; colic of the intestine, ureters, uterus, and blood vessels; tense abdomen, constipation, tremor, numbness, hyperesthesia, muscle fibrillation and cramps, wrist and foot drop, degeneration of nerves and muscles, optic atrophy, lead encephalopathy, sterility in both sexes, miscarriages and degenerate offspring; may be hair loss and urinary excretion of lead, increases of prophyrin and delta-aminolevulinic acid. Lead alkyls produce acute mania, headache, blurred vision, aphasia, and elevated cerebrospinal fluid pressure.

Duration of Symptoms Come and go during intoxication, may disappear months after removal from exposure, convulsive manifestations of encephalopathy may cause death or death may be delayed after a year of toxic manifestations.

Pathology Bone-marrow hyperplasia of the leukoblasts and erythroblasts, decreased fat cells, gum lead line, ulcerative or hemorrhagic changes in the stomach and intestines, peripheral neuritis, degeneration of the anterior horn cells, mengingoencephalitis; Schwann-cell proliferation and degeneration, demyelination, fibrous myositis; arteriosclerosis, chronic interstitial nephritis, degeneration of the germinal epithelium of the testes, and chronic hepatic degeneration.

Diagnosis Acute intoxication requires demonstration of lead in the blood or urine at levels of 0.3–0.9 mg/dl. Chronic intoxication with the above symptoms must be differentiated from gastric crises of syphilis, biliary and renal calculi, appendicitis, intestinal diverticulitis, and vascular spasm. Children show pica in X-ray pictures, increased density beneath the epiphyses of the long bones, and convulsive seizures from their encephalitis. The gum lead lines must be differentiated from the bismuth line and gold and silver sulfide deposits. Increased lead and porphyrin in the urine are diagnostic of lead intoxication.

Treatment Decrease lead intake, improve personal hygiene, and increase bone lead deposition by drinking milk. In acute lead intoxication, administer edetate slowly intravenously, 2–4 g/day over a 12- to 24-h period for a maximum of 5 days. Edetate should not be given prophylactically, as oral administration increases lead absorption. Dimercaprol may be given at a dose of 4 mg/kg every 4–6 h. Higher doses can cause renal tubular necrosis. d-Penicillamine, 0.3–0.5 g orally, 3–5 times daily assists in hastening lead excretion, but beware of the adverse reactions, especially skin rashes. Antispasmodics will control the colic, chlorpromazine will control the emesis, and MgSO₄ will control the constipation. In encephalopathy in children, administration of 1–1.5 g/kg of urea as a 30% solution at 8- to 12-h intervals will reduce the cerebral edema.

Mercury

Source of Exposure Mercuric and mercurous chlorides, tooth amalgams, fur felting, gold mining, laboratory spillage of elemental mercury, fungicides, paints, mercury in various waters, industrial pollution from chloralkali plants, mercury boilers, mirror manufacturing, oxidation catalysts, electric rectifiers, electrolysis, and electroanalysis (Longcope and Luetscher, 1946; Bidstup, 1957; Matthes et al., 1958; Noe, 1960; Smith and Miller, 1961; Copplestone and McArthur, 1966).

Acute Toxicity Symptoms from ingestion include pain, inflammation swelling, whitish necrosis of the oral and pharyngeal mucosa; nausea, vomiting, pain in the abdomen, renal damage, albuminuria, hematuria, oliguira, decreased blood chlorides, increased nonprotein nitrogen, malaise, prostration, shock, bloody stools, anorexia, generalized edema, headache, fatigue, tremor ataxia, deafness, anosmia, scotoma, loss of memory, emotional instability, stupor, manical symptoms, and uremia. Alkyl mercurials, inhaled or ingested, cause central nervous system symptoms. Absorbed by ingestion, dermally, or by inhalation.

Chronic Toxicity Symptoms include severe albuminuria, gingivitis, salivation, metallic taste, loosening of the teeth, tender tongue, diarrhea or constipation, retinal damage with contraction of the visual field, anemia, weight loss, lymphocytosis, increased urinary prophyrins, hepatitis, nephritis, irritability, insomia, anorexia, easy fatiguability, forgetfulness; tremors of the hands, lips, and tongue; unsteady gait, exaggerated reflexes and changes in personality.

Duration of Symptoms Soluble mercurials cause death in 1 h from gastroenteritis and shock; renal death in 10 days; and later deaths due to intestinal damage or hepatitis. In chronic mercurialism, nervous and mental changes including tremor remain after recovery.

Pathology All degrees of necrosis occur in the oral, esophageal, gastric, and other mucosae; local skin damage includes erythema with papular or small pustular lesions; the glomerulus is damaged and cloudy swelling to necrosis of the epithelium of the proximal convoluted tubules is seen and on recovery a mercury-resistant syncytium is formed. The colonic mucosa becomes necrotic and sloughs off, the liver develops cloudy swelling with acute central necrosis, and the myocardium degenerates.

Diagnosis   Severe inflammation of the oral mucosa coupled with oliguria, albuminuria, and prostration occur in mercury and phenol poisoning, and the lack of odor of the latter along with mercury in the urine or stool establishes mercury as the offending agent. At death, the liver, kidney, spleen, urine, and colon contain mercury. In known exposure to mercury, chronic mercurialism is established by gingivitis, loosened teeth, foul breath, and albuminuria. Tremor and personality changes are also indicative.

Treatment   On ingestion, residual mercurial should be removed from the stomach by gastric lavage or emesis. To prevent or treat systemic intoxication use dimercaprol injections as for arsenic. d-Penicillamine orally in doses of 0.3–0.5 g, 3–4 times daily, can be used. In chronic mercurialism, the same treatments are effective, and good oral hygiene is essential to prevent serious consequences from gingivitis.

Nickel

Source of Exposure   Smelting ores, electroplating, storage batteries, electrical contacts and electrodes, spark plugs, alloys, catalysts, vapor plating, and coal gasification (Tolot et al., 1956; Tsuchiya, 1965; Sunderman and Sunderman, 1970; Sunderman, 1971; McConnell et al., 1973).

Acute Toxicity   Symptoms from nickel salts include pruritis, erythematous or follicular skin eruptions, skin ulcers, eczema, pigmented or depigmented skin, plaques, erythemia, dyspnea, decreased pulmonary function, and transient pneumonitis. Symptoms from inhalation of nickel carbonyl include frontal headache, vertigo, nausea, vomiting, substernal and epigastric pain, chest constriction, cough, hyperpnea, cyanosis, profound weakness, gastroenteritis, hyperthermia, leukocytosis, delirium, seizures, and death. Absorbed by ingestion, dermally and by inhalation.

Chronic Toxicity   Symptoms include a permanent sensitivity, and circulating antibodies develop with the possibility of the development of hypersensitivity pneumonitis. Exposure to dusts of nickel, nickel subsulfide, nickel oxide, and nickel carbonyl chronically produce cancer of the paranasal sinuses and lungs.

Duration of Symptoms   Recovery from nickel dermatitis occurs in 7 days to weeks and from nickel carbonyl requires 2–3 months.

Pathology   Pulmonary edema, bronchitis, interstitial pneumonitis, brain edema, and liver and spleen enlargement.

Diagnosis Symptoms include sensitization dermatitis, pneumonitis, fever, headache, vertigo, nausea, vomiting, epigastric pain, substernal pain, constrictive chest pain, cough, hyperpnea, cyanosis, weakness, leukocytosis, bronchiopneumonia, delirium, and seizures. Nickel intoxication must be differentiated from viral upper-respiratory-tract infection, cardiogenic pulmonary edema, viral or bacterial pneumonia, and adult respiratory distress syndrome.

Treatment For mild intoxications, dithiocarb at 2 g orally with sodium bicarbonate followed by dithiocarb at 1 g at 4 h, 0.6 g at 8 h, 0.4 g at 16 h, then 0.4 g every 8 h until symptoms subside. In severe cases, dithiocarb at 26 mg/kg parenterally with a total 24 h dose of 100 mg/kg. Patients should be observed for at least 1 week. Respiratory symptoms should be treated with oxygen inhalation.

Plutonium and Other Actinides

Source of Exposure Occupation exposure occurs by inhalation or cuts during processing used reactor fuel elements (Nenot and Stather, 1979).

Acute Toxicity Symptoms from high-level inhalation, which has never occurred in humans, include pulmonary edema and hemorrhage.

Chronic Toxicity After many years of exposure, symptoms include pulmonary edema, pneumonitis, and fibrosis; lymphopenia, leukemia, and bloodstem-cell neoplasia; bone and hepatic cancer, lymph-node fibrosis and necrosis, and fibrous nodules at the site of dermal penetration. These effects have been reported in various animal species but have not occurred in humans.

Duration of Symptoms Tissue changes, particularly cancer, require many years to develop.

Pathology Alveolar edema, chronic interstitial pneumonia, pulmonary fibrosis, lymphopenia, osteoporosis, necrosis, and various cancers.

Diagnosis History of exposure most important, and the presence of actinides in the urine and at the site of penetrating wounds.

Treatment For wounds, excision and where not possible infiltration with DTPA. For inhalation, bronchiopulmonary lavage or aerosolized DTPA and intravenous DTPA to increase urinary excretion.

Selenium

Source of Exposure Toning baths in photography, glass pigment, arc-light electrodes, rectifiers, photocells, semiconductor fusions mixtures, telephotographic apparatus, vulcanizing agent, and as a dehydrogenation catalyst (McConnell and Portman, 1952; Diplock, 1976).

Acute Toxicity Symptoms include irritation of the nose and throat, vomiting, vague abdominal pain, weight loss, and a garlicky odor of the breath, sweat, and urine. The oxychloride is vesicant. Selenium oxide produces metal fume fever with headache, burning sensation in the nostrils, sneezing, dizziness, bronchospasm, severe dypsnea, bronchitis, and pneumonitis.

Chronic Toxicity Symptoms include yellowing of the skin from decreased ability of the liver to excrete bilirubin into the bile.

Duration of Symptoms Recovery from metal fume fever requires 1 week and from chronic toxicity several weeks.

Pathology Degenerative change sin the parenchymatous organs, rachitic appearance of the long bones, myocardial enlargement, and atrophy of the gonads.

Diagnosis Selenium intoxication is suspected when urinary selenium excretion is 1–6 mg/dl and the breath and urine have a garlicky odor.

Treatment Use gastric lavage or emesis to remove the residual selenium compound and decrease the body burden and increase urinary excretion with dimercaprol as for arsenic.

Tellurium

Sources of Exposure Coloring agent in chinaware, porcelains, enamels, and glass; reagent for black finish on silverware, special alloys of marked electrical resistance, semiconductor research, rubber manufacturing, and as an alloy in steel, tin, silver, and magnesium (Keall et al., 1946; Amdur, 1958; Cherwenka and Cooper, 1961).

Acute Toxicity Symptoms include metallic taste, garlicky odor of the breath, dryness of the mouth, scaly itching patches on the skin, suppression of sweating, and upon inhalation metal fume fever. Absorbed by ingestion and inhalation.

Chronic Toxicity Symptoms include anorexia, nausea, vomiting, dry mouth, blackening of the teeth and tongue, metallic taste, malaise, respiratory depression, circulatory collapse, and damage to the renal tubules and hepatic cells.

Duration of Symptoms   Same as for selenium.

Pathology   Hydropericardium; patchy necrosis of the myocardium, liver, and cerebrum, and dark-appearing kidneys. Tellurium accumulates in the brain grey matter and is found in phagocytic and ependymal cells.

Diagnosis   History of exposure plus the following symptoms: garlicky odor of the breath and sweat, dryness of the mouth, metallic taste, anorexia, somnolence, nausea, loss of sweating function, dermatitis, and a urinary tellurium concentration of at least 0.01 mg/l are indicative of poisoning.

Treatment   Gastric lavage or emesis to remove residual tellurium compounds, followed by dimercaprol (see arsenic) to decrease body burden and increase urinary excretion. Caution must be exercised as dimercaprol can increase tellurium toxicity of the kidney.

Thallium

Source of Exposure   Rodenticides, semiconductor research, alloyed with mercury for switches and closures, catalyst, optical lenser, jewelry, dyes, low-temperature thermometers, pigments, and as a doping agent in scintillation crystals (Munch, 1934; Prick et al., 1955; Richeson, 1958; Stein and Perlstein, 1959; Browning, 1969).

Acute Toxicity   Symptoms include nausea, vomiting, metallic taste, anorexia, dryness of the mouth, soreness of the gums, rhinorrhea, conjunctivitis with puffiness of the eyes and face, diarrhea, abdominal pain, insomnia, deafness, scotoma, tingling, pains in the feet and hands, muscle soreness, severe stomatitis, muscle paralysis, alopecia, white stripes across the nails, gastrointestinal hemorrhage, strabismus, peripheral neuritis, paresthesia in the legs, tremor, retrosternal tightness, and chest pain, prostration, tachycardia, blood-pressure fluctuations, seizures, choreiform movements, and psychosis. Upon recovery, permanent residual effects include ataxia, optic atrophy, tremor, mental abnormalities, and footdrop. Absorbed by ingestion, dermally, and by inhalation.

Chronic Toxicity   Symptoms similar to acute, plusa gingival line, delirium, seizures, and coma.

Duration of Symptoms   Slow recovery with permanent renal and neurological injury, tremor, ataxia, paralysis, scotomas, and blindness.

Pathology   Inflammation of the gastrointestinal mucosae, parenchymatous fatty degeneration of the liver and kidneys, marked alopecia, anemia, organic changes in the brain, and degeneration in the peripheral axons.

Diagnosis History of exposure coupled with alopecia, insomnia, urinary thallium concentration of 150 mg/l, and the symptoms given under acute toxicity. Thallium-induced seizures must be differentiated from idiopathic epilepsy, hypertensive encephalopathy, hypoglycemia, uremia, hypocalcemia, porphyria, hypoxic encephalopathy, viral encephalitis, exposure to convulsants, myositis, mononeuropathy, chronic alcoholism, atherosclerosis, polyarteritis nodosa, diabetes mellitus, pregnancy, acute intermittent porphyria, meningitis, syphillis, Guillain–Barré syndrome, mumps, and vitamin deficiencies.

Treatment Gastric lavage or emesis to remove residual thallium compound and give dimercaprol (see arsenic) to decrease body burden and increase urinary excretion. However, the latter treatment has given inconsistent results. For persistent tremor, antiparkinsonism drugs such as trihexylphenidyl (2.5 mg) can be given. Control seizures with intravenous diazepam, 5–10 mg every 2–4 h as necessary. This drug is given over a period of 1 min to prevent apnea and cardiac arrest. Sodium phenobarbital (200 mg) is also effective.

Asbestosis

Source of Exposure Manufacturing of cement pipes, sheets, shingles, floor tiles, millboards, roofing felt, pipe covering, insulation paper, flooring felts, friction and packing material, paints, roof coatings, caulks, sealants, safety clothing, curtains, brake linings, clutch facing spray insulation, asphalt paving, welding-rod coatings, and filter mediums in the pharmaceutical and beverage industries (Haley, 1975).

Acute Toxicity No clear symptoms, as this is a chronic condition.

Chronic Toxicity Symptoms include asbestos bodies or fibers in the sputum, progressive dyspnea, radiological changes in the lungs, finger clubbing, nonspecific interstitial fibrosis of the perihilar region; granular ground-glass type of infiltration, fibrosis of the lungs and pleura; marked emphysema with blebs and bulba, pleural diphragmatic plaques, calcification of the parietal pleura, thickening of the alveolar walls and intraalveolar septa, alterations in the capillary network, macrophages containing asbestos fibers, alveolar dilation with cuboid metaplasia, squamous-cell carcinoma of the lower lobes, and malignant mesothelioma of the lungs, pleura, and peritoneum. Absorbed orally, intravenously, and by inhalation.

Duration of Symptoms Asbestosis requires 20–30 years to develop and terminates fatally, 2 years after diagnosis.

Pathology Fibrous membrane on the costal surface of the visceral pleura of the lower lobe, diffuse interstitial fibrosis with collagenization, ground-glass appearance of parenchymal tissues, macrophages containing asbestos fibers, thickened pleura with calcified plaques, squamous-cell carcinoma and adenocarcinoma of the lungs, mesotheliomas of the lungs and pleura with metastases to the spine and chest wall, tubopapillary pattern containing cuboidal or flattened cells with masses of collagen; the mesothelioma cell is large and polygonal with amphophilic cytoplasm and a clear membrane, with a large nucleus with loose vesicular chromatin and a large eosinophilic nucleolus and multiple nucleoli.

Diagnosis History of asbestos exposure, fibers or bodies in the sputum, progressive dyspnea, radiological changes in the lung, clubbing of the fingers, marked emphysema with blebs and bulba, pleural diaphragmatic plaques, biopsy showing asbestos fibers or bodies; check vital capacity, 1-sec vital capacity, and lung compliance; asbestos in pleural effusion, decreased diffusion capacity; determine blood gases, whole-body plethysmograph and spirography; diminished breathing sounds, basilar crepitations, limited chest expansion, cor pulmonale, pulmonary endarteritis with intimal hyperplasia, pulmonary hypertension; bronchioelectasia with ECG changes consisting of left-axis deviation, partial or complete bundle branch block, and right ventricular hypertrophy. Asbestosis must be differentiated from chronic bronchitis, viral pneumonia, lymphacitic carcinoma, Hamam–Rich syndrome, and various pneumonoconioses. A history of cigarette smoking is essential, because lung-cancer incidence increases 8.05 times in smokers.

Treatment There is no treatment for asbestosis.

Acetominophen

Source of Exposure Use of over-the-counter analgesic capsules and tablets (Proudfeet and Wright, 1970; Clark et al., 1973; Prescott et al., 1976; Peterson and Rumack, 1977; Stewart et al., 1979; Allen et al., 1979; Symposium Monograph, 1979).

Acute Toxicity Symptoms include erythromatous or urticarial skin rash, drug fever, mucosal lesion, neutropenia, pancytopenia, leukopenia, hypoglycemic coma, fatal hepatic necrosis, renal tubular necrosis, methemoglobinemia, thrombocytopenia, nausea, vomiting, anorexia, abdominal pain, elevated serum transaminase and lactic dehydrogenase activity, increased serum bilirubin, prolongation of the prothrombin time, encephalopathy, transient azotemia, glucosuria, metabolic acidosis or alkalosis, cerebral edema, myocardial depression, and death. Absorbed orally or rectally.

Chronic Toxicity Similar to acute toxicity, but hepatic necrosis more pronounced.

Duration of Symptoms Related to dose, and varies from 1 day to months.

Pathology   Centralobular hepatic necrosis not involving the periportal areas, brain edema, and renal tubular necrosis.

Diagnosis   History of drug ingestion, blood acetaminophen with a half-time of 4–12 h, elevated serum transaminase and lactic dehydrogenase activity, and increased serum bilirubin. Must be differentiated from other chemicals producing the same symptoms.

Treatment   Gastric lavage or emesis to remove residual drug, vigorous supportative therapy and hemodialysis in the first 12 h for patients with plasma drug concentration of 120 mg/ml or more. Acetylcysteine, a loading dose of 140 mg/kg orally, followed by 70 mg/kg orally for 17 additional doses, is an effective treatment for acetaminophen intoxication.

Antihistamines

Source of Exposure   Prescription and over-the-counter products including sleep aids (Haley, 1948, 1982, 1983; Allen et al., 1979).

Acute Toxicity   Symptoms include drowsiness, dizziness, skin rash, urticaria, dry mouth, pylorospasm, colonic spasm, vesicle neck spasm, blurred vision, ataxia, lethargy, somnolence, interference with judgment, palpitation, tachycardia, mammary-gland swelling with milk secretion, fixed and dilated pupils, muscular twitching, medullary and cord seizures, opisthotonus, coma, nervous system and circulatory collapse, and death by respiratory failure. Children are most susceptible. Absorbed orally and dermally.

Chronic Toxicity   Similar to acute.

Duration of Symptoms   Seizures may persist for 24 h and coma for 2 days.

Pathology   Bone-marrow depression with agranulocytosis, thrombocytopenia, pancytopenia, hemolytic anemia, photosensitization, acute labyrinthitis, and upper-nephron nephrosis.

Diagnosis   History of drug taking, an empty bottle, or finding the drug in the urine or blood is necessary for diagnosis.

Treatment   A short-acting anesthetic will control the seizures, but caution should be exercised because when the antihistamine-induced excitement phase ends, a sedative phase begins and the combination of two sedatives could be fatal.

Antimalarials

Source of Exposure   Therapeutic use in malaria, giardiasis, extraintestinal amebiasis, lupus erythematosus, and rheumatoid arthritis (Alving et al., 1946; Craige et al., 1948; Dewer and Mann, 1954; Scherbel et al., 1958; Bernstein et al., 1963; Hart and Nauton, 1964).

Acute Toxicity   Highly variable depending on the compound; symptoms include dizziness, vertigo, headache, nausea, vomiting, tinnitus, skin rash, abdominal cramps, anorexia, difficulty in swallowing, diarrhea, cardiopulmonary arrest in children, nervousness, insomnia, and pruritis. Absorbed orally.

Chronic Toxicity   Symptoms include actinic pigmentation; blue-grey deposits on the nails, oral mucosa, and cornea; dry skin, graying or bleaching of the hair, blurred vision, central scotoma, photophobia, retinal vascular spasm, pallor, disturbances in accommodation, irreversible corneal infiltration, atrophy of the second and eighth cranial nerves, respiratory depression, circulatory collapse, desquamation of the skin, lymphedema of the forearms and hands, leukopenia, fatty infiltration of the skeletal muscles, vertigo, irregular pulse, green blindness, tachycardia, extrasystoles from several foci, acute yellow atrophy of the liver, agranulocytosis, hemoglobinuria, and hemolytic anemia in the colored races.

Duration of Symptoms   From a few hours for most acute symptoms to 2 months for the cardiac effects, and the corneal pigmentation may be permanent.

Pathology   Acute yellow atrophy of the liver, agranulocytosis, hemoglobinuria, and hemolytic anemia from a deficiency of glucose-6-phosphate dehydrogenase.

Diagnosis   History of taking the compound, special symptoms, and demonstration of the drug in stomach contents, blood, liver, and urine.

Treatment   Stop ingestion of the drug, gastric lavage to remove residual drug from the stomach, bed rest, external heat to combat the hypothermia, maintain blood pressure by infusion of 50 mg methoxamine in 5% dextrose solution or intravenous injection of 15 mg mephentermine and oxygen with 5% carbon dioxide to maintain blood oxygenation.

Monoamine Oxidase Inhibitors

Source of Exposure   Therapeutic use in treating depression (Crisp et al., 1961; Moser et al., 1961; Kraines, 1964; Goldman and Braman, 1972; Sievers and Herrier, 1975; Nelson et al., 1983).

Acute Toxicity   Symptoms include overstimulation, increased anxiety, agitation, manic symptoms, restlessness, insomnia, weakness, drowsiness, dizziness, dry mouth, nausea, diarrhea, abdominal pain, constipation, tachycardia, anorexia, edema, palpitations, blurred vision, chills, impotence, headache, hepatitis, skin rash, tinnitus, muscle spasms and tremors, paresthesia, urinary retention, mental confusion, incoherence, hypotension, delayed hypertension, shock, hyperpyrexia, and twitching or myoclonic fibrillation of skeletal muscles. Absorbed orally.

Chronic Toxicity Symptoms include hepatitis, hypersensitivity, jaundice, hallucination, excessive perspiration, tremors, insomnia, confusion, seizures, orthostatic hypotension, inhibition of ejaculation, peripheral neuropathy, and hypertensive crises brought on by cheese or other drugs.

Duration of Symptoms Up to 1 week.

Pathology Hepatitis with cells showing marked ballooning and profound dissociation of the cytoplasmic contents, peripheral neuropathy, cardiovascular-system damage, and cerebrovascular accidents have been reported.

Diagnosis History of drug-taking essential, and demonstration of the drug in blood, tissues, or urine essentials to establish exact drug involved. Must be differentiated from viral hepatitis, as drug-induced hepatitis is similar.

Treatment Gastric lavage to remove residual drug from the stomach, close observation of vital signs, external cooling for hyperpyrexia, short-acting barbiturate to control the myoclonic reactions, regulated infusion of a pressor agent to treat shock, and slow intravenous injection of 5 mg phentolamine to check exaggerated pressor response and hypertensive crises.

Narcotics

Source of Exposure These natural and synthetic analgesics are drugs of abuse, usually obtained from illicit sources, and maybe contaminated with other chemicals or diluents; they also are prescription drugs (Goldfrank and Kirsten, 1978; Treback, 1982).

Acute Toxicity All of these agents produce similar symptoms of acute toxicity, and morphine will be discussed as a model compound. Symptoms include dizziness, ataxia with brisk reflexes, augmented cord reflexes, shallow respiration or sighing of Cheyne–Stokes respiration, unconsciousness, and cold skin; loss of reflexes, muscular relaxation, miosis followed by mydriasis; bradycardia followed by irregular, rapid, and weak pulse; marked hypotension; may have asphyxial seizures, and respiratory slowing with death from paralysis of the respiratory center. During recovery, the following occur: mental and physical fatigue, constipation, pylorospasm, tonic contraction of the colon, and spasm of the sphincter of the urinary bladder. Some individuals show the following symptoms; cerebral excitement, nausea, headache, vomiting, and delirium. Absorbed orally, rectally, and intravenously.

Chronic Toxicity These compounds produce psychic or physical dependence with the following symptoms: simultaneous stimulation and depression of the central nervous system, euphoria, miosis, constipation, mental dullness, anorexia, hypersensitivity to sudden stimuli, dry skin, decreased salivary secretion; pale, hollow-cheeked, shifty eyes, ill-kempt; menses diminished or suspended and increased libido. Sudden withdrawal produces the following symptoms: feeling of anxiety, restlessness, mydriasis, furtiveness, abdominal pain, pain in muscles and joints, gooseflesh, accentuated mucous secretions, diarrhea, increased libido, anorexia, lack of thirst, weight loss, hemoconcentration, hypoglycemia, and menorrhagia.

Duration of Symptoms In acute cases, a quarter of an hour lapses before the development of symptoms from an oral dose, but it is very rapid from an intravenous one and death occurs in 3–12 h. In chronic cases, the onset is similar to the acute one but the duration is variable and usually requires more drug to sustain the effect.

Pathology In acute cases, the appearance of the tissues is characteristic of asphyxia. In chronic cases, no gross or microscopic tissue changes are characteristic of addiction but there are multiple skin scars at the points of injection, and addicts may have both infectious hepatitis and malaria from using infected hypodermic equipment.

Diagnosis In acute intoxication, needle marks coupled with miosis and unconsciousness are distinguishing features but must be differentiated from other central depressants, alcohol, ether, barbiturates, etc. and cerebral disorders, trauma, tumors, and abcesses. In chronic intoxications, multiple scars and the induction of withdrawal symptoms on confinement are characteristic but must be differentiated from other drugs (barbiturates, imipramine, etc.) that produce the same symptoms. Injection of nalorphine at 1–2 mg or levallorphan at 0.5–1 mg produces a withdrawal syndrome if a narcotic has been taken within 12–24 h.

Treatment All narcotic antagonistics counteract the respiration depression that is the cause of death, but the drug of choice is naloxone hydrochloride. It is given intravenously at a dose of 2 mg and repeated in 5 min, and as soon as narcotic antagonism is evident, give 4 mg naloxone in 5% aqueous dextrose at a rate of 100 ml/h and, to sustain its effect, 2 mg intramuscularly. The respiratory depression can also be counteracted by giving carbogen (95% oxygen plus 5% carbon dioxide) by endotracheal tube. Heat loss from vasodilation must be controlled by warming.

Nicotine and Tobacco

Source of Exposure Liquid alkaloid from *Nicotina tabaccum* and other *Nicotiana* species, smoking and chewing tobacco, dipping snuff, and insecticides (vonAhn, 1952; Oberst and McIntyre, 1953; Freund and Ward, 1960; Larson et al., 1961; Spain and Nathan, 1961; Silvette et al., 1962).

Acute Toxicity Symptoms include stimulation of the brain and visceral ganglia, dizziness, nausea, vomiting, cold perspiration, pallor, excitement, general weakness, purging, bradycardia or tachycardia, increased cardiac output, mental confusion, respiratory embarrassment, fibrillary twitching, loss of consciousness; severe irritation of the mouth, esophagus and gastric mucosae; death by medullary or respiratory muscle paralysis. Absorbed from all mucous membranes, pulmonary alveolae, and skin.

Chronic Toxicity Symptoms include angina pectoris, endarteritis obliterans, atherosclerotic heart disease, palpitation, arrhythmia, exaggeration of symptoms of Buerger's disease, amblyopia, deafness, nose and throat irritation, decreased ciliary activity in the bronchi, changes in esophageal epithelial cells, basal-cell hyperplasia, hyperactive esophageal glands, pulmonary emphysema, chronic bronchitis, hepatic cirrhosis, gastric ulcer, cancer of the esophagus, lips, lungs, mouth, and urinary bladder, and death by sudden myocardial infarction.

Duration of Symptoms Acute death occurs in 3 min to 72 h after ingestion of nicotine, but acute toxicity from tobacco is over in 24 h. Chronic tobacco usage requires years to cause cancer, pulmonary emphysema, or myocardial complication to develop. Cessation of tobacco smoking results in weight gain.

Pathology Acute inflammation of the gastric mucosa, congestion of the cerebral vessels, cardiac dilatation, asphyxia, kidney congestion, atherosclerosis of the blood vessels; areas of desquamation and morphological epithelial changes in the bronchi, esophagus, lips, tongue, and urinary bladder; and an increase in goblet cells in the bronchi.

Diagnosis Odor of stale tobacco on the breath or in the vomitus, along with burning pain in the mouth, anxiety, excitement, respiratory effort, nausea, vomiting, blanching of the skin, bradycardia followed by tachycardia, clonic and tonic seizures, respiratory failure, and flaccidity of the muscles are characteristic of acute nicotine intoxication.

Treatment Gastric lavage, artificial respiration, chest compression of the xiphoid or direct cardiac massage may restart the heart, 1 mg atropine sulfate will prevent the inhibitory effect of nicotine on the myocardium, maintain body heat with warm blankets, and increase blood pressure by subcutaneous injection of 40 mg ephedrine hydrochloride. Cautious doses of pentobarbital (0.2 g) or amytal (0.2–0.2

g) orally or intravenously will control the excitement phases of mild intoxication, and cessation of smoking and nitrites or niacin will relieve tobacco amblyopia.

Phenothiazine Tranquilizers

Source of Exposure   Prescription drugs used for psychoses (Ayd, 1961, 1963; Zelickson and Zeller, 1964; Hollister, 1966; Barry et al., 1973; Cain and Cain, 1979).

Acute Toxicity   Symptoms include extrapyramidal symptoms, including parkinsonian syndrome, tremors, rigidity, akinesia, shuffling gait, postural abnormalities, pill-rolling movements, mask-like facies, excessive salivation, torticollis, oculogyric crises, akathisia, motor restlessness, agitation, tardive dyskinesia, pallor, hyperpyrexia, perioral spasms, mandibular tics, difficulties in speech and swallowing, hyperextension of the neck and trunk, and clonic contractions of the muscles. Absorbed orally and parenterally.

Chronic Toxicity   Symptoms include all of the above plus leukopenia, granulocytopenia, agranulocytosis, purpurea, pancytopenia, cholestatic hepatitis with intrahepatic obstructive jaundice, bilirubinuria, icterus, drowsiness, dizziness, fatigue, adrenergic blockade, orthostatic hypotension, reflex tachycardia, ECG alterations, dryness of the mouth, blurred vision, urinary retention, constipation, weight gain, photosensitivity, allergy, dark purplish-brown skin pigmentation, opacities of the lens and cornea, and melanosis of the internal organs and the retina.

Duration of Symptoms   Most of the symptoms disappear upon discontinuing the drug, but the blood dyscrasias, jaundice, and extrapyramidal symptoms remain for 4–6 weeks and the retinal pigmentation is permanent.

Pathology   Plugging of the bile capillaries with inspicated bile, little hepatocellular damage, bone-marrow degeneration, and pigmentation of the lens, cornea, and retina.

Diagnosis   History of drug-taking; finding an empty bottle or spilled tablets; and demonstration of the drug in the blood or urine. Must be differentiated from acute encephalitis, meningitis, tetanus, other neurological disorders, jaundice from hepatitis, cardiovascular disease, various dermatoses, and other types of retinopathy.

Treatment   Discontinue use of the drug, administer norepinephrine or angiotension amide to control blood pressure, trihexylphenidyl to counteract the parkinsonian symptoms; seizures can be controlled by cautious administration of thiopental and the jaundice with 250 mg dehydrocholic acid every 3–4 h.

Salicylates

Source of Exposure   Therapeutic use of aspirin, sodium salicylate, and methyl salicylate (Gross and Greenberg, 1948; Segar and Holliday, 1958; Done, 1959, 1960; Smith, 1960; Tschetter, 1963; Beaver, 1965, 1966; Hill, 1973; Anderson et al., 1976).

Acute Toxicity   Symptoms are dose-dependent and include severe acidosis, hyperpnea, coma, pulmonary edema, nephrosis, fatty infiltration of the liver, hyperventilation, alkalosis, low blood CO_2, acne, gastric irritation with possible hemorrhage, increased ascorbic acid excretion, excess potassium excretion, and, in children, ketosis, dangerous dehydration, and hyperthermia. In asprin idiosyncrasy, the following occur: sudden weakness, sweating, faintness, collapse, cyanosis, edema of the glottis, angioneurotic edema, skin rash, and fatal paroxysm of asthma. Absorbed orally and dermally.

Chronic Toxicity   Symptoms include lethargy and episodic hypernea in children and respiratory alkalosis, mental confusion, decreased blood prothrombin concentration, and tinnitus in older children and adults.

Duration of Symptoms   From hours to weeks, terminating in recovery or death.

Pathology   Gastric ulceration with hemorrhage and asphyxial changes.

Diagnosis   History of drug ingestion with the above symptoms and chemical identification of the drug in gastric contents, blood, liver or urine.

Treatment   Gastric lavage or emesis to remove residual drug from the stomach; use sodium bicarbonate orally or sodium lactate solution intravenously to combat acidosis; use external heat to correct the hyperthermia; respiratory distress is counteracted with oxygen plus 5% CO_2, bed rest; 15 mg mephentermine by intravenous infusion will correct the hypotension. Hemodialysis or peritoneal dialysis is effective in removing salicylate from the blood.

Tricyclic Antidepressants

Source of Exposure   From therapeutic use in treatment of depression (Kramer et al., 1961; Kristiansen, 1961; Sulser and Brodie, 1961; Newton, 1975; Tobis and Das, 1976; Bigger et al., 1977; Biggs et al., 1977; Woodhead, 1979; Rudorfer, 1982).

Acute Toxicity   Symptoms include hypotension, tachycardia, hypertension, palpitations, myocardial infarction, arrhythmias, heartblock, stroke, confusional states, disturbed concentration, disorientation, delusions, hallucinations, excitement, anxiety, restlessness, insomnia, nightmares, numbness, tingling, paresthesis of the extremities, peripheral neuropathy, incoordination, ataxia, tremors, seizures, alterations in the EEG patterns, extrapyramidal syndrome, tinnitus, inappropriate antidiuretic hormone (ADH) secretion, dry mouth, blurred vision, increased intraocular pressure, constipation, paralytic ileus, urinary retention, dilatation of the urinary tract, skin rash, urticaria, photosensitization, edema of the face and tongue, agranulocytosis, leukopenia, eosinophilia, purpura, thrombocytopenia, nausea, vomiting, epigastric distress, anorexia, stomatitis, peculiar taste, diarrhea, parotid swelling, testicular swelling and gynecomastia in the male, breast enlargement with galactorrhea in the female, increased or decreased libido, elevation and lowering of blood-sugar levels, dizziness, fatigue, weakness, headache, weight gain or loss, increased perspiration, urinary frequency, mydriasis, drowsiness, and alopecia. Absorbed orally and intramuscularly.

Chronic Toxicity   Any or all of the acute symptoms and, upon abrupt cessation of treatment, nausea, headache, and malaise.

Duration of Symptoms   Most symptoms continue for 2 weeks, and an ECG should be taken to monitor cardiac function for at least 5 days.

Pathology   Myocardial infarction, congestive heart failure, bone-marrow depression, and hepatic damage with obstructive jaundice.

Diagnosis   History of drug-taking essential, and chemical analysis of the urine essential to establish exact agent involved. Must be differentiated from anticholinergics and tranquilizers, which produce similar symptoms.

Treatment   Gastric lavage or emesis to remove residual drug from the stomach, hospitalize as soon possible and initiate ECG monitoring, maintain open airway, assure an adequate fluid intake and regulate body temperature. Intravenous physostigmine salicylate, 1–3 mg, will reverse the effects of tricylic antidepressant toxicity. Convulsions can be controlled with diazepam, phenytoin or paraldehyde, but barbiturates are contraindicated.

NONSPECIFIC ANTIDOTAL THERAPY

General Principles

Nonspecific therapy is based on the utilization of chemical and physical methods for decreasing the tissue content of the intoxicating agent and aiding its excretion. Nursing care is focused on the maintenance of vital body functions. Fever is reduced by tepid or cold baths, while hypothermia is treated with warm blankets or hot water bottles. If the cough reflex is depressed or coma persists for 24 h or more, antibiotics should be given to prevent pneumonia. Suction should be used to remove collections of throat mucus and the position of the patient changed every 1–2 h. Oxygen therapy should be instituted during coma and respiratory insufficiency. Hypotension may be treated by bandaging the limbs and elevating the foot of the bed to force blood into the head and chest. Body fluids with the proper ion balance may be maintained by giving fluids rectally, intravenously, or by hypodermoclysis. Where oral intake of carbohydrate and protein is not possible, dextrose 5% and protein hydrolysate may be given intravenously. Quiet and rest are essential for recovery from a chemical intoxication, and good oral hygiene is important.

Emesis and Absorbing Agents

Syrup of ipecac is the emetic agent of choice: 30 ml for adults, and 10–15 ml for children. Apomorphine is also effective, having a more rapid onset of action, but its narcotic depressant effects, which are not always counteracted by naloxone, require judgment concerning its use. Furthermore, it is extremely toxic to children. Emesis should not be used in patients that are comotose, have no gag reflex, or are convulsing. Emesis is contraindicated when strong acid or alkali have been ingested.

Gastric lavage using large-bore tubes (36–40 French) utilizing 10–20 l warm saline for adults or 5–10 l for children will rapidly remove residual drug from the stomach (Matthew and Lawson, 1975).

Administration of a slurry of 100 g activated charcoal via the gavage tube will effectively bind most drugs, thereby decreasing absorption, but this treatment should be done within 30 min to be most effective (Decker and Corby, 1970; Chin et al., 1970; Hayden and Comstock, 1975; Comstock et al., 1982). The use of superactivated charcoal, 20 g in 120 ml of 10% fructose solution, has been shown to have a greater absorbing capacity than ordinary activated charcoal (Chung et al., 1982). Recently it has been shown that charcoal in 70% sorbital suspension enhanced the antidotal potency of the charcoal and had the additional advantage that it could be stored for 1 year without losing its potency (Picchioni et al., 1982).

Osmotic Diuresis

Most poisons are passively resorbed in the proximal tubules, where they are concentrated in the filtrate because of salt and water resorption. When water resorption is inhibited, their rate of excretion is increased. Infusion of 10–20 g/h of mannitol or urea after loading with a dose of 25–50 g achieves urine volumes up to 1 l/h. Additional water and electrolytes must be supplied at the same time. The effectiveness of osmotic diuretics in increasing renal excretion has been demonstrated for salicylates, barbiturates, meprobamate, glutethimide, and pentachlorophenol, and should be effective for all ultrafiltered toxicants that are passively resorbed. Passive back-diffusion of some poisons can be inhibited by altering the urinary pH, because renal tubular epithelium is more permeable to unionized molecules than ionized ones. Sodium bicarbonate and sodium lactate solution infusion will alkalinize the urine, but excessive electrolyte disturbances or systemic alkalosis must be prevented. Osmotic diuresis is contraindicated in congestive heart failure, shock, or renal failure (Haley, 1977; Young and Haley, 1977).

High-Ceiling Diuretics

Ethacrynic acid and furosamide cause greater peak diuresis than other diuretics and have a prompt onset of action, inhibit sodium and chloride transport in the ascending loop of Henle, and their action is independent of acid–base balance changes. Ethacrynic acid is secreted by the organic-acid-secretory mechanism of the proximal tubule, and intravenous doses of 40 mg cause an increased urine flow. Ethacrynic acid and furosamide cause the following adverse reactions: fluid and electrolyte imbalance, hyperuricemia, gastrointestinal disturbance with possible hemorrhage, attack of gout, skin rashes, paresthesias, and hepatic dysfunctions. In addition, furosamide also causes allergic interstitial nephritis, decreased carbohydrate tolerance, and deafness. Thus, diuretic therapy in poisonings must be carefully considered prior to its use (Beyer and Baer, 1961).

Peritoneal Dialysis

An indwelling plastic catheter is placed into the peritoneal cavity by paracenteris, and dialysis is fluid introduced and left in place for 20–60 min, during which time solute diffuses from the blood across the peritoneal membrane into the dialysate. This process is repeated 30–40 times, with the dialysate being monitored for drug content each time. As the blood content is reduced, signs of recovery from the intoxication should become evident. This method of treatment can be complicated by infection, protein loss into the peritoneal cavity, pain, and occasional hemorrhage. Large-molecule, nondialyzable poisons cannot be removed by this procedure, and a high degree of protein binding or lipoid solubility decreases its efficiency. Albumin-bound poisons can be successfully removed by adding 5% albumin to the dialysis fluid. Poisons that are dialyzable only in the undissociated form may be dialyzed by changing the pH of the dialyzing fluid sufficiently greater or less than pH 7.4. Dialysis has been used successfully to remove barbiturates, borate, bromide, chlorate, dimercaprol, phenytoin, ethanol, ethlychlorynol, ethinamate, gluthethimide, glycols, isoniazid, methanol, salicylate, sulfonamides, and thiocyanate, and should increase removal of any toxin not irreversibly bound to tissue (Barbour, 1960; Berman and Vogelsang, 1964; Blommer, 1965; Micerli et al., 1979; Lazarus and Nelson, 1979).

Exchange Transfusion

Very useful in children but of limited usefulness in adults because of the large volume of blood required. Works well in removing poisons not highly tissue-bound or lipid-soluble, and is very useful in removing nondiffusible and highly albumin-bound poisons (J. T. Adams et al., 1957).

Hemodilysis

Cannulas are surgically placed in a leg or arm artery and vein and connected to a bypass. The bypass is removed, the arterial cannula is connected to the inflow end of an artificial kidney, and the venous cannula is connected to the outflow end of the apparatus, so that the dialyzed blood can be returned to the patient. The dialysis fluid must be monitored for the intoxicating agent, and as it is reduced, signs of recovery should become evident. This method for treating drug intoxication is complicated by infection, blood clotting, and possible contamination of the dialysate. Furthermore, even moderate sodium depletion may cause orthostatic hypotension 24 h later. This is the most effective method for removing dialyzable poisons. Dialysis solutions containing albumin or lipids accelerate the rate of removal of certain poisons (Berman et al., 1956; Chadler et al., 1959; Cruz et al., 1967; Locket, 1970; Mandelbaum and Simon, 1971; Konighausen et al., 1979).

Hemoperfusion

Utilizing the Sledinger technique, a Teflon catheter (40 cm long, 1.8 mm ID with 7 cm of its length provided with 5 holes of 1 mm diameter) is inserted into the inferior vena cava via the femoral vein. The inflow line of the Extracorporeal S.A. is connected to this catheter, and the outflow with its bubble trap is connected to a cannula inserted in an arm vein. Blood-sampling tubes are provided on both the inflow and outflow lines. Blood-sampling tubes are provided on both the inflow and outflow lines. Blood is pumped through the lines and the hemoperfusion column (Haemocol, Smith and Nephew Research, Ltd., or XR-004 Hemoperfusion System, Extracorporeal Medical Specialities, Inc., or any other charcoal or resin column) at a constant flow rate between 200 and 300 ml/min. Before connecting the patient to the system, it is flushed with 2 l saline containing 100 mg heparin, and the patient receives another 100 mg heparin intravenously. Monitoring the Lee–White coagulation time hourly is essential, and further heparin is administered to maintain the coagulation time above 20 min. If required, 7–10 ml protamine is injected slowly at the end of the perfusion. It is essential to monitor electyrolytes, creatinine, urea, calcium, phosphate, alkaline phosphatase, aspartate aminotransferase, bilirubin, proteins, platelets, protein loss, possible pyrogen reaction, and leukopenia during the perfusion. Drug removal must be checked hourly, to evaluate the efficiency, and along with clinical signs to determine the status of the patient. The utilization of this procedure does not preclude the use of gastric lavage and charcoal to decrease the gastrointestinal absorption of the chemical (McDonald et al., 1963; DeMyttenaere et al., 1967; Bismuth et al., 1979; Cooney, 1979; deGroot et al., 1979; Hampel et al., 1979; Iverson et al., 1979; Konighausen et al., 1979; Larcan et al., 1979).

REFERENCES

Adams, D. A., Goodman, R., Maxwell, M. H., and Latta, H. 1964. Nephrotic syndrome associated with penicillamine therapy of Wilson's disease. *Am. J. Med.* 36:330–336.

Adams, J. T., Bigler, J. A., and Green, O. C. 1957. A case of methylsalicylate intoxication treated by exchange transfusion. *JAMA* 165:1563–1565.

Allen, M. D., Greenblatt, D. J., and Noel, B. J. 1979. Self-poisoning with over-the-counter hypnotics. *Clin. Toxicol.* 15:151–158.

Alles, G. A. 1959. Some relations between chemical structure and physiological action of mescaline and related compounds. In *Fourth Conference on Neuropharmacology,* ed. H. A. Abramson. New York: Josiah Macy, Jr., Foundation.

Altman, J., Wakim, K. G., and Winkelmann, R. K. 1962. Effects of edathamil disodium on the kidney. *J. Invest. Dermatol.* 38:215–218.

Alving, A. S., eichelberger, L., Cragie, B., Jr., Jones, R., Jr., Whorton, C. M., and Pullman, T. N. 1946. Studies on chronic toxicity of chloroquine (SN-7618). *J. Clin. Invest.* 27:60–65.

Amdur, M. L. 1958. Tellurium oxide. An animal study in acute toxicity. *Arch. Ind. Health* 17:665–667.

Anderson, R. J., Potts, D. E. Gabow, P. A., Rumack, B. H., and Schrier, R. W. 1976. Unrecognized adult salicylate intoxication. *Ann. Int. Med.* 85:745–748.

Autor, A. P., ed. 1977. *Biochemical Mechanisms of Paraquat Toxicity.* New York: Academic.

Ayd, F. J. 1961. Toxic somatic and psychopathologic reactions to antidepressant drugs. *J. Neuropsychiatr.* 2:S119–S122.

Ayd, F. J. 1963. Chlorpromazine: Ten years experience. *JAMA* 184:51–54.

Balint, G. A. 1974. Ricin: The toxic protein of castor oil seeds. *Toxicology* 2:77–102.

Bannerman, R. M., Callender, J. T., and Williams, D. L. 1962. Effect of desferrioxamine and DTPA in iron overload. *Br. Med. J.* 2:1573–1577.

Barbour, B. H. 1960. Peritoneal dialysis in the management of dialysable poisons. *Clin. Res.* 8:114.

Barry, D., Meyskens, F. L., Jr., and Becker, C. E. 1973. Phenothiazine poisoning: A review of 48 cases. *Calif. Med.* 118:1–5.

Beaver, W. T. 1965. Mild analgesics: A review of their clinical pharmacology. *Am. J. Med. Sci.* 250:577–604.

Beaver, W. T. 1966. Mild analgesics: A review of their clinical pharmacology. *Am. J. Med. Sci.* 251:576–599.

Belknap, E. L. 1961. Modern trends in the treatment of lead poisoning. A review of the literature on the use of edathamil calcium-disodium. *J. Occup. Med.* 3:380–391.

Berger, A. R., and Ballinger, J. 1947. The relative toxicity of atropine and novatropine in man. *Am. J. Med. Sci.* 214:156–158.

Berman, L. B., and Vogelsang, P. 1964. Removal rates for barbiturates using two types of peritoneal dialysis. *N. Engl. J. Med.* 270:77–80.

Berman, L. B., Jeghers, H., Schreiner, G. E., and Pallotta, A. J. 1956. Hemodialysis, an effective therapy for acute barbiturate poisoning. *JAMA* 161:820–827.

Bernstein, H. N., Zvalifler, N. J., Rubin, M., and Mausour, A. M. 1963. The ocular disposition of chloroquine. *Invest. Ophthalmol.* 2:384–392.

Beyer, K. H., and Baer, J. E. 1961. Physiological basis for the action of newer diuretic agents. *Pharmacol. Rev.* 13:517–562.

Bidstrup, P. L. 1957. *Toxicity of Mercury and Its Compounds.* New York: Elsevier.

Bigger, J. T., Kantor, S. J., Glassman, A. H., and Perel, J. M. 1977. Is physostigmine effective for cardiac toxicity of tricyclic antidepressant drugs? *JAMA* 237:1311.

Biggs, J., Spiker, D., Petit, J., and Ziegler, V. 1977. Tricyclic antidepressant overdose—Incidence of symptoms. *JAMA* 238:135–138.

Bismuth, C., Conso, F., Wattell, F., Gosselin, G., Lambert, H., and Genestal, M. 1979.

Coated activated charcoal hemoperfusion. Experience of French antipoison centers about 60 cases. *Vet. Hum. Toxicol. Suppl.* 21:2–4.

Bismuth, C., Garnier, R., Dally, S., Fournier, P. E., and Scherrman, J. M. 1982. Prognosis and treatment of paraquat poisoning: A review of 28 cases. *J. Toxicol. Clin. Toxicol.* 19:461–474.

Bloomer, H. A. 1965. Limited usefulness of alkaline diuresis and peritoneal dialysis in pentobarbital intoxication. *N. Engl. J. Med.* 272:1309–1313.

Bloomquist, E. R. 1968. *Marijuana.* Beverly Hills, Calif.: Glencoe.

Boehm, R. M., Jr., and Czajka, P. A. 1979. Hexachlorophene poisoning and the ineffectiveness of peritoneal dialysis. *Clin. Toxicol.* 14:257–262.

Bowman, W. C., and Sanghvi, I. S. 1963. Pharmacological actions of hemlock (*Conium maculatum*) alkaloids. *J. Pharm. Pharmacol.* 15:1–25.

Braun, H. A., Lusky, L. M., and Calvery, H. O. 1946. The effect of 2,3-dimercaptopropanol (BAL) in the therapy of poisoning by compounds of antimony, bismuth, chromium, mercury and nickel. *J. Pharmacol. Exp. Ther. Suppl.* 87:119–125.

Brown, S. S., ed. 1977. *Clinical Chemistry and Chemical Toxicology of Metals,* vol. 1. Amsterdam: Elsevier/North Holland.

Browning, E. 1969. *Toxicity of Industrial Metals,* 2d ed. London: Butterworth.

Burnibel, R. H. 1962. Barium granuloma: An anorectal complication of barium enema x-ray studies. *Dis. Colon Rectum* 5:224–227.

Burns, R. S., and Lerner, J. E. 1976. Perspectives: Acute phencyclidine intoxication. *Clin. Toxicol.* 9:477–501.

Cadmium 77. 1978. *Edited Proceedings First International Cadmium Conference,* San Francisco, Calif.

Cain, N. N., and Cain, R. M. 1979. A compendium of antidepressants. *Clin. Toxicol.* 14:545–574.

Castellani, S., Giannini, A. J., Boeringa, J. A., and Adams, P. M. 1982. Phencyclidine intoxication: Assessment of possible antidotes. *J. Toxicol. Clin. Toxicol.* 19:313–319.

Cavanaugh, J. B. 1973. Peripheral neuropathy caused by chemical agents. *CRC Crit. Rev. Toxicol.* 2:365–417.

Chandler, B.F., Meroney, W. H., Czarnecki, S. W., Herman, R. H., Cheitlin, M. D., Goldbaum, L. E., and Herndon, E. G. 1959. Artificial hemodialysis in management of glutethimide intoxication. *JAMA* 170:914–917.

Chen, K. K., and Rose, C. L. 1956. Treatment of acute cyanide poisoning. *JAMA* 162:1154–1155.

Chenoweth, M.B., Kandel, A., Johnson, L. B., and Bennett, D. R. 1951. Factors influencing fluoroacetate poisoning: Practical treatment with glycerol monoacetate. *J. Pharmacol. Exp. Ther.* 102:31–49.

Cherwenka, E. A., and Cooper, W. C. 1961. Toxicology of selenium and tellurium and their compounds. *Arch. Environ. Health* 2:189–200.

Chin, L., Picchioni, A. L., and Duplisse, B. R. 1970. The action of activated charcoal on poisons in the digestive tract. *Toxicol. Appl. Pharmacol.* 16:786–799.

Chung, D. C., Murphy, J. E., and Taylor, T. W. 1982. In-vivo comparison of the absorption capacity of "superactive charcoal" and fructose with activated charcoal and fructose. *J. Toxicol. Clin. Toxicol.* 19:219–224.

Clark, R., Borirakehanyavat, V., Davidson, A. R., Thompson, R. P. H., Widdop, B., Goulding, R., and Williams, R. 1973. Hepatic damage and death from overdosage of paracetamal. *Lancet* 1:66.

Cohen, S. 1964. *Beyond Within: The LSD Story.* New York: Atheneum.

Comstock, E. G., Boisaubin, E. V., Comstock, B. S., and Faulkner, T. P. 1982. Assessment of the efficiency of activated charcoal following gastric lavage in acute drug emergencies. *J. Toxicol. Clin. Toxicol.* 19:149–165.

Connell, P. H. 1958. *Amphetamine Psychosis.* London: Chapman and Hall.

Cooney, D. O. 1979. Rates of heparin adsorption in hemoperfusion devices. *Clin. Toxicol.* 15:287–291.

Copplestone, J. R., and McArthur, D. A. 1966. Vaporization of mercury spillage. *Arch. Environ. Health* 13:675.

Costa, E., and Garattini, S., eds. 1970. *International Symposium on Amphetamines and Related Compounds.* New York: Raven.

Craige, B., Jr., Eichelberger, L., Jones, R., Jr., Alving, A. S., Pullman, T. N., and Whorton, C. M. 1948. The toxicity of large doses of pentaquine (SN-13276), a new antimalarial drug. *J. Clin. Invest.* 27:17–24.

Crisp, A. H., Hays, P., and Carter, A. 1961. Three amino oxidase inhibitor drugs in the treatment of depression: Relative value and toxic effects. *Lancet* 1:17–18.

Cruz, I. A., Cramer, N. C., and Parrish, A. E. 1967. Hemodialysis in chlordiazepoxide toxicity. *JAMA* 202:438–440.

Cullumbine, H., McKee, W. H. E., and Creasy, N. 1955. The effects of atropine sulphate upon health male subjects. *Q. J. Exp. Physiol.* 40:309–319.

Daqirmanjian, R., and Boyd, E. S. 1962. Some pharmacological effects of two tetrahydrocannabinols. *J. Pharmacol. Exp. Ther.* 135:25–33.

Dean, G. 1950. Seven cases of barium carbonate poisoning. *Br. Med. J.* 2:817–818.

Decker, W. J., and Corby, D. G. 1970. Activated charcoal as a gastrointestinal decontaminant: Experience with experimental animals and human subjects. *Clin. Toxicol.* 3:1–4.

deGroot, G., Maes, R. A. A., and van Heijst, A. N. P. 1979. An evaluation of the use of hemoperfusion in acute poisoning. *Vet. Hum. Toxicol. Suppl.* 21:8–11.

Deichmann, W. B., Witherup, S., and Dierker, M. 1952. Phenol studies; Percutaneous and alimentary absorption of phenol by rabbits with recommendations for removal of phenol from the alimentary tract or skin of persons suffering exposure. *J. Pharmacol. Exp. Ther.* 105:265–272.

DeMyttenaere, M. H., Maher, J. F., and Schreiner, G. E. 1967. Hemoperfusion through a charcoal column for glutethimide poisoning. *Trans. Am. Soc. Artif. Intern. Organs* 13:190–198.

Dewar, W. A., and Mann, H. M. 1954. Chloroquine in lupus erythematosus. *Lancet* 1:780–781.

Dimond, E. G. 1957. *Digitalis.* Springfield, Ill.: Thomas.

Diplock, A. T. 1976. Metabolic aspects of selenium action and toxicity. *CRC Crit. Rev. Toxicol.* 4:271–329.

Done, A. K. 1959. Uses and abuses of antipyretic therapy. *Pediatrics* 23:774–780.

Done, A. K. 1960. Salicylate intoxication. Significance of measurements of salicylate in blood in cases of acute ingestion. *Pediatrics* 26:800–807.

Dubnow, M. H., and Burchell, H. B. 1965. A comparison of digitalis intoxication in two separate periods. *Ann. Int. Med.* 62:956.

DuBois, K. P. 1958. Insecticides, rodenticides, herbicides; Household hazards. *Postgrad. Med.* 24:279–288.

Durham, P. 1979. Review of toxicity of household products. *Vet. Hum. Toxicol. Suppl.* 24:40–42.

Eastman, J. W., and Cohen, S. N. 1975. Hypertensive crisis and death associated with phencyclidine poisoning. *JAMA* 231:1270–1271.

Eveloff, H. H. 1968. The LSD syndrome: A review. *Calif. Med.* 109:368–373.

Fernando, P. R. 1979. Attempted homicide with arsenic. *Clin. Toxicol.* 14:575–577.

Fisher, R. S. 1949. Barbiturate toxicity. *New Engl. J. Med.* 240:295.

Foreman, H., Finnegan, C., and Lushbaugh, C. C. 1956. Nephrotoxic hazard from uncontrolled edathamil calcium disodium therapy. *JAMA* 160:1042–1046.

Freeman, J. W., and Couch, J. R. 1979. Prolonged encephalophy with arsenic poisoning. *Neurology* 28:853–855.

Fregert, S., and Rossman, H. 1964. Allergy to trivalent chromium. *Arch. Dermatol.* 90:406–411.

Freund, J., and Ward, C. 1960. The acute effect of cigarette smoking on the digital circulation in health and disease. *Ann. NY Acad. Sci.* 90:85–101.

Friberg, L., Piscator, M., Nordberg, G. F., and Kjellstrom, T. 1974. *Cadmium in the Environment.* Cleveland, Ohio: CRC.

Friberg, L., Nordberg, G. F., and Vouk, V. 1979. *Handbook on the Toxicology of Metals.* Amsterdam: Elsevier/North Holland.

Gerarde, H. W. 1960. *Toxicology and biochemistry of aromatic hydrocarbons,* pp. 97–108. New York: Elsevier.

Gerhardt, R. E., Hudson, J. B., Rao, R. N., and Saobel, R. E. 1978. Chronic renal insufficiency from cortical necrosis induced by arsenic poisoning. *Arch.Int. Med.* 138:1267–1269.

Glaser, H. H., and Massengale, O. N. 1962. "Glue sniffing" in children. Deliberative inhalation of vaporized plastic cements. *JAMA* 181:300–303.

Goldberg, A., Smith, J. A., and Lockhead, A. C. 1963. Treatment of lead-poisoning with oral penicillamine. *Br. Med. J.* 1:1270–1275.

Goldfrank, L. R., and Kirsten, R. 1978. *Toxicology Emergencies: A handbook in problem solving.* New York: Appleton-Century-Crofts.

Goldman, A. L., and Braman, S. S.1972. Isomiazidia review with emphasis on adverse effects. *Chest* 62:71–77.

Goodman, L. S., and Gilman, A., eds. 1965. *The Pharmacological Basis of Therapeutics,* 3d ed., p. 298–299. New York: Macmillan.

Grant, K. L. 1983. Pharmacist's guide to poison prevention. *Am. Pharm.* NS23:114–118.

Gross, M., and Greenberg, L. A. 1948. The salicylates: A critical bibliographic review. New Haven, Conn.: Hillhouse.

Gross, S. B., Yeager, D. W., and Middendorf, M. A. 1976. Cadmium in liver, kidney, and hair of humans, fetal through old age. *J. Toxicol. Environ. Health* 2:153–167.

Grossman, C. M., and Malbin, B. 1954. Mushroom poisoning: A review of the literature and report of two cases caused by a previously undescribed species. *Ann. Int.Med.* 40:249.

Haley, T. J. 1948. The antihistamine drugs—A review of the literature. *J. Am. Pharm. Assoc. Sci. Ed.* 37:383–408.

Haley, T. J. 1956. Insecticides: Hazards in industry and home. *Calif. Med.* 84:248–264.

Haley, T. J. 1969. A review of the toxicology of lead. Air Quality Monographs, 69-7. New York: American Petroleium Institute.

Haley, T. J. 1971. Saturnism, pediatric and adult lead poisoning. *Clin. Toxicol.* 4:11–29.

Haley, T. J. 1975. Asbestosis: A reassessment of the overall problem. *J. Pharm. Sci.* 64:1435–1449.

Haley, T. J. 1977. Human poisoning with pentachlorophenol and its treatment. *Ecotoxicol. Environ. Safety* 1:343–347.

Haley, T. J. 1978a. Piperonyl butoxide, α-[2-(butoxyethoxy) ethoxy]-4,5-methylenedioxy-2-propyltoluene: A review of the literature. *Ecotoxicol. Environ. Safety* 2:9–31.

Haley, T. J. 1978b. A review of the literature of rotenone; 1,2,12,12a-Tetrahydro-8,9-

dimethoxy-2-(1-methyletheny 1)-1-benzopyrano[3,5-*b*] furo[2,3-*h*]-1-benzopyran-6(6*H*)-one. *J. Environ. Pathol. Toxicol.* 1:315–337.

Haley, T. J. 1979. Review of the toxicology of paraquat (1,1'-dimethyl-4,4'-bipyridinium chloride). *Clin. Toxicol.* 14:1–46.

Haley, T. J. 1980. Review of the physiological effects of amyl, butyl and isobutyl nitrites. *Clin. Toxicol.* 16:317–329.

Haley, T. J. 1982. Review of the literature of doxylamine. *Dangerous Properties of Industrial Materials.* 2:17–20.

Haley, T. J. 1983. Physical and biological properties of pyrilamine. *J. Pharm. Sci.* 72:3–12.

Hall, R. F. 1983. Herbicides: Liberators or poisoners of humankind? *Vet. Hum. Toxicol.* 25:92–95.

Hampel, G., Wiseman, H., and Widdop, B. 1979. Acute poisonings due to hypnotics: The role of haemoperfusion in clinical perspective. *Vet. Hum. Toxicol. Suppl.* 21:4–6.

Hart, C. W., and Naunton, R. F. 1964. The ototoxicity of chloroquine phosphate. *Arch. Otolaryngol.* 80:407–412.

Hayden, J. W., and Comstock, E. G. 1975. Use of activated charcoal. *Clin. Toxicol.* 8:515–533.

Hayes, W. J., Jr. 1975. *Toxicology of Pesticides.* Baltimore: Williams & Wilkins.

Henderson, F., Vietti, T. J., and Brown, E. B. 1963. Desferrioxamine in the treatment of acute toxic reaction to ferrous gluconate. *JAMA* 186:1139–1142.

Hill, J.B. 1973. Salicylate intoxication. *N. Engl. J. Med.* 288:1110–1113.

Hock, P. H., Cattell, J. P., and Pennes, H. H. 1952. Effects of mescaline and lysergic acid (*d*-LSD-25). *Am. J. Psychiatr.* 108:579–584.

Hollister, L. E. 1966. Overdoses of psychotherapeutic drugs. *Clin. Pharmacol. Ther.* 7:142–146.

Holmstedt, B. 1959. Pharmacology of organophosphorus cholinesterase inhibitors. *Pharmacol. Rev.* 11:567–568.

Hoogwerf, B., Kern, J., Bullock, M., and Comty, C. M. 1978. Phencyclidine-induced rhabdomyolysis and acute renal failure. *Clin. Toxicol.* 14:47–53.

Inaba, D. S., Gay, G. r., Newmeyer, J. A., and Whitehgead, C. 1973. Methaqualone abuse. "Luding out." *JAMA* 224:1505–1509.

Ishikawa, S. 1973. Epidemiological, clinical and experimental study of optico-neuropathy of chronic organophospahte poisoning. *Nihon Ganka Gakkai Zasshi* 77:1835–1886.

Iverson, B. M., Willassen, Y., Bakke, D. M., and Wallem, G. 1979. Assessment of barbiturate removal by charcoal hemoperfusion in overdose cases. *Clin. Toxicol.* 15:138–149.

Johnson, M. K. 1975. The delayed neuropathy caused by some organophosphorus esters: Mechanism and challenge. *CRC Crit. Rev. Toxicol.* 3:289–316.

Kaelbling, R. 1960. Agranulocytosis due to chlordiazepoxide hydrochloride. *JAMA* 174:1863–1865.

Kay, S. 1954. Tissue reaction to barium sulfate contrast medium. Histological study. *AMA Arch. Pathol.* 57:279–284.

Keall, M. H. H., Martin, N. H., and Turnbridge, R. E. 1946. Three cases of accidental poisoning by sodium tellurite. *Br. J. Ind. Med.* 3:175–176.

Kolansky, H., and Moore, W. T. 1971. Effects of marihuana on adolescents and young adults. *JAMA* 216:486–492.

Konighausen, T., Altrogge, C., Hein, G., Grabensee, B., and Putter, D. 1979. Hemodialysis and hemoperfusion in the treatment of most severe INH-poisoning. *Vet. Hum. Toxicol. Suppl.* 21:12–15.

Koppanyi, T. 1957. Acute barbiturate intoxication. *J. Forensic Med.* 4:65.

Kraines, S. H. 1964. The public interest and drug recall. *JAMA* 188:612.

Kramer, J. C., Klein, D. F., and Fink, M. 1961. Withdrawal symptoms following discontinuation of imipramine therapy. *Am. J. Psychiatr.* 118:549–550.

Kristiansen, E. S. 1961. Cardiac complications during treatment with imipramine (Tolfranil). *Acta Psychiatr. Neurol. Scand.* 36:427–442.

Kyle, P. A., and Pease, G. L. 1965. Hematologic aspects of arsenic intoxication. *New Engl. J. Med.* 273:18–23.

Lander, J. J., Stanley, R. J., Sumner, H. W., Boswell, D. C., and Aach, R. D. 1975. Angiosarcoma of the liver associated with Fowler's solution (potassium arsenite). *Gastroenterology* 68:1582–1586.

Larcan, A., Lambert, H., and Ginsbourger, F. 1979. Acute intoxication by phenformine hyperlactatemia reversible with extra-renal purification. *Vet. Hum. Toxicol. Suppl.* 21:19–22.

Larson, P. S., Haag, H. B., and Silvette, H. 1961. Tobacco experimental and clinical studies. Baltimore: Williams & Wilkins.

Lauwerys, R. R., Bucket, J. P., Roels, H. A., Brouwers, J., and Stanescu, D. 1974. Epidermiological sruvey of workers exposed to cadmium. *Arch. Environ. Health* 28:145–148.

Lawton, J. J., Jr., and Malmquist, C. P. 1961. Gasoline addiction in children. *Psychiatr. Q.* 35:555–561.

Lazarus, H. M., and Nelson, J. A. 1979. Peritoneal lavage with low morbidity. *Clin. Toxicol.* 15:129–138.

Lidbeck, W. L., Hill, T. B., and Beeman, J. B. 1943. Acute sodium fluoride poisoning. *JAMA* 121:826–827.

Liden, C. B., Lovejoy, F. H., Jr., and Costello, C. E. 1975. Phencyclidine—Nine cases of poisoning. *JAMA* 234:513–516.

Locket, S. 1970. Haemodialysis in the treatment of acute poisoning. *Proc. R. Soc. Med.* 63:427–430.

Longcope, W. T., and Luetscher, J. A., Jr. 1946. The treatment of acute mercury poisoning with BAL. *J. Clin. Invest.* 25:557–567.

Longcope, W. T., and Leutscher, J. A. 1949. The use of BAL(British antilewisite) in the treatment of the injurious effects of arsenic, mercury and other metallic poisons. *Ann. Int. Med.* 31:545–554.

Mandelbaum, J. M., and Simon, N. M. 1971. Severe methyprylon intoxication treated by hemodialysis. *JAMA* 216:139–140.

Marbury, T. C., Sheppard, J. E., Gibbons, K., and Lee, C.-SC. 1982. Combined antidotal and hemodialysis treatments for nitroprusside induced cyanide toxicity. *J. Toxicol. Clin. Toxicol.* 19:475–482.

Marcus, S. M. 1982. Experience with D-penicillamine in treating lead poisoning. *Vet. Hum. Toxicol.* 24:18–20.

Matthes, F. T., Kirshner, R., Yow, M. D., and Brennan, J. C. 1958. Acute poisoning associated with inhalation of mercury vapor. Report of four cases. *Pediatrics* 22:675–688.

Matthew, H., and Lawson, A. A. 1975. *Treatment of Common Acute Poisoning,* 3d ed. London: Livingston.

McCawley, E. L., Brummett, R. E., and Dana, G. W. 1962. Convulsions from *Psilocybe* mushroom poisoning. *Proc. West. Pharmacol. Soc.* 5:27–33.

McConnell, K. P., and Portman, O. W. 1952. Excretion of dimethyl selenide in the rat. *J. Biol. Chem.* 195:277–282.

McConnell, L. H., Fink, J. N., Schluster, D. P., and Schmidt, M. G., Jr. 1973. Asthma caused by nickel sensitivity. *Ann. Int. Med.* 78:888–890.

McDonald, D. F., Greene, W. M., Kretchmar, L., and O'Brien, G. 1963. Experiences in acute glutethimide (Doriden) intoxication. Superiority of extracorporeal dialysis over peritoneal dialysis. *Invest. Urol.* 1:127–133.

McEnery, J. T., and Greengaard, J. 1966. Treatment of acute iron ingestion with deferoxamine in 20 children. *J. Pediatrics* 68:777–779.

Micerli, J. N., Bidani, A., and Aronow, R. 1979. Peritoneal dialysis of theophylline. *Clin. Toxicol.* 14:539–544.

Mikolich, J. R., Paulson, G. W., and Cross, C. J. 1975. Acute anticholinergic syndromes due to jimson weed ingestion. *Ann. Int. Med.* 83:321–325.

Modell, W., Gold, H., and Cattell, McK. 1946. Pharmacological observations on BAL by intramuscular injection in man. *J. Clin. Invest.* 25:480–487.

Morse, D. L., Harrington, J. M., Housworth, J., Landrigan, P. J., and Ketter, A. 1979. Arsenic exposure in multiple environmental media in children near a smelter. *Clin. Toxicol.* 14:389–399.

Mortality Statistics. 1978. Special Reports, Accident Fatalities. Division of Vital Statistics, National Center for Health Statistics, Health Resources Administration, US Department of Health, Education and Welfare, Washington, D.C.

Moser, M., Brodoff, B., Bakan, H., and Miller, A. 1961. Experience with isocarboxazid. *JAMA* 176:276–280.

Munch, J. C. 1934. Human thallitoxicosis. *JAMA* 102:1929.

National Clearinghouse for Poison Control Centers. 1978. Food and Drug Administration, Rockwell, Md.

Nelson, M. V., Baille, G. R., and Krenzelok, E. P. 1983. Central nervous system stimulation from isoniazid therapy. *Vet. Hum. Toxicol.* 25:90–91.

Nenot, J. C., and Stather, J. W. 1979. CEC The Toxicity of Plutonium, *Americium and Curium.* New York: Pergamon.

Newton, R. 1975. Physostigmine salicylate in the treatment of tricyclic antidepressant overdosage. *JAMA* 231:941–943.

Nishimura, T., and Tamura, C. 1967. Antidotes in anticholinesterase poisoning. *Nature (Lond.)* 214:706–708.

Noe, F. E. Chronic mercurial intoxication. A review. *Ind. Med. Surg.* 29:338–340.

Oberst, B. B., and McIntyre, R. A. 1953. Acute nicotine poisoning. *Pediatrics* 11:338–340.

Oehme, F. W., ed. 1978. *Toxicity of Heavy Metals in the Environment,* part 1. New York: Dekker.

Oehme, F. w. 1979. *Toxicity of Heavy Metals in the Environment,* part 2. New York: Dekker.

Passo, B., and Harrison, D. C. 1975. A new look at an old problem: Mushroom poisoning. *Am. J. Med.* 58:505–509.

Passow, H., Rothstein, A., and Clarksen, T. W. 1961. The general pharmacology of the heavy metals. *Pharmacol. Rev.* 13:185–224.

Payne, R. B. 1963. Nutmeg intoxication. *N. Engl. J. Med.* 269:36–38.

Pearlson, G. D. 1981. Psychiatric and medical syndromes associated with phencyclidine (PCP) abuse. *Johns Hopkins Med. J.* 148:25–33.

Peterson, R. G., and Rumack, G. H. 1977. Treating acute acetaminophen poisoning with acetylcysteine. *JAMA* 237:2406–2407.

Picchioni, A. L., Chin, L., and Gillespie, T. 1982. Evaluation of activated charcoal-sorbitol suspension as an antidote. *J. Toxicol. Clin. toxicol.* 19:433–444.

Prescott, L. E., Sutherland, G. R., and Park, J. 1976. Cysteamine, methionine and penicillamine in the treatment of paracetamal poisoning. *Lancet* 2:109–113.

Prick, J. C., Sillevio-Smith, W. G., and Muller, L. 1955. *Thallium Poisoning.* New York: Elsevier.

Princi, F. 1957. Toxicology, diagnosis and treatment of chlorinated hydrocarbon insecticide intoxications. *Arch. Ind. Health* 16:333–336.

Proudfoot, A. T., and Wright, N. 1970. Acute paracetamal poisoning. *Br. Med. J.* 2:557.

Puharich, A. 1959. *The Sacred Mushroom: Key to the Door of Eternity.* New York: Doubleday.

Radeleff, R. D. 1970. *Veterinary Toxicology,* 2d ed., chapter 4. Philadelphia: Lea and Febiger.

Richeson, E. M. 1958. Industrial thallium intoxication. *Ind. Med. Surg.* 27:607.

Robson, A. O., and Jelliffe, A. M. 1963. Medicinal arsenic poisoning and lung cancer. *Br. Med. J.* 2:207–209.

Rudorfer, M. V. 1982. Cardiovascular changes and plasma drug levels after amitriptyline overdose. *Clin. Toxicol.* 19:67–78.

Santo, A. S., and Piscotta, A. V. 1964. Acute iron intoxication: Treatment with desferriosamine (Ba-29837). *Am. J. Dis. child.* 107:424–427.

Schafir, M. 1961. The management of acute poisoning by ferrous sulfate. *Pediatrics* 27:83–94.

Scherbel, A. L., Harrison, J. W., and Ateljian, M. 1958. Further observations on the use of 4-amioquinoline compounds in patients with rheumatoid arthritis or related diseases. *Clev. Clin. Q.* 25:95–111.

Segar, W. E., and Holliday, M. a. 1958. Physiological abnormalities of salicylate intoxication. *N. Engl. J. Med.* 259:1191–1198.

Seppalainen, A. M., Tola, S., Hernberg, G., and Kock, B. 1975. Subclinical neuropathy at "safe" levels of lead exposure. *Arch. Environ. Health* 30:180–183.

Shubin, H., and Weil, M. H. 1965. The mechanism of shock following suicidal doses of barbiturates, narcotic and tranquilizer drugs, with observations on the effect of treatment. *Am. J. Med.* 38:853–863.

Sievers, M. L., and Herrier, R. N. 1975. Treatment of acute isonizaid toxicity. *Am. J. Hosp. Pharm.* 32:202–206.

Silvette, H., Hoff, E. C., Larson, P. S., and Haag, H. B. 1962. The action of nicotine on central nervous system function. *Pharmacol. Rev.* 14:137–173.

Smith, P. K. 1960. The pharmacoloyg of salicylates and related compounds. *Ann. N.Y. Acad. Sci.* 86:38–63.

Smith, A. D. M., and Miller, J. W. 1961. Treatment of inorganic mercury poisoning with N-acetyl-D,L-penicillamine. *Lancet* 1:640–642.

Soderman, W. A. 1965. Diagnosis and treatment of digitalis toxicity. *N. Engl. J. Med.* 273:35, 93.

Spain, D. M., and Nathan, D. J. 1961. Smoking habits and coronary artherosclerotic heart disease. *JAMA* 177:683–688.

Sprince, N. L., Kanarek, D. J., Weber, A. L., Chamberlin, R. I., and Kazemi, H. 1978. Reversible respiratory disease in beryllium workers. *Am. Rev. Respir. Dis.* 117:1011–1017.

Stein, M. D., and perlstein, M. A. 1959. Thallium poisoning. *AMA J. Dis. child.* 98:80.

Stein, M., Blayney, D., Feit, T., Georgen, T. G., Micik, S., and Nyhan, W. L. 1976. Acute iron poisoning in children. *West. J. Med.* 125:289–297.

Stevenson, D. S., Suarez, R. M., Jr., and Marchand, E. J. 1948. The use of BAL in heavy metal poisoning with particular reference to antimonial intoxication. *P. R. J. Public Health Trop. Med.* 23:533–553.

Stewart, D. M., Dillman, R. D., Kim, H. S., and Stewart, K. 1979. Acetaminophen overdose: A growing health care hazard. *Clin. Toxicol.* 14:507–513.

Sulser, F., and Brodie, B. B. 1961. On mechanism of the antidepressant action of imipramine. *Biochem. Pharmacol.* 8:16.

Sunderman, F. W., Jr. 1971. Metal carcinogenesis in experimental animals. *Food Cosmet. Toxicol.* 9:105–120.

Sunderman, F. W., and Sunderman, F. W., Jr., ed. 1970. *Laboratory Diagnosis of Diseases Caused by Toxic Agents.* St. Louis, Mo.: Warren Green.

Symposium Monograph. 1979. Aspirin and acetaminophen. *Clin. Toxicol.* 15:313–340.

Temple, A. R., and Veltri, J. C. 1979. Ingestions of soaps, detergents, household products. *Vet. Hum. Toxicol. Suppl.* 21:31–32.

Tepper, L. B. 1972. Beryllium. *CRC Crit. Rev. Toxicol.* 1:261–281.

Thienes, C. H., and Haley, T. J. 1972. *Clinical Toxicology,* 5th ed., pp. 243–244. Philadelphia: Lea and Febiger.

Tobis, J., and Das, B. N. 1976. Cardiac complication in amitriptyline poisoning—Successful treatment with physostigmine. *JAMA* 234:1474–1476.

Tolot, F., Brodem, P., and Neulat, G. 1956. Asthmatic forms of lung disease in workers exposed to chromium, nickel and aniline inhalation. *Arch. Mal. Prof. Med. Trav. Secur. Soc.* 18:288–293.

Tong, T. G., Benowitz, N. L., Becker, C. E., Forni, P. J., and Boerner, U. 1976. Phencyclidine poisoning. *JAMA* 234:512–513.

Trebach, A. S. 1982. *The Heroin Solution.* New Haven: Yale University Press.

Tschetter, P. N. 1963. Salicylism. *Am. J. Dis. Child.* 106:334–346.

Tsuchiya, K. 1965. The relation of occupation to cancer, especially cancer of the lung. *Cancer* 18:136–144.

Tu, J., Blackwell, R. Q., and Lee, P. 1963. *DL*-Penicillamine as a cause of optic axial neuritis. *JAMA* 185:83–86.

Vallee, B. L., Ulmer, D. D., and Wacher, W. E. C. 1960. Arsenic toxicology and biochemistry. *AMA Arch. Ind. Health* 21:132–151.

vonAhn, B. 1952. Paroxymal auricular fibrillation in acute nicotine poisoning. *Cardiologia* 21:765–772.

Wassen, R. g. 1959. The hallucinogenic mushrooms of Mexico. An adventure in ethnomycological exploration. *Trans. N.Y. Acad. Sci.* 21:325.

Weintraub, S. 1960. Stramonium poisoning. *Postgrad. Med.* 28:364–371.

Weiss, G. 1960. Hallucinogenic and narcotic-like effects of powdered myristica (nutmeg). *Psychiatr. Q.* 34:346–356.

Wieland, T., and Wieland, O. 1959. Chemistry and toxicology of the toxins of *Amanita phalloides. Pharmacol. Rev.* 11:87–107.

Wolstenholme, G. E. W., ed. 1965. *Hashish: Its Chemistry and Pharmacology.* Ciba Foundation Study Group 21. Boston: Little, Brown.

Woodhead, R. 1979. Cardiac rhythm in tricyclic antidepressant poisoning. *Clin. Toxicol.* 14:499–505.

Wyeth Laboratories. 1966. *The Sinster Garden.* New York: American Home Products Corporation.

Young, J. F., and Haley, T. J. 1977. Pharmacokinetic study of a patient intoxicated with 2,3-dichlorophenoxyacetic acid and 2-methoxy-3,6-dichlorobenzoic acid. *Clin. Toxicol.* 11:489–500.

Zbinden, G., Bagdon, R. E., Keith, E. F., Phillips, R. D., and Randall, L. O. 1961. Experimental and clinical toxicology of chlordiazepoxide (Librium). *Toxicol. Appl. Pharmacol.* 3:619–637.

Zelickson, A. S., and Zeller, H. C. 1964. A new and unusual reaction to chlorpromazine. *JAMA* 188:394–396.

Index

Vessels (*Cont.*):
  fishing, 485
  lymphatic, 77, 124, 559
  venous, 76
Vinblastine, 200, 205, 208, 312, 315, 318, 333, 334, 342, 346, 347, 351
Vincristine, 313, 315, 318, 333, 334, 342, 350, 351
Vinegar, 460, 516, 597
Vinylacetate, 533
Vinylbromide, 531
Vinylchloride, 34, 90, 99, 101, 208, 242, 529–534, 537, 582, 583
Vinylidene chloride, 34, 535–537, 583
  copolymer, 536
Viperidae, 441, 442, 445, 448
Vipers, 441
Virus, 120, 138, 348, 375, 561, 562, 571, 581, 597, 621, 623–626, 630, 634
  granulosis, 375
  influenza A/PR-8, 138
  nuclear polyhedrosis, 375
Viscosity, 221
Viscera, 604
  greenish, 485
Vision, 474, 516, 525
  blurred, 509, 517, 619, 627, 636, 637, 640, 642
  dimmed, 605
  far, 605
  near, 615
  yellow or green, 603, 616
Vitamins, 285, 432
  A, 196, 271, 432
  B_{12}, 90, 493
  D, 412, 432
  E, 97, 102, 103, 137, 142, 143
Vitiligo, 537
Vocalizing, 614
Voice, 473
Volume:
  air, 116
  blood, 131
  body-compartment, 157
  cells, 129
  closing, 131, 482
  ejaculate, 216
  forced expiratory, 135, 474, 482, 492
  lung, 124, 129, 130, 138, 491
  minute, 124, 483
  residual, 116, 117, 129
  semen, 210
  static lung, 130, 489
  tidal, 116, 129, 483, 490

total chamber, 119–121
urine, 168, 169
Vomiting, 7, 147, 319–322, 324, 325, 327–329, 331, 332, 334–336, 339–341, 369, 374, 376, 337, 406, 457, 458, 461, 465, 478, 482, 484, 506, 513, 515, 518, 520, 522, 524, 596–608, 610–613, 617, 618, 620, 621, 623, 624, 626–631, 634, 636, 637, 639, 642
Vulcanization, rubber, 621
Vulnerability, host, 81
VX, 47, 52

Walls:
  airway, 123
  alveolar, 127, 138, 528, 609
  chest, 116, 130, 633
  thoracic, 131
Wallpaper, 530
Warfarin, 31, 240, 284
  resistant, 378
Washing, 448, 607, 609, 623, 626
Wasps, 462, 464
Wastage, fetal, 268
Water, 24, 161, 163, 166, 175, 365, 367, 401, 486, 513, 521, 522, 524, 525, 527, 530, 535, 537, 576, 597, 600, 602, 609, 619, 621, 623, 625, 627, 628, 643
  brown, 460
Waves, inverted T, 477
Weakness, 45, 333, 335, 340, 369–371, 476, 478, 479, 484, 509, 513, 520, 598, 599, 601, 603, 605, 616, 617, 619, 620, 623, 626, 629, 630, 639, 641, 642
  muscle, 448, 480, 536
Weaning, 259, 263, 411
Weeds, 364, 378
Weevils, banana-borer, 367
Welding, 135, 623
Wheat, treated, 382
Wheezing, 369, 475, 487, 494, 624, 625
Weight:
  accessory sex-gland, 217, 221
  body, 254, 347, 475, 491, 520, 639, 640
  decreased testicular, 211
  kidney, 514, 531
  liver, 514, 531
  loss, 598, 599, 606, 607, 610, 619, 622, 623, 628, 631, 638, 642
  lung, 490, 491
  spleen, 337, 491
  thymus, 337, 581
  uterine, 227